22nd ANNUAL EDITION 1989 - 2010

— THE

Calorie, Fa

EXTRA DIET GUIDES & COUNTERS

Weight Control Tips

Eat Sensibly

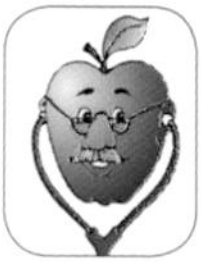

- Avoid fad diets. Eat 3 sensible meals daily with adequate fruit and vegetables.
- Limit portion size. Limit fats and high-fat foods, sugar, soda and alcohol. *(Sample Meal Plan ~ Page 11)*

Exercise Daily

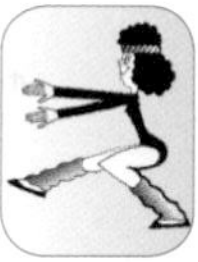

- Get active and exercise every day!
- Include muscle-strengthening exercises. You'll lose more fat and keep it off. You'll also feel and look better, and you can eat a little more! *(Exercise Guide ~ Page 12)*

Reshape Eating Behaviors

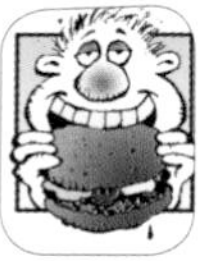

- Be aware of eating habits and behaviors that lead to overeating.
- Also focus on social and emotional situations that lead you to snack compulsively. *(Extra Notes ~ Page 14)*

Keep a Food & Exercise Journal

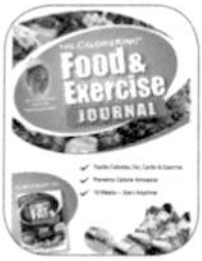

- A journal helps you see exactly what you eat and drink, and how much you exercise. *(Extra Notes ~ Page 15)*
- An excellent motivator and proven weight loss aid. Keeps you honest!

Arrange Moral Support

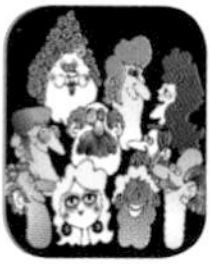

Gain the support of family and friends. Get extra professional help if required, from your doctor, dietitian, psychologist, exercise trainer, or diet club. Beware of family saboteurs who discourage you from adopting a healthier lifestyle!

DOCTOR CHECK-UP

Ask your doctor to check your blood pressure, blood sugar and blood cholesterol levels.

HEALTHY WEIGHTS ~ MEN & WOMEN ~ (Over 18 Years)

Based on weights with least risk of disease or death from heart disease, diabetes, stroke and cancer.

Based on Body Mass Index of 20-25

BMI calculated as: $\frac{\text{Weight (kg)}}{\text{Height (m)}^2}$

Height (No Shoes) Ft Ins		Healthy Weight Range (Pounds)
4'7"	~	86-108
4'8"	~	88-110
4'9"	~	92-114
4'10"	~	97-121
4'11"	~	99-123
5'0"	~	101-127
5'1"	~	105-132
5'2"	~	110-136
5'3"	~	112-140
5'4"	~	114-145
5'5"	~	119-149
5'6"	~	123-156
5'7"	~	127-158
5'8"	~	129-162
5'9"	~	134-167
5'10"	~	138-173
5'11"	~	143-178
6'0"	~	145-182
6'1"	~	149-187
6'2"	~	156-193
6'3"	~	158-198
6'4"	~	162-202
6'5"	~	170-211
6'6"	~	172-215
6'7"	~	175-220

Body Fat Distribution & Health

Moderate amounts of body fat do not compromise health. However, excess fat above the hips carries a far greater health risk than fat on or below the hips - better to be a 'pear-shape' than an 'apple-shape'.

Abdominal obesity greatly increases the risk of developing diabetes, heart disease, high blood fats, hypertension, stroke, sleep apnea, arthritis and some cancers. So-called **'cellulite'** carries no extra health risk.

Waist Circumference directly reflects the increased health risk of abdominal obesity. Waist size associated with a high health risk:
Men ~ Over 40 inches **Women** ~ Over 35 inches

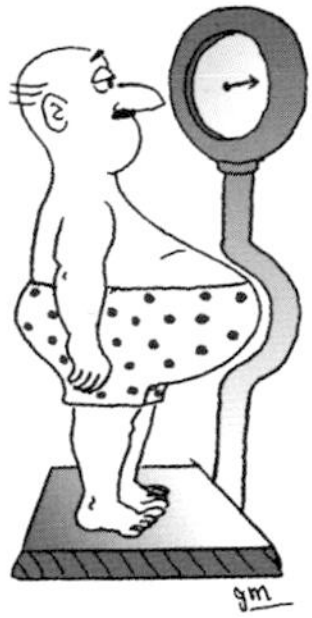

Abdominal obesity greatly increases the risk of ill-health and earlier death.

Body Mass Index (BMI)

BMI is a general (but not specific) indicator of body fatness. Although BMI alone is not diagnostic, the higher the BMI, the greater the health risk of developing diabetes, high blood pressure and heart disease. BMI does not apply to heavily muscled persons. BMI is used in a different way for children.

Check Your BMI: Find your height (no shoes) - look across the row to the weight nearest your own. Then track down to BMI.

Ht	WEIGHT (LBS) ~ ADULTS												
5'1"	100	106	111	116	122	127	132	137	143	148	153	158	185	211
5'2"	104	109	115	120	126	131	136	142	147	153	158	164	191	218
5'3"	107	113	118	124	130	135	141	146	152	158	163	169	197	225
5'4"	110	116	122	128	134	140	145	151	157	163	169	174	204	232
5'5"	114	120	126	132	138	144	150	156	162	168	174	180	210	240
5'6"	118	124	130	136	142	148	155	161	167	173	179	186	216	247
5'7"	121	127	134	140	146	153	159	166	172	178	185	191	223	255
5'8"	125	131	138	144	151	158	164	171	177	184	190	197	230	262
5'9"	128	135	142	149	155	162	169	176	182	189	196	206	236	270
5'10"	132	139	146	153	160	167	174	181	188	195	202	207	243	278
5'11"	136	143	150	157	165	172	179	186	193	200	208	215	250	286
6'0"	140	147	154	162	169	177	184	191	199	206	213	221	258	294
6'1"	144	151	159	166	174	182	189	197	204	212	219	227	265	302
6'2"	148	155	163	171	179	186	194	202	210	218	225	233	272	311
6'3"	152	160	168	176	184	192	200	208	216	224	232	240	279	319
6'4"	156	164	172	180	189	197	205	213	221	230	238	246	287	328
BMI	19	20	21	22	23	24	25	26	27	28	29	30	35	40

BMI Classification:

BMI Below 19
Underweight

BMI 19-24.9
Healthy Weight
(Low Health Risk)

BMI 25-29.9
Overweight
(Moderate Health Risk)

BMI 30-40
Obese (High Health Risk)

BMI Over 40
Morbid Obesity
(Very High Risk)

Interactive BMI Calculator
www.calorieking.com

Calories & Weight Loss

Calories in Food

Calories in food are derived from protein, fat and carbohydrate. Alcohol also provides calories. Vitamins, minerals and water provide no calories.

Calorie Values Per Gram

Fat/Oil	~ 9 Calories
Carbohydrate	~ 4 Calories
Protein	~ 4 Calories
Alcohol	~ 7 Calories

Note that fats have over double the calories of protein and carbohydrate. The higher the fat content of food, the higher the calories.

Sample Calculation

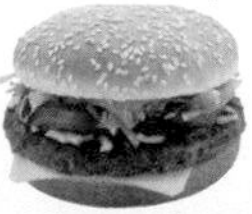

QUARTER POUNDER® WITH CHEESE has 510 calories derived from:

26g Fat (x 9 cals/gram)	=	234
40g Carbohyd.(x 4 cals/gram)	=	160
29g Protein (x 4 cals/gram)	=	116
Total Calories	=	510

Calorie Levels for Weight Loss

Start with a calorie-controlled diet that allows a moderate weight loss of 1/2 - 1 pound per week. Weight loss is usually much greater in the first few weeks due to extra fluid losses.

Note: It is better to increase exercise rather than lessen food calories too drastically.

Suggested Calories for Weight Loss

Women:	Non-active	1000 - 1200
	Active	1200 - 1500
Men:	Non-active	1200 - 1500
	Active	1500 - 1800
Teenagers:		1200 - 1800

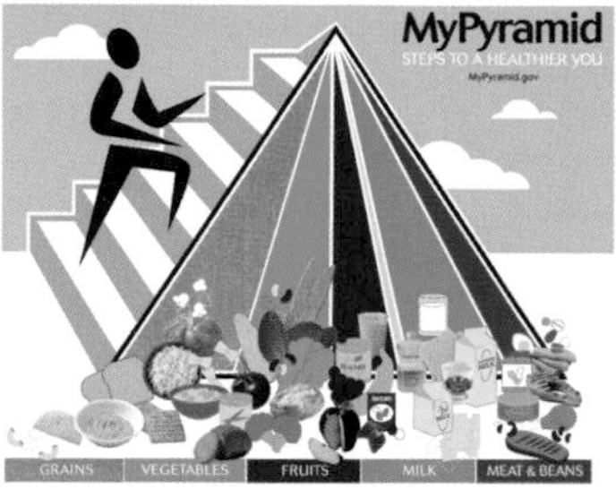

The MyPyramid symbol represents the recommended proportion of foods from each food group and focuses on the importance of making smart food choices in every food group, every day. Daily physical activity is also important. *(More info: www.MyPyramid.gov)*

Examples of Single Serving Sizes

Grains (Eat 6 servings per day):

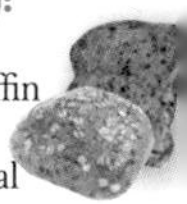

- 1 slice whole-grain bread (1 oz)
- 1/2 bun, small bagel or English muffin
- 4 small crackers or 1 tortilla
- 1 oz ready-to-eat whole-grain cereal
- 1/2 cup cooked cereal, rice or pasta

Vegetable (Eat 3-5 servings per day):

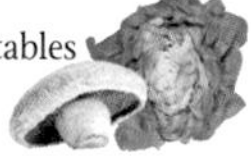

- 1 cup raw leafy vegetables
- 1 1/2 cups raw chopped vegetables
- 1/2 cup cooked vegetables
- 1/2 - 3/4 cup vegetable juice

Fruits (Eat 3-5 servings per day):

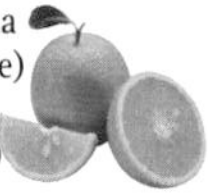

- 1 medium apple, orange, banana
- 1/2 cup canned fruit (in own juice)
- 1/4 cup dried fruit
- 3/4 cup fruit juice (unsweetened)
- 1/4 medium avocado

Milk (2-3 servings per day):

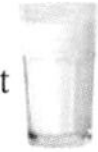

- 1 cup (8 fl.oz) milk/soy (enriched)/yogurt
- 1 1/2 oz cheese or 1/2 cup cottage cheese

Meat & Beans (Eat 2-3 servings per day):

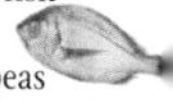

- 2-3 oz (cooked) lean meat/poultry/fish
- 2 eggs **or** 7 oz tofu **or** 1/4 cup nuts
- 1 cup (cooked) dried beans **or** chickpeas
- 4 Tbsp peanut butter **or** 1/2 cup nuts/seeds

Portion Size Counts!

Food portion size is critical to controlling calorie intake for weight control.

Super-sized food servings have become more common when eating out and in the home. This can mean a day's worth of calories being consumed in one meal; or a snack being equivalent to a full meal.

It is easy to underestimate portion size of foods and drinks, and unwittingly consume excess calories – even if the fat content is low or even zero!

To more accurately estimate portion size of different foods, weigh and measure your food with food scales, measuring spoons and cups. Better control of calories will result.

For a visual idea of portion sizes, visit www.CalorieKing.com. See examples (fries and cola) on this page.

Allow for Extra Calories in Packaged Food

The actual weight of packaged foods is usually 5-10% more than the label net weight (the minimum legal weight) - and in some cases up to 50% more. However, manufacturers calculate the calories based on the net weight. For actual calories, weigh the product and calculate the extra calories.

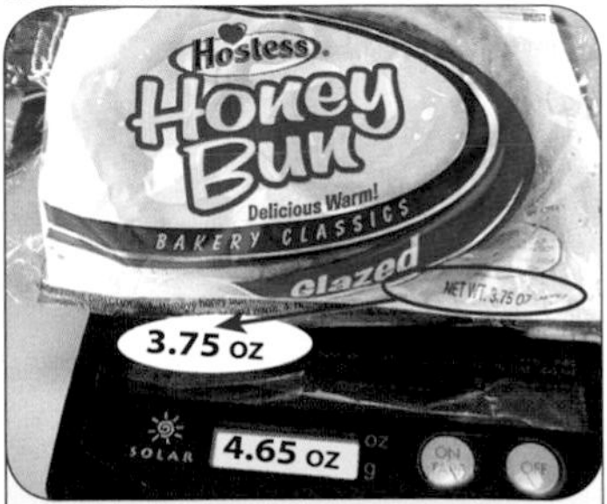

Actual weight of this bun is 24% more than the stated net weight.

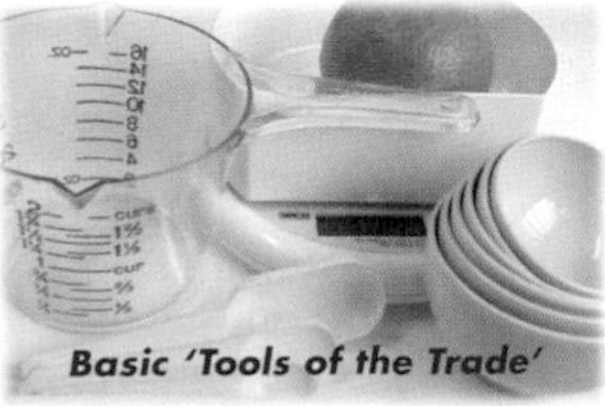

Basic 'Tools of the Trade'

CALORIEKING PORTION WATCH

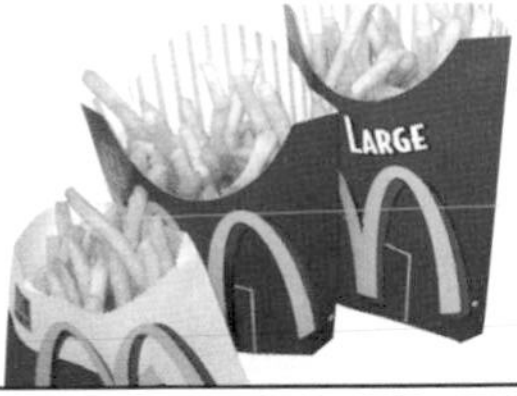

Fries	Cal	Fat	Carb
Small	250	13	30
Medium	380	20	47
Large	570	30	70

CALORIEKING PORTION WATCH

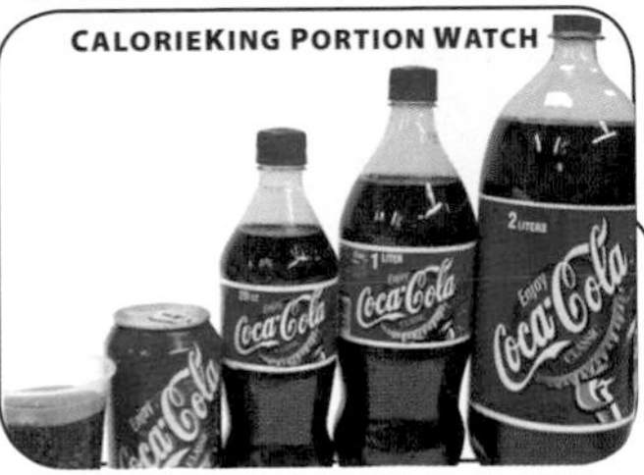

Cola	Cal	Fat	Carb
8 fl.oz Cup	100	0	25
12 fl.oz Can	150	0	37
20 fl.oz Bottle	250	0	63
1 Liter Bottle	400	0	100
2 Liter Bottle	800	0	200

Recommended Fat Intake

Americans consume too much fat with many getting over 40% of total daily calories from fat – either as fat or oil, or as fat in foods and drinks. A range of 20-30% is healthier.

Fat Intake - Healthy Ranges

Children	~	30-60g
Teenagers (Active)	~	40-80g
Women	~	30-60g
Men: Active	~	40-80g
Heavy Activity/Athlete	~	80-120g

MAXIMUM DESIRABLE FAT INTAKE (Daily)

Calories	Fat	% Fat Cals
1200 cals	30g fat	23%
1500 cals	40g fat	24%
1800 cals	50g fat	25%
2000 cals	60g fat	27%
2200 cals	70g fat	28%
2500 cals	80g fat	29%
3000 cals	100g fat	30%
4000 cals	135g fat	30%

Percentage Fat Calories Formula:

$$\frac{\text{Grams of Fat Per Serving x (900)}}{\text{Total Calories Per Serving}}$$

Fat Percent Content

(Grams of fat per 100 grams of food)

Don't be fooled by promotion of foods claiming to have a low percentage of fat. **It's serving size and total grams of fat that count.**

Examples: **Whole Milk with 3.5%** fat sounds low (3.5g fat/100ml) but an 8 fl.oz cup contains 8g fat; and 2 cups contain 16g fat.

Ice cream with 10% fat seems high, yet a regular scoop (3 fl.oz) has only 5g fat.

(**Low-fat ice cream** has less than 2g fat/serving.)

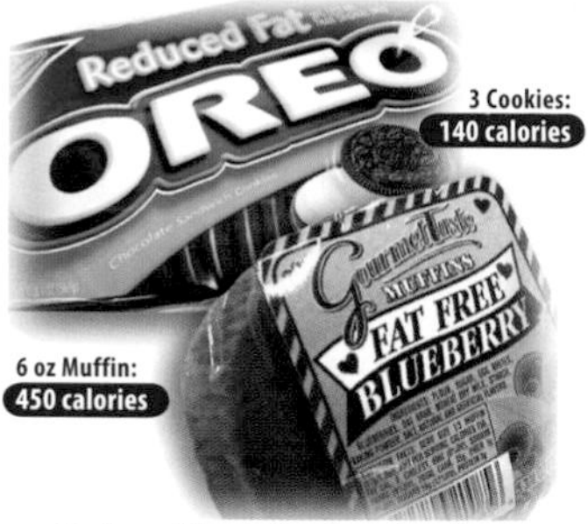

Reduced fat & fat-free foods are not necessarily low calorie. Portion size is still important.

It is a mistake to think that eating low-fat or fat-free foods allows you to eat double the quantity. You can end up with even more calories than eating smaller amounts of regular fat products.

Also fat-free but high in calories are soda drinks, fruit juices, beer, alcoholic spirits, sugar and candy. Bread, rice and pasta also have negligible fat.

Total Calories Count!

Ultimately, **it is food portion size and total calories that count** whether from fat, carbohydrate or protein. Remember, cows get fat on grass!

FOOD LABEL MEANINGS

FDA Nutrition Claim Definitions
(All are on a Per Serving Basis)

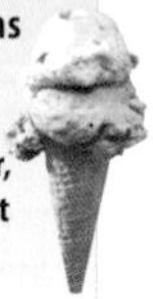

Low Calorie: **40 Calories or less**
Light or Lite: **One third fewer calories or, 50% or less fat than regular product**
Fat-Free: **Less than half a gram of fat**
Low-Fat: **3 grams or less of fat**
Reduced Fat: **25% less fat than regular product**
Fewer or Less Calories: **At least 25% fewer calories than regular product**

Meats, Poultry, Fish

- Choose **lean cuts** of meat with little marbling. **Trim all visible fat** from meat and remove the skin from poultry. Removal of fat after cooking, is okay (to prevent dryness). Choose 'extra lean' ground beef.
- **Avoid high-fat meat products** such as salami, bacon, sausage and franks.
- **Broil or bake. Avoid frying in oil.** Allow casseroles to cool and skim off surface fat.
- **Avoid fried fish**, frozen fish in batter and canned fish in oil.

Fats & Oils

- **Use minimal amounts** of all types of fat and oil. All are high in calories.
- **Choose** 'light' and 'reduced fat' spreads but still use sparingly.
- Use minimal amounts of oil when stir-frying. Use no-stick sprays like Pam.

Salad Dressings & Sauces

- **Avoid regular mayonnaise and oil dressings.** Choose 'light', 'reduced fat' or 'fat-free' brands.
- **Choose** low-fat or fat-free sauces (mainly tomato-based). Avoid 'pesto', 'alfredo', 'cheese' and 'creamy' sauces.

Milk, Cheese

- **Choose** low-fat or nonfat milks and yogurts. **Avoid** full-cream milk, cream, Half & Half.
- **Cheese:** Choose fat-free, and low-fat cheese. Part-skim ricotta is still high in fat. Low-fat cottage cheese is a good choice. Cheese substitutes can still be high in fat.

Snacks, Cookies, Candy

- **Avoid** high-fat snacks such as potato chips, corn/tortilla chips, cheese puffs, buttered popcorn, chocolate and carob bars.

Desserts/Sweets

- **Avoid high-fat desserts**, such as cake, pie, pastries, cheesecake, full-fat puddings.
- **Choose** fresh fruits, fresh fruit salad, canned fruit in water pack, low-fat ice cream. Use low-fat yogurt in place of cream.

Fast-Foods & Take-Out

Check the Fast-Foods Section of this book for actual fat and calorie counts.

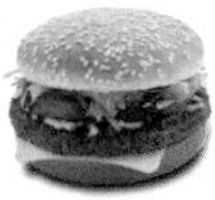

- **Avoid deep-fried chicken**, french fries, and onion rings.
- **Pizzas:** Avoid sausage/pepperoni. Choose vegetarian topping and modest quantity of cheese. Eat a moderate serving. Eat extra salad and fresh fruit.
- **Hamburgers:** Choose medium size, lower fat burgers. Avoid bacon. Have a side salad (with fat-free dressing).
- **Delis:** Choose sandwiches/bread rolls, pitas with low-fat fillings and plain salad. Limit meat/cheese to small portions.
- **Coffees:** Avoid large sizes of latte and frappuccino. Request nonfat milk and no whipped cream. Avoid cookies and pastries.

Extra Information: www.CalorieKing.com

FRYING ADDS FAT!

The greater the surface area of potato exposed to fat or oil, the higher the fat content and calories.

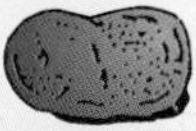

Whole Potato (3 oz)
0g Fat, 65 Cals

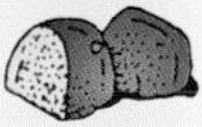

Roast Potato (3 oz)
5g Fat, 155 Cals

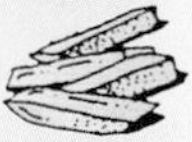

Fries (Large cut, 3 oz)
12g Fat, 220 Cals

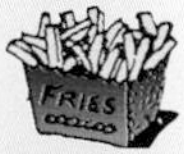

Fries (Small, 3 oz)
15g Fat, 265 Cals

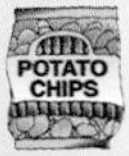

Potato Chips (3 oz)
30g Fat, 450 Cals

Naturally-Friendly Carbs

- **Carbohydrate foods in their more natural forms** (not overly processed) are essential to good health. They are the main source of fuel for the body, and also provide important vitamins, minerals, antioxidants and fiber – all of which help protect against heart disease, diabetes, hypertension, constipation-related ailments and many other diseases.
- Carbohydrates even help the body produce serotonin, the 'feel good' brain chemical that helps control appetite and overeating. Too little serotonin can lead to mood swings and depression.

Carbohydrates are found in different forms in food as:

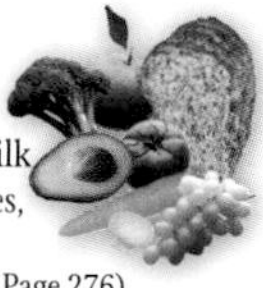

- Sugars in fruit, sugar cane, milk
- Starches in whole grains, legumes, nuts, seeds and vegetables
- Dietary fiber (See Fiber Guide ~ Page 276)

Glycemic Index & Diabetes ~ Page 20

RECOMMENDED CARBOHYDRATE INTAKE

Calories (Daily)	Carbohydrate (Grams)	Percent Carbohydrate Calories
1200 cals	120g	40%
1500 cals	170g	45%
1800 cals	210g	47%
2000 cals	250g	50%
2500 cals	345g	55%
3000 cals	450g	60%

How Much Do We Need?

- As shown in the chart, well-balanced diets above 2000 calories contain 50-60% of total calories from carbohydrates.
- At lower calorie levels used for weight control (1200-1500 calories), carbohydrates account for as little as 40% of total calories. This is because protein calories have nutritional priority.
- Carbohydrates & Diabetes ~ *See Page 20*

Low-carb diets only work if total calories are reduced.

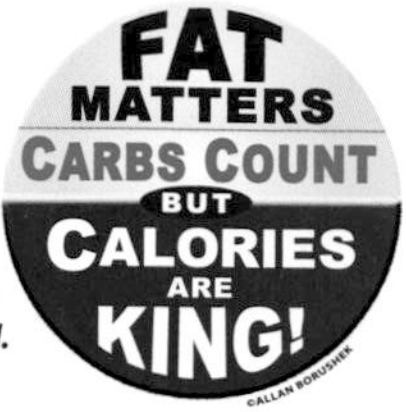

Low-Carbohydrate Diets

- Popular low-carbohydrate diets are extreme in their recommendations to initially cut carb intake to as little as 20 grams per day – the amount in 1 thick slice of bread, or 1 medium apple, or 1 small potato.
  This greatly increases the risk of nutritional deficiencies and compromises health, particularly if fat intake is excessive through fatty meats, high-fat dairy products, and fried foods.
- While overweight Americans do need to reduce carbohydrate intake, it should be done **sensibly as part of reducing portion size and total calories.**
- Simply eating 'low-carb' food products without regard to portion size, calories or fats, will do little to promote weight loss or good health.
- **Low-carb diets (and indeed any diet) only work if total calories are reduced.**
- Refined sugars should be one of the first targets in moderating carb intake.

Extra Info ~ www.CalorieKing.com

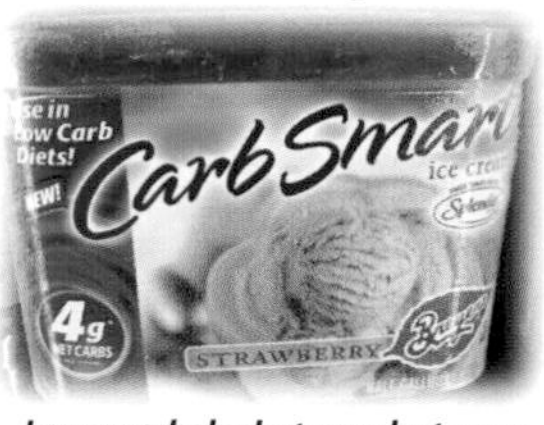

Lower carbohydrate products may still be high in calories and fat.

- Many overweight, inactive people consume over 500 calories of refined sugars per day, either self -added or as part of food products. This is equivalent to over 30 level teaspoons – a significant amount in weight control terms. Halving this amount would be reasonable and worthwhile.

  Note: Naturally occurring sugars in fruits, vegetables and milk are fine when consumed in normal recommended amounts. These foods are also rich in other nutrients.

  Refined sugar is referred to as having 'empty calories' because it supplies calories but negligible nutrients and no fiber.
- **Most sugar in our diet is 'hidden'** in processed foods such as soft drinks, fruit drinks, candy, cookies, cake, jam, sauces, ice cream, desserts, canned foods, and breakfast cereals.

  Certainly enjoy moderate quantities of these foods, but for serious weight control, look for 'low calorie', 'diet' or 'sugar-free'.

  However, be careful not to substitute sugar-rich foods with high-fat foods which might boost calories even more!
- Be aware that sugar comes in different forms such as sucrose, glucose, fructose, malt, high-fructose corn syrup, molasses, honey and maple syrup. Check the label.
- **Sugar alcohols such as sorbitol,** mannitol and maltitol are carb-based and have ½ - ¾ the calories of regular sugar. While not counted as sugar on food labels, they do add to the carb count. Excess amounts can cause bloating, gas and diarrhea.
- **Sugar-free sweeteners** such as *Equal, DiabetiSweet, NutraSweet, Splenda, Sweet'n Low* and *Stevia* make it easy to reduce sugar in drinks and recipes. Use only in moderation.

  Note: Most recipes can be adapted to contain less sugar with little effect on taste or quality.

Extra Info ~ www.CalorieKing.com

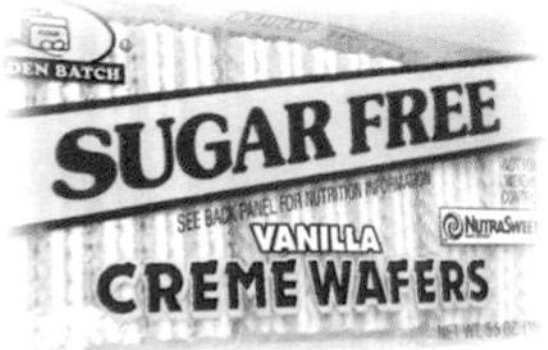

Sugar-free snacks and foods may be higher in fat and calories than the regular product.

Example ~ Creme Wafers (3):
Regular ~ 115 cals, 6g fat
Sugar-Free ~ 160 cals, 10g fat

SUGAR CONTENT OF SOME COMMON FOODS

	Teaspoons of Sugar
Coca Cola or *Pepsi*, 12 fl.oz	10
20 fl.oz size	17
Iced Tea, sweetened, 12 fl.oz	8
Chocolate Milk, 12 fl.oz	6
Honey Smacks Cereal, 1 oz	4
Popcorn, caramel, 1 cup	3.5
Chocolate Bar, 1.5 oz	6
M&M's 1.7 oz pkg	7
Muffin, large, 4 oz	6
Choc Chip Cookie, 1 oz	2
Donut, iced	6
Apple Pie, 1 piece	7
Jell-O, ½ cup	4.5
Jam, 1 Tbsp, 20g	2.5
Syrup, maple, 1 Tbsp	3

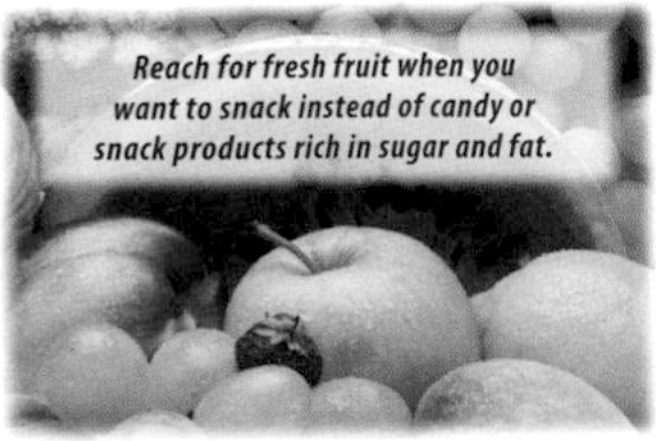
Reach for fresh fruit when you want to snack instead of candy or snack products rich in sugar and fat.

Tips For Overweight Kids & Parents!

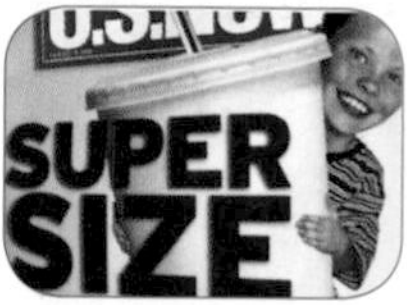

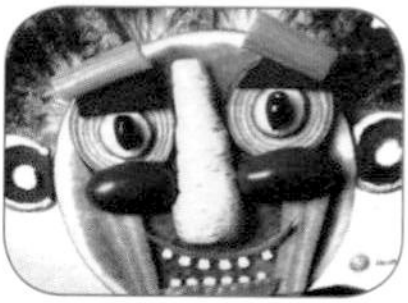

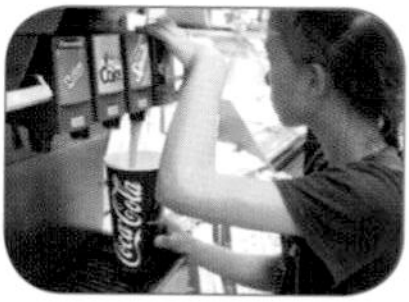

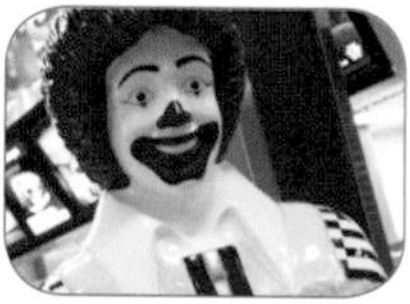

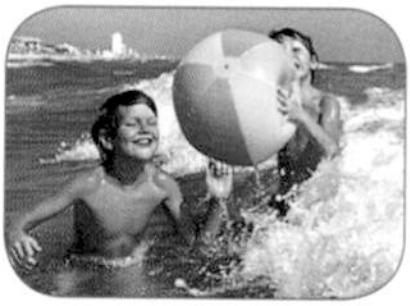

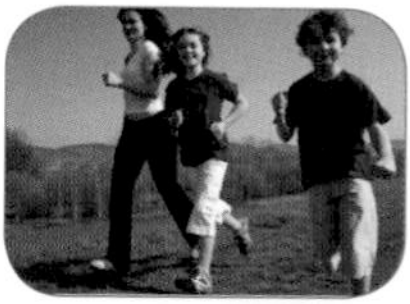

The XL Generation

Some 15% of American kids and adolescents are overweight; and childhood obesity has doubled over the last 20 years. Diabetes, high blood pressure and high cholesterol are major problem areas for overweight children and adolescents, as are depression, low self-esteem, sleep apnea and bone joint problems.

To address this problem, cooperation is required between kids, parents, schools and government. Weight control is a family and community affair.

Five Simple Tips To Get Started:

❶ Watch Soda Intake

Limit soda and sugary drinks to one serving on the weekends. Soda should not be an everyday beverage – water should be. When at restaurants or using a soda fountain, choose small servings with ice or choose diet soda instead. Schools should provide water and restrict access to soda as should parents when eating out or in the home!

❷ Cut back on Fast-Foods and Eating Out

Many more calories are consumed when you eat out. Healthy meals prepared at home are best for the whole family.

❸ Say "No" to Super-Sizing

When meals are upsized, loads more calories are consumed. Choose sensible portion sizes when eating out and at home. Use smaller plates and choose smaller packages.

❹ Limit Between-Meal Snacking

Watch out for high-fat and high-calorie snacks – they can have more calories than a meal! Keep your eye on portion sizes and limit salty snack foods and candy to parties and special occasions. Choose fresh fruit, vegetables, nuts and low-fat milk instead.

❺ Get Moving ~ Watch Less TV

Kids need at least 60 minutes of physical activity every day. It's critical for their fitness, and greatly lessens the risk of obesity.

Encourage kids to be active out of school hours. Wearing a pedometer can be highly motivational for kids to move more – as can playing dance video games such as *Dance Dance Revolution. Wii Fit (Nintendo)* is also useful as a fitness motivator.

Limit TV and non-active computer games to just one hour per day. Also limit the accompanying snacks! Include exercise in family activities.

Extra information and tips ~ www.CalorieKing.com

Sample Meal Plan - 1400 Calories

For Healthy, Overweight Persons ~ Not for Persons With Any Medical Condition ~ Please Check With Your Doctor & Dietitian ~

Breakfast (approx. 300 cal)

	1 Small Fruit or ½ oz Dried Fruit
Plus	Cereal: 1½ oz Dry (high fiber)
	or 1 cup cooked Oatmeal
Plus	½ oz Almonds/Seeds
Plus	Milk (from daily allowance) or Yogurt (low-fat)

Daily Milk Allowance (approx.160 calories)
2 cups Non-Fat Milk or 1½ cups Low-fat (1%) Milk
or equivalent Soy Drink, Yogurt, Cheese, Tofu

Fat Allowance (140 calories; 15g Fat)
4 tsp Fat or 6-8 tsp Diet Margarine or 3 tsp Oil
or 1½ Tbsp Mayonnaise or ½ medium Avocado
or 1½ Tbsp Peanut Butter or 30g Nuts/Seeds

Breakfast ~ Choice 2

	1 Small Fruit
Plus	2 Eggs (no added fat)
	or 2 oz Cheese (low-fat)
	or 4 oz Cottage Cheese (low-fat)
	or 2 oz Lean/Canadian Bacon
Plus	1 Tomato
Plus	1 Slice Whole-Grain Toast

Lunch (approx. 440 calories)

	2 slices Whole-Grain Bread (2 oz)
	or 4 Crispbreads/Crackers or 6" Pita
Plus	2 oz lean Meat, Chicken or Turkey
	or 3½oz Tuna (in water) or 2½ oz Salmon
	or 1 oz Cheese or ½ cup (4 oz) Cottage Cheese
	or ½ cup (4 oz) Ricotta Cheese (low-fat)
	or ½ cup (4 oz) Fruit Yogurt (low-fat)
	or ½ cup (4 oz) Bean Salad
Plus	Large Salad (Oil-free dressing)
Plus	1 small Fruit or ½ oz Dried Fruit

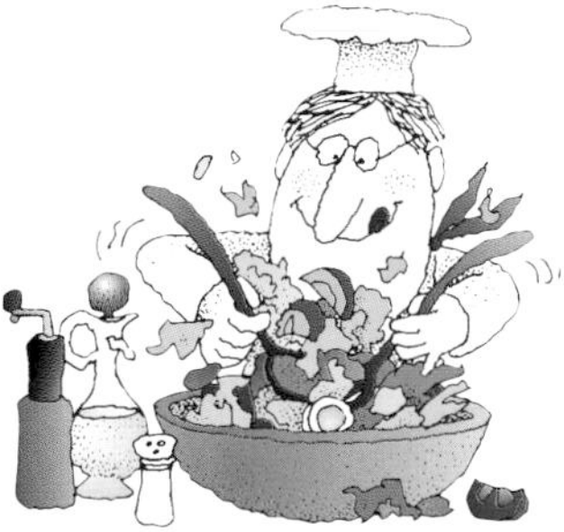

Dinner (approx. 360 calories)

	Soup (fat-free)
Plus	3 oz lean Meat (cooked weight)
	or 4 oz Chicken Breast (no skin)
	or 3 oz Chicken Thigh/Leg (no skin)
	or 5 oz Fish (grilled, no fat)
	or ¾ cup (6 oz) Beans (Soy, Kidney, Pinto etc)/Lentils
	or Low-fat Entree (e.g. Lean Cuisine)
Plus	1 small Potato or ½ cup Rice/Pasta/Sweet Corn
	or 1 slice Whole-Grain Bread
Plus	2-3 servings Vegetables/Salad
Plus	1 small Fruit + Diet Gelatin Dessert

Between Meals

Water, Coffee, Tea, Diet drinks, Fruit from main meals; Raw vegetable pieces, Milk from Daily Allowance

Exercise & Weight Control

- Persons who exercise regularly lose more weight and keep it off longer than non-exercisers.
- Exercise also improves general health and well-being. Mood, confidence and self-esteem are enhanced by a sense of control and accomplishment.
- **Exercise increases the metabolic rate** of the body even for hours after exercise - a good way to 'wake up' a sluggish metabolism and burn extra fat. Exercise compensates for any decrease in metabolic rate with increasing age and also in some heavy smokers who stop smoking.
- **Strength training** further builds muscle and aids body reshaping. You can also eat a little more food! Note: Each extra pound of muscle burns an extra 50 calories daily ~ even while you sleep! Weight from exercised muscles is okay. It is surplus fat (particularly abdominal fat) that is potentially harmful to health.
- **Avoid injury** by beginning with walking, low impact aerobics, or weight-supported exercise (e.g. swimming, cycling). Avoid competitive sports.
- **How Much?** Start with 10 - 20 minutes/day and progress to 30 - 60 minutes/day.
  Also walk up stairs instead of using elevators. Take a brisk walk at lunch. Use an exercise bike, treadmill or stair machine while watching TV. Walk the dog.
- **How Often?** While aerobic fitness requires only 3 - 4 sessions weekly, **weight control is a daily event which requires daily exercise.**

TV CAN BE FATTENING!

- **Many adults and children spend over 20 hours per week watching TV or at the computer (playing games or 'surfing') – at the same time as eating high-calorie snacks and drinks.**
- **Are you a TV couch potato or computer addict? Limit your TV and computer hours and plan healthy physical activities.**
- **At home, limit kids to just one hour daily for TV and computers. Kids need at least 60 minutes of physical activity every day.**

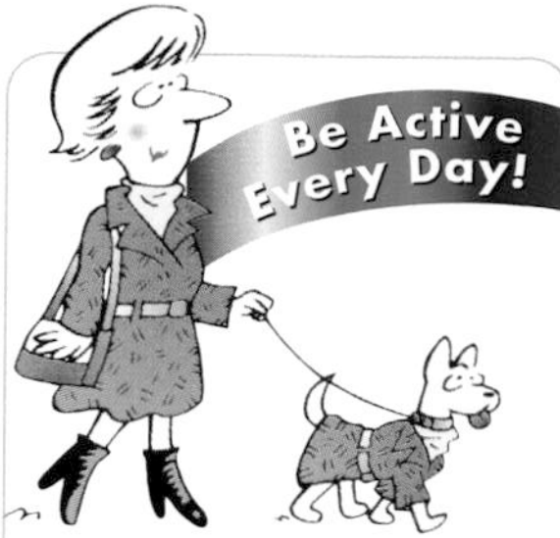

Brisk walking each day is a safe and effective way to keep trim and fit. Try it – you'll like it!

Strength-training with light weights helps to retain or rebuild muscle tissue. It enhances weight control.

FATNESS VS FITNESS

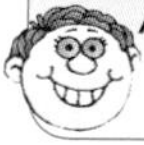

An overweight but fit person can be healthier than a thin, unfit person.

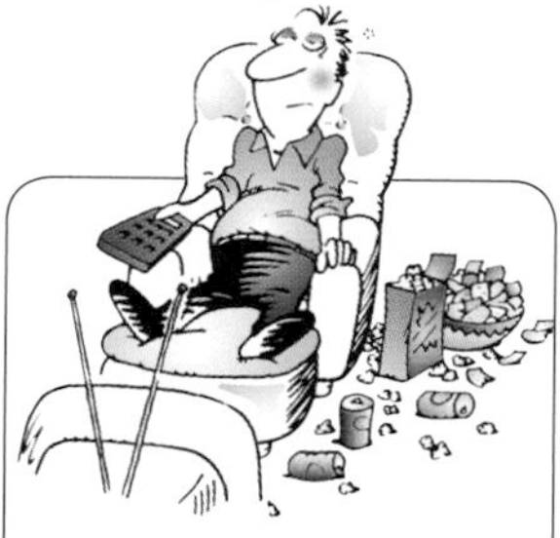

Too little exercise and too much food are the main contributors to middle-age spread.

Daily exercise and sensible eating can minimize middle-age spread. Include some strength-training to retain or build muscle.

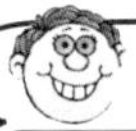

Calories Used in Exercise

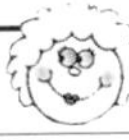

LIGHT

130 lbs ~ 3 Cals/Min

170 lbs ~ 4 Cals/Min

220 lbs ~ 5 Cals/Min

- Walking, slow
- Cycling, light
- Frisbee playing
- Gardening, light
- Golf, social
- Tennis, doubles
- Housework, cleaning
- Calisthenics, light
- Bowling
- Ping-pong, social
- Ice Skating, light
- Aquarobics, light
- Skate Boarding
- Line/Square Dancing
- Tai Chi, Yoga
- Volleyball

MODERATE

130 lbs ~ 5 Cals/Min

170 lbs ~ 6 Cals/Min

220 lbs ~ 7 Cals/Min

- Walking, brisk
- Cycling, moderate
- Swimming, crawl
- Weight-training, light
- Tennis, moderate
- Racquetball, beginners
- Aerobics, light
- Football, touch
- Basketball, Baseball
- Walking Downstairs
- Snow Skiing (downhill)
- Shovelling snow
- Dancing (ballroom)
- Rowing, moderate
- Volleyball, competitive

HEAVY

130 lbs ~ 8 Cals/Min

220 lbs ~ 12 Cals/Min

170 lbs ~ 10 Cals/Min

- Walking (power), Jogging
- Cycling (vigorous), Spinning
- Swimming, strenuous
- Weight-training, heavy
- Wrestling/Judo, advanced
- Racquetball, advanced
- Tae Bo, Kick Boxing
- Football, training
- Basketball (Pro)
- Climbing Stairs
- Skipping Rope
- Skiing (cross country)
- Aquarobics, advanced
- Dancing (strenuous), Zumba
- Rowing, vigorous
- Martial Arts

Note: Only those sports or activities that are sustained over a period of time (e.g running) qualify for heavy exercise. Stop-start sports such as tennis are considered 'moderate'.

Interactive Calculations ~ www.CalorieKing.com/tools

WALKING PROGRAM

USE DISTANCE, STEPS OR TIME

Weeks	Distance	Steps (Pedometer)	Time
1-2	1 mile	2000	20 mins
3-5	1.5 miles	3000	18 mins
6-8	2 miles	3500	35 mins
9-10	2.5 miles	4500	45 mins
11+	3.5 miles	6000	60 mins

10,000 STEPS PER DAY

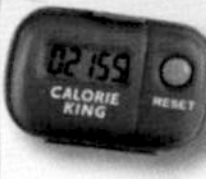

A pedometer can motivate you to be more active. It clips to your belt or waist band and registers each step.

Aim for 8,000 - 10,000 steps per day, instead of an average of only 3,000 - 4,000 steps.

For Extra Information:
www.CalorieKing.com

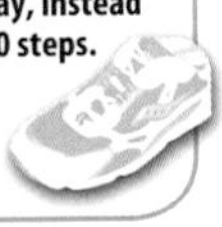

Reshaping Eating Behaviors

- Eating is a behavior that is largely controlled by people with whom we live or socialize, places in which we carry out our lives, and our emotions. Become aware of those situations that commonly lead to extra food being eaten.
- We may also be unaware of 'bad' eating habits that can lead to excess calorie intake; e.g. eating quickly, large mouthfuls, eating when tense or bored, finishing a large serving of food when not hungry.

Tips to help uncover and correct those 'bad' eating habits:

- **Don't eat while engaged in other activities;** for example, watching TV, reading. Eat only at the table, not at the fridge or while standing.
- **Don't eat quickly.** Chewing slowly allows time to register a feeling of fullness. Don't use fingers, only utensils. Cut food into smaller pieces. Don't load your fork until the previous mouthful is finished.
- **Don't purchase problem high calorie foods.** Shop from a set list to prevent impulse buying. Avoid shopping with children.
- **Buy snack foods** in the smallest package. The larger the serving size or package, the more you are likely to eat or drink.
- **Plan meals in advance. Stick to a set menu.**
- **Plan a strategy to avoid uncontrolled eating** and drinking at social events, or when your emotions urge you to binge.

  Rehearse repeatedly in your mind exactly what you will do in such situations. Remind yourself several times each day that you are in charge of your actions and that you can be strong-willed. Seek counseling or coaching on various strategies.
- **Promise yourself** that when you feel the urge to snack, you will engage in some activity that will distract you away from food (e.g. go for a walk, brush your teeth, phone a friend.)

  If you eat out of boredom, find some new hobby or interest that gets you out of the house. Even enroll in an adult education class.

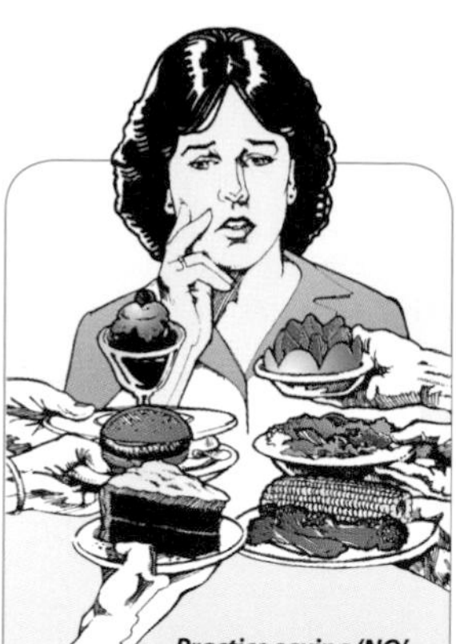

Practice saying 'NO' politely but assertively.

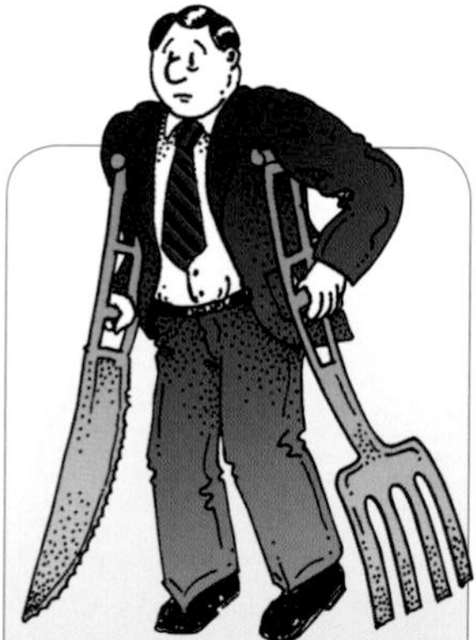

Do you use food as an emotional crutch? If so, professional counseling may be helpful.

The food journal is the most powerful proven aid for dieters. Persons who keep a food and exercise journal not only lose more weight, they also keep it off. Here are some of the reasons:

- **Recording your eating and exercise habits** jolts you into realizing just what you do eat and drink each day; and also whether you exercise sufficiently.
- **Helps you identify problem foods** and drinks with excessive calories and fat.
- **Helps identify moods,** situations and events that lead to excessive eating of unwanted calories. You can then plan to overcome or avoid them.
- **Prevents 'calorie amnesia',** the forgetfulness that leads to rebound weight gain after successful weight loss. Recording puts you back on the right track.
- **Helps you develop greater self-discipline.** You will think twice about overindulging if you have to record it - especially if someone checks your journal regularly. It certainly keeps you honest!
- **Motivates you** to carefully plan your meals and to exercise each day.
- **Serves as a check system** for your doctor, dietitian or counselor to assess your progress and make recommendations.

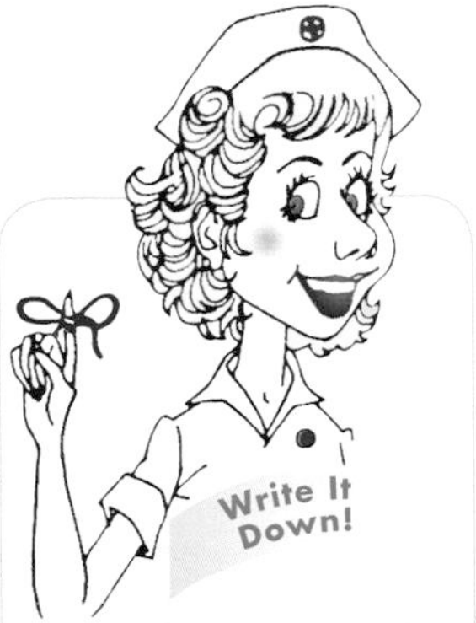

"Keeping a journal gives me feedback on exactly what I eat and drink each day.

It helps prevent 'calorie amnesia' and reminds me to exercise each day.

It's a 'must' for successful weight control!"

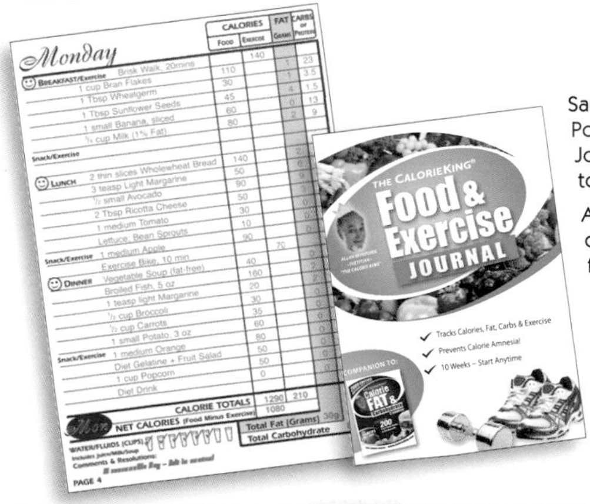

Sample Page from The Pocket Food & Exercise Journal, a 10-week journal to record food and exercise.

At day's end, exercise calories are deducted from food calories.

Includes Weekly Summary Page & Progress Checklist.

EXTRA DETAILS

~ SEE PAGE 302

What is Diabetes?

Diabetes is a disorder whereby the body cannot use carbohydrates (sugar and starches) properly.

- **After digestion**, sugar and starches are changed into **glucose** – the simplest form of sugar vital for body energy and growth.
- **Insulin** is the hormone which acts like a key that opens the door to body cells and allows glucose to enter.
- **Without enough insulin**, glucose builds up in the blood and passes into the urine. High blood glucose levels lead to frequent urination, extreme thirst, and tiredness.
- **Untreated diabetes increases the risk of damage to nerves and blood vessels.** This, in turn, increases the risk of heart disease, stroke, blindness, kidney damage, foot ulcers and gangrene (with amputation), impotence and other complications.

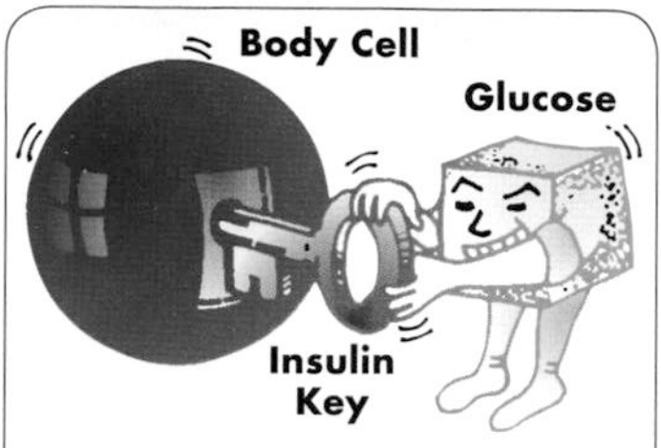

Insulin acts like a key. It opens the door to body cells and allows glucose to enter.

People with type 1 diabetes and some with type 2 have too few or no keys and require insulin injections.

Others (primarily type 2) make enough insulin but the body doesn't use it as well as it should – particularly if obese and inactive.

SYMPTOMS OF DIABETES

- Frequent urination
- Extreme thirst
- Unusual hunger
- Rapid weight loss
- Extreme fatigue
- Blurred vision
- Skin infections that are slow to heal
- Tingling/numbness in feet

Note: Diabetes can be present even with no symptoms.

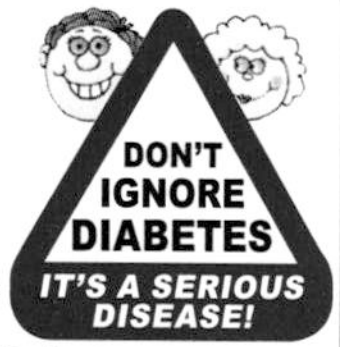

TYPE 2 DIABETES

- Occurs in 90% of diabetes cases
- Occurs mainly in adults - particularly in overweight and inactive persons
- Insulin is produced but body cells resist its action and glucose cannot enter cells
- Usually treated with meal planning and physical activity. Sometimes requires medication (pills or insulin)

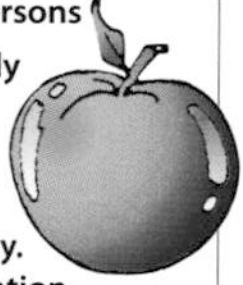

TYPE 1 DIABETES

- Occurs in 10% of diabetes cases
- Usually in children and young adults
- Pancreas produces little or no insulin. Daily insulin injections (or use of an insulin pump) are necessary, as well as:
  - Matching pre-meal insulin to the amount of carbohydrate eaten
  - Weight control and regular physical activity

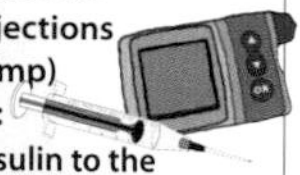

GESTATIONAL DIABETES

- Occurs in some women during pregnancy
- Usually disappears after the baby's birth
- Women who have had gestational diabetes still have a high risk of developing type 2 diabetes within 5 to 10 years
- Requires weight control, a healthy lifestyle and regular medical checks

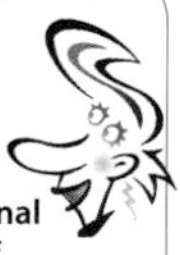

Are You At Risk for Diabetes?

Pre-Diabetes ~ An Early Warning!

Pre-diabetes means that your blood glucose levels are higher than normal, but not high enough to be called diabetes.

If you have pre-diabetes, you have a higher risk for getting diabetes later on.

The good news is that you can start taking steps to prevent diabetes by making healthy lifestyle changes – such as losing weight if overweight, and being more physically active.

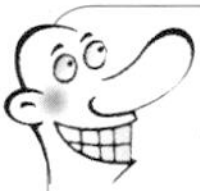

WHAT'S YOUR RISK?

Find out if you're at risk for diabetes by answering the following questions:

- ☐ I have been told I have pre-diabetes
- ☐ I have a family history of diabetes
- ☐ I am African American, Latino American, Asian American, Native American or a Pacific Islander
- ☐ I have had gestational diabetes (diabetes during pregnancy)
- ☐ I am over age 45
- ☐ I am overweight
- ☐ I get little or no physical activity
- ☐ My waist is larger than: 35 inches (for a woman) or 40 inches (for a man)
- ☐ My blood pressure is higher than 130 over 85
- ☐ My HDL (good cholesterol) is too low
- ☐ My triglycerides (blood fats) are too high

✔ CHECK YOUR RESULT

- **If you've put a check mark in two or more of the boxes,** you may be more likely to develop type 2 diabetes.
- **Talk with your healthcare provider** to see if you should have a blood test for diabetes.

BLOOD GLUCOSE CLASSIFICATION OF DIABETES

Normal:	**Below 100 mg/dl***
Pre-Diabetes:	**100-125 mg/dl***
Diabetes:	**Over 125 mg/dl***

(*Fasting Blood Glucose)

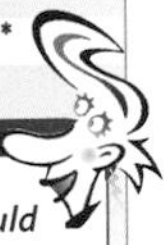

KNOW YOUR BGL

(Blood Glucose Level)

Everyone over the age of 45 should have a blood glucose test every three years

Importance of Weight Control

- **Type 2 diabetes** is more common in people who are overweight.
- **Being overweight** means that your insulin doesn't work as well to control blood glucose levels.
- **Losing just 10 to 20 pounds** can help you better manage your diabetes and lower your risk for heart disease.
- **Keys to weight control include:**
  - Following a healthy eating plan
  - Controlling food portions
  - Being physically active most days of the week
  - Keeping food records
  - Setting realistic goals
- **Work with a registered dietitian** who can help you reach a weight that's good for you.

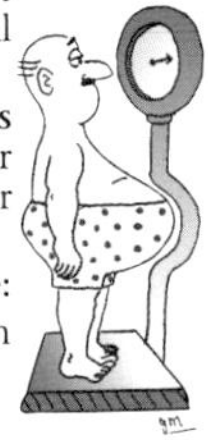

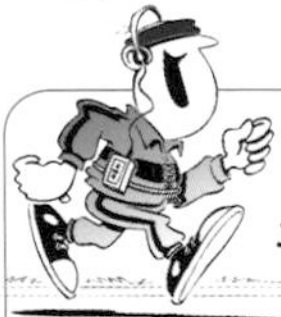

KEEP MOVING!

Every day, do at least 30 minutes of moderate intensity exercise.

(even in 5-minute sets)

It's the key to improving insulin action.

Add muscle strength training 3-4 times a week to double the benefits.

Managing Diabetes

Don't battle diabetes alone. Establish a partnership with your doctor, dietitian, certified diabetes educator, and pharmacist.

Extra Support: • *Joslin Diabetes Center*
- *American Diabetes Association*
- *American Association of Diabetes Educators*
- *Juvenile Diabetes Research Foundation*
- *National Diabetes Education Program*

Hints to keep blood glucose within safe limits:
- **Control your food intake.** Know what and when you will eat. Seek referral to a dietitian for expert advice.
- **Exercise regularly.** It assists weight control and can improve sensitivity of body cells to insulin. Plan physical activity into your daily routine.
- **Monitor your blood glucose** at home and work with a blood glucose meter. It will help you become familiar with your blood glucose patterns, and the effects of food, activity and medication.
- **Take insulin or oral medication as prescribed.** If on insulin, know what action to take if hypoglycemia (low blood glucose) occurs. Also educate your family and friends.

More Info: www.joslin.org

Be Heart Smart ~ Know Your ABC's

If you have diabetes, you are at a higher risk for heart attack and stroke than someone without diabetes. But you can fight back!

Be smart about your heart!

Take control of the ABC's of diabetes and live a long and healthy life. Talk to your healthcare provider about your ABC targets.

Be Smart About Your Heart
Control the ABCs of Diabetes
– A1C
– Blood Pressure
– Cholesterol

National Diabetes Education Program

A is for A1C

The A1C (A-one-C) test – short for hemoglobin A1C – measures your average blood glucose (sugar) over the last 3 months.

Suggested target: below 7%

B is for Blood Pressure

High blood pressure makes your heart work too hard. **Suggested target: below 130/80**

C is for Cholesterol

Bad cholesterol, or LDL, can build up and clog your arteries. **Suggested target: below 100**

Joslin Diabetes Center

RESEARCH • EDUCATION • CARE

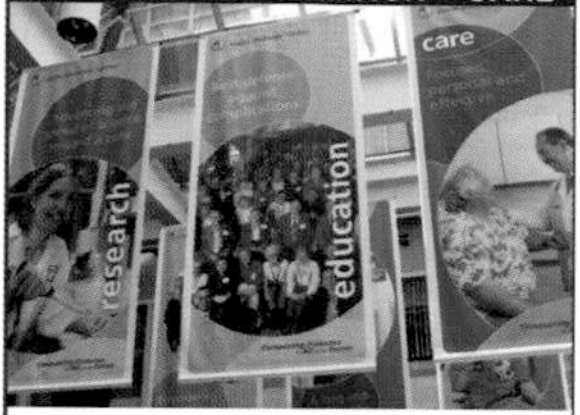

Joslin Diabetes Center, an affiliate of Harvard Medical School, is the world's largest diabetes research center, diabetes clinic and provider of diabetes education.

MORE INFORMATION

www.joslin.org or call 800-344-4501

Blood glucose meters and insulin pumps can greatly improve control of diabetes

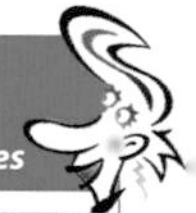

BLOOD GLUCOSE METERS (EXAMPLES)

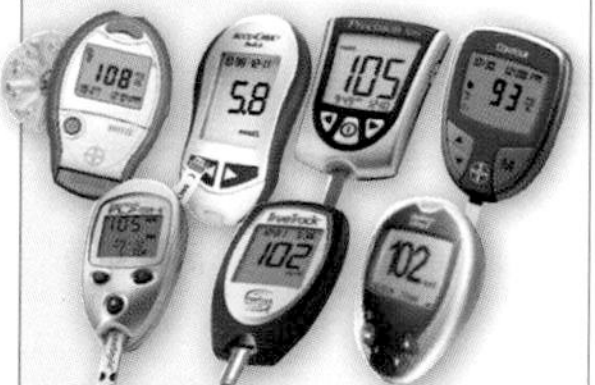

INSULIN PUMPS (EXAMPLES)

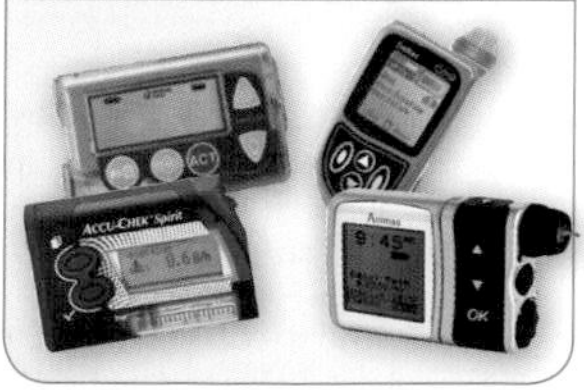

Guidelines for choosing a healthy diet apply equally to people with or without diabetes. Eating a wide variety of foods that are mainly low in fat, low in refined sugars, and high in fiber, is recommended.

However, actual food quantities, as well as when you eat, will also influence control of blood glucose. Your dietitian will individualize a meal plan to suit your food preferences, lifestyle and medical status. Here are a few tips:

- **Maintain a healthy weight.** If overweight, even a modest weight loss plus daily physical activity can help manage blood glucose in type 2 diabetes.
- **Don't skip meals.** If you take insulin or an oral hypoglycemic agent, regular meals are important.
- **If on insulin,** eat meals at the same time each day. Eat a similar amount of food at each meal. Eating about the same amount of carbohydrate over the day will make best use of insulin and prevent wide variations in blood glucose levels.
- **Know how much carbohydrate you should eat** at your meals and snacks each day.
- **Choose whole-grain breads, cereals and pasta.** Eat fresh fruits, vegetables and legumes. These foods contain more fiber and slow the release of glucose into your blood after a meal.

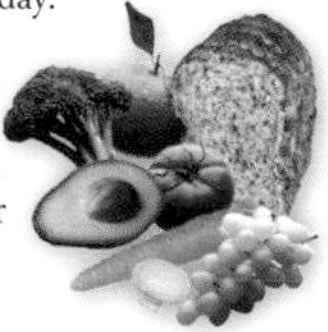

- **Limit foods high in saturated fat, trans fat and cholesterol.** Enjoy fish, soy foods, and other foods rich in omega-3 fats. *(Extra Notes: Page 271)*
- **Limit sugars and foods high in added sugar** particularly if overweight. Small amounts of sugar as part of a meal may occasionally be okay. Check with your dietitian. *(Extra Notes: Page 9)*
- **Read the Nutrition Facts label** on foods. Check the serving size, total fat and total carbohydrate.

Eat a well-balanced diet with foods high in fiber and low in saturated fat.

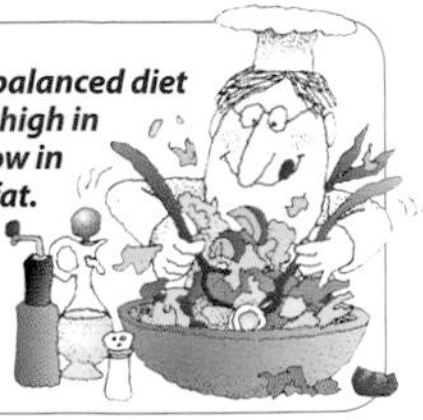

The Plate Method is an easy way to eat healthfully. (See next page)

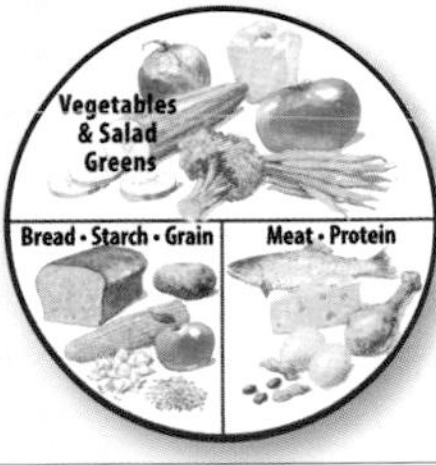

ALCOHOL TIPS

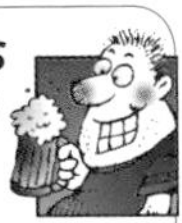

- **If you drink alcohol, have only moderate amounts:**
  Men ~ 1-2 drinks/day
  Women ~ 1 drink/day
  For some people, safe drinking will mean no alcoholic drinks at all.
  (Also see Alcohol Guide ~ Page 25)
- **Drink along with your food** – especially if you use insulin or diabetes pills.
- **Do not omit any carb food** in exchange for an alcoholic drink. However, non-alcoholic beers (12 fl oz) count as one carb exchange.
- **Alcohol increases the risk of hypoglycemia** (low blood sugar) and drug interactions if you take insulin and certain types of diabetes pills.
- **Check with your doctor and dietitian.**

Extra Info: www.joslin.org

The Plate Method – An Easy Way to Eat Healthfully

The plate method is a helpful tool to guide your food choices until you see a dietitian for your own meal plan.

For a healthy meal:

- **Fill half of your plate** with non-starchy vegetables (broccoli, green beans, carrots).
- **Fill a quarter of your plate** with carbohydrate (whole-grain bread, pasta, potato, brown rice).
- **Fill the other quarter of your plate** with 3-4 ounces of lean meat, poultry, or fish.
- **Use 1-2 teaspoons of tub margarine** or a heart-healthy vegetable oil.
- **Add** a small piece of fruit or 8 ounces of skim/low-fat milk or yogurt.

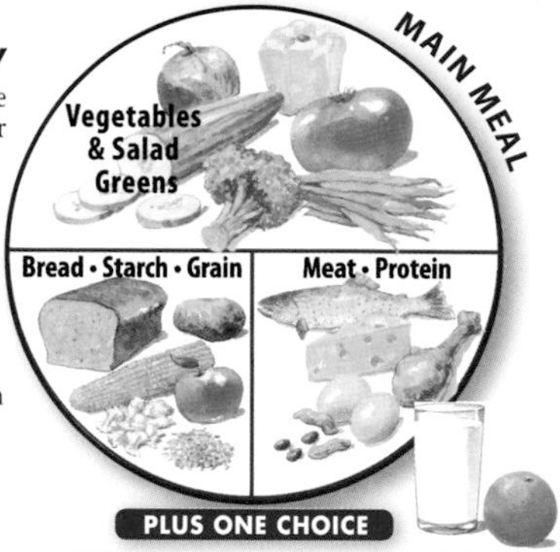

Milk, Fruit, Dessert or other Carb Food

How Much Carbohydrate Should You Eat?

A dietitian can best determine how much carbohydrate you need at each of your meals, based on your lifestyle, food preferences, and overall diabetes control.

Until you see a dietitian, aim to keep the amount of carbohydrate you eat the same at each of your meals.

CARB CHOICES MEAL PLAN
One Carb Choice = 15 Grams of Carb

The amount in: 1 slice Bread
or ¾ cup Cereal (unsweetened)
or 1 small Potato **or** 1 small Fruit

Breakfast

- Eat 2-3 carb choices (30-45 grams)
- Include a low-fat protein source such as egg whites or skim milk.

Lunch and Dinner

- Eat 3-4 carb choices (45-60 grams carb)
- Include fruit and non-starchy vegetables. Choose small portions of low-fat protein foods.

Snacks: If needed, eat 1-2 carb choices (15-30 grams carb).

Carb Type Affects Blood Glucose

The various forms of carbohydrate affect blood glucose levels in different ways. It is difficult to predict the effect of particular foods, sugars, or meals, simply by their carbohydrate content.

Thus the same amount of carbohydrate from different foods may affect blood sugar levels very differently. Many factors affect the rate of digestion and absorption – particularly the type of sugar, starch, and fiber; the degree of processing and cooking (which increases digestion rate); and the amount of protein and fat (which slow stomach emptying and digestion).

Glycemic Index (GI)

The GI is a method of ranking carbohydrate foods on a scale (0-100) according to how they affect blood glucose levels. (See next column). The higher the GI value, the greater the food's ability to rapidly raise blood glucose levels, and the more insulin needed by the body (not desirable).

Eating low-GI foods may lead to better control of blood glucose and insulin levels (which in turn lowers the risk of damage to blood vessels and nerves). The slower digestion of low-GI foods may also help to delay hunger pangs and benefit weight control.

Note: **Choosing low-GI foods is not a license to eat unlimited amounts. Calorie restriction and portion control for weight control is of prime importance.**

- **GI is not meant to be used by itself without regard to portion size,** and other dietary recommendations for healthy eating. Foods are not good or bad on the basis of their GI.
- **While GI may be a helpful tool for some people with diabetes, what is most important is to control the total amount of carbohydrate that you eat.**

Extra Info: *www.joslin.org*
www.glycemicindex.com

LOWER-GLYCEMIC FOODS

Slower-Acting Carbohydrates

These foods are more slowly digested and absorbed. They help maintain more even blood glucose levels, as long as excessive amounts are not eaten. Use these foods regularly but still limit portion size for weight control.

Examples:

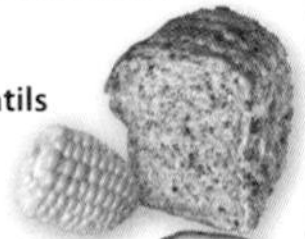

- Dried beans, peas, lentils
- Nuts and seeds
- Whole-grain breads
- Bran cereals, oats
- Sweet corn, barley, buckwheat
- Whole-grain pasta, basmati rice
- Fresh fruit: apples, avocados, bananas (firm), cherries, grapefruit, grapes, olives, oranges, peaches, pears, plums. Fresh juices.
- Vegetables: broccoli, yam, sweet potatoes, salad greens
- Milk, yogurt, soy drinks
- Dark chocolate
- Sugar alcohols (sorbitol, maltitol)

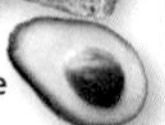

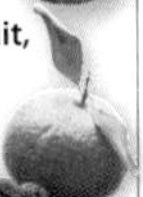

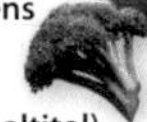

HIGHER-GLYCEMIC FOODS

Quicker-Acting Carbohydrates

These foods more rapidly raise blood glucose levels. Eat only in moderation.

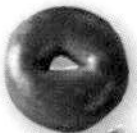

- White bread, rice cakes, bagels, croissants, doughnuts
- Low-fiber cereals: Cornflakes, *Rice Krispies, Froot Loops*
- White potatoes, white rice
- Watermelon, ripe bananas, cantaloupe, pineapple
- Soda, sugar-sweetened sports and energy drinks
- Sugar, candy, popcorn (plain)
- Ice cream (low-fat), frozen yogurt

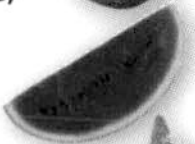

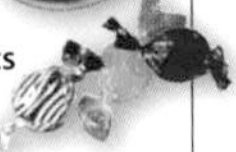

High-GI fruits and potatoes are still healthy choices when eaten in moderate amounts.

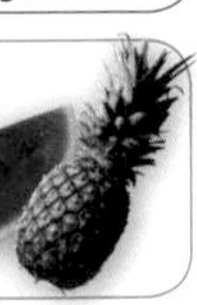

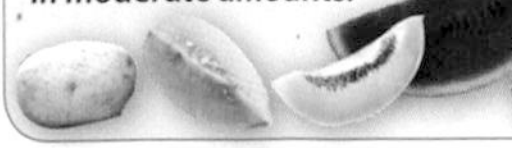

Calcium & Osteoporosis Guide

Calcium's Role in the Body

Calcium plays a vital role in nerve and muscle function, clotting of blood, enzyme regulation, insulin secretion and overall bone strength. Bones and teeth store 99% of the body's calcium.

The calcium level in blood is kept at a steady level by the continual exchange of calcium between blood and bone. When insufficient calcium is obtained from food the body draws calcium out of the bones.

This bone loss over a period of years may lead to **osteoporosis** – thinning of the bones (porous bones).

The bones become weak, brittle and easy to fracture, particularly the bones of the wrist, hips and spine. Loss of height and curvature of the spine may also result, as may periodontal disease - the deterioration of the jaw bones that support the teeth.

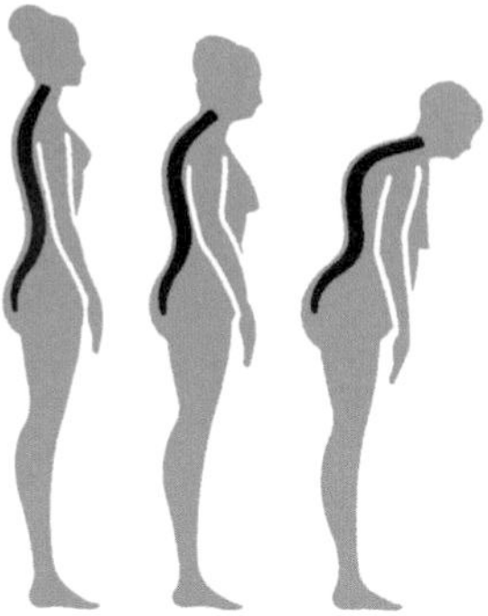

As osteoporosis progresses after menopause, vertebrae may collapse causing the spine to curve and shoulders to hunch.

Common in Women & Men

While osteoporosis also occurs in men, women are particularly vulnerable (1 in 4 by age 60). They have about 30% less bone than men, and a greater bone loss at menopause when oestrogen levels drop. Slender framed women are at greater risk. (A woman in her eighties can have lost up to two thirds of her skeleton.)

Insufficient dietary calcium during pregnancy and breastfeeding will see bone reserves drawn upon, increasing the risk of osteoporosis in later years.

Hip fractures account for 300,000 hospitalizations each year. One in 5 older Americans with hip fracture die within a year – and 1 in 5 end up in a nursing home.

Causes of Osteoporosis

The major factors associated with the bone loss of osteoporosis appear to be:

- hormone changes of menopause
- inadequate dietary intake of calcium and other bone nutrients such as magnesium, vitamin D, zinc and protein
- insufficient exercise (weight bearing - such as walking, cycling ~ 30-60 minutes daily)
- family history of osteoporosis

Other contributing factors may include:

- excessive cola (regular or diet) and alcohol intake
- cigarette smoking
- some drug medications (e.g. steroids, thyroid)

RECOMMENDED DAILY INTAKE OF CALCIUM

Children:	1-3 yrs	~ 500mg
	4-8 yrs	~ 800mg
	9-12 yrs	~ 1300mg
Teenagers:	13-18 yrs	~ 1300mg
Adults:	19-50 yrs	~ 1000mg
	51+ yrs	~ 1200mg
Women:		
Pre-menopausal		~ 1000mg
Menopausal (beginning)		~ 1200mg
Post-menopausal		~ 1500mg
Pregnant & Breast-feeding	14-18 yrs	~ 1300mg
	19+ yrs	~ 1000mg

Early Prevention Important

Gradual loss of bone begins in the thirties after maximum bone mass is reached. The stronger the bones at that time, the less trouble is likely to occur later. The earlier that prevention or treatment begins the greater the benefit. **The key to prevention is to build strong, dense bones early in life. By age 16, some 80% of peak bone mass is already reached.**

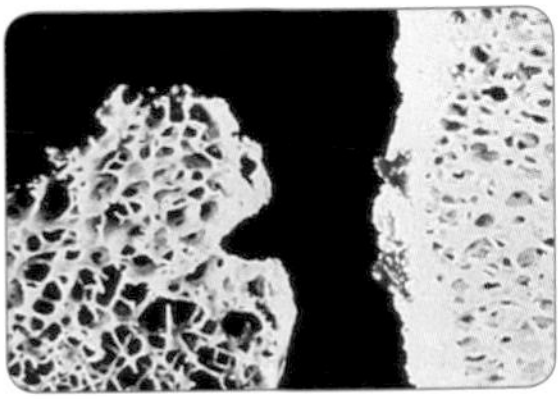

▲ *Osteoporotic Fragile Bone* ▲ *Healthy Dense Bone*

Young women may lessen the risk by:

- eating high-calcium foods as well as adequate fruits, vegetables, whole grains and nuts
- drinking less soda, and more milk
- not engaging in extreme dieting that results in menstrual period cessation (via less estrogen)
- taking regular exercise and not smoking

Good Dietary Sources of Calcium

(Eat 3-4 servings a day of calcium-rich foods)

- Milk, Yogurt, Cheese
- Flavored Milk Drinks & Fruit Smoothies
- Ice Cream (low-fat), Frozen Yogurt (low-fat)
- Soy Drinks (calcium-enriched)
- Orange Juice (calcium-fortified)
- Tofu (with calcium coagulant), Miso, Tempeh
- Canned Salmon or Sardines (with edible bones)
- Breakfast Cereals (calcium-enriched): *Total, Wheaties*
- Broccoli, Dried Beans, Baked Beans
- Almonds, Brazil nuts, Hazelnuts, Seeds

Calculating Calcium From Food Labels

The calcium content of packaged foods and drinks is shown in the Nutrition Facts label as a percentage of the DRI (dietary reference intake) of 1000 mg calcium.

To convert this percentage into milligrams of calcium, simply multiply the percent figure by 10 (or add a zero). Examples: 5% = 50 mg calcium; 35% = 350 mg calcium.

Food Calcium Counter ~ www.CalorieKing.com

Calcium Supplements

Because absorption of dietary calcium decreases with age, prescribed high doses of calcium (1500-2000mg/day) may benefit persons with osteoporosis - as well as vitamin D (preferably in D3 form, not D2), vitamin K, magnesium and zinc. Check with your doctor.

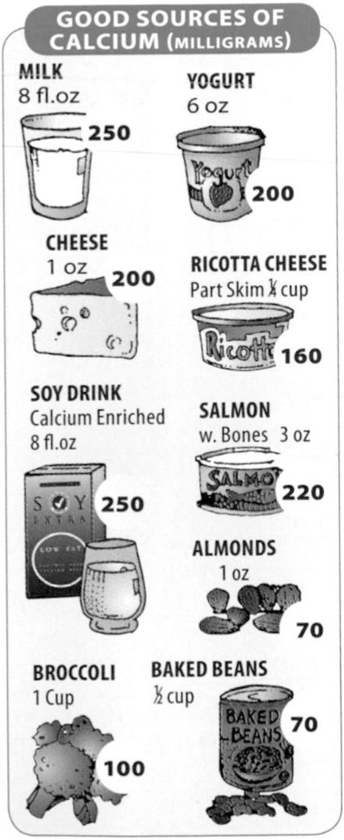

» **Calorie and fat values have been rounded off.**
Calories ~ to the nearest 5 or 10 calories.
Fat ~ to nearest half gram. **Note:** Trace amounts of fat (less than 0.3 grams) have been treated as zero.

» **Carbohydrate figures** in this book are for total carbohydrate, and not **Net Carbs** (which deducts fiber, polydextrose and sugar alcohols from total carbs).

» Because manufacturers' figures on labels are rounded off, figures in this book may differ slightly from the label. Serving sizes may also vary.

IMPORTANT DISCLAIMER

* The authors and publishers of this book are not physicians and are not licensed to give medical advice. This book is not a substitute for professional advice. Users should consult their medical professional before making any health, medical or other decisions based on the material contained herein.

* This book is a compilation of original material from other sources intended for educational purposes only. Because food manufacturers constantly change their products, only they are the authoritative source for food's most current nutritional information.

* Persons using the information herein for any medical purposes, such as matching insulin dosage to carbohydrate intake, should not rely solely on the accuracy of figures herein and should independently check food labels or contact the food manufacturer for the latest data.

* Because nutrition data for food products is subject to change, users should consult the most recent edition of this book, and the author's website www.calorieking.com for the most up-to-date information.

* **WARRANTY DISCLAIMER:**
THE AUTHOR AND PUBLISHER DISCLAIM ANY LIABILITY ARISING DIRECTLY OR INDIRECTLY FROM THE USE OF THIS BOOK. THE INFORMATION HEREIN IS PROVIDED "AS IS" AND WITHOUT ANY WARRANTY EXPRESSED OR IMPLIED. ALL DIRECT, INDIRECT, SPECIAL, INCIDENTAL, CONSEQUENTIAL OR PUNITIVE DAMAGES ARISING FROM ANY USE OF THIS INFORMATION IS DISCLAIMED AND EXCLUDED.

This information is also provided subject to Family Health Publications' Terms and Conditions found at the website, www.calorieking.com/terms and incorporated herein.

C ~ **Calories**
F ~ **Fat (grams)**
Cb ~ **Carbohydrate (grams)**

Abbreviations

tsp	=	teaspoon
Tbsp or T	=	Tablespoon
oz	=	ounce(s)
c	=	cup
fl.oz	=	fluid ounce(s)
g	=	gram(s)
avg	=	average
pkg	=	package

Volume Measures

(All measures are level)

3 tsp	=	1 Tbsp
2 Tbsp	=	1 fl.oz
½ cup	=	4 fl.oz
1 cup	=	8 fl.oz
2 cups	=	1 Pint
2 Pints	=	1 Quart

Note: 8 oz weight is not the same as 8 fl oz volume (space occupied). Dense foods weigh more per set volume. Examples:

1 cup popcorn weighs ½ oz
1 cup milk weighs 8½ oz
1 cup pudding weighs 10 oz

Metric Conversion

½ oz	=	14 grams
1 oz	=	28.4 grams
2 oz	=	57 grams
3½ oz	=	100 grams
1 fl.oz	=	30 mls
1 cup (8 fl.oz)	=	240 mls
33 fl.oz	=	1 liter (volume)

INFORMATION SOURCES

- U.S. Dept. of Agriculture
- Food Manufacturers
- Food Industry Boards & Councils
- Author extrapolations

FEEDBACK WELCOME!

Please contact the author with your queries and suggestions.
feedback@calorieking.com

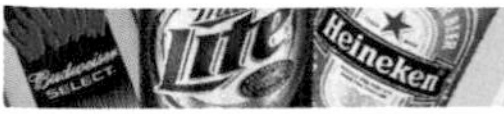

- **Health Hazards:** Excessive alcohol intake contributes to obesity, high blood pressure, stroke, heart and liver disease, some cancers, and even impotence. **Concentration and short-term memory** are reduced as well as athletic performance.

  Other alcohol hazards include fetal alcohol syndrome, stomach upsets, menstrual problems, depression, snoring, sleep problems, work absenteeism, impaired judgement, and social/family problems.

- **Alcohol contributes to obesity** through its high calories and by lessening the body's ability to burn fat. Fat storage is promoted, particularly in the belly - a health danger zone. Alcohol can also stimulate the appetite.

- **Alcohol is potentially more harmful while dieting.** Blood sugar levels may drop with resultant fatigue and further impairment of concentration, reflexes and driving skills - and maybe even the dieter's resolve!

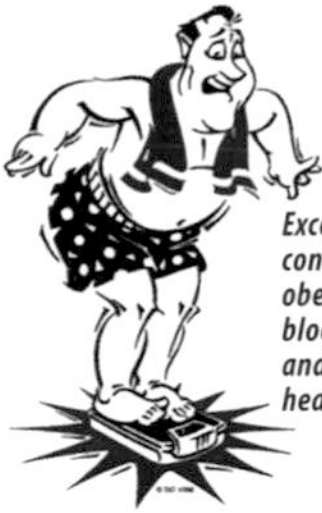

Excess alcohol contributes to obesity, high blood pressure and many other health problems

LOWER RISK ALCOHOL LIMITS

WOMEN:
No more than **1 drink** per day

MEN:
No more than **2 drinks** per day
(Over 65 ~ 1 drink)

(At least 2 days a week should be alcohol-free)

1 DRINK CONTAINS 14 GRAMS ALCOHOL
- **12 fl.oz Regular Beer** (5% Alc.)
- **OR 14 fl.oz Light Beer** (4.2% Alc.)
- **OR 5 fl.oz Wine** (12% Alc.)
- **OR 1½ fl.oz Spirits** (80 Proof)

Note: You cannot save daily drinks for one occasion. Binge drinking is particularly harmful ~ 4 drinks for males or 3 drinks for females (within 2 hours).

For some people, **safe drinking** means no alcohol at all. Even one drink may impair driving skills, particularly if tired. For women who drink frequently, breast cancer risk is increased by 9% for each drink after the first drink.

- **It is advisable not to drink at all if you are:**
  - pregnant, trying to conceive or breastfeeding
  - taking medication or have liver or heart disease (unless approved by your doctor or pharmacist)
  - planning to drive, use machinery or play sports
  - studying or needing to concentrate
  - a child or adolescent

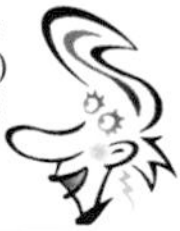

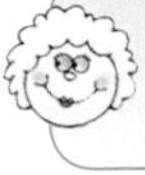

Women and adolescents are more prone to alcohol's ill-effects due to their lower body weight, smaller livers and lesser capacity to metabolize alcohol. As we age, our ability to handle alcohol decreases.

HOW TO CALCULATE ALCOHOL CONTENT

Percent alcohol on label refers to alcohol volume (ml alcohol/100ml). Note: 100ml = 3½ fl.oz

To convert to grams (weight) of alcohol, multiply the percent volume by 0.8 – since 1 ml of alcohol weighs only 0.8 grams.

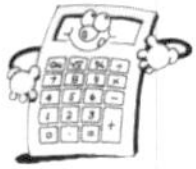

EXAMPLE:
12 fl.oz Can Beer (5% alcohol)

5% alc. volume
= 5% of 12 fl.oz = 0.6 fl.oz
= 18ml alcohol (Note: 1 fl.oz = 30ml)
Weight (18ml x 0.8) = 14.4g alcohol

GOVERNMENT WARNINGS!

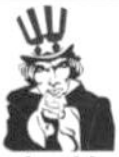

(1) According to the Surgeon General, women should not drink alcoholic beverages during pregnancy because of the risk of birth defects.

(2) Consumption of alcoholic beverages impairs your ability to drive a car or operate machinery, and may cause health problems.

EXTRA INFORMATION

Alcohol & Diabetes ~ *See Page 19*
Alcohol & The Heart ~ *See Page 274*
Tips to Avoid Harmful Drinking ~ *p. 31*

Quick Guide

Alc ~ Alcohol (Grams)
Cb ~ Carbohydrate

Beer

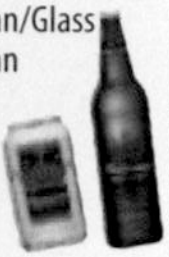

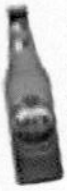

Beer Contains Zero Fat	C	Alc	Cb
Regular Beer (5% Alc. Vol.)			
7 fl.oz Glass	80	8.5	4
12 fl.oz Bottle/Can/Glass	140	14	10
16 fl.oz Bottle/Can	185	19	13
22 fl.oz Bottle	260	26	18
24 fl.oz Can	280	28	20
32 fl.oz Bottle	370	38	28
40 fl.oz Bottle	470	47	35
50 fl.oz Football	590	59	50
Light Beer (4.2% Alc. Vol.)			
7 fl.oz Glass	65	7	4
12 fl.oz Bottle/Can/Glass	110	12	7
16 fl.oz Bottle/Can	145	16	9
22 fl.oz Bottle	200	22	13
24 fl.oz Can	220	24	14
Non-Alcoholic Brews			
(Less than 0.5% alcohol by volume)			
Average All Brands, 12 fl.oz	70	1	14

Beer Brands

Per 12 fl.oz Serving
Percentage alcohol listed is by volume - not by weight.

Alc ~ Alcohol (Grams)

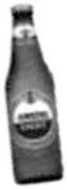

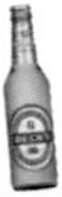

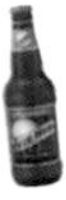

	C	Alc	Cb
Aguila (4%)	125	11	11
Amstel Light (3.5%)	95	10	5
Anchor: Porter (5.6%)	210	15	23
Steam (4.9%)	165	14	14
Asahi: Kuronama (5.3%)	150	14	11
Select (4.7%)	140	13	11
Super Dry (4.9%)	150	14	11
Augsburger Bock (4.9%)	170	14	17
Bass (5.1%)	155	14	12
Beck's: Original (5%)	145	14	12
Premier Light (2.3%)	65	7	4
Big Sky (4.8%)	150	14	12
Black Label (5.6%)	155	16	11
Blackhook Porter (5.2%)	165	15	14
Blatz: Original (4.6%)	145	13	13
Light (3.9%)	110	11	8
Blonde (4.3%)	140	12	10
Blue Moon: Belgian (5.4%)	165	15	13
Pumpkin Ale (5.8%)	180	17	14
Spring Ale (5.4%)	160	15	12
Summer Ale (5.1%)	155	14	13
Winter Ale (5.5%)	180	15	15

Brands (Cont)

Alc ~ Alcohol (Grams)

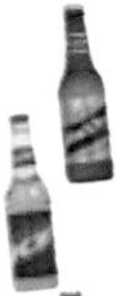

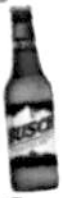

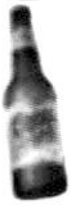

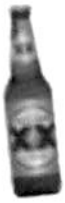

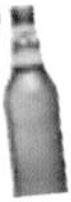

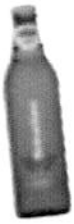

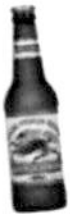

Per 12 fl.oz Serving	C	Alc	Cb
Budweiser: Original	145	14	11
American Ale (5.3%)	180	15	18
Chelada (5%)	185	14	20
Chelada Light (4.2%)	150	12	16
Dry (5%)	130	14	8
Ice (5.5%)	125	16	4
Ice Light (4.2%)	115	14	4
Light Lime (4.2%)	115	12	8
Select (4.3%)	100	12	3
Select 55 (2.4%)	55	6	2
Busch: Original (4.6%)	130	13	10
Ice (5.9%)	170	17	13
Light (4.1%)	95	12	3
Carlsberg (5%)	135	14	10
Castlemaine XXXX (4.7%)	140	13	9
Cerveza Aquila (3.9%)	125	11	11
Colt 45 Malt (6.1%)	175	17	11
Coors: Original (4.9%)	150	14	12
Extra Gold (5%)	150	14	13
Light (4.2%)	100	12	5
Corona: Original (4.45%)	150	14	13
Light (4.1%)	105	12	5
Dos Equis (5%)	130	14	9
Fosters: Lager (5%)	145	14	11
Premium Ale (5.5%)	145	16	12
Genesee: Regular (4.5%)	150	13	14
Genny Light (3.6%)	95	10	6
George Killian's Irish Red (5%)	160	14	15
Grolsch: Blonde (2.8%)	120	18	16
Light (3.6%)	95	11	6
Premium (5%)	145	14	10
Guinness: Draught (4%)	125	12	10
Extra Stout (6%)	175	17	14
Hamm's: Original (4.7%)	145	13	12
Golden Draft (4.7%)	145	13	12
Special Light (3.9%)	110	12	8
Harp (5%)	150	13	13
Heineken: Original (5%)	150	14	12
Special Dark (5%)	165	14	15
Premium Light (3.5%)	100	10	7
Icehouse: Original (5%)	135	14	9
Light (5%)	125	14	7
Keystone: Ice (5.9%)	140	17	6
Light (4.2%)	105	12	5
Premium (4.4%)	110	13	6
Killian's Irish Red (5%)	160	14	15
King Cobra (6%)	135	17	5
Kirin: Ichiban (5%)	150	14	12
Light (3.3%)	95	9	8

Brands (Cont) **Beer Contains Zero Fat**

Per 12 fl.oz Serving

	C	Alc	Cb
Labatt: Blue (4.7%)	**125**	14	9
Blue Light (4%)	**110**	11	8
Leinenkugel's: Original (4.6%)	**150**	13	14
Light (4.2%)	**110**	12	6
Lone Star: Original (4.7%)	**135**	14	12
Light (3.9%)	**110**	11	9
Lowenbrau Original (5.2%)	**160**	15	15
Magic Hat #9 (4.6% alc)	**155**	13	14
Magnum Malt Liquor (5.6%)	**160**	16	11
Michelob: Original (5%)	**165**	14	15
Golden Draft (4.7%)	**125**	14	8
Golden Draft Light (4.1%)	**110**	12	7
Honey Lager (4.9%)	**180**	14	19
Light (4.3%)	**125**	12	9
Pale Ale (5.6%)	**185**	16	9
Porter (5.9%)	**195**	17	18
Ultra (4.2%)	**85**	12	3
Ultra Amber (5%)	**115**	14	4
Ultra Amber Fruit (4.2%)	**105**	12	6
Mickey's Malt Liquor (5.6%)	**160**	16	11
Miller: Chill, 100 Cal, (4.2%)	**100**	12	4
Genuine Draft: (4.7%)	**145**	13	13
High Life (4.7%)	**145**	13	13
High Life Light (4.2%)	**110**	12	7
Lite (4.2%)	**95**	12	3
Milwaukee's Best: (4.3%)	**130**	12	12
Ice (5.9%)	**145**	17	7
Light (4.2%)	**100**	12	4
Minnesota's Best, Original (4.9%)	**140**	14	10
Molson: Canadian/Golden (5%)	**135**	14	11
Ice (5.6%)	**160**	16	12
Light (4%)	**115**	11	10
Molsons XXX (7.3%)	**210**	21	15
Moosehead Lager (5%)	**140**	14	11
Natural: Ice (5.9%)	**160**	17	9
Light (4.2%)	**95**	12	3
Negra Modela (5.3%)	**175**	15	16
Newcastle Brown Ale (4.5%)	**140**	13	13
Old English,"800" (5.9%)	**160**	17	11
Old Milwaukee: Original (4.6%)	**145**	13	13
Light (3.9%)	**110**	11	8
Ice (5.9%)	**180**	17	15
Old Style: Original (4.7%)	**135**	13	12
Light (3.8%)	**110**	11	8

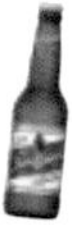
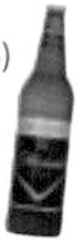
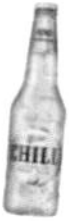
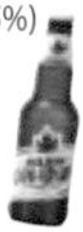
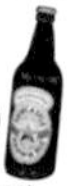
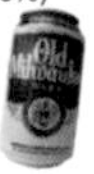

Alc ~ Alcohol (Grams)
Cb ~ Carbohydrate

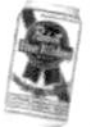

	C	Alc	Cb
Olympia Gold Light (2.2 %)	**70**	6	6
Pabst: Blue Ribbon (4.7%)	**145**	13	12
Light (3.9%)	**110**	11	8
Pete's Wicked Ale (5.3%)	**175**	15	17
Piels (4.7%)	**125**	13	9
Pilsner Urquell (4.4%)	**155**	13	16
Red Dog (5%)	**150**	14	14
Red Hook: ESB (5.8%)	**185**	16	16
India Pale Ale (4.7%)	**190**	13	19
Red Stripe Jamaican Ale (4.7%)	**155**	14	14
Rolling Rock (4.5%)	**130**	13	10
Samuel Adams: Lager (4.9%)	**180**	14	19
Summer Ale (5.3%)	**160**	15	13
Sam Adams Light (4%)	**120**	13	10
Sapporo Premium (3.9%)	**135**	11	14
Schaefer: Original (4.6%)	**145**	13	12
Light (3.9%)	**110**	11	8
Schlitz: Original (4.6%)	**145**	13	12
Light (3.9%)	**110**	11	8
Schmidt's: Original (4.6%)	**145**	13	13
Light (3.9%)	**110**	11	8
Sheaf Stout (5.8%)	**190**	16	19
Sierra Nevada: Bigfoot (9.6%)	**295**	27	25
Pale Ale (5.6%)	**175**	16	14
Pale Bock (7%)	**220**	18	21
Porter (5.6%)	**195**	16	19
Sol Cerveza Especial (4%)	**125**	11	11
Southpaw Light (5%)	**125**	14	7
St Pauli Girl Lager (4.9%)	**150**	14	9
Sparks: Original (6%)	**255**	17	35
Light (6%)	**135**	17	4
Steel Reserve: High Gravity (8.1%)	**220**	23	16
Steel 6 (6%)	**160**	17	11
Stella Artois (5.2%)	**155**	15	12
Stroh's (4.6%)	**145**	13	12
Stroh's Light (3.9%)	**115**	11	7
Tecate: Original (4.7%)	**155**	13	16
Light (3.7%)	**110**	10	8
Tsingtao (4.7%)	**155**	13	16
Warsteimers: *Per 11.2 fl.oz*			
Dunkel/Verum (4.8%)	**140**	14	12
Weinhard's: Pale Ale (4.6%)	**150**	13	13
Hefewéizen (4.9%)	**155**	14	12
Widmer: Hefeweizen (4.7%)	**165**	14	13
Zeigenbock Amber (4.9%)	**145**	14	11

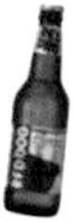

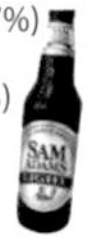
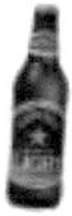
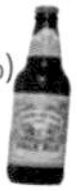
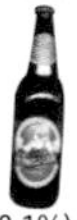
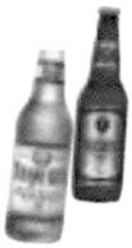
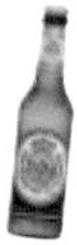

Home-Brewed Beer: Similar to regular beers, according to alcohol content.

Updated Nutrition Data ~ www.CalorieKing.com
Persons with Diabetes ~ See Disclaimer (Page 24)

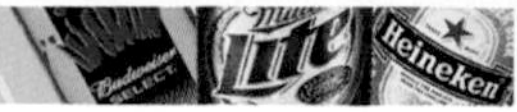

Alc ~ Alcohol (Grams) Cb ~ Carbohydrate

Non-Alcoholic Brews

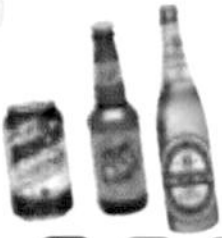

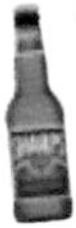

Less Than 0.5% Alcohol
Average All Brands
(Busch NA, Coors NA, Haake Beck, Kaliber, Kingsbury, O'Douls, Old Milwaukee NA, Pabst NA, Stroh's NA, Texas Select)

	C	Alc	Cb
12 fl.oz Can/Bottle	**70**	1	14
O'Doul's Amber, 12 fl.oz	**90**	1	18
Sharp's 12 fl.oz	**60**	1	12

Cider (Alcoholic)

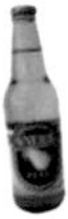

Per 12 fl.oz	C	Alc	Cb
Ace Cider, (5%), av. all flavors	**155**	14	12
Ace Joker (6.9%)	**135**	19	12
Hornsby's: Draft Cider (6%)	**170**	16	16
Hard Apple Cider (5.5%)	**200**	15	27
Woodchuck: Amber (5%)	**200**	14	21
Dark & Dry (5%)	**180**	14	17
Granny Smith (5%)	**165**	14	11
Pear (4%)	**150**	12	18
Raspberry (4%)	**170**	12	22
Wyder's: Apple (5%)	**150**	14	21
Pear (4%)	**140**	12	22
Raspberry (4%)	**120**	12	17

Quick Guide

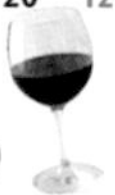

Table Wines
Average All Varieties (11.5% Alc.)
(Wine Contains Zero Fat)

	C	Alc	Cb
4 fl.oz 1 small wine glass OR ½ large wine glass	**100**	11	3
6 fl.oz (¾ large wine glass)	**145**	16	4
8 fl.oz (1 large wine glass)	**195**	21	7
½ Carafe/Bottle, 12 fl.oz	**310**	34	10
1 Bottle, 750ml, 25.4 fl.oz	**620**	68	20

Table Wines

	C	Alc	Cb
Red: *Per 4 fl.oz*			
Burgundy/Cabernet/Merlot, av.	**100**	11	4
White: *Per 4 fl.oz*			
Dry (Chenin; Fume Blanc; Chardonnay)	**95**	11	4
Sparkling, 4 fl.oz	**95**	11	4
Zinfandel Sweet (Moselle/Sauterne), 4 fl.oz	**85**	11	2

Table Wines (Cont)

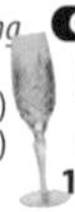

	C	Alc	Cb
Champagne: *Per 4 fl.oz Serving*			
Average 1 glass,	**85**	11	2
w. Orange Jce (3:1 orange)	**75**	8	4
w. Orange Jce (1:1 orange)	**65**	5	7
Cold Duck 4 fl oz	**110**	11	8
Korbel (12%): Brut	**90**	11	3
Extra Dry	**90**	11	4
Mulled Wine *(Gluhwein)*, 4 fl.oz	**180**	14	20
Non-Alcoholic Wine, avg., 4 fl.oz	**50**	0	12
Reduced Alcohol Wine (6%):			
Average all types, 4 fl.oz	**50**	6	12
Sake, *Gekkeikan*, (16%), 4 fl.oz	**120**	15	5

Flavored Wines

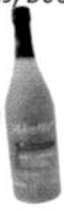

Average All Brands (6% alcohol)
(Examples: Arbor Mist, Wild Vines, Boones)

	C	Alc	Cb
1 small wine glass, 4 fl.oz	**80**	6	10
1 large wine glass, 8 fl.oz	**160**	11	20
1 bottle, 750 ml (25.4 fl.oz)	**510**	35	64

Dessert Wines

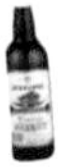

	C	Alc	Cb
Madeira (18% alc), 2 oz	**85**	9	5
Marsala (18%), 2 oz	**110**	9	11
Port, Muscatel (18%), 2 oz	**85**	9	5
Sherry (15%), 2 oz			
Dry, 1 Sherry glass	**90**	7	7
Sweet/Cream, average	**90**	7	8
Vermouth, *Martini & Rossi:*			
Extra Dry (18%), 2 oz	**65**	9	2
Martini Rosso (16%), 2 oz	**90**	10	8

Cooking Wines

Holland House:	C	Alc	Cb
Marsala (14%), 1 fl.oz	**45**	4	4
Red (10%), 1 fl.oz	**20**	2	1
1 cup, 8 fl.oz	**160**	24	8
Sherry (17%), 1 fl.oz	**45**	5	2

COOKING WITH WINE

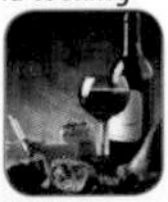

For alcohol to evaporate, sufficient heat and cooking time (at least 30 minutes) is required.
Red and white table wines would then contain negligible residual calories.
Sweetened wines (marsala/sherry) would contain 10 calories per 1 fl.oz.
Flambé Desserts: Only surface alcohol is burned off, so negligible reduction in alcohol or calories.

Quick Guide

Alc ~ Alcohol (Grams)

Spirits/Liquors

Includes Bourbon, Brandy, Gin, Rum, Scotch, Tequila, Vodka, Whiskey.

Note: All spirits with same alcohol proof have similar calories and zero fat.

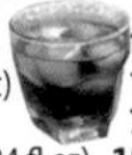

Average All Brands	C	Alc	Cb
80 Proof (40% Alcohol by Volume):			
1 fl.oz	**65**	9.5	0
1½ fl.oz (1 shot)	**100**	14	0
3 fl.oz (Double shot)	**195**	28	0
½ Bottle, 350 ml	**770**	113	0
1 Bottle, 700 ml (24 fl.oz)	**1540**	227	0
86 Proof (43% Alc): 1 fl.oz	**70**	10	0
1½ fl.oz (1 shot)	**105**	15	0
1 Bottle, (24 fl.oz)	**1670**	244	0
100 Proof (50% Alc): 1½ fl.oz	**125**	18	0
Shochu (Soju) ~ Izakaya Lounges			
Average all types (25% alc), 2 fl.oz	**65**	12	0

Flavored Spirits

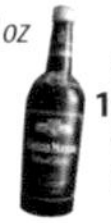

	C	Alc	Cb
Captain Morgan: *Per 1.5 fl.oz*			
Original (35%)	**85**	12	0.5
Black Label (40%)	**100**	14	0
Parrot Bay (21%)	**90**	7.5	10
Silver Spiced (35%)	**90**	12	2
Malibu Rum: *Per 1.5 fl.oz*			
Original/Banana (21%)	**80**	7.5	30
Pineapple (21%)	**75**	7.5	22
Southern Comfort, (35%), 1.5 fl.oz	**100**	12	3

Hard Lemonade & Sodas

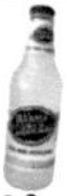

	C	Alc	Cb
Mike's Hard Lemonade: *Per 11.2 fl.oz*			
Original (5%), av. all flavors	**235**	14	32
Light (4%)	**100**	11	6
Mike's Hard Tea: *Per 11.2 fl.oz*			
Original (4.1%)	**175**	11	27
Light (3.5%)	**95**	9	7
Mike's Hard Punch (5.5%), 11.2 fl oz	**210**	15	28
Twisted Tea: *Per 12 fl.oz*			
Original (5%) av., all flavors	**210**	14	31
Light (4%)	**115**	11	9

Alcoholic Energy Drinks (with Caffeine)

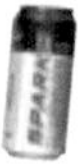

	C	Alc	Cb
Sparks: *Per 12 fl.oz*			
Original (6%)	**255**	17	35
Light (6%)	**135**	17	4
Plus (6%)	**260**	17	35
Tilt: Green (6%), 12 fl.oz	**255**	17	35
Orange (6%), 12 fl.oz	**285**	17	42

Updated Nutrition Data ~ www.CalorieKing.com
Persons with Diabetes ~ See Disclaimer (Page 24)

Coolers & Premix Cocktails

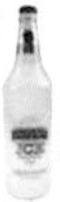

Ready-To-Drink Zero Fat Unless Indicated	C	Alc	Cb
Arbor Mist: Blenders, all flavors (6%), 8 fl.oz	**155**	11	20
Bacardi Silver: *Per 12 fl.oz*			
Lemonade/Sangria, av. (6%)	**270**	17	41
Raz/Strawberry/Watermelon (5%)	**240**	14	36
Mojito: Original (5%)	**230**	14	34
Mango/Pomegranate (5%)	**235**	14	35
Ready to Pour: *Per 4 fl.oz*			
Bahama Mama (10%)	**130**	13	16
Hurricane (12.5%)	**145**	12	16
Rum Island Ice Tea (12.5%)	**150**	12	16
Bartles & Jaymes			
Malt Based Coolers (3.9%): *Per 12 fl.oz*			
Classic Original; Blue Hawaiian	**185**	11	28
Exotic Berry; Juicy Peach	**210**	11	34
Luscious Blackberry; Mango	**230**	11	40
Margarita	**260**	11	46
Strawberry Cosmo; Daiquiri	**220**	11	37
Wine Cooler (5%): *12 fl.oz*			
Classic Original	**200**	14	29
Blue Hawaiian; Exotic Berry, avg.	**230**	14	33
Other flavors, average	**245**	14	38
Captain Morgan Parrot Bay (5%), Average all flavors, 12 fl.oz	**245**	14	39
Daily's (6.9%):			
Bag-In-Box Cocktails (6.9%), 4.4 fl.oz	**110**	7	14
Single Serve Bottles, all flavors, 8 fl.oz	**220**	12	30
Jack Daniels Country Cocktails (5%):			
Average all flavors, 10 fl.oz	**245**	12	40
Jack Daniels Hard Cola (5%) 12 oz	**234**	14	34
Jose Cuervo Margaritas			
Original (10%), 6 fl.oz	**200**	14	27
Mini (10%), 6 fl.oz	**210**	14	24
Seagram's Escapes Coolers (3.2%)			
Bahama Mama, 12 fl.oz	**150**	9	39
Strawberry Daiquiri, 12 fl.oz	**170**	9	44
Average all other flavors, 12 fl.oz	**180**	9	45
Smirnoff Ice (3.2%), 11.2 fl.oz			
Light	**95**	9	12
Triple Black	**175**	9	31
Average all other flavors	**200**	9	36
TGI Friday's: *Per 6 fl.oz*			
On The Rocks: Margarita (7.5%)	**240**	14	39
Long Island Ice Tea (15%)	**190**	14	24
Mudslide (10%)	**365**	14	31
Blenders (12.5% alc): *Per 4.8 fl.oz*			
Orange Dream; Pina Colada, av.	**360**	14	36
Strawberry Shortcake	**365**	14	41

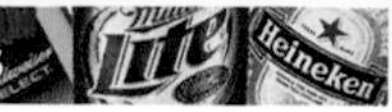

Coolers & Premix Cocktails (Cont)

Ready-To-Drink	C	Alc	Cb
The Club Premix Cocktails: *Per 3.4 oz Serving (½ can)*			
Censored on Beach; Margarita (7.5%)	**105**	6	17
Gin/Vodka Martini, av. (21%)	**155**	17	0.2
Long Island Ice Tea(15%)	**145**	12	16
Manhattan (17%)	**115**	14	5
Mudslide/Pina Colada (10%) av.	**200**	8	16
Screwdriver (7.5%)	**95**	6	14
Whiskey Sour (10%)	**95**	8	11

Shooters

Alc ~ Alcohol (Grams)

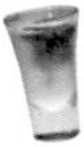

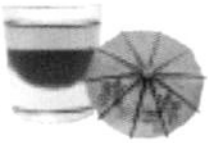

Alabama Slammer	**110**	14	2
Amaretto Sour	**120**	6	19
B52	**145**	14	11
Beam Me Up Scotty	**145**	13	13
Blue Tequila	**160**	18	6
Jager Bomb	**205**	8	30
Jager Bomb (w. Sugar-Free Red Bull)	**155**	8	18
Jell-O Shot, 3 oz (w.1½ oz Vodka)	**180**	14	19
w. Diet Jell-O, 3 oz	**110**	14	0
Kamikaze	**75**	8	3
Kool-Aid	**160**	15	14
Orgasm	**100**	12	6
Peppermint Patty	**195**	8	11
Stinger	**170**	18	12
Surfer on Acid	**90**	7	11

Cocktail Mixers

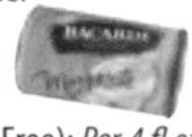

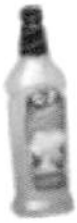

Non Alcoholic ~ No Alcohol Added			
Bacardi: *Per 8 fl.oz Prepared from 2 fl.oz concentrate*			
Daiquiris, Rum runner	**120**	0	32
Margarita	**90**	0	25
Mojito	**110**	0	30
Pina Colada	**170**	0	36
Baja Bob's (Sugar Free): *Per 4 fl.oz*			
Cosmo Martini	**10**	0	2
Pina Colada	**30**	0	4
J.Cuervo: Margarita, 4 fl.oz	**105**	1	28
Strawberry Margarita, 4 fl.oz	**115**	1	20
All other flavors	**0**	0	0
Mr & Mrs T: *Per 4 fl.oz*			
Bloody Mary: Original	**25**	0	5
Bold & Spicy	**35**	0	7
Mai Tai	**130**	0	32
Margarita	**100**	0	26
Pina Colada	**170**	0	44
Strawberry Daiquiri	**180**	0	46
TGI Fridays: Mudslide, 2.3 fl.oz	**110**	0	3
Cosmo; Berrytini, 2 fl.oz	**80**	0	20
Strawb. Daiquiri; Margarita, 4 fl.oz	**190**	0	46

Cocktails

Alc ~ Alcohol (Grams)

Made to Standard Recipes (Standard Size)

(Main Reference: The New American Bartender's Guide)

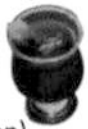

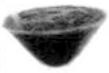

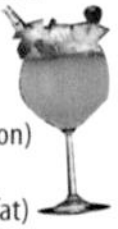

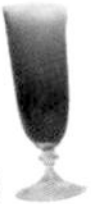

Zero Fat Unless Indicated	C	Alc	Cb
Bacardi & Coke (w. 1½ oz Bacardi)	**160**	14	17
Bellini, av., 4.5 fl.oz	**95**	11	7
Bloody Mary (w. 1½ oz Vodka)	**125**	10	7
Blushin' Russian (20g fat)	**405**	14	23
Bourbon & Soda (w. 2 oz Bourbon)	**130**	19	0
Brandy Alexander (10g fat)	**300**	20	15
Chi Chi's: Long Island Iced Tea, 4 fl.oz	**145**	12	17
Mexican Mudslide, 4 fl.oz (8g fat)	**240**	1.5	42
Mojito, 4 fl.oz	**160**	11	21
Pina Colada 4 fl.oz (6g fat)	**240**	4	42
White Russian 4 fl.oz (7g fat)	**245**	1.5	43
Chupa Naranjas (w. 1½ oz Tequila)	**150**	16	8
Cosmopolitan	**215**	24	12
Daiquiri (w. 2 oz Rum) avg. all types	**140**	19	4
Frozen Daiquiri (w. 2 oz Rum):			
no fruit	**155**	19	6
with fruit (w. 1½ oz Rum)	**145**	14	11
Gin Martini (w. 2 oz alcohol)	**140**	19	0
Grasshopper	**260**	17	28
Harvey Wallbanger (2 oz Alc.)	**200**	19	17
Highball (1½ oz Whiskey)	**100**	14	0
Irish Coffee (contains 10g fat)	**205**	14	2
Kahlua Mudslide: w.milk (3g fat)	**145**	11	12
w. cream (12g fat)	**230**	11	10
Leon Drop, 4 fl.oz	**130**	14	10
Long Island Iced Tea (w. 3 oz Cola)	**270**	19	32
with Diet Cola (w. 3 oz Cola)	**235**	19	22
Mai Tai (with 2 oz Rum)	**290**	24	33
Manhattan	**130**	17	5
Margarita	**160**	18	7
Mint Julep (w.2½ oz Bourbon)	**180**	24	4
Moscow Mule	**185**	14	24
Pina Colada (contains 10g fat)	**325**	19	26
Red Bull & Vodka	**210**	14	28
with Sugar Free Red Bull	**105**	14	3
Screwdriver	**160**	14	15
Sex On The Beach	**235**	19	25
Spritzer (with 3 oz Wine)	**65**	8	2
Tequila Sunrise	**200**	14	25
Tom Collins (w. 2 oz Gin)	**210**	19	18
Vodka Soda (w. 1½ oz Vodka)	**100**	14	0
Vodka Tonic (w. 1½ oz Vodka)	**165**	14	18
Whiskey Sour (w. 2 oz Whiskey)	**155**	19	7
White Russian (w. 10g fat)	**240**	19	7
Non-Alcoholic:			
Cinderella	**45**	0	11
Shirley Temple (w. 6 oz Ginger Ale)	**140**	0	34

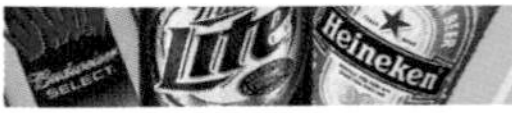

Liqueurs/Cordials

Per 1 fl.oz	C	Alc	Cb
Advocaat (36 Proof; 2g fat)	**85**	4	9
Alizé: Cognac (80 Proof)	**70**	9	2
Gold/Red Passion (32 Proof)	**105**	4	11
Amaretto (56 Proof)	**100**	7	14
Baileys Irish Cream (34 Proof; 5g fat)	**95**	4	7
Lite (30 Proof; 2g fat)	**75**	4	7
Benedictine (80 Proof)	**90**	9	5
Chambord (33 Proof)	**105**	4	11
Chartreuse (80 Proof)	**100**	9	9
Cherry Brandy (48 Proof)	**80**	6	9
Coffee Liqueur (53 Proof)	**115**	6	16
Cointreau (80 Proof)	**95**	9	7
Creme de Cacao (54 Proof)	**100**	6	15
Creme de Menthe (72 Proof)	**125**	9	14
Curacao (70 Proof)	**95**	8	6
Drambuie (80 Proof)	**105**	9	9
Frangelico (40 Proof)	**65**	5	12
Galliano (86 Proof)	**100**	10	8
Grand Marnier (80 Proof)	**100**	9	7
Kahlua (40 Proof)	**90**	5	15
Kirsch (68 Proof)	**80**	8	6
Midori (42 Proof)	**80**	5	11
Ouzo (80 Proof)	**105**	9	11
Pernod (80 Proof)	**75**	9	11
Sambuca (84 Proof)	**100**	10	11
Schnapps (100 Proof)	**115**	12	9
Southern Comfort (70 Proof)	**65**	8	3
Starbucks Liqueur:			
Coffee (40 Proof)	**80**	3	13
Cream (30 Proof)	**85**	3	9
Tia Maria (53 Proof)	**120**	9	15
Triple Sec (48 Proof)	**60**	6	10

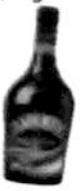

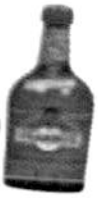

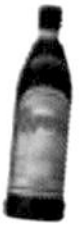

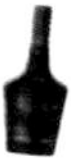

Liqueur Coffee & Hot Drinks

Per Standard Drink	C	Alc	Cb
Liqueur Coffee, avg. all types	**200**	10	10
Hot Toddy, w. 1½ oz liquor, av. all	**170**	9	19
Irish Coffee, 1½ oz whiskey & 1 oz whip	**205**	9	4
Mulled Wine (Glühwein), 4 fl.oz, av	**195**	14	25

"The doctor told him to cut down to just one glass a day."

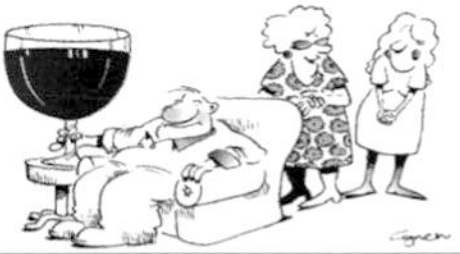

TEN HINTS TO AVOID HARMFUL DRINKING

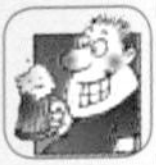

1. **Add up the alcohol** you typically drink each day and on social occasions. How does this compare with 'low risk' amounts? (*See page 25*)
2. **Compare the alcohol content** of different drinks and select the lowest. Request half ounces of alcohol in cocktails and mixed drinks. Dilute them and keep topping off with non-alcoholic drinks.
3. **Go easy on 'Light' beers.** At 4% alcohol, on average, they are still high in alcohol compared to regular beer (5% alcohol).
4. **Try low alcohol or non-alcohol** alternatives such as fruit juices and mineral water. Take your own to parties.
5. **Before drinking alcohol,** quench your thirst with water and non-alcoholic drinks – particularly after vigorous exercise or sports.
6. **Slow the rate of drinking.** Chugging or drinking fast is the major cause of illness and death from alcohol poisoning.
7. **Avoid drinking in 'rounds'.**
8. **Have a non-alcoholic 'spacer'** between drinks (e.g. mineral water, orange juice).
9. **Don't drink on an empty stomach.** Food slows the rate of alcohol absorption.
10. **Keep track of the number of drinks** and know when to stop. Stick to a set limit.

Note: • Alcohol can be very dangerous when taken with prescription or street drugs, or when you are very tired.

Extra Info: www.CalorieKing.com

Cocktail Mixers & Extracts

	C	Alc	Cb
Angostura Bitters, ¼ tsp	**2**	0	0.5
Grenadine, ½ tsp	**6**	0	2
Lime/Lemon Juice, 2 Tbsp, 1 oz	**10**	0	2
Maraschino Cherry, 1 small	**8**	0	2
Simple Syrup, 1 Tbsp, av.	**50**	0	14
Sweet & Sour Mix, 2 Tbsp, 1 oz	**30**	0	7
Tonic Water, 8 fl.oz	**80**	0	22
Flavor Extracts *(McCormick)*:			
Pure Lemon (83%), 1 tsp	**0**	3.5	0
Pure Vanilla (35%), 1tsp	**0**	1.5	0

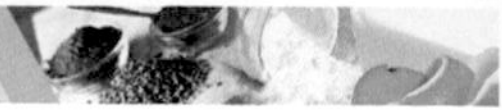

Baking Ingredients

	C	F	Cb
Almond Paste:			
(Marzipan), 2 Tbsp	170	7	24
Apple Pie Filling,			
Sweetened, 9.4 oz	240	0	60
Also See Page 136			
Baking Powder: Regular, 1 tsp	5	0	2
Cream of Tartar, 1 tsp	10	0	2
Baking Mix *(Bisquick)*:			
Original, ⅓ cup, 1½ oz	160	5	26
Heart Smart, ⅓ cup, 1½ oz	140	2.5	27
Batter Mix *(Golden Dipt)*, ¼ c. mix	100	0	23
Blueberries, 1 cup, 5 oz	85	0.5	21
Butter/Margarine, ½ c., 4 oz	815	92	1
Stick, *Land O' Lakes,* ½ oz	100	11	0
Carob Flour, ½ cup	115	0.5	46
Chocolate Baking Bars: *Average all Brands*			
Sweet *(Baker's)*:			
1 oz portion	120	7	16
4 oz bar	470	28	64
Semi-sweet, 1 oz	140	9	16
Bittersweet, 1 oz	140	12	14
White Baking 1 oz	160	9	16
Unsweetened, 1 oz	140	14	8
Grated, 1 cup, 4½ oz	660	69	39
Chocolate Baking Chips: *Average all Brands*			
Milk Choc./Semi Sweet 1 oz	140	8	18
½ cup, 3 oz	420	24	54
1 cup, 6 oz	840	48	108
Mini Kisses (*Hershey*), 1 pce	5	0.5	1
Cocoa Powder, Baking: *Nestle*, 1 T.	15	1	3
⅓ cup, 1 oz	85	5	17
Hershey's, 1 Tbsp	20	0.5	3
⅓ cup, 1 oz	115	3	17
Coconut, dried:			
Unsweet., 1 oz	190	18	7
Sweetened/flaked, 1 oz	130	8	15
½ cup, 1.3 oz	195	12	22
Toasted *(Baker's)*, 1 oz	170	13	13
Coconut Cream/Milk: *See Page 91*			
Cornstarch, 1 Tbsp	30	0	7
Eggs: Large (1)	75	5	0
Jumbo (1)	90	6	0.5
Egg White: 1 Egg White	15	0	0
½ cup (4 egg whites), 4 oz	60	0	1
Flour, white:			
1 Tbsp, 0.3 oz	25	0	5.5
1 cup, 4.2 oz	400	1	88
Whole Wheat, 1 cup, 4.2 oz	400	2	84

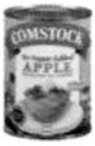

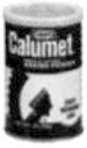

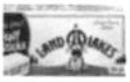
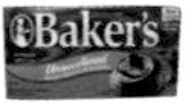

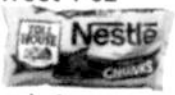

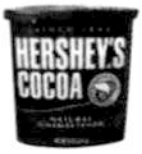

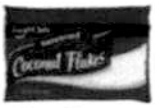

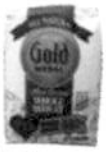

	C	F	Cb
Flavor Extracts: *Average all Brands*			
Imitation, 1 tsp	10	0	2
Pure Extract, 1 tsp	10	0	0.5
Almond, Vanilla, 1 tsp	10	0	0.5
Fruit Pectin: Swtnd, ¼ tsp	5	0	1
Unsweetened, ¼ tsp	0	0	0
Gelatin, dry, ¼ oz pkg	20	0	0
Golden Dipt, Batter Mix			
¼ cup mix, 1 oz	100	0	23
Honey, ½ cup, 6 oz	515	0	140
Lemon/Orange Peel, ¼ cup	25	0	6
Lighter Bake *(Sunsweet)*			
(Butter & Oil replacement)			
1 Tbsp, ½ oz	35	0	9
¼ Cup, 2.7 oz	140	0	36
Milk: Whole, 1 cup, 8 fl.oz	150	8	12
2%, 1 cup, 8 fl.oz	120	5	12
1%, 1 cup, 8 fl.oz	100	2.5	12
Fat-Free, 1 1 cup, 8 fl.oz	90	0.5	13
Pastry ~ *See Page 136*			
Pie Crusts ~ *See Page 136*			
Pie Fillings:			
Fruits ~ *See page 136*			
Lemon Creme, ⅓ cup	130	1.5	28
Mincemeat, 3½ oz	190	5	45
Pumpkin, 1 cup, 9.3 oz	270	1.5	60
Prune Puree, ¼ cup, 3 oz	220	0	55
Raisins, ½ cup, 2.8 oz	240	0.5	63
Rennin, 1 pkg (11g)	10	0	2
Soy Milk ~ *See Pages 48-49*			
Sprinkles, all types, 1 tsp	20	1	3
Sugar: 1 Tbsp, ½ oz	55	0	14
1 oz	110	0	28
1 cup, 7 oz	775	0	195
1 lb, 16 oz	1760	0	454
Sweeteners & Sugar Substitutes ~ *See Page 164*			
Vinegar, avg. all types, 1 oz	5	0	1
Whey, sweet, dry, 1 oz	100	0.5	21
Yeast: Active, dry, ¼ oz pkg	21	0	3
Bakers, compressed, 1 oz	30	0.5	5
Fleischmann's, 0.6 oz pkg	0	0	0

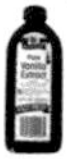
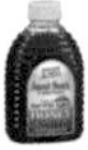
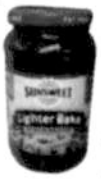

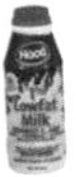
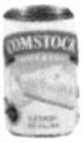

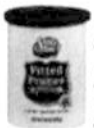
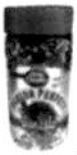
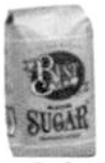

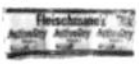

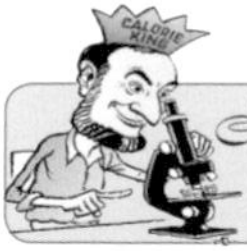

For Full Nutritional Data & Product Updates ~ See Author's Website www.CalorieKing.com

Note: Actual weight of bars is usually 5-10% more than label Net Weight. Weigh bar and allow extra calories.

Breakfast Bars

Per Bar	C	F	Cb
Atkins:			
Day Break: Cinnamon Bun	160	8	18
Apple Crisp; Fruit Crumble, average	125	5	17
Choc. Chip Crisp; Cranberry, av.	140	6	16
Peanut Butter Fudge Crisp	150	7	14
Barbara's Bakery: Nature's Choice, av.	150	2	28
Fruit & Yogurt, 1.1 oz, average	150	3	28
dotFIT: *Per 2 oz Bar*			
Iced Oatmeal Blueberry 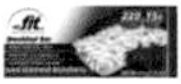	220	5	29
Iced Oatmeal Strawberry	220	5	29
Note: Carb figures include 11 grams of sorbitol and maltitol sweeteners			
General Mills: Milk 'n Cereal Bars,			
Cinnamon Toast Crunch, 1.6 oz	180	4	33
Honey Nut Cheerios, 1.6 oz	160	4	28
Health Valley:			
Cobbler Cereal Bars, average, 1.3 oz	140	2.5	27
Toaster Tarts, all flavors, 1.4 oz	150	3	29
Kashi, Cereal Bars, average, 1.2 oz	110	3	21
Kellogg's: Cinnabon Bars, av., 1.3 oz	150	4.5	27
Fiber Plus, Antioxidants, av. 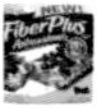	125	5	25
Pop Tarts:			
Fruit/Frosted, av., 1.8 oz	200	5	36
Low-Fat, all flavors, 1.8 oz	185	3	39
Splitz, average all flavors, 1.7 oz	200	6	36
Market Pantry *(Target)*, Bar, 1.4 oz	140	3	26
Nature's Path,			
Toaster Pastries, 1.8 oz, average	210	5	40
Nutri-Grain Bars			
Cereal Bars, average, 1.3 oz	130	3	24
Strawberry Yogurt Bar, average, 1.3 oz	140	3.5	25
Quaker: Breakfast Cookies (1), 1.7 oz	175	4.5	33
Morning Minis, 1 pouch, av., 1.3 oz	135	4	25
Muffin Bars, average, 1.3 oz	135	3.5	26
Granola Bars: *See Page 36* 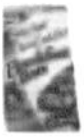			
Slim-Fast: Fruit Crisp, 1.3 oz	180	4.5	29
Muffin Bar, average, 1.2 oz	135	5	20
South Beach Living *(Kraft)*			
High Protein Cereal Bars, av., 1.25 oz	145	5	15
Special K Cereal Bars, average, 0.8 oz	90	1.5	18
Bliss Bar, Mocha 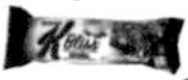	90	2	17
Toaster Strudel:			
Fruit flavors, average	190	9	26
Boston Cream Pie	210	9	29
Cream Cheese	200	11	23
Trader Joe's: Fig, 1.3 oz	120	2	24
Apple, Blueb./Strawberry, average	140	2.5	28

Sports & Diet Bars

Per Bar	C	F	Cb
ABB, Steel Bar, average, 2.3 oz	270	5	35
AdvantEdge *(EAS)* 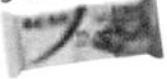			
Carb Control:			
Crisp Bar, average, 2.1 oz	240	8	27
Nutrition Bar, average, 2.1 oz	230	8	27
Anytime Health: 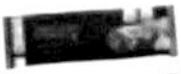			
Meal Replacement:			
Cookies N' Cream, 2.8 oz	310	9	42
P'nut Butter Choc Chip, 2.8 oz	310	9	42
Snack Bars: S'mores, 1.75 oz	190	6	26
Triple Choc., 1.75 oz 	190	6	26
Apex:			
Fit: Choc. Chip Cookie Dough	210	5	30
Cookies 'N Cream	220	6	30
Fruit Fuel Bars: Apple Pie, 1.3 oz	200	2	37
Strawberry Strudel	200	2	36
Fix Crisp Bar: Peanut Butter, 1.4 oz	160	4	21
Oatmeal Raisin, 1.03 oz	150	3	23
Atkins:			
Advantage: Caramel varieties, av.	170	10	21
Choc. Peanut Butter 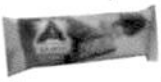	240	12	22
Granola flavors, av.	200	8	18
Marshmallow Mudslide	210	10	19
S'Mores	220	9	27
Endulge: Caramel Nut Chew	130	8	17
Choc. Peanut Butter Cups (2)	160	13	18
P'nut Caramel Cluster	140	9	12
Attune Bars:			
Chocolate Probiotic Wellness Bars: *Per 0.7 oz Bar*			
Blueberry Vanilla	100	7	9
Chocolate Crisp 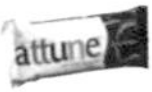	90	6	12
Dark Chocolate	80	6	11
Mint Chocolate	90	6	12
Granola Probiotic, average, 1.4 oz	170	7	23
Balance: Original, average, 1.76 oz	200	7	23
Carb Well, average, 1.7 oz	195	8	23
Gold, average, 1.75 oz	210	6	23
Pure, average all fl. 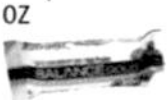	180	7	22
Barbara's Bakery:			
Crunchy Granola (2), average, 1.5 oz	190	8	27
Bariatrix Proti-Bar: (15g Protein)			
Average all flavors, 1.4 oz	155	5	15
Biochem: Greens & Whey Bar, 2.1 oz	280	12	26
Raw Foods & Whey Bar, 2.1 oz	200	4	37
CarbRite Diet *(Doctor's)*, av., 2 oz	195	3.5	23
Cascadian Farms *(General Mills)*			
Chewy Granola: Choc. Chip, 1.25 oz	140	4	25
Harvest Berries, 1.25 oz	130	2	26

Updated Nutrition Data ~ www.CalorieKing.com
Persons with Diabetes ~ See Disclaimer (Page 24)

B Bars ~ Granola ◆ Nutrition

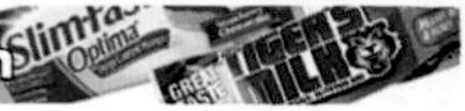

Note: Actual weight of bars is usually 5-10% more than label Net Weight. Weigh bar and allow extra calories.

Sports & Diet Bars (Cont)

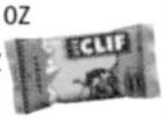
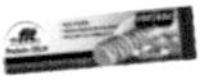
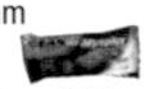
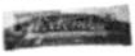
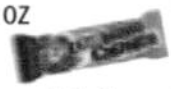

Per Bar	C	F	Cb
Clif Bars:			
Original: Apricot, 2.4 oz	**230**	3	45
Chocolate Chip, 2.4 oz	**240**	5	44
Builder's, average, 2.4 oz	**270**	8	30
Kid Z, average, 1.26 oz	**125**	3.5	23
Mojo: Avg., 1.58 oz	**200**	10	20
Detour: Original, 3 oz	**365**	11	33
Biker, average, 1.76 oz	**210**	6	32
Lean Muscle, average, 3.17 oz	**380**	14	33
Lower Sugar, 3 oz	**340**	9	34
Oatmeal Whole Grain, av., 4.28 oz	**450**	10	59
Runner, average, 1.76 oz	**205**	5	27
Yoga,1.6 oz	**170**	2	28
dotFIT: *Breakfast Bars ~ Page 33*			
dotSTICK: Protein Stick (12g Prot.):			
Iced Peanut Butter Delight	**190**	6	26
Iced Lemon Vanilla Cream	**190**	6	26
EAS			
AdvantEDGE, Carb Control, av., 2.12 oz	**245**	8	27
Myoplex: Deluxe Bar, average, 3.17 oz	**335**	9	35
Lite , Chocolate Chip Crisp, 1.9 oz	**190**	4.5	26
Carb Control,			
Choc Peanut Butter, 2.46 oz	**260**	8	27
(Carbs include 17g sugar alcohol)			
Elevate Me!, average, 2.33 oz	**235**	4	33
Extend Bar, av., 1.4 oz	**150**	3	25
First Endurance, EFS Bar, 2.32 oz	**250**	6	40
General Mills:			
Fiber One Chewy, average, 0.8 oz	**90**	2.5	17
1.4 oz, average all flavors	**140**	4.5	28
GeniSoy: Genisoy Bars, av., 2.2 oz	**240**	5.5	32
Organic Bars, 1.6 oz	**160**	3	25
Protein Crunch, 1.6 oz	**150**	5	18
Ultra Bar, 1.6 oz, 1.6 oz	**160**	2	27
Glenny's:			
Slim Carb, Peanut Caramel, 1.3 oz	**130**	2.5	19
100 Calorie, Slim 1, av. all flav.,1.06 oz	**100**	3	20

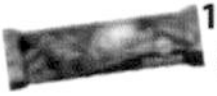
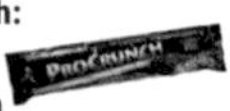
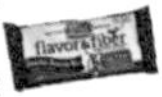

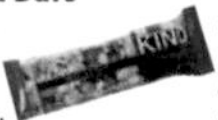
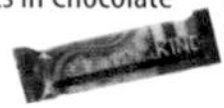

Per Bar	C	F	Cb
Glucerna: Meal Bars, average, 2 oz	**220**	7	34
Snack Bar, 1.3 oz	**150**	4	25
Mini Snack Bar (1)	**80**	2.5	12
GNC ProCrunch:			
Choc Crisp	**260**	7	34
Cookies n' Cream	**250**	4.5	36
Peanut Butter Crunch, 2.3 oz	**260**	7	34
Pro Crunch Lite, 1.2 oz	**140**	4	15
Gnu Foods:			
Banana Walnut, 1.6 oz	**140**	4	30
Cinn. Raisin; Orange Cranb., 1.6 oz	**130**	3	32
Choc. Brownie; P'nut Butter, av., 1.6 oz	**140**	4.5	30
Health Valley Chewy Granola, av.	**110**	1.5	22
Herbalife, Protein Deluxe!, 1.25 oz	**140**	4	15
Hershey's Smart Zone, av., 1.75 oz	**205**	7	22
HMR Benefit Bars, average, 1.4 oz	**160**	4	25
Jenny Craig: S'mores, 1.2 oz	**130**	4	22
Chocolate Caramel Peanut, 1.2 oz	**150**	5	19
Choc Chip Snack Bar, 1.21 oz	**140**	3	23
Joy Ride Bars, average, 2.8 oz	**340**	12	27
Kashi, GoLean Chewy, av., 2.75 oz	**290**	6	48
GoLean Crunchy!:			
Chocolate Almond	**170**	5	27
Chocolate Peanut	**180**	5	30
Average other flavors	**160**	4	27
GoLean Roll!, average, 1.95oz	**190**	5	28
TLC: Crunchy Granola Bars, 0.7 oz	**90**	3	13
Chewy Granola Bar, average, 1.3 oz	**135**	5	19
Fruit & Grain Bars, average, 1.15 oz	**120**	3	22
Keribar, Apple Peanut Butter, 1.4 oz	**160**	6	21
Kind Fruit & Nut Bars			
Almond & Apricot	**170**	11	16
In Yogurt	**210**	13	19
Almond & Coconut	**190**	14	14
Fruit & Nut in Yogurt	**210**	13	20
Macadamia & Apricot	**190**	14	15
Sesame & Peanuts in Chocolate	**230**	15	19
Walnut & Date	**150**	7	22
Kind Plus:			
A, C & E, Cranberry & Almond	**190**	12	19
Omega-3, Almond & Cashew	**150**	9	18
Protein, Almond, Walnut, Macadamia	**210**	15	11

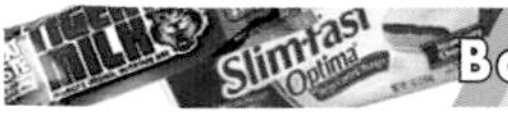

Sports & Diet Bars (Cont)

Per Bar	C	F	Cb
Kudos: Chocolate Chip, 1 oz	120	3.5	20
Peanut Butter, 1 oz	130	6	18
M&M's; Snickers, average, 0.84 oz	100	3	17
Larabar:			
Apple Pie, 1.6 oz	180	10	23
Banana Bread, 1.8 oz	220	11	28
Cherry Pie, 1.7 oz 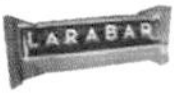	190	8	28
P'nut Butter & Jelly	210	10	27
Tropical Fruit Tart	210	12	25
Lean Body: Cookie Bar, S'mores	360	13	30
Gold, Caramel Peanut, 3 oz	330	9	32
Granola Bar, average, 2.85 oz	345	12	38
Rockin' Roll, Peanut, 2.5 oz	290	16	25
Lindora: Cinnamon Crisp	160	4.5	16
Other varieties, av. 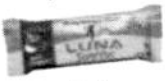	150	5	17
Luna: Bars, av., 1.7 oz	180	4.5	27
Sport, Moons Chews, av., 1.1 oz	100	0	24
Sunrise, average, 1.7 oz	175	4.5	27
Marathon *(Snickers)*: Energy, 2 oz	215	7	26
Nutrition, average, 1.55 oz	150	4.5	22
Protein, average, 2.8 oz	285	10	38
Market Pantry *(Target)*			
Chewy Granola, 1 oz, average	100	3	17
Sweet & Salty Bar, 1.3 oz, average	150	6	23
Medifast: Crunch, 1.13 oz	110	3	12
Maintenance Bar, 1.5 oz	170	5	20
Met-Rx: Big 100, average, 3.5 oz	370	5	52
Big 100 Colossal: 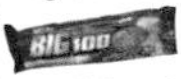			
Crispy Apple Pie	400	10	47
P'nut & Butter: Caramel Crunch	400	12	44
Pretzel	420	12	48
Super Cookie Crunch	410	14	43
Big 100 Brownies, average	400	13	41
MLO Bio Protein: Average, 2.85 oz	315	6.5	43
Xtreme, Chocolate, 3.2 oz	320	6	44
Mojo Bars: *See Clif*			
Muscle Milk, 2.57 oz 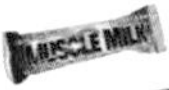	300	11	28
Muscle Tech:			
Nitro-Tech Hardcore: 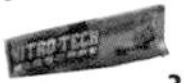			
Choc. Caramel Nut	310	8	29
S'mores; Peanut Butter	270	6	31
Strawberry Cheesecake	290	7	32
Nabisco:			
100 Calorie Granola Bars:			
Chips Ahoy, 1 oz 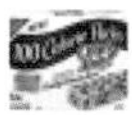	100	1.5	22
Nutter Butter, 1 oz	100	1.5	21
Oreo, 1 oz	100	2	21

Per Bar	C	F	Cb
Nature Valley			
Crunchy Granola Bars			
Apple Crisp, 1.25 oz 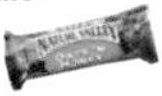	160	6	26
Cinnamon, 1.25 oz	180	6	29
Chewy: w/ Yogurt coating, av., 1.4 oz	140	3.5	26
Trail Mix, average, 1.25 oz	140	4	25
Nature's Path			
Granola Bars, average, 1.25 oz	150	5	26
Optimum Energy, av., 1.98 oz	220	6	36
Nutiva: Hempseed, 1.4 oz	210	14	11
Flax Choc., 1.4 oz 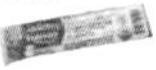	200	13	17
NutriSystem:			
Dessert Bars: Blueberry Lemon	160	5	25
Chocolate Peanut Butter	170	8	17
Nutrilite *(Quixtar):*			
Meal Bars: Blueberry Crunch, 1.8 oz	200	7	26
Cherry Almond, 1.8 oz 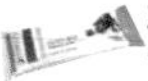	200	6	26
Chocolate Crisp, 1.8 oz	190	6	26
Lemon Twist, 1.8 oz	200	7	27
Snack Bar: Caramel Creme, 0.9 oz	100	2.5	16
Cranberry Crunch, 0.9 oz	100	3	15
Fudgy Brownie w/ Almonds, 0.9 oz	100	3.5	9
Odwalla Energy Bars 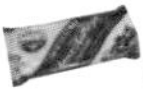			
Choc. Chip Peanut, 2 oz	230	8	33
Strawberry Pomegranate, 2 oz	200	2	42
Protein, Choco-walla, 2 oz	210	5	39
Superfood, 2 oz	200	3.5	39
Other varieties, average, 2 oz	210	6	39
Oh Yeah! *(ISS)*, average, 3 oz	375	18	31
One Way, average 3 oz	340	12	29
Optifast, P'nut Butter 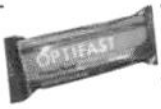			
1.6 oz bar	160	4	23
PowerBar: Energize, average	220	3.5	43
Harvest Whole Grain 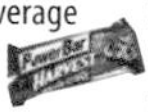	245	5	42
Nut Naturals, av., 1.6 oz	210	10	20
Ride, Chocolate Caramel, 1.95 oz	210	9	23
Performance, Cookies & Cream, 2 oz	230	3	41
Pria Bars, 110 Plus, average, 1.7 oz	110	3	16
Protein Plus: Choc. Fudge Brownie	250	6	21
Cookies & Cream, 2.3 oz	260	5.5	20
PR Bar: Lemon Drop, 1.8 oz	160	7	22
Granola Crunch, 1.8 oz	210	8	20

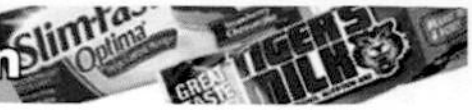

Sports & Diet Bars (Cont)

Per Bar	C	F	Cb
Premier Nutrition:			
Premier Protein, average, 2.5 oz	**280**	**9**	23
Twisted Bar, average, 1.6 oz	**190**	**6**	21
Promax:			
Classic: Cookies 'N Cream, 2.64 oz	**270**	**5**	38
Choc Peanut Crunch, 2.64 oz	**280**	**6**	38
Double Fudge, 2.6 oz 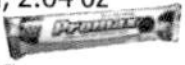	**280**	**7**	37
70 Calorie Bars, 0.66 oz	**70**	**1.5**	10
Proti 15, Choc P'nut, 1.48 oz	**160**	**5**	16
Pure Protein: 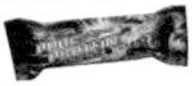			
1.75 oz Bars, av.	**180**	**5**	18
2.75 oz Bars, average	**300**	**8**	30
Pure Fit, average, 2 oz bar	**230**	**6**	26
Quaker:			
Chewy Granola Bars 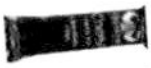			
Regular, average, 0.85 oz	**100**	**3**	18
Dipps: Chocolate Chip, 1 oz	**140**	**5**	22
Peanut Butter, 1 oz	**150**	**7**	19
Omega-3, average, 1.25 oz	**150**	**4**	26
25% Less Sugar, average, 0.85 oz	**100**	**3.5**	17
90 Calories, average, 1 oz	**90**	**1.5**	19
True Delights, average, 1.25 oz	**140**	**4.5**	24
Morning Minis: *Per 1.25 oz Pouch*			
Cinnamon Sugar & Oats	**130**	**4**	25
Peanut Butter	**140**	**4.5**	24
Rebar: Original, 1.75 oz	**160**	**0**	38
Perfect 10 Energy, Lemon, 1.75 oz	**210**	**12**	24
Elev8me, Banana Nut Bread, 2.3 oz	**230**	**4.5**	34
Revival Soy Bars *(Direct)*:			
Chocolate Temptation	**270**	**7**	32
Apple Cinnamon; Marshm. Krunch	**225**	**3**	30
Peanut Pal	**240**	**6**	28
Low Carb, average all flavors	**235**	**8**	31
Slim-Fast Bars:			
Original Breakfast & Lunch Bars:			
Dutch Chocolate, 1.2 oz	**140**	**5**	20
Peanut Butter, 1.2 oz	**150**	**6**	19
Meal Bar, Choc. Cookie Dough, 2 oz	**220**	**5**	36
High Protein: 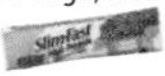			
Meal Bar, av., 1.7 oz	**195**	**7**	20
Snack Bar, average, 1 oz	**105**	**3.5**	15
Lower Carb, Snack Bars, av., 1 oz	**120**	**4.5**	18
Optima: Meal Bars, av.	**220**	**5**	35
Snack Bar, av., 1 oz 	**120**	**4**	20
Snickers, Marathon	**210**	**7**	28
South Beach Living 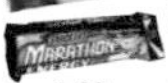			
Fiber Fit Granola Bars, av., 1.23 oz	**120**	**4**	25
High Protein Cereal Bars, av., 1.23 oz	**145**	**5**	15
South Beach Living (Cont)			
Snack Bars, average, 1 oz 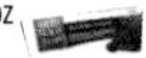	**100**	**4**	14
Meal Replacement, average all flavors, 2.1 oz	**220**	**7**	26
SoyJoy Bars, average, 1 oz	**135**	**6**	16
Solo GI, average, 1.75 oz	**200**	**7**	26
Special K 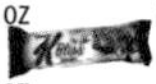			
Bliss Bars, average, 0.8 oz	**90**	**2**	17
Protein Meal, average, 1.6 oz	**180**	**5**	25
Protein Snack Bars, average 0.9 oz	**110**	**3**	16
Spiru-tein *(Nature's Plus)*:			
Original, Carob Coated, 1.4 oz	**140**	**4**	18
Supreme, Banana Split, 1.75 oz	**170**	**4.5**	22
Steel Bar *(ABB)*, average, 2.47 oz	**270**	**5**	35
Supreme Protein:			
Original, Caramel Nut Choc., 3.45 oz	**390**	**16**	34
Carb Conscious, Peanut Butter Crunch	**400**	**18**	26
think Bars:			
thinkPink Protein, average, 1.23 oz	**130**	**3.5**	22
thinkThin: Protein, average, 2 oz	**230**	**8**	27
Bites, average, 0.88 oz	**100**	**4**	7
Tiger's Milk: 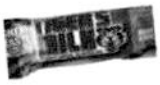			
Protein Rich, 1.2 oz	**140**	**5**	18
Peanut Butter, 1.2 oz	**150**	**6**	18
King Size, average, 1.9 oz	**225**	**9**	28
Trader Joe's:			
Chewy Granola Bars, 6-Packs: 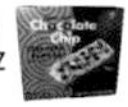			
Chocolate Chip, 1.23 oz	**140**	**4**	25
Vanilla Almond, 1.23 oz	**130**	**4**	21
Fruit & Nut Bars: 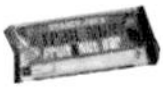			
Choc. Chip, 1.6 oz	**170**	**5**	31
Trail Mix, 1.6 oz	**200**	**6**	37
Tri-O-Plex: average, 4.2 oz	**420**	**13**	45
Duo: Peanut Butter, 3.5 oz	**300**	**10**	26
Caramel Peanut Butter, 3.5 oz	**340**	**8**	45
U-Turn Protein, 2.8 oz	**300**	**8**	26
Usana:			
Nutrition Bar: Oatmeal Raisin, 2 oz	**190**	**3**	32
Peanut Butter Crunch, 1.5 oz	**160**	**5**	19
Vyo-Pro *(AST)* Choc. Brownie, 2.2 oz	**220**	**7**	27
Zoe's, Omega-3's, Chocolate Delight	**190**	**7**	27
Zone Perfect			
Classic, average, 1.76 oz	**210**	**7**	24
Dark Chocolate, average, 1.6 oz	**190**	**6**	22
Fruitified: Apple Cinn., 1.76 oz	**180**	**2**	27
Banana Nut, 1.8 oz 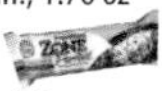	**200**	**6**	24
Blueberry, 1.8 oz	**190**	**4**	25
Indulgence, average, 1.6 oz	**185**	**6**	21

Cocoa & Hot Chocolate

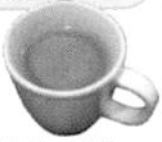

	C	F	Cb
Cocoa (8 fl.oz cup):			
with Whole Milk	205	8.5	22
with Nonfat Milk	145	1	23
Tall (12 fl.oz): with Whole Milk	280	12	26
with Nonfat Milk	185	1	28
Hot Chocolate:			
8 fl.oz cup: With Whole Milk	180	7	26
with Nonfat Milk	140	2	17
Tall (12 fl.oz): With Whole Milk	260	10	36
with Nonfat Milk	190	2	37
Cinnabon, Mochalatta Chill, 16 oz	450	18	66
Swiss Miss Mixes, average, 1 packet	120	2.5	22

Cocoa - Chocolate Mixes

Add extra cals/fat/carbohydrate for milk

Carnation Breakfast Drinks: *See Page 50*

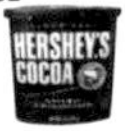

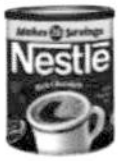

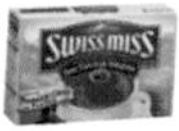

	C	F	Cb
Ghirardelli			
Choc Mocha, 4 Tbsp, 1.2 oz	135	1.5	33
Double Chocolate, 4 Tbsp, 1.4 oz	140	1.5	34
White Mocha, 2 Tbsp, 0.8 oz	100	0	24
Hershey's			
Cocoa, Natural, 1 T, 0.18 oz	10	0.5	3
Horlicks, Malt Extract, 1 oz	90	1	18
Land O' Lakes: *Per 1¼ oz Package*			
Mint/Raspberry/Supreme	140	3.5	26
Nestle: *Per Single Serve Package*			
Dark Milk Chocolate	80	1	17
Carb Select: Fat-Free Hot Cocoa	25	0	5
with Marshmallows	35	0	8
Rich Milk Chocolate	80	3	15
No Sugar Added	50	0	10
Supreme Cocoa, 1 oz	120	2	22
Nesquik Powder *(Nestle): Per 2 Tbsp*			
Choc.; Strawberry, 25% less sugar	60	0	15
Chocolate; Strawb., No Added Sugar	35	1	7
Ovaltine Cocoa Mixes, average, 4 Tbsp	80	0	19
Swiss Miss: *Per Single Serve Package*			
Milk Chocolate: Made with water	120	2	23
Made with milk	210	6	31
With Marshmallows, made w/ water	120	2	23
Made with milk	210	6	33
French Vanilla	110	2	23
Marshmallow	120	2	24
Marshmallow Lovers	140	2.5	29
Rich Chocolate	110	1.5	23
Fat-Free	50	0	10
Marshmallow Lovers	70	0	13

Updated Nutrition Data ~ www.CalorieKing.com
Persons with Diabetes ~ See Disclaimer (Page 24)

Instant Coffee

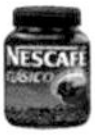

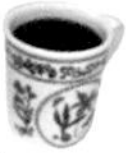

	C	F	Cb
Powder/Granules: Regular or Decaffeinated			
1 level tsp	2	0	0.5
1 rounded tsp	4	0	1
Ground, 3 tsp	7	0	1
Brewed/Percolated, 1 cup, 8 fl.oz	4	0	1
Coffee With Milk/Cream/Creamers:			
Per Cup Coffee (8 fl.oz):			
Black	4	0	1
with Whole Milk: Dash, 1 Tbsp	15	0.5	2
2 Tbsp, 1 fl.oz	25	1	2
with 2% Milk, 2 Tbsp	20	0.5	2
with 1% Milk, 2 Tbsp	20	0.5	3.5
with Fat Free Milk, 2 Tbsp	15	0	3
with Half & Half, 2 Tbsp	50	3	2
with ¼ cup, 2 fl.oz	90	6	3
with Cream (light coffee), 2 Tbsp	65	6	2
with *Coffee Mate:* Liquid, reg., 1Tbsp	20	1	2
Liquid Fat Free, 1 Tbsp	25	0	5
Powder, 1 heaping tsp	15	1	2
Sugar ~ Add Extra: 1 heaping tsp	25	0	6
Single portion, 1 package	25	0	6
Sweeteners: *Equal/Splenda/Sweet N Low*			
Powder, package	0	0	0

Flavored Coffee Mixes

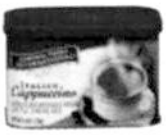

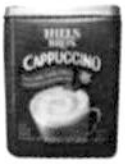

	C	F	Cb
Chicory: Instant Coffee, 1 tsp	5	0	1
Coffee Essence, 1 tsp	15	0	4
Caffé D'Vita: Mixes, 3 tsp	60	1.5	11
Sugar Free Mixes, 2 tsp	35	2	3
General Foods Int'l:			
Average, ½ oz	60	3	10
Sugar-free, av,. 1 tsp	30	2.5	2
Cappuccino Coolers, ½ oz	60	0	15
Hills Bros:			
Cappuccino, Fr. Vanilla 3 Tbsp, 1 oz	120	4.5	19
Jakada *(Folgers):*			
Cappuccino, 3 tsp	80	2	16
Mocha Latte, 3 Tbsp	90	2.5	15
Nescafé: Average all flavors	75	2.5	10

B Beverages ~ Coffee

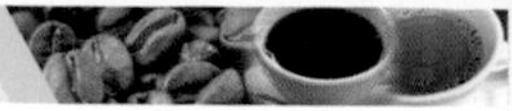

Coffee Shops/Restaurants

Per 8 fl.oz Cup (Unless Indicated)	C	F	Cb
Coffee (Regular/Percolated/Filtered)	**5**	**0**	0
Americano Drip Coffee, 1 cup	**7.5**	**0**	1
Cafe Au Lait: 1 cup, 8 fl.oz	**60**	**3.5**	5
Nonfat Milk, 1 cup, 8 fl.oz	**35**	**0**	5
Caffe Latté:			
8 fl.oz cup: With Whole Milk	**110**	**6**	9
With 2% Milk	**100**	**3.5**	9
With Nonfat Milk	**70**	**0**	10
12 fl.oz: With Whole Milk	**180**	**9**	14
With Nonfat Milk	**100**	**0**	15
16 fl.oz: With Whole Milk	**220**	**11**	18
With Nonfat Milk	**130**	**0**	19
Cafe Mocha (Mochaccino): 1 cup	**150**	**6**	20
12 fl.oz	**230**	**9**	31
16 fl.oz	**290**	**12**	41
Cappuccino:			
8 fl.oz cup: With Whole Milk	**90**	**3.5**	7
With 2% Milk	**80**	**3**	8
With Nonfat Milk	**50**	**0**	8
12 fl.oz: With Whole Milk	**110**	**6**	9
With 2% Milk	**90**	**3.5**	9
With Nonfat Milk	**60**	**0**	9
16 fl.oz: With Whole Milk	**140**	**7**	11
With 2% Milk	**120**	**3.5**	11
With Nonfat Milk	**80**	**0**	12
Mocha (with cream):			
8 fl.oz: With Whole Milk	**200**	**11**	22
With Nonfat Milk	**160**	**6**	22
12 fl.oz: Whole Milk	**290**	**15**	33
With Nonfat Milk	**230**	**8**	34
Iced Mocha (no cream):			
12 fl.oz: With Whole Milk	**170**	**6**	26
With Nonfat Milk	**130**	**2**	27
Espresso: Single (Solo)	**5**	**0**	1
Doppio (Double)	**10**	**0**	2
Espresso con Panna,			
(with dollop whipped cream), solo	**30**	**2.5**	2
Espresso Macchiato, solo	**10**	**0**	1
Frappuccino: Tall, 12 fl.oz	**180**	**2.5**	37
Grande, 16 fl.oz	**240**	**3**	48
Frappuccino Mocha			
(with Cream): Tall, 12 fl.oz	**280**	**11**	43
Grande, 16 fl.oz	**380**	**15**	57

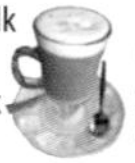

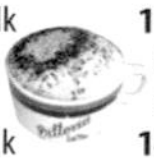

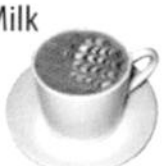

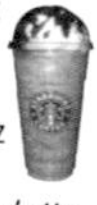

Iced Latte: *Similar to Caffe Latte*

Starbucks: *See Fast-Foods Section*

Coffee Substitute Mixes

	C	F	Cb
Roasted Cereal Beverages: (No Caffeine)			
Cafix Instant Beverage, 1 tsp	**5**	**0**	1
Kaffree Roma *(Morningstar Farms)*, 1 tsp	**10**	**0**	2
Revival Soy "Coffee", 1 Tbsp	**0**	**0**	0
Teeccino Caffe, 1 tsp	**10**	**0**	2

Irish & Liqueur Coffees

	C	F	Cb
Irish Coffee (no sugar)	**175**	**10**	0
Liqueur Coffee, average 1 fl.oz	**100**	**5**	7

Coffee Extras

	C	F	Cb
Chocolate (Cocoa) Topping, ½ tsp	**5**	**0**	1
Flavored Syrups: Regular, 2 Tbsp	**80**	**0**	20
Sugar-free, 2 Tbsp	**0**	**0**	0
Half & Half Cream, 2 Tbsp	**40**	**3.5**	1
Single Serve Cup, ⅜ fl.oz	**15**	**1.5**	0.5
Light Whipped Cream, 2 Tbsp	**15**	**1.5**	1
Marshmallows, miniature (2)	**5**	**0**	1
Sugar: 1 package, 0.18 oz	**20**	**0**	5
1 level tsp, 0.14 pz	**15**	**0**	4
1 heaping tsp, 0.21 oz	**25**	**0**	6
Equal/Splenda/Sweet 'N Low, pkt	**0**	**0**	0

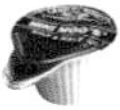

Coffee Shop ~ Cakes, Cookies

Cookies:	C	F	Cb
Biscotti, 1 oz	**140**	**6.5**	18
Chocolate Chip, 3 oz	**350**	**15**	54
Oatmeal Raisin, 3 oz	**350**	**12**	56
Peanut Butter, 3 oz	**410**	**25**	39
White Chocolate Macadamia, 3⅓ oz	**420**	**20**	55
Cakes/Pastries:			
Almond Croissant, 5 oz	**620**	**35**	67
Apple Danish, 5 oz	**450**	**18**	67
Banana Walnut, 4½ oz	**410**	**17**	60
Brownie, 3 oz	**390**	**24**	42
Bundt, Chocolate, 4 oz	**440**	**21**	61
Carrot Cake, 4 oz	**400**	**22**	45
Chocolate Cake, 5 oz	**530**	**28**	65
Crumble Coffee Cake, 4½ oz	**500**	**25**	65
Cupcake, 3 oz	**330**	**16**	43
Pound Cake, 3 oz	**330**	**17**	40
Cinnamon Roll, 6 oz	**500**	**15**	83
Doughnuts: Sugared, 1¾ oz	**220**	**11**	27
Glazed, 2 oz	**250**	**12**	34
Pretzel, large, 4 oz	**290**	**5**	52

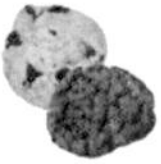

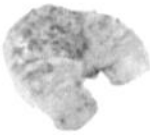

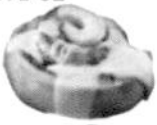

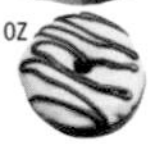

Bottled Coffee (Chilled)

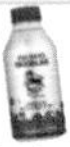

Ready-To-Drink: *Per Bottle*			
Caribou: Espresso, 12 fl.oz	100	0.5	22
Regular; Vanilla, 12 fl.oz	120	1.5	24
Deerfield Farms: *Per 11 oz Bottle*			
Chai Latte, Regular/Vanilla, average	220	6	37
Full Throttle Coffee & Energy ~ *See Page 50*			
Java Monster Energy ~ *See Page 51*			
Kahlúa Cappuccino Shake 10.5 fl.oz	130	2	24
Main St Cafe,			
French Vanilla Ice Latte, 11 fl.oz	260	3	52
Shock Coffee: Triple Latte, 15 fl.oz	140	2	27
Triple Mocha, 15 fl.oz can	140	2	27
Starbucks: *Per Bottle*			
Frappuccino: Caramel, 9.5 fl.oz	200	3	37
Coffee: 9.5 fl.oz	200	3	37
13.7 fl.oz bottle	290	4.5	53
Mocha: Regular, 13.7 fl.oz	260	4.5	47
Dark Choc., 13.7 fl.oz	280	4.5	51
Light, 9.5 fl.oz	100	3	12
Vanilla: 9.5 fl.oz	200	3	37
13.7 fl.oz bottle	295	4.5	55
DoubleShot: Espresso & Cream, 6.5 fl.oz	140	6	18
Light Espresso & Cream, 6.5 fl.oz	70	4	6
Energy + Coffee,			
all flavors, 15 fl.oz	210	2.5	18
Iced Coffee, 11 fl.oz can	100	1	23
Tully's: *Per 12 fl.oz*			
Caramel	620	15	118
Creme	390	14	63
Espresso	380	14	60
Mocha	460	14	78

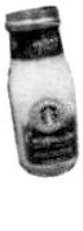

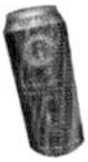

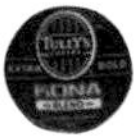

CALORIE KING TIP!

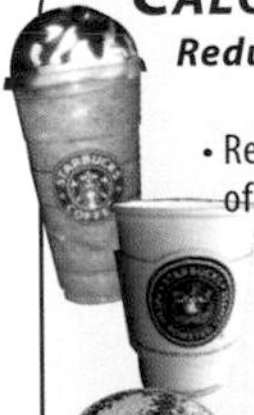

Reduce the Calories in Your Coffee:

- Request non-fat milk in place of whole or 2% milk
- Downsize to 8 fl.oz or 12 fl.oz
- Avoid cream on frappuccinos
- Replace sugar with *Equal, Splenda Stevia* or *Sweet 'N Low*
- Avoid syrup add-ons

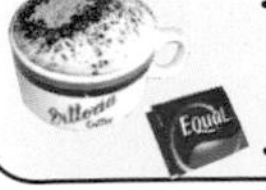

CAFFEINE COUNTER

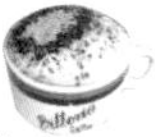

Moderate caffeine intake is not harmful to healthy adults. However, frequent large amounts (over 350mg/day) may cause dependency ('caffeinism') and adversely affect health. To be safe, limit caffeine to 200mg/day. Avoid if pregnant; breast feeding; a child under 8; have sleep problems or heart arrhythmia.

	Caffeine (mg)
Coffee: Instant, weak, 1 level teaspoon	30
Medium, 1 rounded teaspoon	60
Strong, 1 heaping teaspoon	100
Decaffeinated, 1 round teaspoon	2
Bags *(Folgers)*, 1 bag (6-8 fl.oz)	115
Ground, 1 Tbsp, 0.2 oz	60
Bottled (Ready-To-Drink), 9.5 fl.oz	70
Coffee Shop: Brewed, 8 fl.oz	110 -150
Cappuccino: 1 cup, 8 fl.oz	75
Tall, 12 fl.oz	110
Large, 16 fl.oz	150
Decappuccino (decaffeinated)	5
Espresso: Regular/Solo	75
Double (Doppio) Espresso	150
Iced Coffee, 12 fl.oz	140
Latte, 1 cup, 8 fl.oz	75
Mocha, 1 cup, 8 fl.oz	90
Hot Chocolate, 8 fl.oz	15
Tea (Black/Green): Weak, 1 cup	20
Medium Strength, 1 cup	40
Strong, 1 cup	70
Decaffeinated Tea	0-5
Herbal Tea	0
Iced Tea, tall glass/can, 12 fl.oz	25-30
Soft Drinks: *Per 12 fl.oz Can*	
Coca-Cola, Pepsi (Regular/Diet)	35
Diet Coke; TAB; RC Cola (Regular)	45
Dr. Pepper (Reg./Diet) *Sunkist* Orange	40
Pepsi One; Mountain Dew; Mellow Yellow; Surge	55
Pepsi Max (Regular/Diet) *Sun Drop* (Reg/Diet)	70
7-Up, Fanta, Sprite, Fresca, Diet Rite Cola	0
Energy Drinks (with added caffeine): *(AMP, Adrenaline Rush, Full Throttle Monster, No Fear, Red Bull, Rockstar)*	
Average all brands: 8 fl.oz	80
16 fl.oz	160
Chocolate Bars: Milk Chocolate, 2 oz	20
Dark Chocolate, 2 oz	30
Cocoa/Hot Choc. Mix, 1 oz packet	5
Chocolate Milk, 1 cup, 8 fl.oz	2
Choc Chip Cookies, 2 medium, 2 oz	6
Chocolate Syrup, 2 Tbsp, 1.4 oz	5
Medicinals: *Excedrin,* Extra Strength (2)	130
NoDoz Maximum, 1 tablet	200

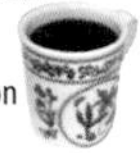

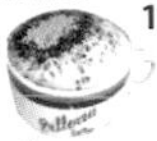

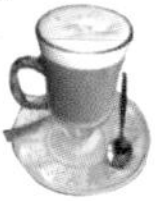

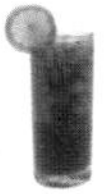

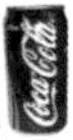

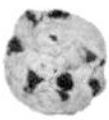

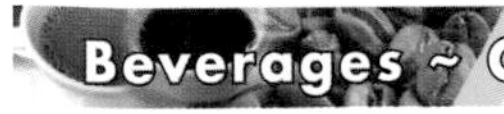

Extensive Caffeine Counter ~ www.CalorieKing.com

Quick Guide

Orange Juice

Average ~ Fresh or Sweetened:	C	F	Cb
½ Cup, 4 fl.oz	55	0	13
Small Glass, 6 fl.oz	85	0	19
Regular Glass, 8 fl.oz	110	0.5	26
8¾ fl.oz Box	120	0.5	28
10 fl.oz Bottle	140	0.5	32
11½ fl.oz Can	160	0.5	37
16 fl.oz Bottle	225	1	52
20 fl.oz Bottle	280	1	64
64 fl.oz, ½ Gallon	895	4	206

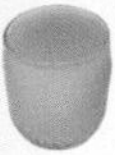

Juices ~ Generic

Average All Brands: Per 8 fl.oz Unless Indicated

	C	F	Cb
Aloe Vera Juice, unsweetened, 2 oz	10	0	0
Apple Juice: 8 fl.oz	120	0	29
10 fl.oz Bottle	145	0.5	36
16 fl.oz	235	0.5	58
Carrot Juice: Fresh, 6 fl.oz	35	0	8
Sweetened, 6 fl.oz	75	0	17
Cranberry Juice, Cocktail/Blend	140	0	34
Fruit Blends, average, 8 fl.oz	110	0	27
Fruit Nectars, average, 8 fl.oz	140	0	36
Grape Juice, 8 fl.oz	155	0	38
Grapefruit Juice, 8 fl.oz	95	0	22
Lemon/Lime Juice: 1 Tbsp	3	0	1
1 cup, 8 fl.oz	50	0.5	16
Concentrate, 1 tsp	0	0	0
Noni Juice: *Tahitian*, 2 Tbsp, 1 fl.oz	5	0	1
Tahiti Traders, 1 fl.oz	20	0	5
Passion Fruit Juice (Fresh):			
Purple, 1 cup, 8 fl.oz	125	0	34
Yellow, 1 cup, 8 fl.oz	80	1.5	14
Papaya/Peach Nectar, av., 8 fl.oz	140	0	36
Pear Nectar, 8 fl.oz	150	0	40
Pineapple Juice, 8 fl.oz	130	0	32
Pomegranate Juice, 8 fl.oz	160	0	40
Prune Juice, 8 fl.oz	180	0	45
Strawb./Raspberry Juice, 8 fl.oz	100	0	23
Tangerine Juice, 8 fl.oz	105	0.5	25
Tomato Juice, 8 fl.oz	40	0	10
Vegetable Juice, 8 fl.oz	45	0	11
Wheat Grass Juice: 1 fl.oz 'Shot'	5	0	1
2 fl.oz 'Shot'	15	0	2

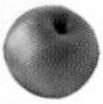
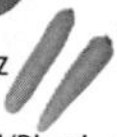
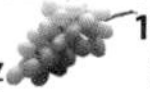
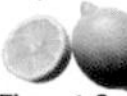
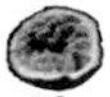

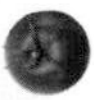

Quick Guide

Fruit Smoothies (Jamba Juice; Smoothie King)

Average All Brands	C	F	Cb
Fruit Only: 8 fl.oz	115	0.5	29
12 fl.oz	175	1	43
16 fl.oz	230	1	58
24 fl.oz	350	1	78
Fruit + Non-Fat Milk/Soy:			
12 fl.oz	135	0	29
16 fl.oz	155	0	37
24 fl.oz	265	1	59
Fruit + Non-Fat Frozen Yogurt/Sherbet:			
12 fl.oz	200	0	47
16 fl.oz	265	0	63
24 fl.oz	395	0	95

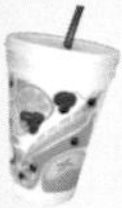

Juice Brands

Per 8 fl.oz Unless Indicated

	C	F	Cb
Apple & Eve			
Naturally Cranberry	130	0	32
Cranberry Grape	140	0	34
Fruitables, average all flavors, 6.75 fl.oz	70	0	16
Bolthouse			
100% Juices: Carrot, 8 fl.oz	70	0	14
Clementine	110	0	29
Vedge	60	0	12
Lemonade, Prickly Pear	130	0	34
Fruit Smoothies:			
Berry Boost	110	0	30
Blue Goodness	180	0	45
C-Boost	150	0	36
Green Goodness	140	0	33
Strawberry Banana	125	0	29
Bossa Nova: *Per 10 fl.oz Bottle*			
Acai Juice: Original	120	0	29
With Blueb./ Mango/Raspb./P'Fruit	110	0	27
Other Juices,			
Acerola/Goji/Mangostein, average	105	0	26
Bright & Early *(Minute Maid)*			
Orange Juice (Chilled/Frozen)	110	0	29
Campbell's			
Tomato Juice: 5.5 fl.oz can	30	0	7
8 fl.oz	50	0	10
Capri Sun			
Juice Drink, 25% Less Sugar: *Per 6.75 fl.oz Pouch*			
Coastal Cooler; Mountain Cooler	70	0	19
100% Juice, average, 6.75 fl.oz	100	0	24

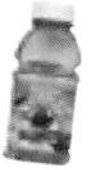
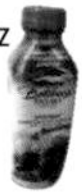
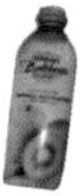
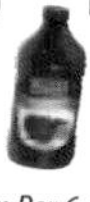

Juice Brands (Cont)

Per 8 fl.oz Unless Indicated

Item	C	F	Cb
Chiquita Smoothies:			
Average all flavors,			
4 oz concentrate (8 oz reconst'd)	120	0	28
12 oz Can (concentrate)	360	0	84
Clamato			
Tomato Cocktail, average	50	0	11
Crystal Geyser			
Juice Squeeze: *Per Bottle (12 fl.oz)*			
Blackberry Pomegranate	170	0	43
Ruby Grapefruit	150	0	36
Average other flavors	140	0	32
Dannon			
Frusion Smoothie, av., 7 fl.oz	180	2.5	35
Light & Fit, 7 fl.oz bottle	70	0	14
Dole			
Chilled, 100%: *Per 8 fl.oz*			
Orange Peach Mango	120	0	29
Pina Colada	120	0	29
Pineapple Juice	130	0	30
Pineapple-Orange Banana	120	0	30
Strawberry Kiwi	120	0	31
Average other flavors	120	0	29
Frozen Concentrates 100%:			
Average all flavors, ¼ cup	125	0	31
Single Serve, 100%: *Per 15.2 fl.oz Bottle*			
100% Apple, no sugar added	210	0	51
100% Blends:			
Ruby Red Grapefruit	260	0	63
Strawberry Kiwi	230	0	58
Grape, no sugar added	300	0	74
Orange, no sugar added	210	0	51
Five Alive *(Minute Maid):*			
Frozen Concentrate, prepared, 8 fl.oz	110	0	29
Florida's Natural			
Orange	110	0	29
Ruby Red Grapefruit	90	0	22
Frützzo: *Per 12 fl.oz Bottle*			
(No Added Sugar)			
Pomegranate 100%	210	0	52
With Acai; Cherry	210	0	51
With Blueberry; Raspberry	195	0	48
Yumberry 100%			
Natural	150	0	33
Organic	120	0	25
with Blueberry; Pomegranate	165	0	39

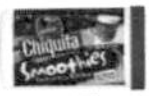
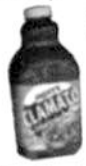
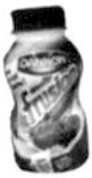
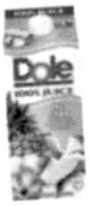
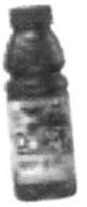
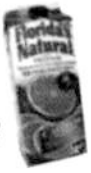
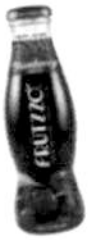

Updated Nutrition Data ~ www.CalorieKing.com
Persons with Diabetes ~ See Disclaimer (Page 24)

Item	C	F	Cb
Fuze: *Per 16 fl.oz*			
Refresh, average all flavors	180	0	48
Slenderize, average all flavors	15	0	3
Vitalize, all flavors	200	0	50
Goya Nectar			
5% Juice: Guanabana, 12 fl.oz	230	0	57
Passion & Pineapple, 12 fl.oz	220	0	55
Hansen's			
Juice Slam: *Per 6.75 fl.oz Box*			
Awesome Apple	90	0	23
Other flavors	120	0	29
Organic, 1 Pouch	100	0	24
Junior Juice, 4.23 oz box	60	0	15
Natural (64 fl.oz Bottles): *Per 8 fl.oz*			
Apple, Strawberry	120	0	28
Black Grape, Pomegranate Cocktail	160	0	39
White Grape	140	0	36
Organic Blends, average	110	0	27
Fruit Smoothies, average, 12 fl.oz	175	0	44
Low-Carb, average, 12 fl.oz	40	0	9
Light Juice Cocktails, average, 8 fl.oz	40	0	9
Hawaii's Own			
Frozen Concentrate: *Per 8 fl.oz, Prepared*			
10% Juice, average all varieties	110	0	28
Hi-C Juice Drinks:			
6.75 fl.oz box, average	90	0	26
Blast, 6.75 fl.oz pouch	100	0	26
Hood: Apple, 8 fl.oz	120	0	31
Fruit Punch; Orange	120	0	30
Jamba Juice: *See Fast-Foods Section*			
Juicy Juice (Nestle): *Per 6.75 fl.oz Box*			
Grape	100	0	25
Average other flavors	100	0	24
4.23 fl.oz box, average	60	0	15
Kerns All Nectars			
Nectars: *Per 11.5 fl.oz Can*			
Pear	220	0	54
Pineapple Coconut	280	8	53
Average other flavors	215	0	52
Kool Aid			
Jammers, 6.75 oz, average	90	0	24
Jammers 10	10	0	2
Kroger Smoothies, average, 10 fl.oz	280	3.5	53
L & A: *Per 8 fl.oz*			
All Cherry	180	0	45
All Prune Juice	180	0	41
Mixed Berry	120	0	30

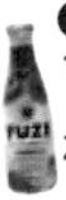
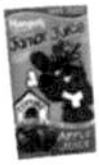
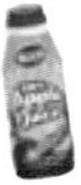

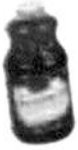

Juice Brands (Cont)

	C	F	Cb
Lakewood Organic: *Per 8 fl.oz*			
Acai Amazon Berry	125	0	28
Banana Strawberry	115	0	28
Blueberry Blend	120	0	30
Cranberry Lemonade	80	0	20
Fruit Garden: Summer/Green, average	100	0	20
Blue/Purple/Red Pomegr., average	110	0	24
Goji	90	0	20
Lemonade	85	0	21
Pomegranate Blend	125	0	32
Pure: Apple	105	0	26
Blueberry	90	0	24
Carrot	90	0	20
Pink Grapefruit	90	0	22
Prune	170	0	42
Super Veggie	55	0	12
Light: Lemonade	40	0	15
Other flavors, average	60	0	21

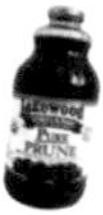
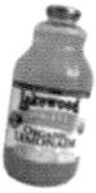

(Note: Carbs include Erythritol natural sweetener)

	C	F	Cb
Langers: *Per 8 fl.oz*			
100% Juice (No Sugar Added):			
All Pomegranate	140	0	34
Apple Cider	120	0	28
Apple Juice	120	0	28
Mixed Berry	120	0	30
Pineapple Coconut	140	3	28
Red/White Grape Juice	160	0	40
Diet Low-Carb (25-50% Juice):			
Apple Juice Cocktail	60	0	14
Cranberry	30	0	8
Pomegranate	40	0	9
Juice Cocktails (27% Juice)			
Blueberry Cranberry	135	0	34
Cranberry Berry	135	0	34
Cranberry Grape	165	0	41
Cranberry Raspberry	150	0	36
Pomegranate	140	0	34
Pomegranate Blueberry/Cranberry	140	0	34
Strawberry Peach (20% Juice)	120	0	30
White Cranberry	120	0	28
White Cran-Raspberry	120	0	28

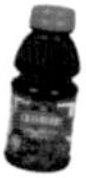

Minute Maid	C	F	Cb
Orange Juice: 100%, 8 fl.oz	110	0	27
15.2 fl.oz bottle	210	0	51
Light, 42%, 8 fl.oz	50	0	13
Fruit Punch, 6.75 fl.oz	100	0	24
Pineapple Orange, Apple, 8 fl.oz	120	0	29
Kids+Orange Juice, 6.75 fl.oz	100	0	23
Enhanced: *Per 8 fl.oz*			
Pomegranate Blueberry	120	0.5	31
Pomegranate Lemonade	110	0	31
Boxed Juices, average, 6.75 fl.oz	100	0	22
Soft Frozen: Limeade, 3 fl.oz	70	0	19
MonaVie Acai Blends			
Original; Active, 4 fl.oz	120	2	20
Mott's			
100% Apple Juice: *Per 8 fl.oz*			
Original	120	0	29
Natural	110	0	27
100% Juice Singles: *Per 14 fl.oz*			
Apple	200	0	48
Fruit Punch	230	0	16
Sunkist Orange Sensation	210	0	12
Veggie Blend	90	1	15
100% Juice Boxes: Average all flavors			
6.75 fl.oz box	100	0	24
4.23 fl.oz box	60	0	15
Mott's Plus Light,			
Apple, 8 fl.oz	130	0	15
Mott's Plus for Kids, average, 8 fl.oz	125	0	31
Mott's For Tots (47-54% Juice),			
All flavors, 6.75 fl.oz box	50	0	13
Naked Juice: *Per 8 fl.oz Unless Indicated*			
Antioxidants:			
Cherry Pomegranate Power	140	0	34
Pomegranate	150	0	37
Bare Breeze, av. all flavors	130	0	31
Probiotics, Tropical Mango, 10 fl.oz	180	0	43
Protein Zone: Mango	220	1	35
P'apple, Coconut & Banana	220	2	34
Pure Juice (100%): O-J	110	0	27
Chai Spiced Cider	120	0	30
Well Being: Berry Blast	130	0	29
Black & Blueberry	130	0	31
Mighty Mango	150	0	36
Strawberry Banana	120	0	29
Tropical	130	0	31

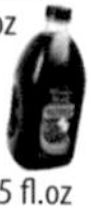
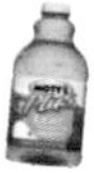
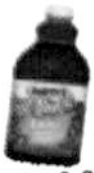
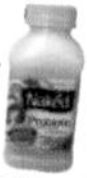
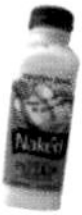

Juice Brands (Cont)

	C	F	Cb
Naked Juice (Cont)			
Superfood Smoothies:			
Acai Machine	160	3	31
Blue Machine	170	0	40
Gold/Green Machine, av.	140	0	32
Power C	120	0	29
Red Machine	170	4.5	31
Nantucket Nectars			
Juice Cocktails: *Per 17.5 fl.oz Bottle*			
Big Cranberry	285	0	70
Carrot Orange Mango	260	0	60
Grapeade	305	0	72
Other varieties, average	260	0	65
100% Juice: *Per 17.5 fl.oz Bottle*			
Peach Orange	285	0	70
Pineapple Orange Banana	305	0	74
Pomegranate Cherry	265	0	63
Premium Orange Juice	240	0	57
Pressed Apple	260	0	65
Nectar Lemonade, 17.5 fl.oz	240	0	61
Newman's Own			
Lemonade, Regular; Pink, 8 fl.oz	110	0	27
Fruit Juice Cocktail: Gorilla Grape	140	0	34
Orange Mango Tango	130	0	33
Razzma Tazz Raspberry	120	0	28
Northland			
100% Juice: *Per 8 fl.oz*			
Cranberry; Blackberry; Raspberry	140	0	34
Cranberry Grape	140	0	36
Ocean Spray: *Per 8 fl.oz*			
Juice Cocktails:			
Cranberry Juice Cocktail	120	0	30
With Calcium	130	0	31
Ruby Tangerine	120	0	31
Ruby Red Grapefruit	110	0	28
100% Juice Blends:			
Cranberry & Concord Grape	150	0	37
Cranberry Blueberry	140	0	36
Cranberry Blends	140	0	35
Juice Drinks:			
CranApple	130	0	32
CranGrape	120	0	31
CranRaspberry/Strawberry	110	0	27
Light Juice Drinks, all flavors	40	0	10
Diet Juice Drinks:			
Cranberry Spray	5	0	2
Cranberry Grape Spray	5	0	2

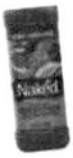

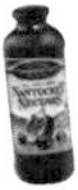

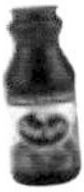
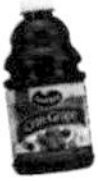
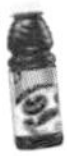

Updated Nutrition Data ~ www.CalorieKing.com
Persons with Diabetes ~ See Disclaimer (Page 24)

	C	F	Cb
Odwalla *Per 16 fl.oz Bottle*			
Carrot Juice	140	0	30
Mo'Beta	300	0	74
Mojito Mambo	100	0	28
PomaGrand Pomegranate	320	0	80
Pomegranate Strawberry	100	0	28
Strawberry Lemonade	220	0	56
Super Protein Original	380	2	70
Smoothies:			
Citrus C Monster	280	0	68
Mango Tango	300	2	68
Strawberry Banana	260	0	62
Strawberry C Monster	320	0	76
Orange Julius			
Originals, Orange:			
Small, 16 fl.oz	130	0.5	33
Medium, 20 fl.oz	160	0.5	41
Large, 32 fl.oz	260	1	65
Smoothies: *See Fast-Foods Section*			
Pom Wonderful			
100% Juice: *Per 8 fl.oz*			
Pomegranate: Blueberry	160	0	40
Cherry	150	0	38
Kiwi	150	0	36
Mango	140	0	35
Nectarine	130	0	31
R.W. Knudsen: *Per 8 fl.oz*			
Natural Juices: 100% Apple	120	0	30
Cranberry Raspberry	130	0	32
Grape	150	0	37
Hibiscus Cooler	100	0	25
Kiwi Strawberry	120	0	29
Mango Peach	130	0	31
Razzleberry	120	0	30
Rio Red Grapefruit	140	0	35
Other varieties, average	120	0	30
Pure Juice: Just Blackcurrant	100	0	15
Just Black Cherry	160	0	36
Just Blueberry	100	0	24
Simply Nutritious: Mega C	140	0	34
Average other varieties	125	0	30
Sparkling Essence: *Per 10.5 fl.oz*			
Average all varieties	0	0	0
Spritzers, 100% Juice: *Per 12 fl.oz Bottles*			
Black Cherry	180	0	46
Mango	170	0	42
Red Raspberry; Tangerine	200	0	47
Very Veggie, Orig, 8 fl.oz	50	0	11

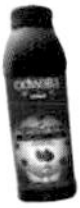
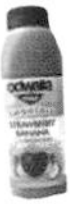

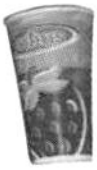
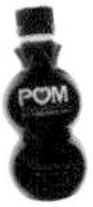

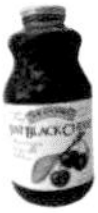
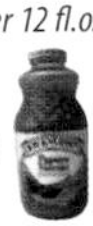

Juice Brands (Cont)

Juice Brands (Cont)	C	F	Cb
Ralphs			
Lemonade (Premium Juice), 8 fl.oz	110	0	29
Pineapple Juice, 8 fl.oz	130	0	33
ReaLemon - ReaLime (Borden)			
Lemon/Lime Juice (from concentrate)			
1 teaspoon	0	0	0
2 Tbsp, 1 fl.oz	8	0	2.5

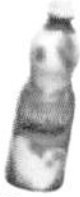

Santa Cruz (Organic)			
100% Juice: *Per 8 fl.oz*			
Apple Juice	120	0	30
Concord Grape; White Grape	160	0	40
Orange Mango	130	0	32
Strawberry Kiwi	120	0	30
25% Juice Drink Boxes: *Per 8 fl.oz*			
Lemon	120	0	29
Orange; Grape, average	100	0	24
Tropical	110	0	27
Champagne Style:			
Sparkling Lemonade	110	0	27
Sparkling Limeade	100	0	26
Nectars: Cranberry	110	0	27
Passionfruit	150	0	40
Average other varieties	120	0	30
Sodas: *Per 12 fl.oz Can*			
Cherry	140	0	34
Concord Grape	150	0	36

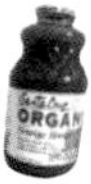

Seismic Super Juices: *Per 12 fl.oz Bottle*			
Citrus/Berry	200	0	49
Low Sugar Cherry	60	0	15
Simply Orange			
Lemonade; Limeade	120	0	30
Orange Juice, av., all varieties	110	0	26

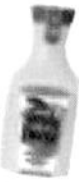

Snap•E•Tom			
Tomato & Chili Cocktail, 6 fl.oz	40	0	7
Snapple			
Juice Drink Blends: *Per 8 fl.oz*			
Grapeade; Orangeade	100	0	26
Average other flavors	110	0	27
Diet: Cranberry Raspberry	10	0	2
100% Juiced, (added vitamins), 11.5 fl.oz	170	0	40
Ssips			
Juice Drinks, average, 6.75 fl.oz box	105	0	26
Stonyfield Farm: *Per 10 fl.oz Bottle*			
Peach Smoothie	230	3	41
Berry; Strawberry Smoothie	230	3	39

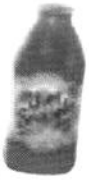

SunnyD	C	F	Cb
Baja Juice: *Per 12 fl.oz Bottle*			
Orange	190	0	46
Orange Berry	190	0	46
Orange Pineapple	190	0	46
Red Punch	170	0	43

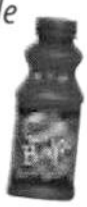

SunnyD Blends: *Per 8 fl.oz*			
Orange Fused, all flavors	80	0	20
SunnyD Original: *Per 8 fl.oz*			
Smooth/Tangy Style	90	0	22
Fruit Punch	80	0	21
Mango	90	0	22
Reduced Sugar	60	0	15

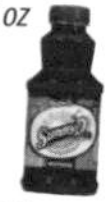

SunnyD Smoothies: *Per 8 fl.oz*			
Orange Whirl; Strawberry Swirl	140	0	34
Sunsweet: *Per 8 fl.oz*			
Prune Juice/with Pulp	180	0	43
Tampico: Citrus Punch	110	0	25
Mango/Tropical Fruit Punch	110	0	28

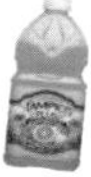

Tang			
Pouches, average all flavors (1)	90	0	24
Mix: *Prepared as Directed*			
Regular (2 Tbsp dry), 6 fl.oz	110	0	27
Sugar Free, 8 fl.oz	5	0	0

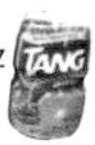

Trader Joe's			
Refrigerated: *Small 16fl.oz Bottle:*			
Carrot Juice	160	2	32
Mango Smoothie	150	0	36
Protein with Pzazz	440	4	68
Strawberry Smoothie	240	0	58
Watermelon Juice	160	0	54

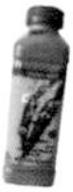

Organic, 32/64 fl.oz Bottle: *Per 8 fl.oz*			
100% Pomegranate	160	0	40
Apple Juice	120	0	30
Concord Grape Juice	160	0	39
Cranberry	70	0	18
Grapefruit Sunset; Lemonade	120	0	30
Mango Nectar	130	0	32
Pink Lemonade	130	0	32
Strawberry Lemonade	120	0	29
White Grape Juice	160	0	40

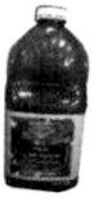

All Natural Pasteurized, 32/64 fl.oz Bottle: *Per 8 fl.oz*			
100% Cranberry	70	0	18
Just Blueberry	100	0	24
Just Pomegranate	150	0	37
Mango PassionFruit	130	0	32
Omega Orange Carrot	110	0	26
Pomegranate Blueberry	140	0	34

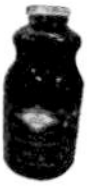

Juice Brands (Cont)

Per 8 fl.oz Unless Indicated	C	F	Cb
Trader Joe's (Cont)			
Joe's Kids: *Per 6.75 oz Box*			
100% Juice: Apple	90	0	23
Apple Grape	100	0	24
White Apple	120	0	30
10% Juice, Lemonade	90	0	22
Sparkling Juices, 750ml/25.4 fl.oz Bottle: *Per 8 fl.oz*			
Blueberry	120	0	30
Cranberry	140	0	35
Pomegranate	130	0	31
Tree Top			
100% Juice From Concentrates			
Apple Berry/Grape	120	0	31
Apple Pear, 6.75 fl.oz	100	0	25
Apple/Spiced Cider	120	0	29
Kiwi Strawberry, 10 fl.oz	130	0	32
Mango Peach, 10 fl.oz	160	0	39
Ochango, 10 fl.oz	170	0	42
Orange Passionfruit	110	0	26
Tropical	120	0	29
100% Juice Fresh Pressed			
3 Apple Blend	120	0	30
Fiber Rich:			
Apple	140	0	35
Apple Apricot/Orange Banana	160	0	38
Trim			
Kiwi Strawberry; Pom. Blackberry	60	0	15
Mango Peach; Tangerine Pineapple	60	0	16
Tropicana			
Coastal Groves Lemonade, av. all flav	120	0	30
Pure Premium Orange Juice	110	0	26
Pure: Indian River Grapefruit	110	0	25
Valencia without Pulp	120	0	27
Twisters: Average, 8 fl.oz	120	0	29
20 fl.oz bottle	300	0	74
V8® Juices & Drinks			
V8 100% Vegetable Juice:			
5.5 fl.oz can	35	0	7
8 fl.oz cup	50	0	10
11.5 fl.oz can	70	0	14
12 fl.oz bottle	75	0	15
V-8 Splash, average	70	0	19
V-8 Splash Smoothies: Strawberry	90	0	20
Tropical Colada	100	0	21
Diet V-8 Splash, all flavors	10	0	3
Fusion, all flavors	115	0	28

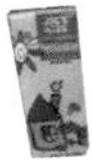
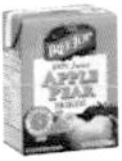
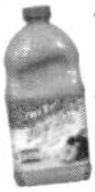
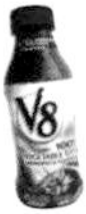

Per 8 fl.oz Unless Indicated	C	F	Cb
Veryfine			
Apple Juice (100%)	110	0	27
Orange Juice (100%)	120	0	28
Walnut Acres: *Per 8 fl.oz*			
Organic: Apple	110	0	29
Apricot; Raspberry	130	0	32
Cherry	140	0	34
Cranberry	110	0	26
Incredible Vegetable	50	0	12
Mango Nectar	120	0	29
Welch's: *Per 8 fl.oz*			
100% Grape: Red Grape	170	0	43
100% Juice: White Grape Cherry	140	0	35
White Grape Peach	160	0	39
Cocktails (Refrigerated, 64 fl.oz Ctn):			
Guava Pineapple	140	0	36
Mango Twist	150	0	38
Strawberry Breeze	130	0	33
Light Juice (52 fl.oz Bottle),			
Grape, 8 fl.oz	50	0	13
Sparkling Juice Cocktail, 8 fl.oz	160	0	40
Concentrates (100% Juice),			
All flavors, ¼ cup, 2 fl.oz	160	0	41

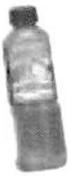
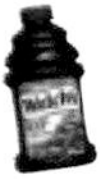
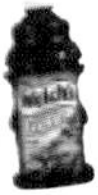

CalorieKing Portion Watch

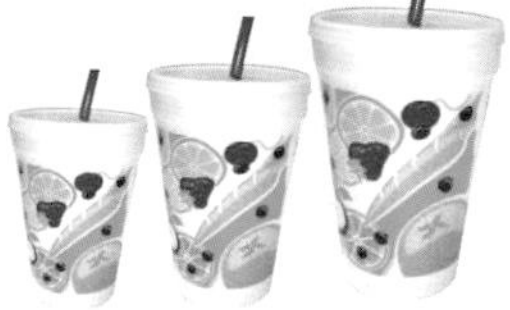

ORANGE JUICE	C	Cb
8 fl.oz	110	26
16 fl.oz	220	52
24 fl.oz	330	78
32 fl.oz	440	104

Quick Guide

	C	F	Cb
Cow's Milk ~ *Average All Brands*			
Whole (3.25% fat):			
2 Tbsp, 1 fl.oz	20	1	1.5
1 Cup, 8 fl.oz	150	8	12
1 Large Glass, 12 fl.oz	220	12	17
1 Pint, 16 fl.oz	295	16	22
1 Quart, 946 ml	590	32	44
Reduced-Fat (2% fat):			
2 Tbsp, 1 fl.oz	15	0.5	1.5
1 Cup, 8 fl.oz	120	5	12
1 Large Glass, 12 fl.oz	180	7.5	18
1 Pint, 16 fl.oz	245	10	23
1 Quart, 946 ml	490	20	46
Light/Low-Fat (1% fat):			
2 Tbsp, 1 fl.oz	13	0.3	1.5
1 Cup, 8 fl.oz	100	2.5	12
1 Large Glass, 12 fl.oz	150	4	18
1 Pint, 16 fl.oz	205	5	25
1 Quart, 946 ml	410	10	49
Fat Free/Skim:			
2 Tbsp, 1 fl.oz	10	0	1.5
1 Cup, 8 fl.oz	90	0.5	13
1 Pint, 16 fl.oz	180	1	26
with Oatrim Fiber (for replacement), 1 cup	85	0	12
Buttermilk: Average All Brands			
Reduced-Fat (2%), 1 cup	120	5	10
Low-Fat (1%): 1 cup	100	2.5	12
Lactose-Free: *Per 8 fl.oz*			
Dairy Ease: Whole	160	9	11
2% Reduced-Fat	130	5	12
Fat-Free	90	0	12
Lactaid 100: Whole	150	8	12
2% Reduced-Fat	130	5	12
1% Low-Fat	110	2.5	13
Fat-Free	80	0	13
Calcium-Fortified	80	0	13
Real Goodness: 2% Fat	120	5	7
Fat Free 0%	80	0	7
Lower Calorie Dairy Drinks: *Per 8 fl.oz Cup*			
Calorie Countdown (Hood):			
2% Reduced-Fat	90	5	3
2% Reduced-Fat, Chocolate	90	5	5
Fat-Free	45	0	3

Goat/Sheep Milk, Kefir

	C	F	Cb
Goat's Milk (Meyenberg):			
Whole, 1 cup, 8 fl.oz	140	7	11
Light/Low-Fat (1%), 8 fl.oz	100	2.5	11
Evaporated, reconst., 8 fl.oz	150	8	11
Kefir (Cultured Milk):			
Nancy's: Plain, 8 fl.oz	110	3	14
Fruit flavors, average, 8 fl.oz	180	2.5	34
Trader Joe's: Plain, 8 fl.oz	110	2.5	8
Strawberry, 8 fl.oz	160	2	21
Sheep's Milk: Whole, 1 cup	265	17	13

Canned & Dried Milk

	C	F	Cb
Condensed: Reg. 2 Tbsp, 1 fl.oz	130	3	23
Low-Fat *(Eagle)*, 2 Tbsp	120	1.5	23
Fat-Free *(Eagle)*, 2 Tbsp	110	0	24
Evaporated: Whole, 2 Tbsp	40	3	3
Whole, ½ cup	170	10	13
Low-Fat *(Carnation)*, 2 Tbsp, 1 oz	25	0.5	3
½ cup, 4 fl.oz	115	2.5	14
Fat-Free, 2 Tbsp, 1 oz	25	0	4
Dried: Whole, ¼ cup, 1 oz	160	9	12
Skim/Non-Fat, ⅓ cup	80	0	12
Made-up, 1 cup, 8 fl.oz	80	0	12
Buttermilk (sweet cream), 1 oz	110	2	14
Non-Fat, 1 Tbsp	25	0	3
Malted *(Carnation)*, dry, 1 Tbsp	30	0.5	6

Soy/Non-Dairy Drinks ~ *See Page 48*

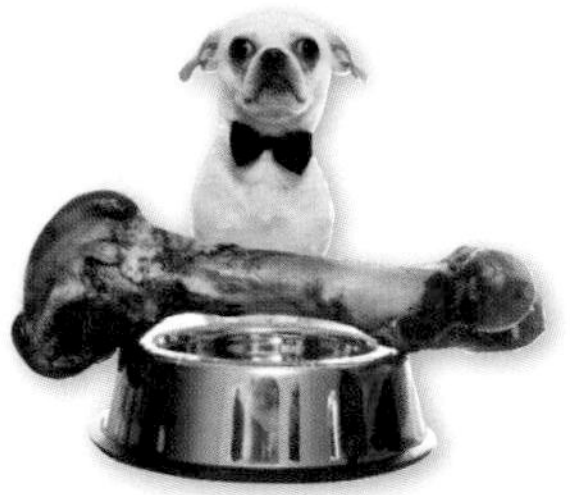

'What ever happened to sensible portion size?!'

Quick Guide

Chocolate Milk

Average All Brands: Per Cup (8 fl.oz)

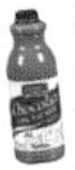

	C	F	Cb
Whole Milk (3.3%): 1 cup	210	8	26
1 Pint	415	17	52
Reduced-Fat (2%), 1 cup	190	5	30
Low-Fat (1%), 1 cup	160	2.5	26

Brands ~ Flavored Milk

Ready-To-Drink: *Per 8 fl.oz Cup Unless Indicated*

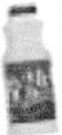

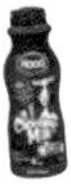

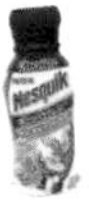

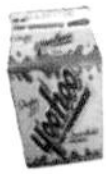

	C	F	Cb
Albertson's, Choc Milk	200	2.5	34
Alta Dena: Chocolate	260	9	37
Low-Fat Chocolate	200	3	32
Dean's, Milk Chug: *Per 12 fl.oz Bottle*			
Chocolate	420	12	68
Vanilla	440	11	75
Hood: Chocolate	230	9	31
Low-Fat (1%), Chocolate	170	3	28
Horizon Organic: Low-Fat Chocolate	170	3	27
Reduced-Fat Vanilla	190	4.5	30
Kroger, Choc Milk, Low-Fat, 1%	180	2.5	33
Muscle Milk (*Cytosport*) (Hi Protein):			
Chocolate, 17 fl.oz	330	16	13
Average other flavors, 17 fl.oz	310	12	16
Nesquik: *Per 16 fl.oz*			
Banana	400	10	60
Chocolate	400	10	65
Fat-Free	320	0	64
Strawberry	400	10	66
Prairie Farms, Choc., 16 fl.oz bottle	440	16	58
Quaker, Milk Chillers, 14 fl.oz bottle	245	9	32
Ralphs, Chocolate, Low-Fat	210	2.5	36
Skinny Cow, Chocolate, Fat-Free	150	0	26
Starbucks, Van.Frappuccino 13.7 fl.oz	290	4.5	53
Yoo-Hoo:			
Chocolate: 6½ fl.oz box	105	1	29
8 fl.oz	130	1	29

Shakes

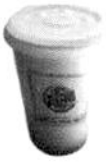

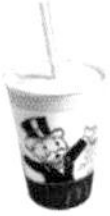

	C	F	Cb
Burger King:			
Chocolate:			
Value, 12 fl.oz	340	9	60
Small, 16 fl.oz	440	11	78
Medium, 22 fl.oz	650	16	119
Large, 32 fl.oz	960	23	176
Other flavors ~ *See Page 193*			
McDonalds:			
Average all flavors:			
12 fl.oz cup	430	10	75
16 fl.oz cup	570	13	101
21 fl.oz cup	760	18	132
32 fl.oz cup	1140	26	200

Nutrition/Meal Shakes ~ *See Page 50*

Smoothies

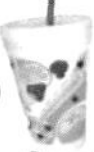

	C	F	Cb
Smoothies			
Made Up Ready-To-Drink			
(8 fl. oz Milk/Soy + Fruit): *Per 12 fl.oz*			
Average all types:			
With Whole Milk	300	8	50
+ Ice Cream, 1 scoop	400	13	62
With Non-Fat Milk	240	0	50

Fruit Smoothies ~ *See Page 40*

Freshens; Jamba Juice; TCBY: **See Fast-Foods**

Bottle Coffee Drinks ~ *See Page 39*

CALORIE KING TIP!

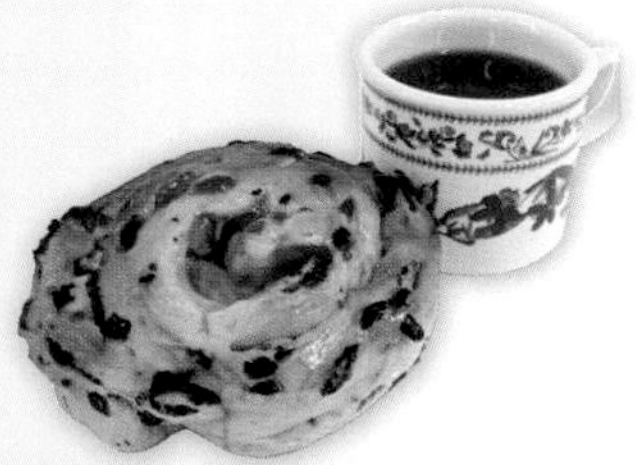

'Low-Fat' does not mean 'Low-Calorie'. This low-fat Apricot Sticky Bun has only 2g fat but has over 400 calories!

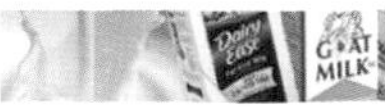

Rice & Cereal Drinks

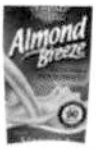
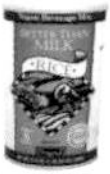

Per 8 fl.oz Cup	C	F	Cb
Almond Breeze *(Blue Diamond)*			
Original	60	2.5	8
Chocolate	120	3	22
Vanilla	90	2.5	16
Almond Dream			
Original Enriched	50	2.5	6
Unsweetened	30	2.5	1
Amazake, Original	150	0	34
Better Than Milk			
Rice Vegan Mix:			
Original, 2 Tbsp powder, 0.67 oz	70	1	16
Vanilla, 2 Tbsp powder, 0.67 oz	75	2	15

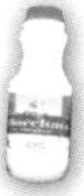
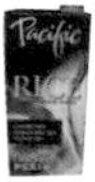

Per 8 fl.oz Cup	C	F	Cb
Cacique,			
Horchata Rice Drink	160	3.5	31
Don Jose:			
Horchata Rice Drink	140	4	25
Cereal Match	100	3	17
EdenBlend, Rice & Soy	120	3	18
Kern's, Horchata	140	3	26
Pacific			
Rice Drinks:			
Low-Fat Plain/Vanilla	130	2	27
Organic Oat: Original	130	2.5	24
Vanilla	130	2.5	25
Nut Drinks: Hazelnut, Original	110	3.5	18
Almond: Original, Low-Fat	60	2.5	8
Vanilla, Low-Fat	70	2.5	11
Organic: Original	60	2.5	8
Chocolate, Single Serve	100	3	19
Vanilla, Single Serve	70	2.5	11

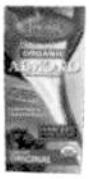
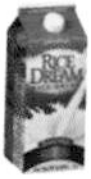
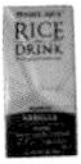
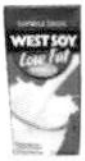

Per 8 fl.oz Cup	C	F	Cb
Rice Dream			
Original/Enriched	120	2.5	23
Carob	150	2.5	30
Heartwise: Original	130	2	27
Vanilla	140	2	30
Horchata	160	2.5	32
Vanilla; Vanilla, Enriched	130	2.5	27
Supreme: Chocolate Chai	160	3	35
Vanilla Hazelnut	140	2.5	29
Trader Joe's:			
Rice Drinks:			
Original, Organic	120	2.5	23
Vanilla	130	2.5	26
Organic Almond, Vanilla	70	2.5	11
WestSoy: Plain Rice	110	2.5	20
Vanilla Rice	110	2.5	20

Note: Rice/Oat/Nut drinks are very low in protein. Unless enriched with protein (and calcium), they are not suitable for infants as a substitute for milk or calcium-enriched soy drinks.

Soy Milk ~ Ready-To-Drink

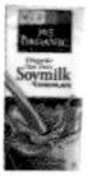
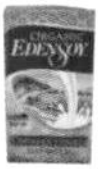

Per 8 fl.oz Cup	C	F	Cb
365 Organic *(Whole Foods):*			
Original	90	3.5	9
Plain, unsweetened	70	4	4
Chocolate	140	3.5	22
Vanilla	90	3.5	10
EdenBlend, Organic	120	3	18
Edensoy: Original	140	5	14
Carob; Chocolate, average	175	4	29
Vanilla	150	3	24
Light: Original	100	2	15
Vanilla	110	1	22
Extra: Original	130	4	13
Vanilla	150	3	23

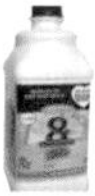
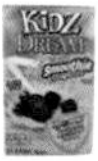

Per 8 fl.oz Cup	C	F	Cb
8th Continent:			
Original	80	2.5	7
Chocolate	140	3	22
Vanilla	100	3	11
Fat-Free: Original	60	0	8
Vanilla	70	0	11
Light: Original	50	2	2
Chocolate	90	1.5	12
Kidz Dream Smoothie			
Berry Blast	100	2	17
Orange Cream	120	2	21

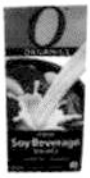
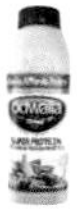

Per 8 fl.oz Cup	C	F	Cb
Lifeway			
SoyTreat Kefir, Peach/Strawberry	160	4	23
O Organics *(Safeway):*			
Plain	90	3.5	8
Chocolate	150	4	23
Vanilla Soy	100	3	9
Odwalla:			
Super Protein: Original	190	1	35
Vanilla Al'Mondo	190	6	25
Protein Monster, Vanilla	200	3.5	24
Pacific			
Select: Plain, Low-Fat	70	2.5	9
Vanilla, Low-Fat	80	2.5	11
Organic, Original, Unsweetened	90	4.5	4
Ultra (Extra Protein/Calcium): Plain	120	4	11
Vanilla	130	4	14

Soy Milk ~ Ready-To-Drink

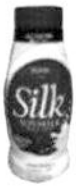
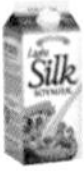
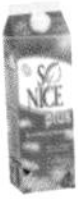
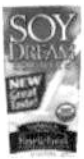
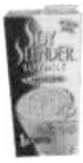
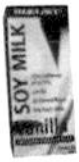
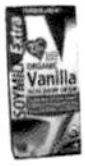
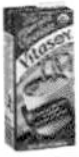

Per 8 fl.oz Cup	C	F	Cb
Silk			
Original	100	4	8
Chocolate	150	3	25
Heart Health	80	1.5	10
Plus DHA Omega-3	110	5	8
Unsweetened	80	4	4
Vanilla	100	3.5	10
Very Vanilla	130	4	19
Light: Original	70	2	8
Chocolate	90	1.5	15
Vanilla	80	2	10
Slim-Fast (Soy-Based) ~ *See Page 52*			
So Nice:			
Fortified: Original	80	3	7
Chocolate	150	3	24
Mocha	150	3.5	24
Natural	80	4	3
Strawberry	110	3	15
Omega+: Original	90	4	8
Vanilla	120	4	16
Soy Dream			
Classic Vanilla	140	4	18
Enriched: Original	100	4	8
Chocolate	150	4	21
Vanilla	120	4	14
Omega Plus: Original	110	4	10
Vanilla	130	4	15
Soy Slender: Plain	60	3	3
Average other flavors	70	3	4
Trader Joe's:			
Soy Milk: Original	110	2.5	17
Vanilla	100	2.5	14
Organic: Original	110	2.5	17
Chocolate	120	3	17
Vanilla	130	3	19
Organic Unsweetened	70	3.5	3
Soy Essential	90	4	6
Chocolate Soy Milk, 8 fl.oz box	130	2.5	23
Vitasoy:			
Chocolate Banana	130	4	21
Peppermint Chocolate	140	4	22
Strawberry Banana	140	4	18

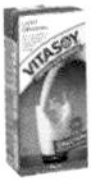

Updated Nutrition Data ~ www.CalorieKing.com
Persons with Diabetes ~ See Disclaimer (Page 24)

Soy Milk ~ Ready-To-Drink (Cont)

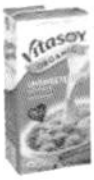
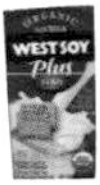
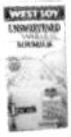
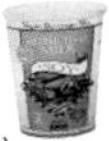

Per 8 fl.oz Cup	C	F	Cb
Vitasoy (Cont):			
Single Serve Bottle: *11.5 fl.oz*			
Plain	140	6	12
Chocolate	230	6	33
Vanilla	160	5	18
Light Plus: Original	60	2	5
Chocolate	100	2	17
Vanilla	70	2	8
Organic: Plain	110	4	11
Unsweetened	90	4.5	5
Chocolate	160	4	24
Vanilla	120	4	13
WestSoy			
Lite: Plain	60	2	6
Vanilla	70	2	8
Low-Fat: Plain	90	1.5	14
Vanilla	120	1.5	21
Non-Fat: Plain	70	0	10
Vanilla	80	0	12
Longevity, Plain	90	3.5	10
Plus: (25% Less Sugar):			
Plain	90	3.5	7
Vanilla	100	3.5	10
Soy Shakes, Chocolate; Vanilla, av.	170	3.5	29
Unsweetened:			
Almond; Organic Plain	90	4.5	5
Chocolate; Vanilla	100	4.5	6

Soy Powder Mix

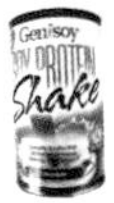
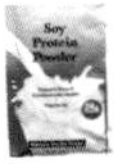
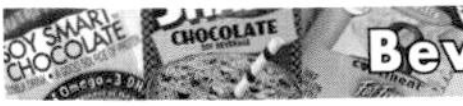

1 oz (¼ cup) mix makes 8 fl.oz Cup	C	F	Cb
Soy Protein Isolate, 1 oz dry	95	1	0
Better Than Milk:			
Original, 2 Tbsp	100	2.5	16
Vanilla, 2¾ Tbsp	80	2	8
Light, 2 Tbsp	75	2.5	7
Genisoy (Powder Shakes):			
Per 3 Rounded Tbsp			
Plain; Natural: 1 oz	110	1.5	0
Ultra-XT, 1.3 oz	130	1.5	5
Chocolate: 1.2 oz	130	0.5	16
Ultra-XT, 1.4 oz	150	1	20
Vanilla: 1.2 oz	130	1	17
Ultra-XT, 1.4 oz	150	1	20
Now, Soy, ¼ cup, 0.78 oz	90	4	5
Revival Soy Shakes: *Per Packet*			
Plain, Unsweetened	100	1.5	2
Vanilla Pleasure	220	2	31
Average other flavors	230	2	33
Whole Foods			
Choc.with Spirulina, 1 oz	110	0	11
Vanilla with Spirulina, 1 oz	100	0	11

Energy/Protein Drinks

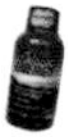
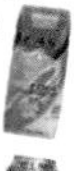
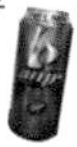
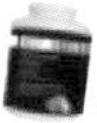

Item	C	F	Cb
5-hour Energy, 2 fl.oz	4	0	1
ABB:			
Anytime, Turbo Tea, 18 fl.oz	150	0	38
Energy: Adrenalyn Stack, 18 fl.oz	25	0	6
Ripped Force, 18 fl.oz	90	0	23
Hi-Pro: Pure Pro, Grape, 22 fl.oz	150	0.5	2
Pure Pro 50, 14.5 fl.oz	240	1.5	7
Recovery Blue Thunder, 22 fl.oz	290	0.5	40
Extreme XXL, 22 fl.oz	980	1	197
Mass Recovery, Grape, 18 fl.oz	380	0.5	60
Accelerade, all flav., 20 fl.oz	200	0	38
AdvantEdge (EAS):			
Carb Control, 11 fl.oz	110	3	4
AllSport, all flavors, 20 fl.oz	150	0	40
AMP: Energy Drink, 16 fl.oz	220	0	58
Overdrive, 16 fl.oz	220	0	58
Relaunch/Elevate, 16 fl.oz	220	0	58
Anytime Health:			
Performance Powder,			
Green Apple/Lemonade,			
2 scoops, 1 pkt, 1.73 oz	160	0	30
Whey Protein Isolate, all flavors, 1 oz	105	0	1
Arizona: All City, 16 fl.oz	200	0	56
Caution Energy, 8.3 fl.oz	120	0	30
Green Tea Energy, 16 fl.oz	200	0	32
Atkins: Advantage Shake, 11 oz can	155	9	3
Bally Total Fitness:			
Whey Pro, Vanilla, 1 scoop	115	1.5	3
Blast, Sugar Free, 8.3 oz	10	0	3
Bariatrix: Shakes, 1 serving	100	2	6
Proti 15 Drinks, average, 1 package	75	1	4
Ready-To-Serve, 1 box	120	4	4
Bawls Guarana, 10 fl.oz	120	0	32
Blue Sky:			
Blue Energy, 8.3 fl.oz	120	0	29
Blue Sport, 16 fl.oz	90	0	24
Body Fuel *(w. NutraSweet)*, 1 scoop	80	0	20
Bolthouse: *Per 15.2 fl.oz*			
Perfectly Protein:			
Mocha Cappuccino	340	5	55
Vanilla Chai Tea	305	6	48
Boost: High Protein, 8 fl.oz	240	6	33
Glucose Control, 8 fl.oz	190	7	16
Nutritional Energy, 8.25 fl.oz	245	9	33
Plus, 8 fl.oz	360	14	45
Kid Essentials, 8.25 fl.oz	245	9	33

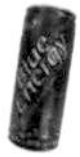
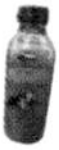
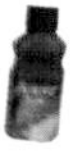

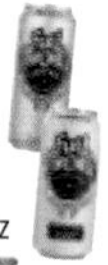
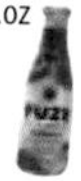
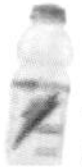
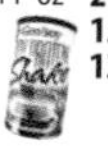

Item	C	F	Cb
Carnation Instant Breakfast			
Powder: All flav., 1 envelope, 1.3 oz	130	1	27
No Sugar Added, average, 0.7 oz	60	1	27
Ready-To-Drink, average, 11.5 fl.oz	260	5	41
Celebrity Juice Diet, 4 fl.oz	60	0	14
CeraSport, EX1, 8.45 fl.oz	20	0	5
Champion Lyte, Sports Drink	0	0	0
Champion Nutrition:			
Heavyweight Gainer 900, 4 scps, 5.4 oz	630	10	101
Ultramet: Original, 1 packet, 2.7 oz	280	2	24
Lite, 1 packet, 2 oz	190	1	17
Low Carb, 1 packet, 2 oz	230	6.5	6
Clif Shot Energy Gel, 1.1 oz packet	100	0	24
Cocaine Energy, 8.4 fl.oz can	70	0	18
Curves Protein Drink:			
Chocolate; Vanilla, 2 scoops, 1 oz	110	1.5	8
made with skim milk, 8 fl.oz	200	12	20
CytoSport Muscle Milk, 2 scoops	300	12	16
Designer Whey Protein, Van. Praline., 1 s.	100	2	3
Drank, Anti Energy, 8 fl.oz serve	110	0	27
EAS ~ *See AdvantEdge/Myoplex*			
Endura *(Unipro)*, 2 scoops, 1.3 oz	120	0	30
Ensure: High Protein, 8 oz	230	6	31
Immune Balance, 8 fl.oz	250	6	41
Plus, 8 fl.oz bottle	350	11	50
Enterex Glucose Control, 8 fl.oz	235	9	27
FRS Energy, Orange, 11.5 fl.oz	140	0	35
Fruit$_2$O *(Veryfine)*	0	0	0
Full Throttle			
Energy: Original, 16 fl.oz	220	0	57
Blue Demon/Fury, 16 fl.oz	225	0	58
Coffee & Energy:			
Caramel; Vanilla, 15 fl.oz	275	0	48
Mocha, 15 fl.oz	295	0	54
Hydration + Energy, 16 fl.oz	140	0	35
Fuze: Slenderize, 8 fl.oz	10	0	2
Refresh, 8 fl.oz	95	0	25
Vitalize, 8 fl.oz	100	0	25
Gatorade			
Thirst Quencher:			
(Lemon/Lime, AM, Fierce, Rain)			
1 Cup, 8 fl.oz	50	0	14
12 fl.oz Bottle	75	0	20
20 fl.oz Bottle	125	0	32
32 fl.oz Bottle	200	0	52
Carbohydrate Energy, 12 fl.oz bottle	320	0	79
Endurance (Powder), made up, 8 fl.oz	50	0	14
G2 (Low Calorie), 1 cup, 8 fl.oz	25	0	7
20 fl.oz bottle	70	0	17
Nutrition Shake, all flavors, 11 oz	360	8	54
Protein Recovery Shake, 11 oz	270	1.5	45
Genisoy: Ultra XT, 3 Tbsp	150	1	20
Protein Powder, 3 Tbsp	130	1.5	5

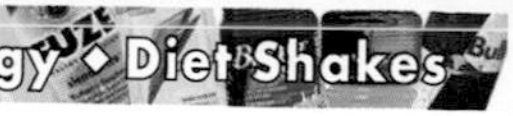

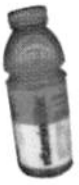
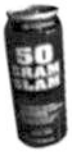

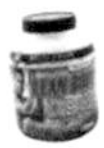
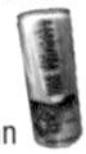

	C	F	Cb
Glaceau:			
Smartwater	0	0	0
Vitaminenergy, 16 oz can	100	0	26
Vitaminwater, 20 fl.oz	125	0	31
Glucerna, Shakes, 8 fl.oz	200	7	27
GNC Lean Shake, 2 scoops	180	2	30
Pro Performance:			
24 Hour Pro Complex, 1.4 oz	150	5	7
100% Whey Protein, 1 oz	120	1.5	5
50 Gram Slam, Van., 15 fl.oz	240	1	8
Mass XXX, Strawb., 7 oz	750	5	126
Weight Gainer 2200 Gold, Choc., 17 oz	1840	30	402
Wheybolic Extreme 60, Van., 2.9 oz	280	1	7
GU Energy Gel, average, 1 packet	100	0	25
Guru Energy: Regular, 8.3 oz can	100	0	25
Lite, 8.3 oz can	10	0	2
Hammer Gel, av. all flavors, 2 T., 1¼ oz	90	0	23
Hansen's: Energy Pro	120	0	32
Rumba, 8 fl.oz	120	0	28
Herbalife: Shapeworks Mix, 1 pkt	70	0	3
with 8 fl.oz non-fat milk	160	1	16
HMR, 70 Plus, 1 package	110	0.5	13
Hollywood Miracle Diet, ½ cup	100	0	25
Jarrow: Whey Protein, av., 1 scoop	100	1	5
Berry High, 1 scoop, 0.2 oz	25	0	5
Muscle Optimeal, 2 scoops, 1.65 oz	180	2	18
Java Monster Energy: *Per 15 fl.oz Can*			
Lo-Ball	95	3	10
Loca Moca; Mean Bean	190	0	48
Original/Irish/Nut-Up/Russian	190	3	34
Jolt: Cola, 16 fl.oz can	200	0	52
Blue Raspberry, 16 fl.oz	240	0	60
Jones, Energy, 16 fl.oz	260	0	64
Knudsen: ReCharge, 8 fl.oz	70	0	18
Simply Nutritious, average, 8 fl.oz	130	0	30
Kombucha, Wonder Drink, 8.5 fl.oz	60	0	16
La Brada			
Drink: Lean Body, RTD, 17 fl.oz	260	9	9
Powders: Lean Body, 2.8 oz	330	8	24
Lean Body Mass 60, 6 oz	615	7	76
Breakfast, 3.25 oz	360	7	35
Carb Watchers, 2.3 oz	250	4.5	12
Lipovitan B3, 8.6 fl.oz	130	0	30
Liquid Ice: 8.3 fl.oz	130	0	29
Sugar Free, 8.3 fl oz	15	0	0
Liquid Lightening, Reg., 8.4 fl.oz	105	0	22
Max Velocity: Reg., 8.45 fl.oz can	130	0	33
16 fl.oz can	240	0	62
Sugar Free: 16 fl.oz can	15	0	1
Met-Rx:			
Colossal RTD 15Z, 15 fl.oz can	380	14	28
Meal Replacement, 1 pkt, average	250	2	21
Protein Plus, Choc., 2 scoops	220	1.5	7

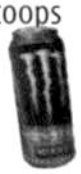
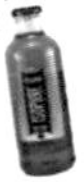
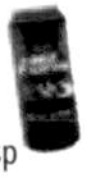
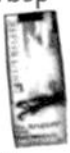
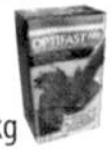

	C	F	Cb
Metabolol:			
Endurance, 2 scoop, 1.83 oz	200	5	24
GlyProXTS, 1 scoop, 0.21 oz	20	0	4
Met, 2 scoops, 2.33 oz	260	3	40
Met Max, mix, 2 scoops, 2.2 oz	230	2.5	11
MLO Mus-L Blast, Choc., 4 scoops	570	3.5	112
Monster Energy: 16 fl.oz can	200	0	54
Lo-Carb, 16 fl.oz can,	20	0	5
M-80, 8 fl.oz can	90	0	23
Mixxd (with Juice), 16 fl.oz	220	0	54
MRM: Low Carb Protein, 1 scoop	120	2.5	2
Iso-bolic, 1 scoop, 1 oz	115	1.5	2
Metabolic Whey, 1 scoop, 1 oz	115	2	2
Muscle Milk *(Cytosport)*: *Per 14 fl.oz Bottle*			
Ready to Drink: Chocolate	240	9	14
Lite	170	4.5	12
Average other flavors	225	9	11
Tetra: Chocolate, 11 fl.oz	230	11	11
17 fl.oz	340	16	17
Muscle Tech: Meso-Tech Comp. 1 pkt	275	3	31
Mass Tech Weight Gain, 5 scoops	870	4	168
Nitro Tech Hard Core, RTD, 15 fl.oz	195	1	6
Myoplex: Original Shake, 17 fl.oz	300	7	20
Carb Control, 11 fl.oz	150	3.5	5
Deluxe Powder, 1 packet, 3.4 oz	330	3	29
Lite, 11 fl.oz	170	2	20
Powder: Deluxe, 1 packet, 3.4 oz	330	3	29
Lite, 1 packet, average, 1.9 oz	180	2	24
Naturade:			
Powders: 100% Whey, Chocolate, 1 oz	110	1	11
100% Soy Protein Booster, 1 oz	110	1	0
Veg Protein Booster, 1 oz	110	1.5	0
Nature's Best:			
Isopure: Original, 20 fl.oz	260	0	25
Endurance, 20 fl.oz	320	0	60
Zero Carb, 20 fl.oz	160	0	0
Carbo Power, 16 fl.oz	400	0	100
Pro Smoothie, 15 fl.oz	240	1.5	17
No Fear: 16 fl.oz	260	0	72
Sugar Free, 16 fl.oz	20	0	2
Noni: Tahitian/Pacific, 2 Tbsp	10	0	3
Noni Juice, 1 fl.oz	10	0	3
Liquid Hawaiian/Tahiti, 1 Tbsp	30	0	8
Nutrament *(Nestle)*, 12 fl.oz	360	10	52
Nutri•15•Fast, 8 fl.oz pkg	160	3	19
Nutrilite			
Protein Shakes, 11.5 fl.oz	170	6	6
Sports Drinks, Regular, 16 fl.oz	120	0	28
Whey Protein, Chocolate, 1.27 oz pkg	130	2	5
Odwalla Serious Energy, 15.2 fl.oz	305	0	74
Optifast 800:			
Ready To Drink Shakes, 8 oz	160	3	20
Powder 800 Formula, 1 pkg	160	3	20
High Protein Powder, 1 pkg	200	6	10

Updated Nutrition Data ~ www.CalorieKing.com
Persons with Diabetes ~ See Disclaimer (Page 24)

Energy/Protein Drinks (Cont)

	C	F	Cb
Optimum Nutr.: 100% Whey, 1 oz	120	1	3
100% Oats & Whey, 1 scoop, 1.85 oz	200	1.5	22
100% Soy Protein, 1.1 oz Scoop	120	1.5	1
Piranha Energy *(EAS)*, 8.4 oz	140	0	35
PowerAde			
Regular: 12 fl.oz bottle	85	0	23
20 fl.oz bottle	160	0	30
PowerAde Zero	5	0	0
PowerBar			
Endurance, 1 scoop, 0.7 oz	70	0	17
Power Gel, average, 1.5 oz package	115	0	27
Pro-Cal 100 *(R-Kane)*, 1 pkt	100	1.5	7
Propel Fitness Water,			
all flavors, 23.7 oz bottle	30	0	6
Red Bull Energy, 8.3 fl.oz	110	0	27
12 fl.oz can	160	0	40
Sugar-Free, 8.3 fl.oz	10	0	3
Redline Energy, 8 fl.oz	0	0	0
Resource *(Nestle)*: Breeze, 8 fl.oz	250	0	54
Diabetishield, 8 fl.oz	150	0	30
Health Shake: 4 fl.oz	200	4	35
No Added Sugar, 4 oz	200	9	22
Shake Plus, 8 fl.oz	480	16	69
Shake, Thickened, 6 fl.oz	270	6	45
Revenge: Sport (Champ. Nutr.), 0.9 oz	90	0	23
Pro-Score 100, Chocolate, 1.4 oz	150	2	3
Revival Soy Mix: Plain Soy, 1 pkg	100	1.5	2
Chocolate Day Dream, 1 package	240	2.5	36
Other varieties, average, 1 package	225	2	33
Rhino's Energy Drink, 100ml	50	0	11
Rip It Energy Fuel, Citrus X, 16 fl.oz	260	0	66
Rockstar:			
Energy Drink: 16 fl.oz	280	0	62
Sugar Free, 16 fl.oz	20	0	0
Punched, 16 fl.oz	260	0	62
Rush Energy: Regular, 8 fl.oz	140	0	31
Lite, 8 fl.oz	0	0	0
Sav-on Nut'l: Plus, 8 oz	350	11	50
Equaline Advance, 8 oz	250	6	40
High Protein, 8 oz	230	6	31
Slim-Fast Shake (Ready To Drink):			
Original, 11 fl.oz	220	3	40
High Protein, 11 fl.oz	190	5	24
Easy To Digest, 11 fl.oz	180	5	25
Optima, 11 fl.oz	185	6	24
Low Carb Diet, average, 11 fl.oz	185	9	6
Powder Shake Mix: Average, 0.9 oz	110	3	18
with 8 fl.oz fat-free milk	200	5	30

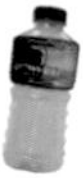
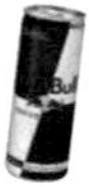
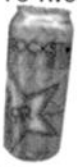
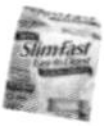

	C	F	Cb
Snapple: Antioxidant Water			
Average all flavors, 20 fl.oz bottle	125	0	31
SoBe: *Per Can/Bottle*			
Adrenaline Rush, 16 fl.oz	260	0	68
Elixir: *Per 20 fl.oz*			
Cranberry Grapefruit	250	0	65
Orange-Carrot	225	0	58
Yumberry Pomegranate	250	0	65
Energy: 20 fl.oz	270	0	67
Lean, all flavors, 20 fl.oz	15	0	2
Life Water: All flavors, 20 fl.oz	100	0	42
0-Cal, all flavours	0	0	6
Lizard Fuel, 20 fl.oz	300	0	75
Power, 20 fl.oz	250	0	63
Tsunami, 20 fl.oz	250	0	63
Sparks (Alcoholic) ~ *Page 29*			
Spiru-Tein: Powder, average, 1.2 oz	100	0	10
Starbucks:			
Doubleshot Energy & Coffee, 15 fl.oz	205	3	34
Steaz: Energy, 12 fl.oz	130	0	34
Diet Berry Energy, 12 fl.oz	60	0	14
The Sports Club/LA, PTS Protein Powder,			
Choc; Mocha; Van., 2 scoops, 1.4 oz	130	4	7
Trader Joe's: Energy, 8 fl.oz can	130	0	33
Enhanced Water, 33.8 fl.oz	0	0	0
Twin Lab:			
Energy Fuel, 250ml can	0	0	0
Ultra Fuel Powder, 4 scoops	400	0	100
Vault: Citrus; Red, 20 fl.oz	290	0	78
Vault Zero, 8 fl.oz	0	0	0
Venom Energy: Average, 16 fl.oz	250	0	58
Low Carb, 16 fl.oz	50	0	8
Verve Energy, 8.3 fl.oz can	70	0	18
Sugar Free	5	0	1
Vitamin Water ~ *See Glaceau*			
Weider (Powders)			
Creatine ATP, ½ cup, 1.7 oz	210	0	37
Mega Mass 4000, 1½ cups, average	570	3.5	105
Muscle Builder, 1½ oz	170	1	22
Pure Pro Shake: Chocolate, 11.5 fl.oz	170	0.5	7
Vanilla, 11.5 fl.oz	160	0	6
Ultra Whey Pro, ⅓ cup, 1 oz	115	1.5	6
Weight Gainer, 4 scoops, 3.4 oz	380	2	71
Worldwide: Carbo Rush, 20 fl.oz	265	0	68
Pure Protein Shakes:			
21g Protein, 11 fl.oz	110	1	5
35g Protein, 11 fl.oz	160	1	2
XS *(Quixtar)*, Energy Drink, 8.4 oz	10	0	1
Zico, Coconut Water, all flavors, 11 fl.oz	60	0	15
Zola Acai: Orig. Juice, 93%, 12 fl.oz	185	2	44
Energy Smoothie, 12 fl.oz	185	1.5	42
Wellness Shot, 1 fl.oz	20	1	4

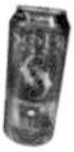
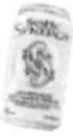
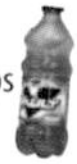
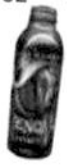

Quick Guide

Cola Drinks

Average All Brands

Includes *Coca-Cola* and *Pepsi*

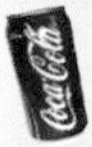
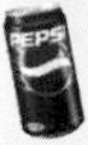

	C	F	Cb
8 fl.oz Cup/Can	100	0	26
12 fl.oz Can	150	0	39
16 fl.oz Bottle	200	0	52
20 fl.oz Bottle	250	0	65
24 fl.oz (Pepsi)	300	0	84
1-Liter Bottle (34 fl.oz)	400	0	100
2-Liter Bottle (68 fl.oz)	800	0	200

Other Soda Drinks *(Average All Brands)*

	C	F	Cb
Club Soda, 12 fl.oz	0	0	0
Cream Soda, 12 fl.oz	190	0	48
Diet/Low Cal Drinks, 12 fl.oz	5	0	1
Ginger Ale, 12 fl.oz	125	0	31
Lemon Lime, 12 fl.oz	150	0	37
Orange, 12 fl.oz	180	0	45
Pink Lemonade, 12 fl.oz	180	0	45
Root Beer, 12 fl.oz	150	0	39
Tonic Water, 12 fl.oz	125	0	2
Mineral Water: Plain, 12 fl.oz	0	0	0
Sweetened/flavored, 12 fl.oz	150	0	37
w. Fruit Juice, 12 fl.oz	120	0	30
Soda Water/Seltzer: Plain/Diet	0	0	0
Sweetened/flavored, 12 fl.oz	155	0	39
w. Fruit Juice, 12 fl.oz	160	0	40
Soft Frozen Lemonade, 12 fl.oz	300	0	75

Fountain, Movie Theater & Take-Out

Average All Flavors

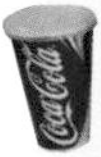

	C	F	Cb
Small Cup, 12 fl.oz: No Ice	160	0	40
With ⅓ Ice	120	0	30
Regular, 16 fl.oz: No Ice	215	0	53
With ⅓ Ice	160	0	40
Medium, 22 fl.oz: No Ice	295	0	73
With ⅓ Ice	220	0	55
Large, 32 fl.oz: No Ice	430	0	105
With ⅓ Ice	320	0	80

(Note: ⅓ Cup of Ice = ¼ Cup Liquid)

Soft Drinks Brands

Per 12 fl.oz Unless Indicated

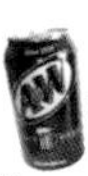

	C	F	Cb
A&W:			
Float, 11.5 fl.oz bottle	230	1.5	55
Root Beer	180	0	48
Diet Cream Soda/Root Beer	0	0	0
Albertson's:			
Super Chill: Cola	165	0	44
Root Beet	180	0	48

Updated Nutrition Data ~ www.CalorieKing.com
Persons with Diabetes ~ See Disclaimer (Page 24)

Soft Drink Brands (Cont)

Per 12 fl.oz Unless Indicated

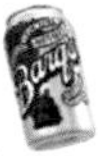
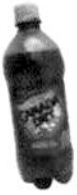
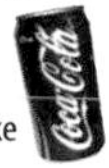
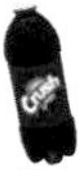
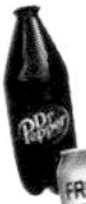
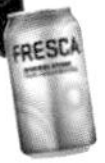
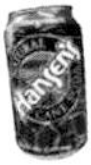

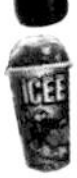

	C	F	Cb
Barq's: Root Beer	165	0	45
Floatz	190	0	51
Big Red, 12 fl.oz	150	0	38
Blue Sky: Cola; Orange Creme	160	0	43
Black Cherry	140	0	37
Grape; Lemon Lime, average	130	0	36
Raspberry; Root Beer, average	165	0	44
Bubble Up, 12 fl.oz	160	0	42
Cactus Cooler, 12 fl.oz	150	0	40
Canada Dry: Club Soda	0	0	0
Ginger Ale	135	0	38
Tonic Water	135	0	36
Capri Sun:			
Sport, all flavors, 6.75 fl.oz	60	0	16
Coca-Cola: *Per 12 fl.oz*			
Classic/Caffeine Free	145	0	41
Diet Coke, all flavors	0	0	0
Cherry Coke/Vanilla Coke	155	0	42
Coca-Cola Zero	0	0	0
Country Time, Lemonade, 12 fl.oz	135	0	36
Crush:			
Orange/Grape: 12 fl.oz	195	0	53
20 fl.oz bottle	320	0	86
Strawberry, 20 fl.oz	290	0	77
Diet Orange, 20 fl.oz	35	0	10
Dad's: Orange Cream Soda, 12 fl.oz	180	0	46
Root Beer, 12 fl.oz	165	0	41
Diet Rite, Pure Zero	0	0	0
Dr Pepper: Regular	150	0	40
Cherry Vanilla	150	0	39
Diet, all flavors	0	0	0
Fanta, all flavors	175	0	48
Fresca: Orig. Citrus	0	0	0
Blackcherry Citrus	0	0	0
Peach Citrus	0	0	0
GuS, average all flavors	95	0	23
Hansen's: Diet Soda	0	0	0
Natural Cane Sugar:			
Creamy Root Beer	160	0	43
Pomegranate	130	0	35
Hawaiian Punch, Fruit Juicy Red	180	0	45
Henry Weinhard's: Root Beer	170	0	43
Cream flavor, average	175	0	42
Hires, Root Beer	170	0	45
IBC: Root Beer	160	0	43
Cherry Limeade	170	0	44
Cream Soda; Black Cherry	180	0	48
Icee: Coca-Cola; Barq's	100	0	27
Minute Maid: Fruit Punch	175	0	48
Lemonade	100	0	25

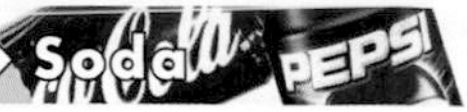

Per 12 fl.oz Unless Indicated	C	F	Cb
Jolt Cola, 16 fl.oz	200	0	52
Cherry Cola, 16 fl.oz	180	0	46
Grape, Orange, 16 fl.oz	210	0	52
Ultra Citrus, 16 fl.oz	10	0	0
Jones Soda: Cola	160	0	40
Whoopass, 16 fl.oz	200	0	52
Other flavors, average	185	0	46
Mello Yello, Regular	175	0	48
Minute Maid: Fruit Punch	160	0	44
Lemonade Regular/Pink			
12 fl.oz can/bottle	150	0	42
20 fl.oz Bottle	275	0	70
Orangeade	160	0	43
Mountain Dew:			
Live Wire; Code Red	180	0	47
Diet flavors	0	0	0
Mug Root Beer	160	0	43
Natural Brew: Draft Root Beer	180	0	44
Ginseng Cola; Outrageous Ginger Ale	170	0	42
Vanilla, Cream	170	0	42
Nehi, Royal Crown Peach	190	0	51
Orangina: 10 fl.oz bottle	120	0	32
Pepsi: Regular/Blue/Caffeine Free	150	0	42
Diet Pepsi; Jazz	0	0	0
One, 12 fl.oz	0	0	0
Wild Cherry; Vanilla	150	0	42
Perrier, Carbonated Water	0	0	0
Pibb, Xtra	145	0	39
RC Cola, Regular	160	0	43
Reed's, Ginger Brew,			
average all varieties	145	0	38
7•UP: Regular	150	0	39
Cherry	150	0	39
Diet varieties, 12 fl.oz	0	0	0
7•UP Plus, 12 fl.oz	15	0	3
Safeway/Vons: Go 2 Cola	160	0	44
Cherry Cola	160	0	43
Ditto Lemon Lime	160	0	40
Parker's Cream Soda	170	0	42
Parker's Root Beer	180	0	47
Santa Cruz, Sparkling, average	135	0	32
Schweppes: Seltzer	0	0	0
Tonic Water; Ginger Ale, average	130	0	35
Shasta: Cream Soda	190	0	47
Cherry Cola	180	0	45
Dr. Shasta	150	0	38
Club Soda; Diet, all flavors	0	0	0
Tiki Punch; Pineapple; Or.	200	0	50
Ginger Ale	130	0	33
Other flavors, average	170	0	41

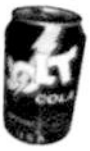
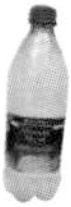
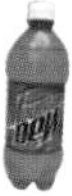
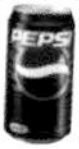
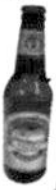

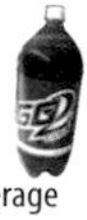

Per 12 fl.oz Unless Indicated	C	F	Cb
Sierra Mist, Lemon Lime	150	0	39
Sprite: Regular	145	0	40
Zero	5	0	0
Squirt, Citrus Burst	150	0	40
Stewarts: Root Beer	160	0	40
Grape; Orange 'n Cream	190	0	48
Sun Drop: Regular, 20 fl.oz bottle	325	0	81
Cherry Lemon, 20 fl.oz bottle	300	0	78
Sunkist: Orange	190	0	52
Diet Sunkist	0	0	0
Sunkist Float, 12 fl.oz	260	1.5	64
TAB, 12 fl.oz	0	0	0
Thomas Kemper: Root Beer	160	0	41
Other flavors, average	160	0	40
Trader Joe's:			
Sparkling:			
French Berry Lemonade,			
1 cup, 8 fl.oz	130	0	31
1 Bottle, 33.8 fl.oz	520	0	124
Lime Ade, 1 cup, 8 fl.oz	110	0	28
1 Bottle, 33.8 fl.oz	440	0	108
Pink Lemonade, 8 fl.oz	130	0	31
1 Bottle, 33.8 fl.oz	520	0	124
Mojito: 8 fl.oz	110	0	26
25.4 fl.oz bottle	340	10	80
Refreshers, Blueberry	150	0	37
Vernor's, Ginger Soda	150	0	39
Virgil's Root Beer	160	0	42
Walgreens:			
Orchard Grape Soda, 20 fl.oz	300	0	84
Cola; Lemon Lime, 20 fl.oz	225	0	65
Root Beer, 20 fl.oz	225	0	75
Welch's: Soda, 12 fl.oz	190	0	51
Sparkling Juice Cocktail	320	0	80
365 Organic *(Whole Foods)*:			
Spritzers, all flavors	110	0	28

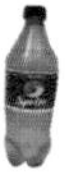
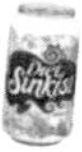
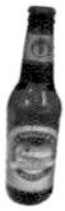

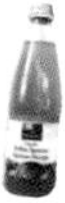

Powdered Soft Drink Mix

Per 8 fl.oz Prepared, Unless Otherwise Stated	C	F	Cb
Capri Sun, Sport, 6.75 fl.oz	60	0	16
Cool Splashers, 8 fl.oz	60	0	16
Country Time: Lemonade	60	0	16
Other flavors, average	80	0	19
Lite	35	0	8
Crystal Light, 8 fl.oz	5	0	0
Flavor Aid, ⅛ package	0	0	0
Kool-Aid: All flavors	60	0	16
Unsweetened, 6 fl.oz	0	0	0
Propel, ½ package	10	0	3
Tang, Regular, 2 Tbsp, 0.9oz	105	0	28

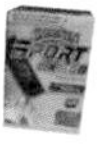
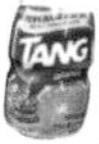

Quick Guide

Teas	C	F	Cb
Regular: Bag, Loose or Instant			
Brewed, 1 cup, 8 fl.oz	2	0	0.5
(Add extra for sugar/milk)			
Herbal: Average all varieties, 1 cup	2	0	0
Bigelow, *all flavors*	0	0	0
Celestial Seasonings:			
All flavors	0	0	0
Bubble Tea, average, 12 fl.oz	175	0	41
Chai Tea: *Cafe D' Vita,* 2 Tbsp	120	3.5	21
Starbucks: *See Fast-Foods Section*			

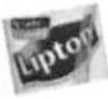

Iced Tea	C	F	Cb
Average All Brands			
Sweetened: 8 fl.oz	100	0	25
12 fl.oz	150	0	38
16 fl.oz	200	0	50
Unsweetened: 8 fl.oz	2	0	0

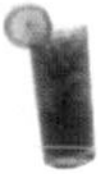

Iced Tea Mixes

Per 8 fl.oz Made-Up

	C	F	Cb
4C Iced Teas:			
Sweetened, average all flavors	70	0	18
Totally Light, all flavors	0	0	0
Crystal Light Sugar Free	5	0	0
Lipton: Instant, unsweetened	0	0	0
Instant Raspberry	80	0	19
Lemon	70	0	18
Peach; Raspberry, Sugar Free	5	0	1
Iced Tea To Go	0	0	0
Nestea			
Lemonade Tea, 1⅓ Tbsp	60	0	15
Lemon flavored Iced Tea, 1⅓ Tbsp	60	0	15
Sugar Free Lemon Iced Tea, 2 tsp	5	0	2
Unsweetened Tea, 2 tsp	0	0	0

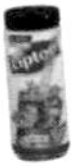

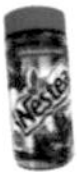

Bottled & Canned Teas

	C	F	Cb
Arizona: *Per 8 fl.oz*			
Black with Ginseng	60	0	15
Green Tea(s)/Asian Plum	70	0	18
Diet Green Tea (with Sorbitol)	5	0	2
Extra Sweet Tea	90	0	23
Peach/Raspberry	70	0	18
24 fl.oz Cans, average all flavors	210	0	54
Fuze, all flavors, 16 fl.oz	120	0	30
Gold Peak, Lem. ,16.9 fl.oz bottle	170	0	44
Hansen's: Green Tea: Reg., 16 fl.oz	120	0	30
Peach; Pomegranae, 16 fl.oz	180	0	44

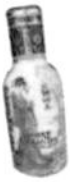

Updated Nutrition Data ~ www.CalorieKing.com
Persons with Diabetes ~ See Disclaimer (Page 24)

Bottled & Canned Teas (Cont)

	C	F	Cb
Honest Tea: *Per 16.9 fl.oz*			
Black Forest Berry/Peach/Lori's Lemon	65	0	17
Lipton Brisk			
Av. all flavors, 12 fl.oz can	130	0	33
20 fl.oz bottle	215	0	55
Lipton Iced Tea			
Lemon; White w/Raspb., 16.9 fl.oz	120	0	32
Green Tea with Citrus:			
16.9 fl.oz bottle	170	0	44
20 fl.oz bottle	200	0	53
Diet, all flavors	0	0	0
Sparkling, average all flavors, 16 fl.oz	120	0	32
Nantucket, Lemon Tea 17.5 fl.oz	175	0	48
Nestea Iced Tea			
Lemon Sweetened: 8 fl.oz	90	0	23
16.9 oz Bottle	180	0	45
20 fl.oz Bottle	210	0	52
Diet Green/Lemon	0	0	0
Minute Maid,			
Pomegranate Tea, 8 fl.oz	40	0	9
Pom Pomegranate:			
Pomegranate Tea, 16 fl.oz	140	0	34
Pomegranate Lychee, 16 fl.oz	140	0	36
Pomegranate Peach Passion, 16 fl.oz	160	0	38
Light flavors, average, 16 fl.oz	70	0	34

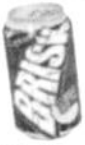

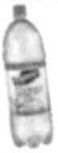

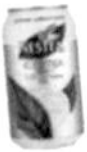

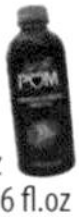

Note: Carbs figure for Light flavors includes Erythritol natural sweetener which has negligible calories.

	C	F	Cb
Sbarro, 16 fl.oz Bottle	180	0	48
Shasta, Lemon, 16 fl.oz	140	0	35
Snapple: Iced Tea Blends, all flav., 16 fl.oz	200	0	50
Black Teas, average, 17.5 fl.oz	75	0	19
Diet/Unsweetened Teas	0	0	0
Green; White, 17.5 fl.oz	130	0	32
Red Tea, 17.5 fl.oz	80	0	14
SoBe: Green, 20 fl.oz	240	0	61
Ssips, Lemon Iced, 6¾ fl.oz	80	0	21
Steaz: Peach/Mint, 16 fl.oz	80	0	20
Sparkling Organic, 16 fl.oz	135	0	35
TeaZazz: Original, 20 fl.oz	50	0	12
Green Tea Lemon, 20 fl.oz	60	0	15
Peach Tea, 20 fl.oz	50	0	12
Trader Joe's: *Per 8 fl.oz*			
Organic Tea & Lemonade	100	0	25
Pomegranate Green Tea	60	0	15
Unsweetened *(Kettle/Green)*	0	0	0
Turkey Hill: Iced Tea, 16 fl.oz	180	0	42
Fruit flavors, average, 16 fl.oz	205	0	50
365 Organic *(Whole Foods):*			
Berry Black Tea, 16 fl.oz	60	0	14
Lemon Green Tea, 16 fl.oz	40	0	10
White Jasmine Tea, 16 fl.oz	30	0	8

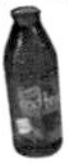

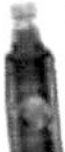

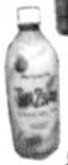

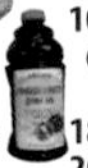

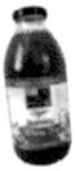

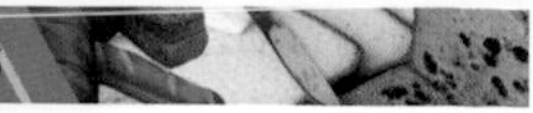

B Bread & Bread Products

Note: Most breads have similar calories on a weight basis. However, volume may vary.

For example, 1 oz of bread may equal 1 slice regular bread or 2 slices of a lighter bread.

It is best to weigh bread used and calculate using: 1 oz bread = 70 calories, 14g carb.

Quick Guide

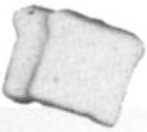

Bread	C	F	Cb
White or Wheat ~ *Average Per Slice*			
Thin or Light, ¾ oz	50	0.5	10
Sandwich slice, 1 oz	70	1	14
Thick or Large slice, 1½ oz	105	1.5	21
Thick/Home-made, 2 oz	140	2	28
Extra Thick/Home-made, 3 oz	210	3	42
Whole Loaf: 16 oz	1120	16	224
24 oz Loaf	1680	24	336
With Seeds or Nuts:			
Sandwich slice, 1½ oz	130	5	18
Thick slice/Home-made, 2½ oz	215	8	30
Toast ~ **Has same calories as bread used**			
1 Slice (1 oz fresh)			
with 2 tsp regular spread	140	9	12
with 2 tsp "light" spread	105	5	12
with 1 Tbsp regular spread	170	12	12
with 1 Tbsp "light" spread	120	7	12

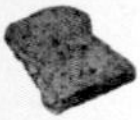

Breads

Per Slice Unless Indicated	C	F	Cb
12-Grain, 1½ oz	110	1.5	22
Batard (8 oz), thick slice, 2 oz	150	0.5	28
Bran style/Dark, 1 oz	70	1	14
Bread with Soy Isoflavones, 1.2 oz	80	2.5	13
Buttermilk, average, 1½ oz	110	1	22
Caraway Rye, 2 oz	150	2	28
Challah, ¾ oz	85	1.5	17
Chapati, 1 oz	110	3	18
Ciabatta, 2 oz	130	1	26
Cornbread, average, 3 oz	220	6	37
Cracked Wheat Sourdough, 1½ oz	130	0.5	27
Croissants: *See Page 113, 173*			
Crustless Bread, regular slice, ¾ oz	40	0.5	8.5
Crusts Only, regular slice, ¼ oz	30	0	7
English Toasting, 2 oz	140	1.5	27
'Enriched' Breads, average, 1 oz	60	1	12
Flax & Grain, 1½ oz	120	3	19
Flax & Sunflower Round, 1.2 oz	90	2	18

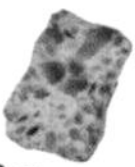

Breads (Cont)

Per Slice Unless Indicated	C	F	Cb
Foccacia: Plain, 2 oz portion	150	2.5	28
Cheese & Garlic; Pesto, 2 oz	160	6	21
Tomato & Olive, 2 oz	150	5	21
French Stick/Baguette, 1 oz	70	1	15
French Toast, 1.6 oz	140	2	26
Sticks *(Aunt Jemima)*,1 oz	90	2	17
Garlic Bread/Toast:			
Small slice + 1 tsp spread, ¾ oz	80	5	7
Med. slice + 2 tsp spread, 1½ oz	160	10	14
Thick slice + 3 tsp spread, 1.8 oz	220	14	20
Pepperidge Farm, 1 slice, 1.4 oz	160	10	15
Hemp Bread, 1.2 oz	95	2	12
Italian Bread, 2 oz	140	1	28
Light Bread, averaage, 0.8 oz	40	0.5	8
Lower Carb (higher Protein/fiber),			
average all brands, 1 oz	60	1.5	9
MultiGrain, 1.5 oz	100	2	21
Nut/Health Nut, 1.35 oz	90	1.5	18
Oatmeal/Oatbran Bread, 1½ oz	90	0.5	19
Pita: Average all types,			
Small (4" diam) 1.1 oz	90	0	18
Large (6½" diam) 2 oz	140	1.5	27
Extra Large (9" diam) 4 oz	300	1.5	60
Popovers (1), no butter	130	2	18
Poppyseed (Vienna), 0.8 oz	55	1	10
Pumpernickel: Large slice, 1.35 oz	80	0	15
Cocktail/Party size	30	0.5	6
Raisin Bread, 1 oz	80	1	15
Raisin Walnut, 1 oz	70	0.5	15
Roman Meal, 1.1 oz	80	1	15
Rye: Average, 1 thin slice, 1 oz	80	1	14
1 thick slice, 2 oz	150	2	25
Cocktail size, 0.4 oz	25	0.5	4
Sandwich Bread, 1 oz	70	1	12
Sandwich Pockets, 2 oz	140	1.5	27
Sourdough, 1½ oz	120	1	25
Sourdough French, 1 oz	75	0	14
Spelt, 1.6 oz	130	1	26
Sprouted 7-Grain, 1.5 oz	110	0.5	18
Squaw, 1.1 oz	85	0.5	13
Sweet Hawaiian Bread, 1.3 oz	110	2	19
Tacos/Tortillas: *See Page 179*			
Turkish/Middle Eastern, 1 oz	80	1.5	16
Wheat-Free Breads: Spelt, 1.6 oz	130	1	26
Brown Rice with Fruit Juice, 1.5 oz	110	2	21
Healthseed Rye, 1.6 oz	90	1	20
Millet, 1.5 oz	100	1	20
Whole Wheat: Thin, 1 oz	70	1	14
Thick, 1.7 oz	130	2	23

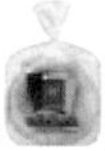

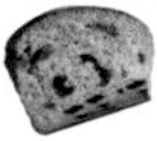

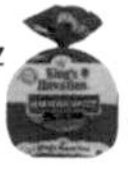

Bread Brands

Per Slice Unless Indicated

Item	C	F	Cb
Ener-G: Gluten-Free Breads			
Brown Rice Bread, 1.3 oz	130	6	18
Light Brown Rice, ¾ oz	50	2	7
Corn Loaf, ¾ oz	40	1.5	8
Light Tapioca, ¾ oz	45	1.5	7
Ezekiel: Low Sodium, 1.2 oz	80	0.5	15
Sesame ,1.2 oz	80	0.5	14
Francisco International			
Sesame French, 1.6 oz	120	1	23
Sourdough, 1¾ oz	110	0	22
Nature's Path:			
Manna: Carrot Raisin; Millet Rice	130	0	27
Cinnamon Date	150	0	29
Fruit & Nut	140	1	27
Sun Seed	160	2	29
Whole Rye	150	0	32
Oroweat:			
100% Whole Wheat, 1.35 oz	90	1	18
9 Grain DHA, 1.35 oz	90	1	17
Country Buttermilk, 1.35 oz	100	1	19
Health Nut, 1.35 oz	100	2	18
Pepperidge Farm: Deli Flats, av.	100	1	19
100% Whole Wheat, Very Thin	110	2	20
15 Grain, Small Slice	70	1.5	13
Farmhouse Soft Hearty White	120	1.5	22
Light Style, average	130	1	26
Frozen Breads, Garlic Bread:			
Crusty Slice, 2.5"	180	8	21
Premium Roasted	170	8	21
Texas Toast, average	145	7	18
Sara Lee:			
45 Calories & Delightful Wheat	45	0.5	9
Honey Wheat, 1 oz	80	1	14
Hearty & Delicious:			
100% Multigrain, 1.5 oz	120	1.5	21
Sunflower Seed, 1.5 oz	130	2	23
Soft & Smooth, 100% Whole Wheat, 1 oz	80	1	13
Schwan's, Frozen: *Per Serving*			
Cheese Stuffed Breadsticks w/ Sce, 2 oz	160	7	18
Five Cheese Garlic French Bread , 3.4 oz	330	20	26
French Baguette Bread, ¼ loaf, 1.7 oz	130	0	25
Southern Style Biscuits , 2.2 oz	190	9	23
Trader Joe's:			
Fat-Free Multi-Grain, 1.1 oz	70	0	15
Gourmet White, 1.5 oz	120	3.5	19
Seeded Harvest, 1 oz	65	1	12
Sprouted Rye, 1.2 oz	90	1	15
Wonder: Classic White Sandwich, 1 oz	70	1	14
Light Wheat, ¾ oz	40	0	9
Smartwhite, 1 slice, 0.92 oz	50	0.5	11

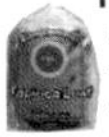
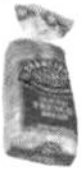
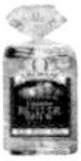
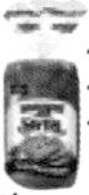
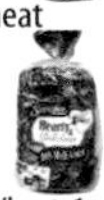
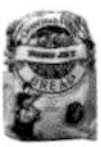

Biscuits, Bread Rolls & Buns

Item	C	F	Cb
6" Roll, Plain, average 2½ oz	200	1	38
Biscuits/Rolls: Average, 2½" diameter			
Commercially Baked	130	6	17
Prepard from Recipe	210	10	27
Refrigerated Dough, Baked	95	4	13
Brown 'n Serve, average, 1 oz	70	1	13
Ciabatta Roll, 3½ oz	230	4	41
Dinner Rolls:			
1 small, 1 oz	90	1.5	17
1 medium (3" diam),1½ oz	110	1	23
Frankfurter/Hot Dog: 1¼ oz	110	1.5	21
1½ oz size	130	2	25
French: 1 med, 1.3 oz	110	1.5	22
1 large, 3 oz	230	2.5	42
Hamburger: Regular, 1½ oz	110	1.5	22
Large, 3 oz	210	3	40
Hoagie/Submarine, Plain, 2⅓ oz	200	1	38
Kaiser Rolls:			
Small, 2 oz	200	2.5	35
Large, 3½ oz	350	4	61
Refrigerated Dough, Baked: *Pillsbury*			
Buttermilk Biscuit (3), 2.25 oz	150	2	29
Crescent Roll, Original, 1 oz	110	6	11
Grands! Flaky Layers Bisc., Original	180	8	25
Traditional Dinner Roll, 1.4 oz	100	1.5	20
Sourdough Roll, 1¼ oz	110	1	21
Wheat Rolls: Small, 1.2 oz	100	1	17
Medium, 1¾ oz	130	1.5	23
Large, 3½ oz	260	3	46

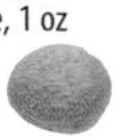
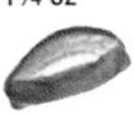
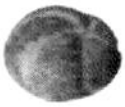
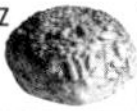

Breadsticks, Croutons

Item	C	F	Cb
Breadsticks: Salt Sticks, plain, 1 oz	110	1	20
Fresh baked (1), 2 oz	180	2.5	34
Stella D'oro: Sesame (1)	50	2	7
Original, 1 piece	45	1	7
Croutons: Seasoned, 2 Tbsp, ¼ oz	35	1.5	4
Zesty Italian (*Pepp. Farm*), 6 croutons	30	1	5

Bread Products

Item	C	F	Cb
Bread Crumbs, dry:			
Plain or seasoned, 1 oz	110	1.5	20
1 cup, 3½ oz	385	5	70
Corn Flake Crumbs, 1.1 oz	120	0	29
Graham Cracker Crumbs, 1 oz	110	2.5	20
Keebler, 3 Tbsp, ½ oz	70	1.5	13
Bread Dough: Frozen, 1 slice, 2 oz	140	2	26
Refrigerated, French, 1" slice	60	1	13
Wheat; White, 1" slice	80	2	14
Coating Mixes: Average, 2 Tbsp., 1 oz	100	0.5	20
Stuffing: Average, dry mix, 1 oz	110	1	10
Prepared, ½ cup, 4 oz	180	9	11

Updated Nutrition Data ~ www.CalorieKing.com
Persons with Diabetes ~ See Disclaimer (Page 24)

Quick Guide

Bagels

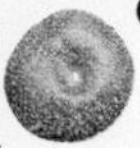

Average All Brands	C	F	Cb
Plain/Onion:			
1 mini/bagelette, 1 oz	**75**	0.5	15
1 small bagel, 2 oz	**145**	1	29
1 medium bagel, 3 oz	**230**	1.5	45
1 large bagel, 4 oz	**285**	2	56
Bagel Chips *(New York Style)*, 4 slices, ¾ oz	**100**	4.5	12
Pizza Bagel Bites, 4 pieces, 3.1 oz	**200**	6	29
Bagel Bites *(Ore-Ida)*, 4 pieces	**200**	6	29
Bagel Crisps *(New York Style)*, 7 pieces	**140**	6	17

Bagel Brands
~ Per Bagel

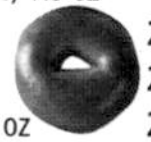

	C	F	Cb
Controlled Carb Gourmet			
High Fiber Bagel, average, 2 oz	**160**	5	22
Individual Wrapped, 2 oz	**80**	6	18
Zero Net Carbs, 2 oz	**120**	2	14
Costco Bakery: Plain, 4 oz	**300**	1	61
Everything, 4 oz	**330**	3.5	62
Enjoy Life, all types, 3.2 oz	**275**	6	50
Lenders: Original, plain, frozen, 2 oz	**140**	0.5	29
New York, plain, frozen, 3.3 oz	**230**	1	48
Premium, plain, refrigerated, 2.9 oz	**210**	1.5	43
Sara Lee: Mini, average, 1.3 oz	**100**	0.5	20
Plain	**270**	1.5	57
Blueberry, 3.7 oz	**290**	1.5	61
Cinnamon Raisin, 3.7 oz	**280**	1.5	60
Everything, 3.7 oz	**300**	4	55
Onion, 3 oz	**230**	1.5	50
Western, The Alternatives, av., 2 oz	**110**	0	25

Fast-Food Stores: *See Page 182*

Bagel Spreads

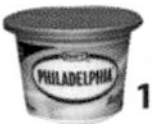

	C	F	Cb
Cream Cheese:			
Plain: 2 Tbsp, 1 oz	**80**	8	2
2 oz mini-tub	**160**	16	4
Reduced Fat: 2 Tbsp, 1 oz	**60**	5	2
2 oz mini-tub	**120**	10	4
Flavors: Lox, 1 oz	**75**	6	1
Raisin Walnut, 1 oz	**90**	6	8
Strawberry, 1 oz	**60**	3	7
Sundried Tomato, 1 oz	**80**	7	2
Vegetable, 1 oz	**60**	6	1

English Muffins

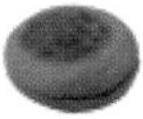

Average All Brands	C	F	Cb
Plain/Whole Wheat:			
Regular, 2 oz	**133**	1.5	26
Heavier, 2.5 oz	**155**	2	31
Super Size, 3.2 oz	**190**	2	38
Raisin-Cinnamon, 2.2 oz	**140**	1	29

Note: Actual weight of packaged muffins can be 10-15% heavier than stated net weight.

Rice Cakes

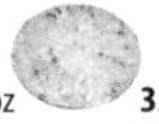

	C	F	Cb
Reg. size, av. 1 cake, 0.32 oz	**35**	0	7.5
Hain, Mini, plain, 10 pieces	**70**	2	12
Lundberg, all types, 0.65 oz	**70**	0.5	14
Quaker, Apple Cinnamon, 0.45 oz	**50**	0	11

Taco Shells & Tortillas

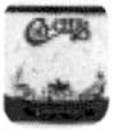

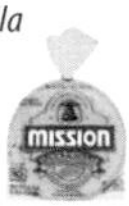

	C	F	Cb
Tacos: Mini Size (1)	**25**	1.5	2
Regular size, all types (1)	**50**	2	7
Large (1)	**90**	4	13
Salad Shell, flour *(Del Oro)*, 1.4 oz	**230**	17	10
Tortilla (Soft Taco), each	**85**	2	15
Corn Tortilla: 6", 1 oz	**55**	0.5	11
Flour Tortilla: 8", 1.75 oz	**145**	3	26
Low-Fat	**110**	1.5	22
Burritos, 1 tortilla, 2.3 oz	**190**	5	32
Low-Fat	**110**	1.5	22
Tostada Bowl (Rio Rancho), 6" 1.25 oz	**180**	9	22
Tostada Shells, (1)	**55**	3	6
La Tortilla Factory			
Fat Free Flour Tortillas:			
Burrito size, 2.5 oz	**120**	0.5	34
Soft Taco, 1.8 oz	**90**	0	24
Low-Fat Low Carb Tortillas:			
Large, 2.2 oz	**80**	3	19
Original; Flavors, 1.26 oz	**50**	2	11
Mission Foods			
Tortillas: *Per 1, 6" Tortilla*			
Carb Balance, 1.5 oz	**120**	3.5	18
Flour, med., 1.73 oz	**150**	3.5	25
Multi-Grain, 1.75 oz	**150**	4.5	23
White Corn, 1.15 oz	**70**	1	14
96% Fat-Free Burrito, 8", 1.75 oz	**130**	1.5	26

Crispbreads & Matzos ~ Page 90

Quick Guide

Cooked Cereals

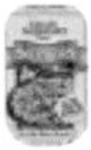
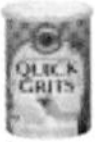

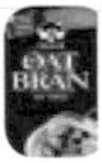

Cooked Cereals	C	F	Cb
Buckwheat Groats, roasted:			
Dry, ½ cup, 3 oz	**285**	2	61
Cooked, 1 cup, 6 oz	**155**	1	34
Bulgur: Dry, ½ cup, 2½ oz	**240**	1	53
Cooked, 1 cup, 6½ oz	**150**	0.5	34
Corn/Hominy Grits:			
Dry: ¼ cup, 1.4 oz	**145**	0.5	31
3 Tbsp, 1 oz	**110**	0.5	23
Cooked, ¾ cup, 6½ oz	**110**	0.5	23
Instant, 1 packet, dry, 0.8 oz	**75**	0	18
With Imitation Bacon Bits, 1 oz	**100**	0.5	22
Cream of Rice, cooked, ¾ cup, 6½ oz	**95**	0	21
Cream of Wheat:			
Regular, cooked, ¾ cup, 6½ oz	**100**	0.5	21
Quick, cooked, ¾ cup, 6½ oz	**95**	0.5	20
Instant, cooked, ¾ cup, 6½ oz	**110**	0.5	24
Farina: Cooked, ¾ cup, 6 oz	**85**	0	18
Millet, dry, ¼ cup, 1¾ oz	**190**	2	36
Oat Bran: Raw, ⅓ cup, 1 oz	**70**	2	19
Cooked, ½ cup, 3¾ oz	**45**	1	13
Oatmeal: Dry, ⅓ cup, 1 oz	**105**	1.5	18
Regular, cooked, ¾ cup, 6 oz	**110**	2	19
1 cup, 8 oz	**145**	2.5	25
Instant: Regular, dry, average, 1 oz	**105**	1.5	18
Flavored, dry, average, 1½ oz	**150**	2	32
Wheat Hearts, 1 oz dry, ¾ cup cooked	**110**	0.5	24

Brans, Wheat Germ, Add-Ons

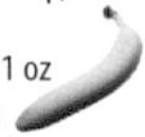

Brans, Wheat Germ, Add-Ons	C	F	Cb
Bran: Wheat, unprocessed,			
1 Tbsp, 0.10 oz	**5**	0	2
Rice Bran: Raw, 1 Tbsp, 0.18 oz	**15**	1	2.5
¼ cup, 1 oz	**95**	6	15
Oat Bran: Raw, 1 Tbsp, 0.18 oz	**10**	0.5	4
⅓ cup, 1 oz	**70**	2	19
Wheat Germ: Raw, 1 Tbsp, ¼ oz	**25**	0.5	4
¼ cup, 1 oz	**105**	3	15
Fruit: Dried, average, 1 oz	**70**	0	18
Banana, ½ medium	**55**	0	14
Prunes in Syrup (5), 3 oz	**90**	0	23
Honey, 1 Tbsp, ¾ oz	**65**	0	17
Lecithin Granules, 1 Tbsp, 0.35 oz	**55**	4	0.5
Nuts, Almonds (6), ¼ oz	**40**	4	1.5
Bee Pollen Granules, 1 Tbsp, 0.28 oz	**25**	1	2
Psyllium Husks, 1 Tbsp, 0.18 oz	**15**	0	4

Hot/Cooked Cereals ~ Brands

Per Serving, Dry Mix only	C	F	Cb
Albers Grits, ¼ cup, 1.4 oz	**140**	0.5	31
Bobs Red Mill,			
10 Grain, ¼ cup, 1.4 oz	**140**	1	28
Country Choice,			
Quick Oats, ½ cup, 1.4 oz	**150**	3.5	27
Dr McDougall's			
Big Cup Organic Oatmeal: *Per Cup*			
Grains: W/ Cranb. Muesli, 3.1 oz	**320**	4	*62*
With Peach Raspberry 3 oz	**300**	4	62
4 Grain with Real Maple, 2.55 oz	**260**	3	52
Organic Instant Oatmeal: *Per Packet*			
Original, 1 oz	**120**	2	21
Light Apple Cinnamon, 1.95 oz	**120**	1.5	24
Light Maple Brown Sugar, 1.34 oz	**150**	2	28
Erewhon: Barley Plus, ¼ cup, 1.7 oz	**170**	1	37
Brown Rice Cream, ¼ cup, 1.6 oz	**170**	1	36
Instant Oatmeal, 1.25 oz pkg, av.	**130**	2.5	25
McCann's Instant Irish Oatmeal			
Apple & Cinnamon, 1.23 oz	**130**	1.5	27
Maple & Brown Sugar, 1.5 oz	**160**	2	32
Original, 1 oz package	**100**	1.5	18
Steel Cut Oats, ¼ cup, 1.4 oz	**150**	2	26
Nabisco: Cream of Wheat, Farina, 1 oz	**120**	0	23
Malt-O-Meal: Orig., 3Tbsp, 1.2 oz	**130**	0.5	27
Maple Brown Sugar, ¼ cup	**170**	0	37
Natures Path:			
Oatmeal: Apple Cinnamin, 1.7 oz	**210**	2.5	40
HempPlus, 1 packet, 1.4 oz	**160**	2.5	40
Maple Nut, 1.7 oz	**200**	4	38
Ocean Spray,			
Oatmeal, all flavors, 1.52 oz	**160**	2	33
Quaker: Oat Bran, 1¼ cup, 2 oz	**210**	3	43
Instant Oatmeal: *Per Packet Unless Indicated*			
Regular, Organic 1 oz	**100**	2	19
Cinnamon & Spice, 1.62 oz	**170**	2	35
Maple Brown Sugar, 1.45 oz	**160**	2	31
Peaches & Cream, 1.23 oz	**130**	2	27
Raisin, Date & Walnut, 1.3 oz	**140**	2.5	27
Take Heart, average, 1.6 oz	**160**	2.5	33
Oatmeal Express, average all flavors	**200**	2.5	42
Old Fashioned Oats, ½ cup, 1.4 oz	**150**	3	27
Quick Oats, ½ cup, 1.4 oz	**150**	3	27
Grits: Instant, all types, 1 oz	**100**	0	22
Quick, ¼ cup, 1.3 oz	**130**	0.5	29
Silver Palate, Oatmeal, 1.4 oz	**160**	3	26

B Breakfast Cereals

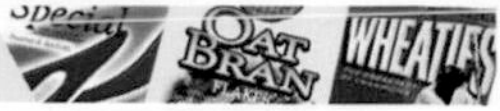

Quick Guide

Cold Cereals *Average All Brands*	C	F	Cb
Bran Flakes, ¾ cup, 1 oz	95	0.5	24
Corn Flakes, 1 cup, 1 oz	100	0	24
Granola, ¼ cup, 1 oz	150	7.5	16
Oat Bran Cereal, ½ cup, 1½ oz	145	3	25
Puffed Rice, 1 cup, ½ oz	55	0	13
Puffed Wheat, 1 cup, ½ oz	45	0	10
Raisin Bran, ½ cup, 1 oz	90	0.5	22
Rice Crisps, 1 cup, 1 oz	105	0.5	24
Shredded Wheat, 1 biscuit, 1 oz	85	0.5	20
Sugar-frosted Flakes, ¾ cup, 1 oz	115	0	28
Wheat Flakes, ¾ cup, 1 oz	105	1	24

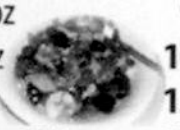

Breakfast/Cereal Bars/Pop Tarts: *See Page 33*

Ready-To-Eat Cereal

	C	F	Cb
Arrowhead Mills : *Per Cup*			
Flakes: Amaranth, 1.2 oz	140	2	26
Ancient Grain, 1. 7 oz	200	4	38
Corn, 1.1 oz	120	0	27
Kamut, 1.1 oz	120	1	25
Multi Grain, 1½ oz	170	2	33
Oat Bran, 1.2 oz	140	2.5	24
Rice, sweetened, 1.7 oz	180	1	40
Spelt, 1.1 oz	120	1	24
Granola, Crunchy Oat Bran, 1.7 oz	210	8	33
Puffed: Corn, ½ oz	60	1	12
Kamut, ½ oz	50	0	11
Millet, ½ oz	60	0.5	11
Rice, ½ oz	60	0	14
Wheat, ½ oz	60	0	12
Shredded Wheat: Original, 1.7 oz	190	1	38
Sweetened, 1.8 oz	200	10	42
Back to Nature: *Per ½ Cup, Unless Indicated*			
Granola: Apple Blueberry, 1.7 oz	200	2.5	39
Cherry Vanilla, 1.7 oz	200	4	38
Choc. Delight, 1.8 oz	220	6	37
Classic Granola, 1.7 oz	200	3	39
Cranberry Pecan, 1.7 oz	220	3	35
Honey Almond with Flax, 1.5 oz	190	7	29
Sunflower & Pumpkin Seed, 1.65 oz	200	7	31
Wild Blueberry Walnut, 1.5 oz	190	6	30

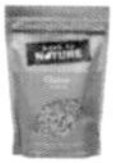

Barbara's Bakery	C	F	Cb
Brown Rice Crisps, sweetened, 1.1 oz	120	1	25
Corn Flakes, sweetened, 1 cup, 1.1 oz	110	1	25
Crispy Wheats, ¾ cup, 1.1 oz	110	0.5	25
Honey Crunch 'n Oats, ⅔ cup, 1.1 oz	110	1.5	25
Organic Breakfast O's, av., ¾ cup, 1 oz	120	2	24
Wild Puffs, av. all flavors, ¾ cup, 1.1 oz	120	1	25
Puffins: Original, ¾ cup, 1 oz	90	1	23
Cinnamon, ⅔ cup, 1 oz	100	1	26
Peanut Butter, ¾ cup, 1 oz	110	2	23
Shredded Oats:			
Cinnamon Crunch, 1 cup, 2 oz	230	3	43
Bite Size: Vanilla Almond, 1 cup, 2 oz	220	3	42
Ultima Organic:			
Flax & Granola, 1 cup, 2 oz	210	3	43
High Fiber, 1 cup, 2 oz	170	1.5	44
Pomegranate, 1 cup, 2 oz	200	1.5	44
Breadshop Granola:			
Honey Gone Nuts, 1.85 oz	240	10	33
Average other flavors, 1.8 oz	220	8	34
Cascadian Farm			
Hearty Morning, ¾ cup, 1.9 oz	200	3	43
Honey Nut O's, 1 cup, 1 oz	120	2	24
Multi Grain Squares, ¾ cup, 1 oz	110	1	25
Oats & Honey Granola, ⅔ cup, 2 oz	230	6	42
Purely O's, 1 cup, 1.1oz	110	1	24
Raisin Bran, 1 cup, 1.9 oz	180	1	43
Dr McDougall's			
Big Cups: Cranberry Muesli, 3 oz	320	4	62
Organic Apple Cinn. Oatmeal	250	3	50
Organic Maple 4 Grain, 3 oz	260	3	52
Peach Raspb. Oatmeal & Barley	300	4	62
Oatmeal: Orig., no added sugar, 1 oz	120	2	21
Light (50% less sugar):			
Apple Cinnamon, 1 packet	120	1.5	24
Maple Brown Sugar, 1 packet	150	2	28
Ener-G, Rice Bran, ½ cup, 2.4 oz	220	14	34
EnviroKidz: *Per 1 oz*			
Amazon Frosted Flakes	120	0	27
Gorilla Munch	120	0	27
Koala Crisp	110	1	25
Leapin Lemur	120	1.5	25
Panda Puffs	130	2.5	24

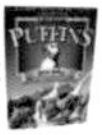

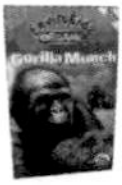

Ready-To-Eat (Cont)

	C	F	Cb
Erewhon			
Aztec Crunchy Corn & Amaranth, 1 oz	110	0	26
Corn Flakes, 1 cup, 2 oz	130	0	30
Crispy Brown Rice: 1 cup	110	0	25
with Mixed Berries, 1 cup	120	0.5	27
Gluten Free, 1 cup, 1 oz	110	0.5	25
Kamut Flakes, ⅔ cup, 1.2 oz	110	0	25
Raisin Bran, 1 cup, 1.8 oz	170	1	40
Rice Twice, ¾ cup, 1 oz	120	0	26
Ezekiel 4.9 Flourless Cereals			
Almond ½ cup, 2 oz	200	3	38
Golden Flax, ½ cup, 2 oz	180	2.5	37
Original, ½ cup, 2 oz	190	1	40
General Mills			
Basic 4, 1 cup, 1.9 oz	200	2	43
Boo Berry, 1 cup, 1.2 oz	130	1	28
Cheerios: *Per ¾ Cup*			
Apple Cinnamon, 1 oz	120	1.5	25
Berry Burst, Triple Berry, 1 oz	100	1	22
Frosted, 1 oz	110	1	23
Fruity, 1 oz	100	1	23
Honey Nut, 1 oz	110	1.5	22
Multi Grain, 1 oz	110	1	23
Oat Cluster Crunch, 1.1 oz	100	1	22
Original, 1 oz	100	2	20
Yogurt Burst, all flavors, 1 oz	120	1.5	24
Chex: Corn, 1 cup, 1 oz	120	0.5	26
Chocolate, ¾ cup, 1.1 oz	130	2.5	26
Honey Nut, ¾ cup, 1.1 oz	120	0.5	28
Multi-Bran, ¾ cup, 1.6 oz	160	1.5	39
Rice, 1 cup, 1 oz	100	0	23
Wheat, ¾ cup, 1.6 oz	160	1	38
Cinnamon Toast Crunch, ¾ cup, 1 oz	130	3	25
Cocoa Puffs, ¾ cup, 1 oz	110	1.5	23
Count Chocula, ¾ cup, 1 oz	110	1	23
Country Corn Flakes, 1 cup, 1.2 oz	120	0.5	28
Fiber One, ½ cup, 1 oz	60	1	25
Fiber One Honey Clusters, 1 cup	160	1.5	42
Golden Grahams, ¾ cup, 1 oz	120	1	26
Honey Nut Clusters, 1 cup, 2 oz	210	1	49
Kix: 1¼ cups, 1 oz	110	1	25
Berry Berry, ¾ cup, 0.9 oz	100	1	22
Lucky Charms, average, ¾ cup, 1 oz	110	1	22
Oatmeal Crisp, Almond, 1 cup, 2 oz	240	4.5	47
Raisin Nut Bran, ¾ cup, 1.75 oz	180	3	38
Reese's Puffs, ¾ cup, 1 oz	120	3	22
Total: Honey Clusters, ¾ cup	170	1	38
Raisin Bran, 1 cup, 1.9 oz	160	1	40
Wheaties, ¾ cup, 1 oz	100	0.5	22

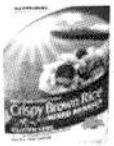

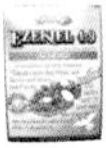

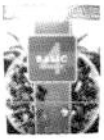

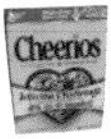

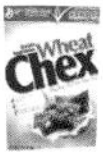

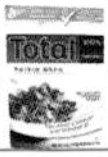

Updated Nutrition Data ~ www.CalorieKing.com
Persons with Diabetes ~ See Disclaimer (Page 24)

	C	F	Cb
Glucerna			
Crunchy Flakes:			
'n Strawb., ¾ cup, 1.1 oz	100	0.5	25
'n Almonds, ¾ cup, 1.1 oz	100	1	24
'n Raisins, ¾ cup, 1.2 oz	110	0.5	28
Health Valley			
Organic Flakes:			
Amaranth Flakes, 1 cup, 1 oz	100	1	23
Blue Corn Flakes, ¾ cup, 1.1 oz	100	0	24
Cranberry Crunch, ¾ cup, 1.8 oz	190	4	38
Fiber 7, Multigrain Flakes, 1 c., 1.7 oz	160	1	37
Golden Flax, 1 cup, 1.75 oz	190	3.5	37
Oat Bran Flakes: 1 cup, 1.75 oz	190	1.5	39
With Raisins, 1 cup, 1.9 oz	200	1.5	43
Crunch-Ems!, Rice; Corn, 1 cup, 1 oz	110	0	27
Heart Wise, 1 cup, 2 oz	200	3	37
Heartland			
Granola: Original, ½ cup, 2.25 oz	240	6	40
Low-Fat Raisin, ½ cup, 2 oz	200	3	40
Kashi			
7 Whole Grain: Flakes, 1 cup, 1.8 oz	180	1	41
Honey Puffs, 1 cup, 1.1 oz	120	1	25
Nuggets, ½ cup, 2 oz	210	1.5	47
Puffs, 1 cup, 0.67 oz	70	0.5	15
Biscuit Cereals:			
Autumn Wheat, 1 cup, 1.9 oz	180	1	43
Cinnamon Harvest, 1 cup, 1.9 oz	180	1	43
Island Vanilla, 1.9 oz	190	1	44
Kashi U, 1 cup, 2 oz	200	3.5	42
GoLEAN, Original, 1 cup, 1.8 oz	140	1	30
Crunch!: Plain, 1 cup, 1.9 oz	190	3	37
Honey Almond Flax, 1 cup, 1.9 oz	200	4.5	36
Good Friends: Orig., 1 cup, 1.9 oz	160	1.5	42
Cinna-Raisin Crunch, 1 cup, 1.8 oz	170	1.5	41
Granola: Apple Orchard, ½ cup, 1.9 oz	220	7	38
Cocoa Beach, ½ cup, 1.9 oz	230	9	36
Mountain Medley, ½ cup, 1.9 oz	220	7	38
Summer Berry, ½ cup, 1.9 oz	220	6	39
Heart to Heart:			
Honey Toasted Oat, ¾ cup, 1.2 oz	110	1.5	25
Oat Flakes & Blueberry Clusters, 1 cup	200	2	44
Warm Cinnamon Oat, ¾ cup, 1.2 oz	110	1.5	24
Mighty Bites, Honey Crunch, 1 cup	120	1.5	23
Vive, Toasted Graham & Van, 1¼ cups	170	2.5	43

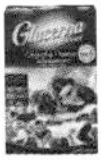

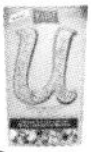

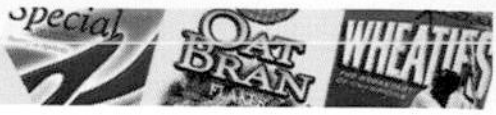

Ready-To-Eat (Cont)

Kellogg's	C	F	Cb
All-Bran: Original, ½ cup, 1.1 oz	80	1	23
Bran Buds, ⅓ cup, 1.1 oz	70	1	24
Complete Wheat Flakes, ¾ cup, 1.1 oz	90	0.5	23
Strawberry Medley, 1 cup, 1.9 oz	170	1.5	44
Apple Jacks, 1 cup, 1 oz	100	0.5	25
Cocoa Krispies, ¾ cup, 1.1 oz	120	1	27
Corn Flakes: Original, 1 cup, 1 oz	100	0	24
Touch of Honey, 1 cup, 1 oz	120	0	27
Corn Pops, 1 cup, 1 oz	110	0	26
Cracklin' Oat Bran, ¾ cup, 1.8 oz	200	7	35
Crispix, Original, 1 cup, 1 oz	110	0	25
Crunch: Raisin Bran, 1 cup, 1.9 oz	190	1	45
Froot Loops: Original, 1 cup, 1 oz	110	1	25
Marshmallow, 1 cup, 1.1 oz	110	1	25
Frosted Flakes, ¾ cup, 1.1 oz	110	0	27
Red. Sugar, 1 cup, 1.1 oz	120	0	28
Granola, Low-Fat:			
with Raisins, ⅔ cup, 2.1 oz	230	3	48
without Raisins, ½ cup, 1.7 oz	190	2.5	40
Honey Smacks, ¾ cup, 1 oz	100	0.5	24
Keebler Cookie Crunch, 1 cup, 1 oz	110	1	26
Mini Swirlz Cinnamon Bun, 1 cup	120	2	25
Mini-Wheats: Frosted Big Bite (5)	180	1	41
Frosted: Bite Size (24), 2.1 oz	200	1	48
Blueberry Muffins (24)	180	1	43
Unfrosted (30), 2.1 oz	200	1.5	46
Mueslix, ⅔ cup, 2 oz	200	3	40
Nutri-Grain Bars: *See Page 33*			
Product 19, 1 cup, 1.1 oz	100	0	25
Raisin Bran: Regular, 1 cup, 2.1 oz	190	1.5	45
Extra, 1 cup, 1.9 oz	190	3	44
Rice Krispies: Orig. 1¼ cups	130	0	29
Frosted, ¾ cup, 1.1 oz	110	0	27
Cocoa, ¾ cup, 1.1 oz	120	1	27
Treats, ¾ cup, 1.1 oz	120	1.5	26
Smart Start, Antioxidants, 1 cup, 1.8 oz	190	0.5	43

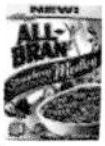

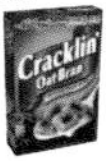

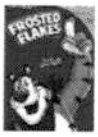

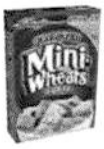

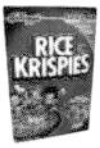

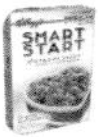

Kellogg's (Cont)	C	F	Cb
Smorz, 1 cup, 1.1 oz	120	2	25
Special K: Original 1 cup, 1.1 oz	120	0.5	23
Blueberry, ¾ cup, 0.9 oz	100	0	23
Fruit & Yogurt, ¾ cup, 1.1 oz	120	1	27
Red Berries, 1 cup, 1.1 oz	120	0	26
Vanilla Almond, ¾ cup	110	1.5	25
Kozy Shack			
Ready Grains: *Per 7 oz Pkg*			
Apple & Cinnamon	210	2	39
Maple Brown Sugar	190	2	33
Original	180	2	30
Strawberry	210	2	38
Malt-O-Meal			
Apple Zings, 1 cup, 1.1 oz	130	1	30
Blueb. Muffin Tops, ¾ cup	130	3.5	24
Cocoa Dyno-Bites, ¾ cup	120	1	26
Coco Roos, ¾ cup, 1 oz	120	1.5	26
Colossal Crunch, ¾ cup, 1.1 oz	120	1.5	26
Frosted Flakes, ¾ cup, 1 oz	120	0	28
Frosted Mini Spooners, 1 cup	190	1	45
Golden Puffs, ¾ cup, 1 oz	110	0	24
Honey Nut Scooters, 1 cup, 1 oz	110	1.5	24
Raisin Bran, 1 cup, 1.7 oz	220	1.5	49
Nature's Path			
Heritage, average, ¾ cup, 1 oz	120	1	24
Honey'd Cornflakes, ¾ cup, 1 oz	120	0	26
Multigr. Oatbran Flakes, ¾ cup, 1 oz	110	1	24
Flax Plus, Multibran ¾ cup, 1 oz	110	1.5	23
Maple Pecan Cr., ¾ cup	220	7	38
Pumpkin Raisin Cr., ¾ cup	210	4.5	40
Raisin Bran, ¾ cup, 2 oz	190	2.5	41
Kamut Puffs, 1 cup, ½ oz	50	0	11
Optimum, Blueberry Cinn. 1 cup 2 oz	200	3	38
New England Natural Bakers			
Muesli, ½ cup, 2.1 oz	220	5	40
Granola: Almond Raisin Crisp, ½ cup	220	9	36
Berry Good, ⅔ cup, 2.1 oz	250	6	44
French Vanilla, ⅔ cup, 2 oz	260	9	38
Grateful Date, ½ cup, 1.7 oz	210	7	33
Honey Crunch; Pecan, ½ cup	285	13	37
Low-Fat Cranberry, ½ cup, 1.7 oz	200	2.5	41

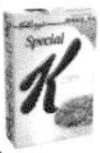

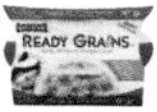

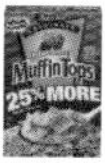

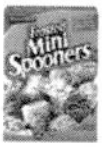

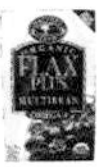

Ready-To-Eat (Cont)

	C	F	Cb
New Morning			
Cocoa Crispy Rice, ¾ cup, 1 oz	120	0.5	26
Fruit-e-O's, Organic, 1 cup, 1 oz	120	1.5	25
Oatios: Original, 1 cup, 1 oz	110	2	22
Apple Cinnamon, 1 oz	120	1	18
NutriSystem: *Per Packet*			
Granola, Low-Fat	160	2.5	31
NutriCinnamon Squares	120	0.5	23
NutriFlakes (40% Bran Flakes)	110	1	23
NutriFrosted Crunch	120	0.5	24
Oatmeal, Apple Cinnamon	130	1.5	26
Peace			
Crisps: *Per 1.95 oz*			
Golden Honey	240	6	40
Maple Pecan	240	6	42
Raspberry Ginger	230	3.5	45
Low-Fat: Mango Peach Passion	230	2.5	46
Very Berry	230	3	46
Granola, French Vanilla, ⅔ cup	240	6	41
Post			
Alpha Bits, 1 cup, 1 oz	110	1	23
Bran Flakes, ¾ cup, 1 oz	100	0.5	24
Grape-Nuts: Original, 2 oz	200	1	48
Flakes, ¾ cup, 1 oz	110	1	24
Honey Bunches of Oats, ¾ cup, 1 oz	120	1.5	25
Just Bunches: Caramel, ⅔ cup, 2 oz	250	7	43
Honey, Roasted, ⅔ cup	250	7	43
Pebbles: Cocoa, ¾ cup, 1 oz	110	1.5	26
Fruity, ¾ cup, 1.1 oz	110	1	26
Raisin Bran, 1 cup, 2.1 oz	190	1	46
Selects: Banana Nut Crunch 2.1 oz	240	6	44
Cranberry Almond Crunch, 1.8 oz	200	3.5	39
Quaker			
100% Natural Granola:			
with Honey, ½ cup, 1.8 oz	210	6	35
with Honey & Raisins, 1.8 oz	210	6	38
Low-Fat: ⅔ cup	210	3	45
Oat Bran, 1¼ cup, 2 oz	210	3	43
Oatmeal Squares, Brown Sugar, 1 c.	210	2.5	44
Captain Crunch: Regular, ¾ cup, 1 oz	110	1.5	23
Crunch Berries, ¾ cup, 1 oz	100	1.5	22
Peanut Butter, ¾ cup, 1 oz	110	2.5	21
Crunchy Corn Bran, 1 cup, 1 oz	90	1	23
Honey Graham Oh's, ¾ cup	110	2	23
King Vitaman, 1½ cup, 1.1 oz	120	1	26
Life, all types, ¾ cup, 1.1 oz	120	1.5	26

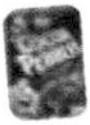

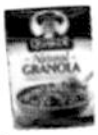

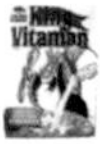

	C	F	Cb
Quaker (Cont)			
Toasted Oatmeal: 1 cup, 1.7 oz	190	2	40
Brown Sugar Bliss, 1 cup, 1.7 oz	190	2	40
Honey Nut Heaven, 1 cup, 1.7 oz	190	2	40
Instant Oatmeal: *See Page 59*			
Bars: *See Page 33*			
Sweet Home Farm			
Honey Nut Granola, ½ cup, 1.9 oz	250	10	37
Low-Fat Granola, ½ cup, 1.9 oz	210	3	44
Trader Joe's			
Clusters: Raisin Bran, 1 cup, 2 oz	190	3	40
Super Nutty Toffee, ¾ cup, 2 oz	250	9	38
Average all other flavors			
⅔ cup, 1.3 oz	145	3.5	26
1 cup, 2 oz	220	5	39
Chocolate Decadence, ¾ cup, 2 oz	250	8	38
Cornflakes, 1 cup, 1.1 oz	110	0	26
Golden Flax Cereal, ¾ cup, 1.7 oz	200	3.5	37
Granola: Mango Passion, 2 oz	240	8	37
Gluten Free, ¾ cup, 2 oz	260	12	35
Trek Mix, ⅔ cup, 2 oz	240	8	37
Honey Nut O's, ¾ cup, 1 oz	120	1.5	24
Joe's O's, 1 cup, 1 oz	110	1.5	22
Morning Lite, 1 cup, 1.85 oz	170	2.5	40
Shredded Wheats, Bite Size, 1 c., 1.7 oz	180	1	38
Soy Flax Clusters, 1 cup, 2 oz	190	3	38
Triple Berry O's, ¾ cup, 1 oz	110	1	25
Toasted Oatmeal Flakes, ¾ cup, 1.1 oz	110	1	23
Wheats, average, 1 cup, 2 oz	200	1	42
Twigs, Flakes & Clusters, 1 cup, 1.9 oz	170	1.5	41
Udi's, Granola, Au Naturel, ½ cup, 2 oz	240	8	38
Uncle Sam			
Cereal with Real Mixed Berries, 1 cup	190	4.5	39
Original, ¾ cup, 1.95 oz	190	5	38
Weetabix: 2 biscuits, 1.3 oz	125	1	26
Crispy Flakes: ¾ cup, 1.1 oz	110	0.5	24
& Fiber, 1¼ cup, 2 oz	170	1.5	44
Whole Foods (365)			
Corn Flakes, 1 cup, 1 oz	110	0	26
Honey Puffed Wheat, 1 oz	110	0	24
Frosted Flakes, ¾ cup, 1 oz	110	0	27
Oat Bran Flakes, 1 cup, 2 oz	220	2.5	44
Raisin Bran, 1 cup, 2 oz	200	0.5	44
Shredded Wheat, 1 cup, 1.7 oz	180	1	38
Frosted, 1 cup, 2 oz	210	1	45

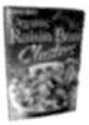

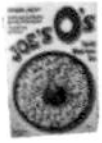

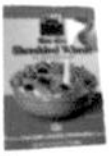

Updated Nutrition Data ~ www.CalorieKing.com
Persons with Diabetes ~ See Disclaimer (Page 24)

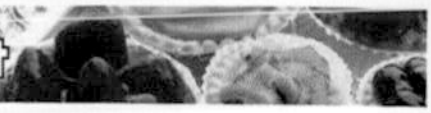

Ready-to-Eat

	C	F	Cb
Angel Food: Plain, w/o oil, 2 oz	145	0	33
Plain with oil, 2 oz	145	1	27
with Cream Frosting	255	7	45
Almond Croissant, 5 oz	620	35	67
Apple Danish, 5 oz	450	18	67
Apple Pie: *See Pies/Tarts Page 136*			
Baklava, 1½" square, 1.75 oz	200	10	27
Banana with Butter Cream, 2 oz	230	9	37
Banana Walnut, 3 oz	270	11	40
Bear Claw, 4½ oz	540	24	71
Black Forest, 3 oz (1/12)	345	11	59
Brownie: Small, 2" Square, 1 oz	130	8	14
Large, 3 oz	390	24	42
Bundt, average all types			
1 slice 3 oz (1/10)	300	13	42
Mini-Bundt, 5 oz	500	22	70
Cannoli	375	17	44
Carrot Cake: Plain, 3 oz	300	16	37
with Cream Cheese Frosting	400	22	48
Cheesecake: Small serving, 3 oz	235	13	26
Large serving, 5 oz	395	21	44
with Low-Fat Cheese/Fruit, 3 oz	170	4	28
Cheesecake Factory: 1 slice	630	45	53
Denny's Cheesecake, 1 slice	580	38	51
Chocolate Cake:			
Plain, w/o frosting, 1/12 of 9", 3½ oz	340	14	51
with chocolate frosting, 4 oz	415	18	62
Chocolate Croissant, 4¼ oz	470	26	54
Chocolate Eclair with Custard, 3½ oz	260	16	24
Chocolate Fudge Cake, 3 oz	270	12	40
Chocolate Meringue, 1/6 pie	320	13	48
Churros, 1 stick, 1½ oz	125	5	18
Cinnamon Crumb Cake, 2½ oz	260	9	40
Cinnamon Roll: Small, 2 oz	220	8	34
Regular, 4 oz	440	16	68
Large, 6 oz	660	24	102
Brands ~ *See Page 69*			
Coffee Cake, 2 oz	180	6	30
Concha: Small, 2 oz	240	9	33
Large (5" diameter), 5½ oz	615	23	85
Cream Puff (custard fill), 4.6 oz	335	20	30
Creme Horns, each, 3 oz	210	5	36
Crumble Coffee Cake, 4½ oz	500	25	65
Danish Pastry:			
Small, 2½ oz	250	14	25
Large, 5 oz	500	28	50
Donuts: *See Page 68*			
Eclair, Choc., Custard fill, 3½ oz	260	16	24
Fig Bars, average, each	160	3	31

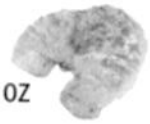

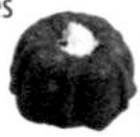

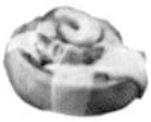

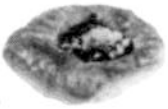

Ready-to-Eat (Cont)

	C	F	Cb
Fruit Cake, Dark/Light, 2 oz	185	5	34
Fudge Nut Brownie, each, 3½ oz	380	18	54
Gingerbread: From mix, 3" square	210	4	41
Honey Bun, each, 2.7 oz	310	15	39
Jelly Roll, 1/12 roll, 1.8 oz	150	2	32
Key Lime Pie, 4.3 oz	400	25	41
Kolacky, Apricot/Raspberry, ½ oz (1)	60	3.5	8
Lady Fingers, 3 oz	310	4.5	59
Lemon Cake, 4 oz	440	24	49
Lemon Poppy Seed Creme, 1.6 oz	180	9	23
Marble Cake, 1 slice, 4 oz	430	23	50
Mississippi Mud Pie, 4 oz	480	22	67
Mud Cake, 1 piece, 4½ oz	380	20	44
Muffins: *See Page 69*			
Palmier Cookie, large, 4½ oz	490	25	62
Pineapple Upside Down, 2½ oz	230	9	36
Peach Melba, 3½ oz	300	8	52
Pecan Sticky Roll, 6½ oz	690	22	91
Pecan Twirls, 1 piece, 1.3 oz	170	7	26
Pies & Tarts: *See Page 136*			
Pound Cake, 3 oz	330	17	40
Raspberry Rugulah,			
1 piece, 1.2 oz	110	9	7
Scone, fruit, 2 oz	200	9	30
Sponge: Plain, 2½ oz	220	10	33
with Cream & Strawberry Jam	390	12	69
with Chocolate Frosting	290	12	45
Strawberry Creme, 4.7 oz	400	27	33
Strudel Bites, ¾ oz	60	2.5	9
Strudel, fruit, average, 4.4 oz	300	17	32
Sweet Roll, average, 1½ oz	150	6	23
Swiss Rolls, (2)	270	12	38
Tiramisu, 4.4 oz	440	22	34
Turnovers, fruit, average, 3 oz	290	15	35

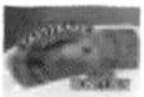

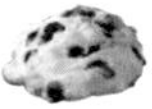

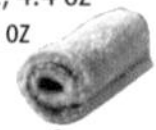

Cupcakes

	C	F	Cb
Average all Varieties			
Regular:			
Cake only, 1½ oz	140	5.5	20
Cake + Icing, 2½ oz	260	13	34
Large *(Muffin Size):*			
Cake only, 2½ oz	235	9	34
Cake + Icing, 5 oz	520	27	67
Mini (2-Bite):			
Cake only, 0.4 oz	40	1.5	5.5
Cake + Icing, 1 oz	110	5.5	13
Icing Only: Per 1 oz	115	7	13
Thick/Tall amount, 2½ oz	290	17	32
Starbucks Cupcakes:			
Triple Chocolate, 3¼ oz	360	20	46
Vanilla, 3 oz	320	16	43

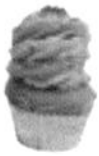

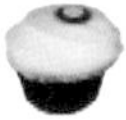

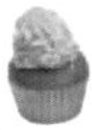

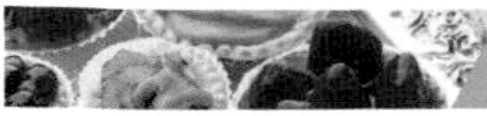

Cakes ~ Brands

	C	F	Cb
Albertson's Bakery			
Choc. Ring Cake, ⅛, 3 oz	300	14	38
Lemon Ring Cake, ⅛, 3 oz	320	15	42
Sock it to me Ring Cake, ⅛, 3 oz	290	12	42
Cake Slices: *Per 1.6 oz Slice*			
Banana Nut Creme Cake	155	8	19
Blueberry Creme Cake	155	8	20
Butter Creme Cake	110	6	20
Cinnamon Butter Streusel Creme	140	9	20
Bimbo			
Concha, avg., 2.1 oz	240	9	33
Homestyle Pound Cake	300	15	37
Pecan Pound Cake, 2.9 oz	330	16	41
Raisin Pound Cake, 2.9 oz	340	16	43
Bon Appetit			
Banana Bread	440	25	49
Cheese Coffee Cake, 4 oz	480	26	56
Walnut Brownie, 3.5 oz	380	18	54
Sliced: Cheesecake, 4 oz	430	24	49
Lemon Cake, 4 oz	430	24	49
Marble Cake, 4 oz	430	24	50
Danish: Apple (1), 5 oz	420	22	50
Bear Claw (1), 5 oz	480	26	54
Cheese & Berries (1), 5 oz	500	28	52
Vienna Cream (1), 5 oz	480	28	54
Claim Jumper: Carrot Cake, 4.6 oz	450	24	54
Choc. Motherload Cake, 5.3 oz	520	27	73
Cheesecake Factory: *See Fast-Foods Section*			
Entenmann's			
Cheese-Filled Crumb Coffee, 1.9 oz	200	10	25
Chocolate Fudge, ⅛ cake, 2.5 oz	270	11	40
Crumb Coffee Cake, 1/10, 2 oz	260	13	34
Gourmet Cinn. Rolls, ½ roll	220	8	34
Louisiana Crunch, 1/9,	330	14	49
Pecan Danish Ring, ⅛	240	15	24
Raspb. Danish Twist, ⅛	220	11	29
Enten-Minis:			
Butterscotch Cakes (2), 2 oz	250	10	37
Carrot Cakes (2), 2.8 oz	330	15	46
Choc. Creme Cupcakes (2), 2 .8 oz	310	11	50
Sponge Creme Cupcakes (2), 2.3 oz	260	12	36
Muffins/Sweet Rolls: *See Page 69*			
Glenny's			
100 Calorie Brownie: *Per Brownie*			
Regular, 1.4 oz	100	4	12
Blondie, 1.4 oz	100	4	15
Peanut Butter, 1.4 oz	100	4	15

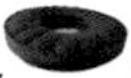
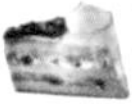
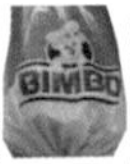

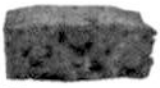
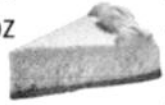
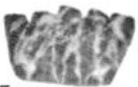
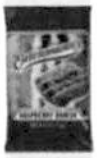

	C	F	Cb
Great American Cookies			
Cookie Cakes: *Per Slice*			
By the Slice, 4.6 oz	580	27	83
Heart Shaped, 3.5 oz	440	21	64
M&M, 1 slice, 4 oz	500	24	73
Hershey's:			
Brownies: Hershey's	380	18	56
Reese's	380	18	54
Hostess:			
100 Calorie Packs,			
Coffee Cakes, Cinn. (3)	100	3	21
Cinnamon Streusel Cake (1)	170	5	29
Chocodiles	240	11	33
Cup Cake: Choc. (1), 1.76 oz	180	6	30
Golden (1), 1.95 oz	180	6	30
Ding Dongs (2), 2.82 oz	360	19	47
Ho Ho's (3), 3 oz	370	17	54
Snoballs (1), 1.7 oz	170	5	32
Suzy Q , 2 cakes, 4 oz	440	18	68
Twinkies, 1 cake, 1.5 oz	150	4.5	27
Fried Twinkie	360	28	26
Zingers:			
Chocolate (1)	150	5	25
Devils Food (1)	150	5	25
Raspberry (1)	160	7	24
Vanilla (1)	160	5	27
Little Debbie			
100 Calories: Choc. Cake (1), 1 oz	100	3	17
Yellow Cake w. Icing (1), 1 oz	100	3	18
Boston Crème Rolls (1), 2.2 oz	270	12	40
Brownies, Fudge (1), 2.15 oz	280	12	40
Choc Chip Snack Cake (2), 2.4 oz	300	14	42
Chocolate Cup Cake	210	8	33
Coffee Cakes (1)	200	6	35
Devil Cremes (1) 1.65 oz	200	9	29
Devil Squares, 2 cakes, 2.2 oz	260	11	38
Fancy Cakes (2)	300	13	44
Frosted Fudge , 1.5 oz cake	190	9	27
Orange Zebra Cup Cake (1)	210	10	29
Star Crunch (1)	150	6	22
Smores (1)	190	7	30
Strawberry Shortcake Rolls, 2.1 oz	240	9	40
Swiss Cake Rolls (2), 2.15 oz	270	12	38
Zebra Cakes, 2 cakes, 2.6 oz	320	14	48
Nemo's			
Banana Cake, 3 oz	300	12	45
Chocolate Cake, 3 oz	300	14	42
Carrot Cake, 3.6 oz	390	21	47

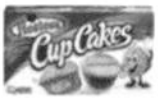

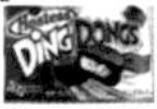

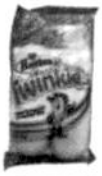
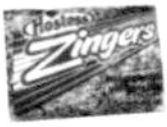

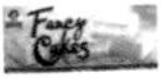
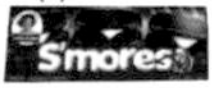

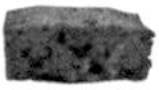

Cakes ~ Brands (Cont)

	C	F	Cb
Oreo			
Cakesters			
2 cake packet, 2 oz	250	12	36
Pepperidge Farm			
3-Layer Cakes:			
Chocolate Fudge, ⅛ cake	230	10	33
Coconut, ⅛, 2.5 oz	240	10	35
Golden, ⅛ cake, 2.5 oz	230	9	34
Dumplings: Apple	230	11	29
Peach	250	11	34
Turnovers (Frozen): Apple, 3.15 oz	270	15	31
Raspberry, 3.15 oz	280	15	34
Safeway Select			
Molten Chocolate Lava Cake, 4½ oz	440	26	50
Sara Lee			
Cheesecake: *Per Slice*			
French Classic, ⅕ cake	410	25	41
French Strawberry, ⅙	320	14	43
New York Style Classic, ⅙ cake	480	30	47
Original Cream Cherry, ¼ cake	320	11	50
Original Cream, ¼ cake	320	17	36
Original Cream Strawberry, ¼ cake	330	12	49
Coffee Cakes: *Per Slice*			
Butter Streusel, ⅙ cake	190	9	24
French Crumb Cake, ⅛ cake	180	4	33
Deluxe Cinnamon Rolls w. Icing (1)	260	12	33
Pecan Cake, ⅙ cake	190	10	22
Layer Cakes: *Per ⅛ Whole*			
Chocolate Gold, ⅛ cake	320	14	46
Layer Coconut, ⅛ cake, 2.7 oz	290	12	44
Layer Double Chocolate, ⅛ cake	290	9	49
Layer Vanilla, ⅛ cake	260	14	32
Pound Cakes: *Per ¼ of Cake*			
All Butter	300	16	35
Free & Light	220	4	41
Strawberry Swirl	225	7.5	38
Bites: *Per* Serving			
Original: (1)	20	1	3
(24)	440	27	43
Choc. Dipped Orig. Cheesecake	100	7	8
Choc. Dipped Praline Pecan (5)	90	6	8
Triple Choc. Fudge Brownie (1)	90	4	12

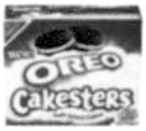

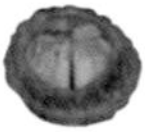
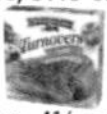

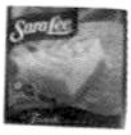

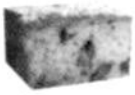
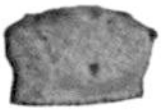

Smart Ones (Weight Watchers)	C	F	Cb
Brownie à la Mode	200	4	36
Chocolate Mousse	180	4	28
Chocolate Eclair	140	4	24
Choc. Chip Cookie Dough Sundae	170	3	32
Double Fudge Cake	220	7	35
Key Lime Pie, 3.3 oz	190	4.5	33
Mint Choc Chip Sundae, 2½ oz	150	3	28
Mocha Fudge Sundae, 2½ oz	160	4	27
Strawberry Shortcake, 3½ oz	170	6	25
Tastykake: Chocolate Jnr, 3.3 oz	340	12	55
Creme Filled Koffee Kakes, 3.15 oz	350	16	50
Koffee Kake Junior, 2.53 oz	280	10	44
Trader Joe's			
Bakery:			
Almond Ring Cake, ⅛, 1.8 oz	250	13	30
Carrot Cake, ⅛, 3.25 oz	480	33	42
Cheesecake Brownie Bites (1)	110	7	9
Danish Tea Cake, 1/13, 1.9 oz	200	9	28
Flourless Choc. Cake, 1 pce, 2 oz	260	17	23
Lemon Cake, ⅛, 3.25 oz	350	19	43
Mini Carrot Cake, 5 oz	450	19	68
Cupcakes: Choc., 3.2 oz	430	23	54
Vanilla, 3 oz	400	20	52
Frozen Dessert:			
Cappuccino Craving Cake, 1 pce	140	9	11
Cheesecake: Plain, 3.5 oz	320	19	30
Choc Chip, 3.5 oz	350	20	36
Triple Choc, 3.5 oz	340	19	34
Tuxedo, 3.5 oz	320	17	34
Chocolate Cloud Cake, ⅛, 1.8 oz	160	10	15
Chocolate Ganache, ⅛, 3.5 oz	390	22	44
Choc Lava Cake (1), 3.8 oz	360	23	40
Ice Cream Cake, 1/9, 5 oz	370	18	48
Karat Cake, ⅛, 2.9 oz	320	19	37
Lemon Tarts (1), 3.3 oz	300	13	40
Mango Passion Torta Cotta, 1 pce	170	12	16
N.Y. Style Cheesecake, 1/7, 4.5 oz	400	28	32
Tiramisu Torte, 1/7, 3.2 oz	230	12	24
Tarts: Apricot Almond, ⅙, 4 oz	450	24	56
Lemon, ⅙, 2.7 oz	280	14	38
Linzer, ⅙, 2 oz	200	7	32
Pear, ⅛, 3 oz	230	10	34

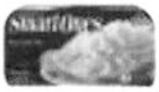
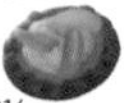
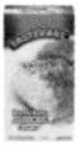
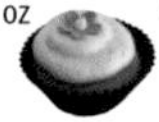
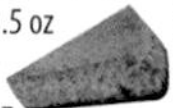
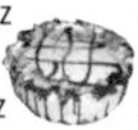
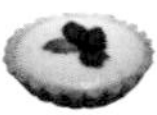
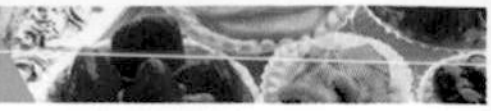

Cakes ~ Mixes

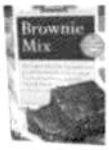

Prepared As Directed	C	F	Cb
Arrowhead Mills			
All Purpose Baking, ⅓ cup	130	1	28
Oatmeal Raisin (1), 0.7 oz	80	0	16
Gluten Free: Brownie, 1/20 pkg	110	2	21
Choc Chip (1), 0.7 oz	80	1	17
Betty Crocker			
Cakes (Super Moist): *Per 1/12 Cake*			
Butter Recipe Yellow	250	12	35
Carrot	260	14	35
Cherry Chip	230	7	35
Chocolate varieties	270	13	34
Devil's Food	260	13	35
White	220	6	35
Other flavors, average	270	13	35

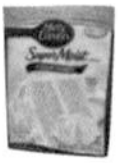

If using No-Cholesterol Recipe, deduct 40 cals and 4g fat.

	C	F	Cb
Other Cakes: Pound Cake, ⅛	260	8	45
Gingerbread Cake, ⅛	220	6	39
Pineapple Upside Down, ⅙	390	13	65
Sunkist Lemon Bar (1)	140	4	24
Brownie Mix: *Per 1/20 Pkg*			
Dark Chocolate Fudge	160	10	24
Fudge	170	6.5	23
Low-Fat Fudge, 1/18 pkg	140	3	28
Supreme: Original	160	7	26
Chocolate Chunk	180	8	25
Peanut Butter; Walnut, average	180	9	23
Triple Chunk	180	8	25
Cookie Mix: *Per 2 Cookies*			
Chocolate Chip	170	8	21
Double Chocolate Chunk	150	6	21
Oatmeal	160	7	22
Oatmeal Chocolate Chip	160	8	21
Peanut Butter	150	8	20
Rainbow Chocolate Candy	160	7	22
Sugar Cookie	160	8	21
Walnut Chocolate Chip	170	9	21
Warm Delights: *Per Bowl*			
Cinnamon Swirl, 3.3 oz	390	10	72
Lemon Swirl Cake, 3.6 oz	380	9	72
Molten Caramel Cake, 3.4 oz	360	10	64
Molten Chocolate Cake, 3.4 oz	370	12	61

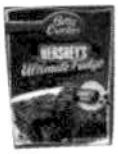

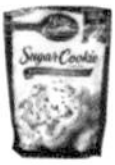

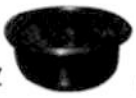

Updated Nutrition Data ~ www.CalorieKing.com
Persons with Diabetes ~ See Disclaimer (Page 24)

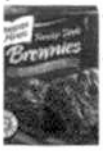

Duncan Hines	C	F	Cb
Brownie Mix: *Per 1 oz Brownie, Prepared*			
Candy Shop Peanut Butter Cup, 1 oz	170	8	23
Choc. Lovers, Turtle	160	7	23
Family-Style, Chewy Fudge	170	8	23
Cake Mix: *Prepared, 1/12 Pkg.*			
Moist Deluxe Cake:			
Ban. Supreme/Yellow Cake	270	12	36
Coconut Supreme	250	11	34
Dark Choc. Fudge/Devil's Food	290	15	35
French Vanilla	270	12	34
Jell-O No Bake Cheesecakes: *Prep'd As Directed*			
Cherry, 1/9 pkg	300	13	48
Homestyle Cheesecake, ⅙ pkg	370	17	50
Real Cheesecake, ⅙ pkg	350	14	48
Strawberry, 1/9 pkg	300	13	48
Krusteaz: Cinn. Crumb Cake, 1"	220	7	38
Lemon/Key Lime Bar, 2" bar	150	3.5	29
Pillsbury			
Moist Supreme: *Per 1/12 Pkg, Dry Mix Only*			
Classic White/Yellow	170	3.5	35
Devils Food	160	2.5	35
Brownie Mix: *Dry Mix Only*			
Caramel Swirl, 1/12 pkt, 1.2 oz	130	2.5	27
Cheesecake Swirl, 1/18 pkt, 0.85 oz	100	2.5	20
Chocolate Extreme, 1/16 pkt, 1 oz	120	3	22
Mint Chocolate, 1/15 pkt, 1 oz	110	2.5	22

Cake Frostings

	C	F	Cb
Betty Crocker			
Drizzlers, 2½ Tbsp	150	6	23
Rich & Creamy, average, 2 Tbsp	140	5	23
Whipped, all flavors, 2 Tbsp	100	4.5	15
Easy Flow Icing, 1 Tbsp	75	3	12
Duncan Hines:			
Creamy Homestyle, av. all flav., 2T.	140	6	23
Whipped, avg., 3 Tbsp	160	9	20
Pillsbury: *Per 2 Tbsp (approx. 1/12 Tub)*			
Creamy Supreme: Choc Fudge	140	6	21
Classic White	140	0	3
Milk Choc	140	6	21
Vanilla; Vanilla Funfetti	150	6	25
Red. Sugar: Milk Choc., 2 Tbsp	100	6	17
Vanilla, 2 Tbsp	120	7	17
Whipped Supreme, avg all flavors	100	5	14

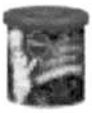

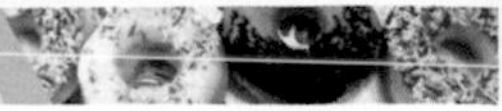

Quick Guide

Donuts
Average All Brands

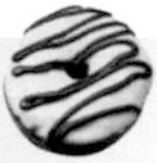

	C	F	Cb
Plain, 1¾ oz	210	12	25
Sugared, 1¾ oz	220	11	27
Glazed, 2 oz	250	12	34
Chocolate Iced, 2 oz	260	14	29

Donuts ~ Brands

	C	F	Cb
Albertson's			
Donut Holes: Assorted	150	8	18
Powdered Sugar (4) 1.7 oz	210	12	24
Gem Donuts: Plain Cake (3) 1.6 oz	190	12	20
Chocolate (3)	260	16	25
Glazed (4), 1.9 oz	260	16	26
Sticky Donuts, 2.2 oz	230	10	32
Bon Appetit			
Cherry Donuts (1) 2 oz	280	18	28
Mini Donuts: Chocolate (4)	270	16	29
Powdered; Crumb, average (4)	245	12	33
Dolly Madison			
Regular, 1¾ oz	270	12	40
Donut Gems,			
Powdered Mini's (4), 2 oz	230	11	31
Dunkin' Donuts			
Apple N' Spice Donut	240	11	32
Blueberry Cake Donut	330	18	38
Boston Kreme Donut	280	12	38
Chocolate Frosted Cake Donut	340	19	38
Chocolate Glazed Cake Donut	280	15	33
Cinnamon Cake Donut	290	18	30
Glazed Cake Donut	320	18	37
Jelly Filled Donut	260	11	36
Old Fashioned Cake Donut	280	18	27
Powdered Cake Donut	300	18	30
Sugar Raised Donut	190	9	22
Vanilla Kreme Filled Donut	320	17	37
Entenmann's			
Frosted Devil's Food	310	18	36
Glazed Buttermilk, 2¼ oz	270	13	37
Milk Chocolate Frosted, 2.4 oz	310	19	35

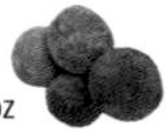

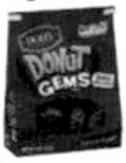

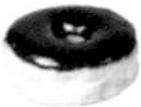

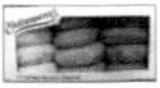

Donuts ~ Brands (Cont)

	C	F	Cb
Entenmann's (Cont)			
Powdered, 1¾ oz	230	14	25
Rich Frosted, 2 oz	300	20	30
Pop'ems (bite size): *Per 4 pieces*			
Glazed (4) 2 oz	240	12	31
Glazed Devil's Food (4) 2 oz	240	11	33
Popettes (bite size), av., 3 pcs, 1.8 oz	240	15	24
Hostess			
Dunkin Stix (3)	490	25	63
Donut Bites, 1 pouch, 2.3 oz	300	15	39
Regular: Plain, 1.4 oz	160	9	18
Choc. Frosted, 2 oz	240	14	27
Powdered, 1.7 oz	190	9	25
Old Fashioned Glazed, 2.1 oz	260	13	33
Donettes: Frosted (4) 2.15 oz	270	17	29
Crumb (3), 2 oz	220	9	32
Crunch (3), 2 oz	220	9	32
Powdered (4) 2.15 oz	240	12	31
Krispy Kreme			
Chocolate Glazed Cruller	290	15	37
Chocolate Iced Glazed	250	12	33
Chocolate Iced Kreme Filled	350	20	39
Chocolate Iced w. Sprinkles	270	12	38
Cinnamon Twist	240	15	23
Glazed Cruller	240	14	26
Glazed Kreme Filled	340	20	39
Maple Iced Glazed	240	12	32
New York Cheesecake	340	20	34
Original Glazed	200	12	22
Powdered Cake	290	14	37
Traditional Cake Doughnut	230	13	25
Glazed Doughnut Holes, Orig., (5)	200	11	25
Little Debbie			
Donut Sticks (2), 1.65 oz	230	14	25
Mini Donuts: Frosted (4), 2.1 oz	280	16	32
Powdered (4)	210	10	29
Tastykake			
Cinnamon, 1.8 oz	210	11	26
Mini: Coated, 3 oz	380	22	42
Powdered Sugar (6) 2½ oz	280	13	37

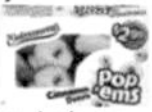

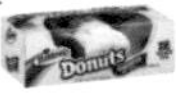

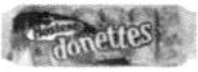

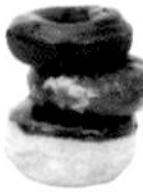

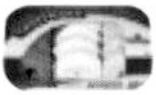

Quick Guide

	C	F	Cb
Muffins: Ready-To-Eat			
Average All Types:			
Small, 1 oz	80	3	12
Medium, 2 oz	160	6	24
Large, 3 oz	240	9	36
Extra Large, 4 oz	320	12	48
Giant, 6 oz	480	18	72
Super Size, 8 oz	640	24	96

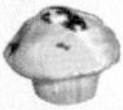
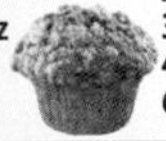

Brands ~ Ready-To-Eat

	C	F	Cb
Albertsons: *Mini Muffins, Per 1.76 oz*			
Banana Nut (2)	200	12	20
Blueberry (2)	180	10	21
Honey Raisin Bran (2)	170	7	24
Awrey's: Blueberry, 2.5 oz	240	12	31
Raisin Bran, 1.5 oz muffin	160	8	23
Controlled Carb Gourmet			
Almond Blueberry Muffins, 3 oz	210	15	27
Entenmann's:			
Little Bites, Blueberry, 1 pkt,	180	8	25
Chocolate Chip, 1 packet	190	9	26
Hostess: Mini, 1 pouch, avg.	260	15	30
Fruit Pie/Tart, avg., 4.5 oz	475	20	68
Hearty Muffin: Blueberry, 6 oz	590	28	78
Banana Nut, 6 oz	620	31	78
Muffin Loaf: Blueberry, 3.8 oz	440	19	62
Banana Nut, 3.8 oz	460	24	56
100 Calorie Packs:			
Banana Streusel (3)	100	3.5	19
Blueb. Streusel (3)	100	3	20
Little Debbie: Banana Nut (1), 1.9 oz	210	9	30
Blueberry (1), 1.9 oz	190	8	27
Chocolate Chip (1), 1.9 oz	210	9	28
My Favorite Muffin:			
Chocolate Chip, 6 oz	630	33	81
Fat-Free, Blueberry; Cherry Pie, 6 oz	325	0	78
Otis Spunkmeyer: *Per Whole Muffin (4 oz)*			
Banana Nut, 4 oz	420	20	54
Chocolate Chip	420	22	52
Wild Blueberry	360	16	52
Starbucks: *See Fast-Foods Section*			
Trader Joe's:			
Banana Chocolate Chip, 4 oz	400	18	57
Triple Berry (1), 4 oz	310	11	49
Mini: Blueberry, 0.8 oz	110	6	12
Bran w. Raisin, 0.8 oz	80	3	13
Weight Watchers: Blueb., 2.5 oz	190	2.5	42
Double Chocolate, 2.5 oz	180	3	41

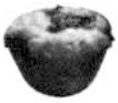
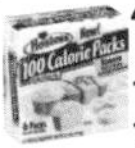

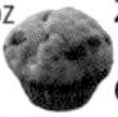
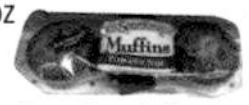

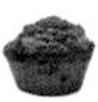

Fast-Food Restaurants: *See Page 183*

Updated Nutrition Data ~ www.CalorieKing.com
Persons with Diabetes ~ See Disclaimer (Page 24)

Muffin Mixes

	C	F	Cb
Prepared: Per Muffin			
Betty Crocker: Apple Streusel	230	8	37
Banana Nut	210	10	27
Choc Chip; Cinnamon Streusel	220	8	30
Wild Blueberry	180	8	26
Water Muffins: Choc Chip	130	3.5	22
Blueb.; Lemon Poppyseed, avg.	120	2.5	23
Cornbread	160	9	24
Krusteaz: Banana Nut	220	3.5	32
Choc Chip	180	4	34
Lem. Poppyseed	170	4	30
Oatbran (1)	180	4.5	31
Pillsbury, Hot Roll Mix (1)	110	1.5	21
Sunmaid: Honey Raisin Bran	220	2.5	47
Trader Joe's: Ban. Muffin Mix	180	11	22

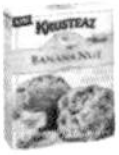

Sweet Rolls & Buns

	C	F	Cb
Note: It is best to weigh for accuracy as actual weight can be 10-50% higher than label weight.			
Bon Appetit: Cinn. Roll, 5 oz	690	40	78
Mammoth Cinnamon Roll, 5 oz	690	40	78
Cinnabon: Classic	815	32	117
Caramel Pecanbon	1100	47	156
Minibon, 1 roll	340	13	49
CinnaPretzel	750	6	156
Cinnabon Stix (5) w/out frosting	410	23	46
with Frosting	590	34	66
Cloverhill Bakery			
Jumbo Honey Bun, 4.75 oz	600	35	64
Entenmann's: Cinn. Bun (1), 4.5 oz	500	22	72
Hostess:			
Cinnamon Sweet Roll (1)	210	7	34
Honey Bun, Glazed:			
Net weight, 3.75 oz	440	25	51
Actual weight, 4.65 oz	550	31	63
Iced/Frosted, 3.5 oz	410	24	42
Little Debbie:			
Honey Buns, 1.76 oz	220	12	26
Pecan Spinwheels, 1 oz	100	4	16
McDonald's: Cinnamon Melts, 4 oz	460	19	66
Pillsbury: Cinnamon Roll, w. Icing	140	5	23
Reduced Fat (1) 1.5 oz	130	3.5	24
Ralph's, Cinnamon Roll, 2.5 oz	290	11	44
7-Eleven, Iced Honey Bun, 4.75 oz	520	24	71
Trader Joe's: Cinn. Roll, 2.35 oz	250	7	41
Low-Fat Cinn. Roll, 2.35 oz	180	2	36
Frosted Cinnamon Bun, 4 oz	380	9	66
Zen Bakery: Cinn. Raisin Roll (1), 3.2 oz	230	2	48

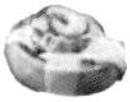
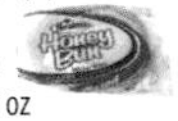

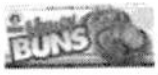

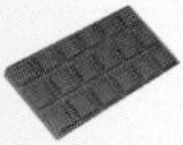

Quick Guide

Chocolate	C	F	Cb
Average All Brands			
Milk Chocolate, regular:			
Plain/Nuts/Fruit, average, 1 oz	155	10	16
1½ oz Bar	225	15	24
2 oz Bar	310	20	32
4 oz Block	620	40	64
8 oz Block	1240	80	128
1 Pound, 16 oz	2480	160	256
Dark/White Chocolate, 1 oz	155	9	17
Sugar Free *(Hershey's)* 1 pce, 0.3 oz	40	2	5
Chocolate-coated:			
Almonds, 5-6, 1 oz	155	9	16
Clusters, Nut, 3 pcs, 1.2 oz	210	14	20
Coffee Beans, 1.4 oz	220	13	22
Creme/Cordial Centers, 1.26 oz	170	6	28
Fudge, 1.5 oz	220	13	27
Macadamias, 10 pcs, 1.4 oz	220	16	21
Mints, 1 med., ½ oz	55	1	11
Nougat & Caramel, 1 oz	150	9	15
Peanuts, 12 med., 1 oz	150	10	15
Raisins, 28 med., 1 oz	110	4	19
Cooking Chocolate:			
Sweet/Semi-sweet, 1 oz	140	9	16
4 oz Bar *(Baker's)*	480	28	64
Chips: 1 Tbsp, ½ oz	70	4	9
½ cup, 3 oz	420	24	54
Unsweetened, 1 oz	140	14	8
Carob: Plain, 1 oz	150	9	16

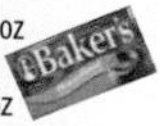

Brands & Generic

Per Piece/Serving	C	F	Cb
3 Muskateers: 1 bar, 2.13 oz	260	8	46
Minis, 7 pieces, 1.4 oz	170	5	32
100 Calorie Bars *(Hershey's)*, 0.6 oz	100	6	11
100 Grand: 1.5 oz bar	190	8	30
Super Size, 2.8 oz	360	14	58
Snack Size (1), ¾ oz	100	4	15
Abba Zabba, 2 oz bar	250	5	48
After Dinner Mints, 1 small	25	1.5	3
After Eight Mint *(Nestlé)*, each	35	1.5	4
Air Head, 1 bar, ½ oz	60	1	15
Almond Joy: 2 bars, 1.6 oz	220	13	26
King Size, 4 bars, 3.22 oz	440	26	52
Snack, 0.6 oz bar	80	4.5	10
Cookies (2), 1 oz	140	8	17
Almond Roca, 3 pcs, 1.27 oz	200	15	17
Almonds, sugar-coated (15), 1.4 oz	190	7	27

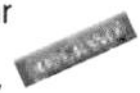

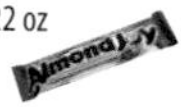

Brands & Generic (Cont)

Per Piece/Serving	C	F	Cb
Almond Clusters *(Trader Joe's)*, 2 pieces, 1.2 oz	210	14	15
Altoids *(C & B)*, 3 pieces	10	0	2
Andes, Thins, av., all flav. (8), 1.4 oz	200	13	22
Anthon Berg: Cognac, each	180	8	25
Creamy Mint (4), 1.4 oz	180	6	31
Marzipan with Madeira, 1.4 oz	175	7.5	26
Marzipan Brod	120	7	13
Atomic Fireball, 1 piece, 0.3 oz	35	0	9
Baby Ruth: King Size, 3.7 oz bar	500	24	66
2.1 oz bar	280	14	39
Fun size, 2 bars	170	8	24
Minis, 4 bars	210	9	30
Baci *(Perugino)*: 1 piece, ½ oz	75	6	7
3 pieces, 1½ oz	230	18	21
Baskin-Robbins: 3 pieces, 0.5 oz	60	1	12
Sugar Free, 4 pieces	40	1	15
Big Hunk, 2 oz	230	3	47
Bit-O-Honey, 1.7 oz	180	3.5	39
Chews, 6 pieces, 1.4 oz	160	3	32
Bliss *(Hershey's)*: Milk/Dark Choc. 6 pcs	210	14	24
Dark Chocolate Bar (1), 1.25 oz	160	12	21
Milk Choc: Meltaway Center, 6 pcs	220	15	24
Bar (1), 1.25 oz	180	12	20
Blow Pops, ea., 0.6 oz	60	0	17
Bon Bons, 3 pieces	65	0	15
Boston Baked Beans, 11 pcs, ½ oz	70	2	11
Brach's: Almond Supremes (11)	220	13	22
Bridge Mix, 16 pieces, 1.4 oz	190	8	26
Chocolate Peanut Cluster, 3 pcs	210	14	19
Double Dippers (15), 1.4 oz	210	12	23
Maple Nut Goodies (8)	190	9	27
Milk Maid Caramel (4), 1.37 oz	160	5	30
Special Treasure Butter Toffee (3)	80	2	15
Star Brites, Peppermint (3), 0.5 oz	60	0	15
Wild 'N Fruity (14), 1.4 oz	140	0	32
Breath Savers, all types, each	5	0	2
Bubble Gum: *See 'Gum' Page 77*			
Bulls Eyes, 3 pieces, 1.2 oz	130	3	23
Buncha Crunch: ⅓ cup, 1.4 oz	180	8	26
Movie Box, 3.2 oz	450	20	65
Burnt Peanuts, 31 pieces, 1.4 oz	170	6	29

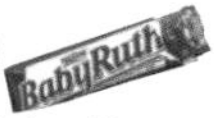

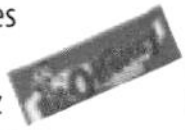

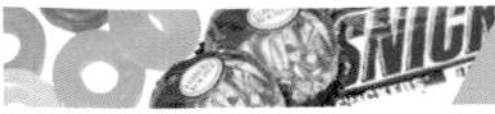

Brands & Generic (Cont)

Per Piece/Serving	C	F	Cb
Butterfinger: 2.1 oz bar	270	11	43
King Size (3), 3.7 oz	480	18	75
Fun Size, (1), 0.75	100	4	15
Giant (5 oz pkg), pieces in choc.,			
½ pkg, 2½ oz	340	16	48
Miniatures: 1 pce, 10g	45	2	7.5
4 pieces, 40g	180	7	29
On The Go, 4 bars, 1.4 oz	180	7	29
Crisp Bar: 1.76 oz bar	250	14	32
King Size, 3.17 oz	440	24	58
Minis, 2 bars	210	11	25
Butter Mints, 7 pcs, 0.46 oz	50	0	12
Butterscotch: 3 pcs	60	0	15
Chips *(Hershey's)*, 1 T.	80	4	10
Discs *(Walgreens)*, 3 pcs, 18g	70	0	17
Cadbury: Caramello Bar, 1.4 oz	200	9	28
Dairy Milk Bar, 7 pcs, 1.4 oz	200	11	23
Mini Eggs, 12 pcs,1.4 oz	190	8	28
Candy Apple, medium, 6.5 oz	280	0	60
Candy Cane, medium, 5", ½ oz	40	0	10
Candy Corn, 24 pieces	150	0	37
Candy Jar Mix *(Jewel)* (3), 0.6 oz	60	0	14
Candy Necklaces, 20g each	80	0	20
Caramels: each, 0.35 oz	40	1	8
Chocolate, each, 6.6g	25	0.3	6
Creams: 3 pcs, 1¼ oz	130	3	23
Caramel Nips: 2 pcs	60	1.5	11
Chocolate Parfait, 2 pcs	60	2	11
Peanut Butter, 2 pcs	60	2	11
Sugar Free Caramel, 2 pcs	60	1.5	12
Caramel Popcorn, ⅔ cup	150	6	23
Caramello Bar *(Cadbury)*, 1.6 oz	220	10	29
Cella's Cherries, 3 pcs, 43g	160	6	27
Certs, Breath Mints, 1 pce	5	0	2
Charleston Chew: 1 bar, 40g	160	4.5	30
Mini (13), 1.4 oz	180	6	33
Charms: Blow Pop	60	0	17
Flat Pop, 15g	50	0	14
Chew-ets Peanut Chews:			
Original, 4 pcs, 47g	230	12	29
Chewz, 1 roll, 30g	120	1	28
Chick O Stick, 2 oz	240	9	42
Chocolate Mints *(Hershey's)*, 3 mints	15	0	3
Chocolate Parfait Nips, 2 pcs	60	2	11

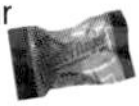
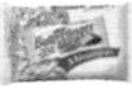
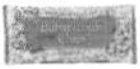
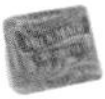

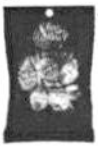

Updated Nutrition Data ~ www.CalorieKing.com
Persons with Diabetes ~ See Disclaimer (Page 24)

Per Piece/Serving	C	F	Cb
Chunky Bar *(Nestlé)*,			
King Size, 2½ oz	370	21	41
Chupa Chups, 1 Pop	50	0	12
Cinn. Buttons *(Walgreens)*, 3 pce	60	0	18
Cinnamon Disks *(Walmart)*, 3 pcs	70	0	18
Circus Peanuts, Marshmallow *(Spangler)*,			
4 pieces, 1.5 oz	150	0	38
CocoaVia, Original, 0.8 oz	100	6	12
Coconut Stacks, 8 pieces	290	13	37
Coffee Go, Candie, 4 pieces	60	1	12
Coffee Rio-Gold, each	15	0.5	3
Conversation Hearts *(Necco)*, 1 lge	10	0	3
Cookie Dough Bites, 1.4 oz	200	10	27
Cote d'Or: Dark 86% Coca, 3.5 oz	605	55	19
Dark 70%, Orange, 3.5 oz	575	46	34
Dark Raspberry, 3.5 oz	580	46	34
Milk Intense, 3.5 oz	575	40	45
Cotton Candy, 1 oz	110	0	28
Cough Drops: *See Page 77*			
Cracker Jack, ½ cup, 1 oz	120	2	23
Creme Savers: *See Lifesavers*			
Crisped Rice, Choc Chip, 1 bar, 1 oz	115	4	20
Crows, 11 pieces, 1.4 oz	130	0	33
Crunch: Original, 1.55 oz bar	220	12	29
Fun Size, 1.34 oz	210	10	29
Miniatures: 6 pce	180	9	25
Dark, 1 pce	50	3	6
Buncha Crunch, ⅓ cup, 1.3 oz	180	8	26
Crunch Crisp, 1.34 oz bar	190	11	24
Dots, 11 dots, 1.4 oz	130	0	33
Double Dip Stick, 1 stick	16	0.5	3
Dove			
Milk Choc: Singles Bar	200	12	22
Large Tablet Bar, 3.53 oz	540	33	60
Choc. Covered Almonds, 13 pieces	220	15	19
Promises: Plain, 1 piece, 0.3 oz	45	2.5	5
with Caramel, 1 piece, 0.3 oz	40	2	5
w. Peanut Butter, 1 piece, 0.3 oz	40	2	5
Dark Choc: Singles Bar, 1.3 oz	190	12	22
Large Tablet Bar, 3.53 oz	510	33	60
Choc. Covered Almonds, 13 pcs	210	15	19
Promises: W/ Raspberry Cream, 1 pce	40	3	5
with Tiramisu, 1 piece, 0.3 oz	40	2	5
Sugar Free, all flavors, 5 pieces	190	15	22
Dum Dum Pops (Spangler), 1 pop	20	0	5

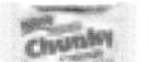
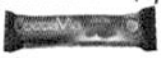

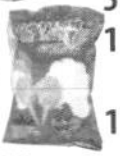
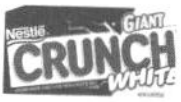

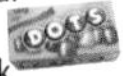
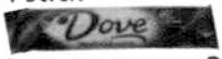

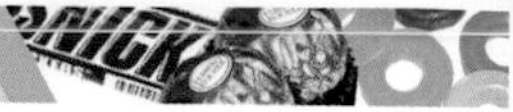

Brands & Generic (Cont)

Per Piece/Serving	C	F	Cb
English Toffee, 1 pce, 12g	**70**	**4**	6
Eda's Sugar Free, all flav., 5, ½ oz	**40**	**0**	15
5th Avenue: 2 oz bar	**260**	**12**	37
King Size bar	**480**	**24**	60
Fannie May: Single Wrapped Pieces			
Mint Milk, 1.55 oz	**190**	**6**	32
Pixie, 2 pcs, 1.6 oz	**240**	**14**	26
Trinidad, 1 pce, 1.15 oz	**160**	**9**	18
Fast Break *(Reese's)*: 2 oz bar	**260**	**12**	35
3.5 oz bar	**460**	**22**	62
Ferrero Rocher: each	**75**	**5**	5
3 pcs, 1.3 oz	**220**	**16**	16
Rondnoir (4), 1.4 oz	**210**	**14**	20
Fifty 50 Snack Bars:			
Peanut Butter, 1.2 oz	**200**	**14**	21
Almond, 7 pieces, 1.4 oz	**210**	**15**	20
Crunch Bar, 7 piece, 1.1 oz	**160**	**11**	17
Dark Choc, 7 pieces, 1.4 oz	**180**	**13**	24
Milk Choc., 7 pieces, 1.4 oz	**200**	**14**	21
Fluffy Stuff *(Charms)*,1.4 oz	**150**	**0**	40
Fondant: Choc-coated, 1.2 oz	**125**	**3**	27
Mint, 1 oz	**105**	**0**	25
Fran's: Gold Bar, 1.6 oz	**250**	**14**	27
Gold Bites (Almonds), 0.8 oz	**120**	**7**	13
Frooties, 12 pieces, 1.4 oz	**160**	**3.5**	32
Fruit Crystals *(Wonka)*, 3 pcs	**70**	**0**	17
Fruit Drops, each, ¼ oz	**20**	**0**	4
Fruit Gems *(Sunkist)*, (4), 1.4 oz	**130**	**0**	33
Fruit Leathers, average, 0.5 oz	**50**	**0.5**	12
Fruit Pastilles *(Rowntree)*, 1 roll	**185**	**0**	45
Fruit Rolls, 1 roll	**80**	**1**	17
Fruit Roll-Ups, ½ oz	**50**	**1**	12
Fruit Runts *(Walgreens)*, 12 pieces	**60**	**0**	14
Fudge: Chocolate/Vanilla (1), 1 oz	**120**	**4**	20
with Nuts (1), 1 oz	**145**	**9**	15
Choco. Marshmallow, 1 oz	**130**	**5**	20
w. Nuts, 1 oz	**135**	**6**	19
Peanut Butter, 1 oz	**115**	**3**	19
Ghirardelli:			
Squares: Dark Choc. (4), 1.6 oz	**220**	**17**	23
Milk & Caramel (3), 1.6 oz	**220**	**12**	28
3.5 oz Bars: Dark Choc., 7.5 pcs	**440**	**34**	46
Other varieties avg., 12 pcs	**440**	**28**	52
Intense Dark: Twilight Delight, 3 pcs	**200**	**17**	17
Evening Dream, 3 pcs	**190**	**15**	20

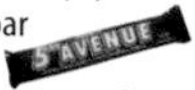

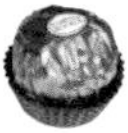

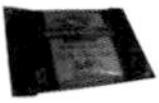

Per Piece/Serving	C	F	Cb
Godiva: Hearts, 7 pieces, 1.4 oz	**210**	**13**	23
Bars: Milk/Dark, av., 1½ oz	**230**	**14**	26
Extra Dark 72%, 1½ oz	**230**	**17**	18
Assorted Chocs, 2 pieces, 1.1 oz	**110**	**7**	11
Chocoiste: (8), 4 oz	**200**	**12**	20
Dark Choc: Almonds	**210**	**17**	16
Cherries (10)	**160**	**7**	28
Praline Pecans (7)	**210**	**41**	21
Whole Cashews (14)	**220**	**15**	19
Go Lightly: Choc Lovers Asst. (2)	**220**	**16**	28
Bags: Assorted Taffy, 5 pieces	**130**	**3**	36
Vanilla Caramels, 5 pieces	**150**	**6**	32
Sugar Free Creme Crunch (4)	**150**	**5**	33
Hard Candy (4), ½ oz	**45**	**0**	15
Goobers Peanuts, 1 pkg, 1.4 oz	**200**	**13**	21
Good & Plenty *(Hershey's)* 1.4 oz	**140**	**0**	35
GooGoo Cluster, 1 bar, 1.75 oz	**230**	**13**	28
Gum Drops: 1 small, 0.1 oz	**15**	**0**	3
5 pcs, 0.63 oz	**75**	**0**	15
Gummi: Bears, 22 bears, 1.4 oz	**150**	**0**	34
Chewy Sweet Tarts (4), 1.5 oz	**160**	**0**	36
Novelties (Walgreens), 7	**140**	**0**	34
Savers, 10 pieces	**130**	**0**	30
Worms (1), 13 pcs, 1.4 oz	**130**	**0**	31
Guylian: Milk Choc., 8 squares, 1 oz	**150**	**9**	16
Dark Choc., 8 squares, 1 oz	**140**	**9**	13
Guylian Twists, 1 piece, 0.25 oz	**45**	**3.5**	3
Seashell Bar, 40g	**210**	**13**	21
Hard Candy: All flavors (3), 0.63 oz	**60**	**0**	16
1 regular piece	**20**	**0**	5
Heath: Original (1), 1.38 oz	**210**	**13**	24
Bites, 15 pcs, 1.38 oz	**210**	**12**	25
King Size, 2.8 oz	**410**	**22**	49
Snack Size, 6 pcs, 1.4 oz	**230**	**14**	27
Hershey's:			
Milk Chocolate: 1.55 oz bar	**210**	**13**	26
Cookies 'n' Creme, 1 bars, 1.2 oz	**220**	**11**	27
King Size, 2.6 oz bar	**370**	**42**	44
7 oz bar, 3 pcs	**180**	**11**	22
with Almonds, 1.26 oz bar	**190**	**12**	20
Cacao Reserve:			
Milk Choc. (35% cacao), 4 blocks, 1.4 oz	**220**	**15**	21
Dark Choc. (65% cacao), 1.3 oz	**160**	**13**	19
Extra Dark (60% cacoa):			
Raspberry, 4 pcs, 1.4 oz	**180**	**14**	21
Pomegranate, 4 pcs, 1.4 oz	**170**	**12**	23
Candy-Coated Eggs:			
Milk Choc (8), 1.2 oz	**170**	**8**	27
with Almonds, (8) 1.2 oz	**200**	**12**	18

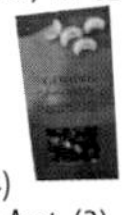

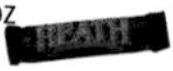

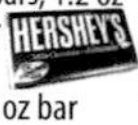

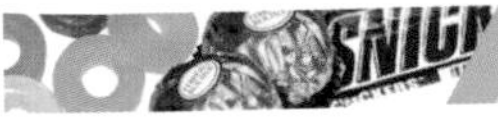

Brands & Generic (Cont)

Per Piece/Serving	C	F	Cb
Hershey's (Cont):			
Pot of Gold Chocolate:			
Nut Assortment, 4 pcs 1.4 oz	210	13	23
Caramel Assort., 4 pcs, 1.4 oz	190	10	25
Chocolate Assortment, 1.4 oz	200	12	23
Truffle Assortment, 1.5 oz	200	9	27
Special Dark Choc.: 1.45 oz bar	180	12	25
King Size, 2.6 oz	330	22	45
Lge, 3 pcs, 1.45 oz	180	12	23
Snack Size, 0.5 oz	220	13	26
Snacksters, 1 pkg, 20g	100	3.5	15
Sugar Free: Milk Choc. 5 pcs, 1.4 oz	160	13	24
Peanut Butter Cups Minis (5)	180	13	27
Special Dark Choc. (5), 1.4 oz	190	15	23
York Peppermint Patties, 3 pcs	120	8	24
Honeycomb: Plain, 1 oz	115	0	27
Choc-coated, 2 pieces	180	7	31
Hot Tamales, 20 pieces, 1.4 oz	150	0	36
Hugs ~ *See Kisses*			
Jawbreakers *(Sathers)*, (15), 0.6 oz	60	0	16
Jellies, 3 medium, 1 oz	130	0	33
Jells, Raspberry *(Joyva)*, 3 pcs, 1.55 oz	160	0	38
Jelly Beans: Small, 37 beans, 1.4 oz	120	0	35
Regular, 13 beans, 1.4 oz	150	0	37
1 bean	10	0	3
Sugar Free, 35 beans	80	0	37
Jumbo, 1 bean	20	0	5
Jewel, 13 beans, 1.4 oz	140	0	36
Sathers/Walgreens, 13 pieces	150	0	38
Wonderbeans, 33 beans	100	0	24
Jelly Bellys: each	4	0	1
35 pcs, 1.4 oz	140	0	37
Sugar Free Beans/Sours (35), 1.4 oz	80	0	37
Jelly Rings *(Jewel)*, 5 pieces, 1.4 oz	110	0	26
Jolly Rancher:			
Gummies, 10 pcs	120	0	28
Hard Candy, 3 pcs	70	0	17
Jelly Beans, 30 pieces, 1.4 oz	140	0	36
Lollipops (1), 0.55 oz	60	0	15
Screaming Sours, 3 pieces, 2 oz	200	0	49
Soft & Chewy, 1pkt, 2 oz	200	0	49
Sour Blasts, 4 pieces, ½ oz	50	0	13
Jujubees, all types (52), 40g	110	0	28
Juju Bears, 5 pieces	130	0	34
Juju Mix *(Sathers)*, 11 pieces, 1½ oz	150	0	36
Jujyfruits, 16 pieces, 1.4 oz	120	0	32

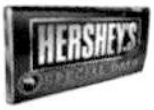

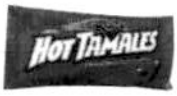

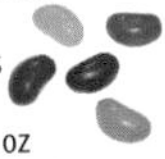

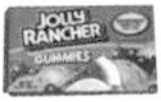

Per Piece/Serving	C	F	Cb
Junior Caramels: 13 pcs, 1.48 oz	190	6	34
Mini, 2 boxes, 1 oz	130	4	23
Junior Mints: 1.83 oz	220	4	45
16 pcs, 1.4 oz	170	3	35
Kissables, 39 pcs, 1.4 oz	180	9	28
Kisses:			
Milk Choc, 1 pce, 0.16 oz	25	1.5	2.5
9 pieces, 1 oz	230	13	24
Caramel Filled 9 pcs, 1.5 oz	190	9	27
Cherry Cordial, 9 pcs, 1.5 oz	180	7	30
Pink Kisses, 9 pcs, 1.4 oz	230	13	24
Special Dark, 9 pieces, 1.4 oz	180	12	25
Kit Kat: 4-piece bar, 1.5 oz	200	11	27
King Size, 8 pce, 3 oz bar	420	22	54
Snack Size, 3 pcs, 1.48 oz	210	11	27
Extra Krispy Bar (1)	220	11	27
White Choc, 4 piece, 1½ oz	220	12	26
Kraft, Caramels (5), 1.4 oz	160	3.5	31
Kudos: *See Page 139*			
Lance, Peanut Bar, 2.3 oz pkg	340	19	29
Lemon Drops (4), 0.6 oz	60	0	16
Sugar Free *(Walgreens)* (3), 0.6 oz	50	0	17
Lemonhead (20), 1 oz	100	0	28
Licorice: Average all types, 1oz	100	0	25
Bites *(Switzer)*, each	10	0	3
Chews *(Panda)*, each	10	0	3
Tid Bits, each	10	0	1.5
Twists: Black/Red, avg. 1 pce	35	0	8
Sugar Free, 1 piece	13	0	2.5
American Licorice Co.: Extinguisher (1)	160	1.5	37
Red Vines, 7 pcs, 1.4 oz	140	0	33
Sip-n-Chew, 1 pkg, 1 oz	100	1	23
Snaps, 4 pcs, 1.4 oz	140	0	34
Sour Punch, 6 pcs, 1.4 oz	150	0.5	34
Super Ropes (1), 2 oz	200	0	46
Superstring, 1⅓ pieces	140	0	34
Sugar Free Red Twists (7)	90	0	25
Lifesavers: Large size, 1 candy	15	0	3
Regular, all flavors, 1 candy	10	0	2.5
1 Roll (14 candies), 1.14 oz	140	0	35
Creme Savers: 3 pieces, 0.5 oz	60	1	11
Sugar Free, 4 pieces	45	1.5	13
Gummies (4), 0.5 oz	45	0	11
Pep-o-mint (4), ½ oz	60	0	16
Fruit Splosion, 10 pcs, 1.4 oz	130	0	31
Sugar-Free Delites: *Per Candy*			
Orchard Fruits; Summer Blend	7	0	2.5
Butter Toffee; European Collect.	10	1	2.5

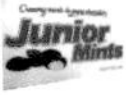

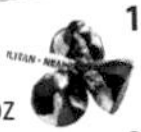

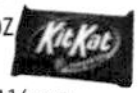

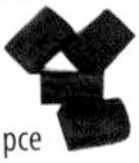

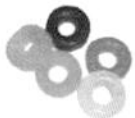

Updated Nutrition Data ~ www.CalorieKing.com
Persons with Diabetes ~ See Disclaimer (Page 24)

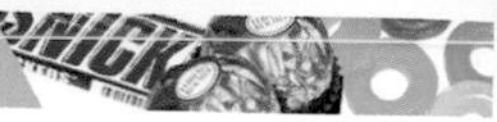

Brands & Generic (Cont)

Per Piece/Serving	C	F	Cb
Lik-m-aid *(Nestlé)*, Wonka Fun Dip, 1 pkg	50	0	13
Lindt: Lindor, Truffles avg. (1)	75	6	5
Milk Chocolate Bars: Raspb. (5)	200	10	25
Truffles, 7 pieces	240	18	18
Classic Recipe, Hazelnut (10)	230	16	20
70% Cocoa, 4 pieces 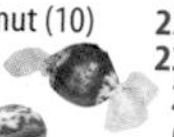	220	17	13
Lollipops: Mini, ¼ oz	25	0	6
Small, ½ oz 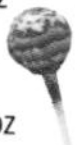	50	0	12
Medium, 1 oz	100	0	25
Giant (4" diam), 7 oz	790	0	198
M & M's:			
Milk Chocolate, 1 pce 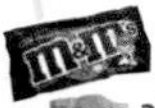	5	0.1	0.5
20 pcs, 0.6 oz	70	3	10
1.7 oz package 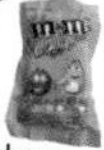	240	10	34
13 pieces, 1.5 oz	210	9	30
Dark Choc.: 1.5 oz pkg	230	14	25
Fun Size, 18g package	90	4	13
Almond Choc., 1.3 oz package	200	11	21
Minis, 1 tube, 1.08 oz 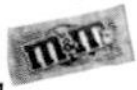	280	13	37
Peanut: 1.74 oz pkg	250	13	30
Fun Size, 18g pkg	90	4.5	11
Peanut Butter, 1.6 oz package	240	14	26
Premiums: Choc. Raspb. Almond			
¼ cup, 1½ oz	240	16	20
Dark; Triple, avg., 1½ oz	230	14	25
Mamba, 9 pcs, 1½ oz	170	2.5	36
Marshmallow Egg, 1 egg, 1 oz	120	3	22
Mary Jane, 5 pieces, 1.4 oz	160	4	32
Marshmallows: Firm/Soft, 1 oz	90	0	23
Regular size, 4 pieces, 30g	100	0	24
Mini-Marshmallow, ⅔ cup, 1 oz	95	0	24
Choc-coat. Twists (Joyva), each	95	2	10
Fluff, 2 Tbsp, 0.63 oz	60	0	15
Kraft: Mini, ½ cup, 1 oz 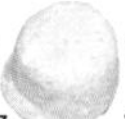	100	0	24
Creme, 2 Tbsp	45	0	11
Jet-Puffed, 5 pcs, 1 oz	100	0	24
Funmallows, ⅔ cup, 30g	100	0	24
Marzipan, 2 Tbsp, 39g	160	4	29
Mauna Loa (10), 1.3 oz 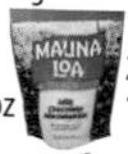	220	16	21
Mexican Hats (7), 1.34 oz	120	0	30
Mentos: Regular (1)	10	0	3
Sugar Free (1) 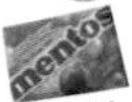	5	0	2.5
Mike & Ike:			
Orig.: 1 pkg, 2.1 oz 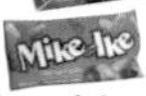	220	0	55
23 pieces, 40g	140	0	36
Milkfulls *(Storck)*, 6 pieces, 1.4 oz	170	3	35
Milk Chocolate: *See Hershey's*			
Milk Duds, 13 pcs, 1.4 oz 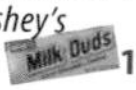	170	6	28

Per Piece/Serving	C	F	Cb
Milky Way:			
Bars: Single, 2 oz	260	10	41
Fun Size (2), 1.2 oz 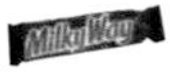	150	6	24
To Go, 1.8 oz	230	9	36
Miniatures (5), 1.52 oz	190	8	30
Midnight Bar (1), 1.76 oz	220	8	36
Mints: Uncoated, 3 pieces	70	0	17
1 mint (¾" diam.)	7	0	1
1 large mint (1½" diam.)	15	0	3
Mon Cheri *(Ferrero)*, 4 pcs, 1.59 oz	260	18	20
Mounds: 1.7 oz bar	230	13	29
Snack, 0.6 oz 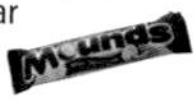	80	4.5	10
King Size, 3½ oz	460	26	58
Minis, 3 pcs, 1.45 oz	190	11	24
Mr Goodbar, 1.37 oz bar	200	13	21
Mrs Fields Choc, 2 pieces, 1.16 oz	160	6	26
Munch Bar, 1.42 oz	220	15	18
Necco Candy Wafers (40) 2 oz	220	0	56
Newman's Own:			
Milk Chocolate, Caramel Cups (3)	160	8	21
Dark Chocolate: Caramel Cups (3)	160	9	21
Peanut Butter Cups (3)	180	12	17
Nibs, all types, 1 pouch, 2.25 oz	220	2	50
Nips, all flavors, 2 pcs, ½ oz	60	2	11
Nougat: 3 pcs, 1.48 oz 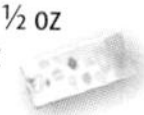	170	1	39
Choc. Covered, 1 oz	125	4	22
Nuggets: Milk Chocolate, 4 pieces	200	12	25
w/ Toffee & Almonds, 4 pcs, 1.3 oz	200	13	21
Special Dark w. Almonds, 4 pieces	180	13	20
Nutrageous Bar *(Reese's)*, 1.8 oz	260	16	28
Oh Henry!, 2.2 oz bar	300	17	26
Orange Slices: *Jewel*, 3, 1½ oz	140	0	35
Walgreens, 4 pcs, 1.6 oz	160	0	39
Pastel Mints *(Walgreens)*, 20 pcs	60	0	14
Patteez *(Sweet n' Low)*, 4 piecs	100	2	29
PayDay Bar: 1.85 oz bar	240	13	27
King Size, 3.4 oz bar 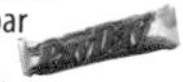	480	24	52
Snack Size, 0.7 oz	90	5	10
Avalanche, 1.8 oz bar	260	14	29
Peanut Bar, 1.6 oz bar	235	15	21
Peanut Butter Cups: *See Reese's; Newman's Own*			
Peanut Brittle: 1 piece, 1½ oz	190	5	32
Sugar Free *(Russell Stover)*			
4 pcs, 1.3 oz	140	10	24
Peanuts, choc-covered, 14 piecs	230	14	23
Pearson's Mint Patties, (5), 1.34 eoz	150	2.5	31
Pecan Roll, ⅓ bar, 1.4 oz	190	10	24
Peppermints, 7 small, 0.5 oz 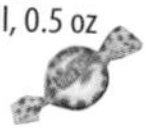	60	0	15
Brach's, 3 pieces	60	0	16

Brands & Generic (Cont)

Per Piece/Serving	C	F	Cb
Pez, 1 roll	35	0	9
Planters: Choc. Peanuts (25) 7 oz	220	15	20
Orig. Peanut Bar, 1.6 oz	230	14	22
Pops ~ *See Lollipops*			
Pop Rocks, 0.34 oz pkg	35	0	9
Pot of Gold:			
Assortment: Caramel, 4 pieces	190	10	25
Nut, 4 pieces	210	13	23
Pretzels: Choc-covered, Mini (6), 38g	200	9	25
White Choc Bites (23), 40g	200	9	25
Pretzel Flipz *(Nestlé)*, 8 pcs, 1 oz	130	5	20
Raisinets: Milk Choc: 1 pkg, 1.6 oz	190	8	30
King Size, 2.8 oz	330	13	56
Movie Pack, 3.5 oz	380	16	64
Dark Choc., ¼ c., 1.6 oz	180	8	32
Reese's			
Clusters, 3 pcs, 1½ oz	220	12	24
Crispy Crunchy Bar: 1.7 oz	260	18	22
2 pcs, 1.2 oz	190	11	18
King Size, 3.1 oz bar	460	26	52
Fast Break, 2 oz bar	260	12	35
Peanut Butter Chips, 1 Tbsp, 15g	80	4	8
Peanut Butter Cups: 2 cups, 1.5 oz	200	12	22
King Size (1), 2.8 oz	400	24	44
Mini, 5 pcs, 1.55 oz	220	13	25
8-Pack, 1 pce, ½ oz	80	4.5	9
Snack Size, 1 pce, 0.74 oz	110	6.5	12
Sugar Free: 5 pcs, avg., 1.38 oz	180	13	27
Caramel Filled (2),1.4 oz	150	11	27
Big Cup: Regular, 1.4 oz	200	12	22
King Size (2), 2.8 oz	400	22	24
White Chocolate (2), 1.5 oz	220	13	22
Pieces: Regular, 51 pcs, 1.4 oz	190	9	25
Mini, 1 Tbsp, ½ oz	70	3	10
Sticks: 1.5 oz	210	13	23
King Size (1), 3 oz	440	26	46
Snack Size (1), 0.6 oz	90	5	9
Snacksters, 1 pkg, ¾ oz	100	4	14
Whipps, (40% less fat). 1½ oz	230	9	37
Rice Krispies Treats *(Kellogg's)*:			
1 bar, average all varieties	100	3	17
Rice Crunchy Bars, 1.4 oz bar	200	11	23
Riesen Choc. Chew, 4 pcs, 1.26 oz	170	6	28
Rocky Road, 2 oz bar	240	11	34
Roca Thins, all flavors, 4 pieces	210	15	23
Rolo: All types, per roll, 1.7 oz	220	10	33
Bites, 7 pieces, 1.4 oz	190	9	29
Root Beer Barrels (3) 0.63 oz	60	0	17

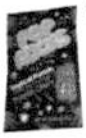
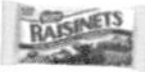

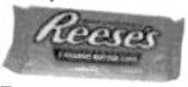

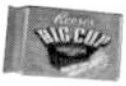

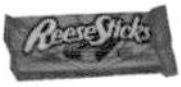

Per Piece/Serving	C	F	Cb
Russell Stover Candy:			
Boxed Chocolates: Chocolate Coated			
Assorted (2), 1.13 oz	150	6	23
Cherry Cordials (3), 1.34 oz	150	5	25
Dairy Cream Caramels (2), 1.16 oz	150	7	22
Elegant Assortment, 3, 1.59 oz	210	10	28
French Choc. Mints, 4, 1.34 oz	220	13	22
Nut, Chewy & Crisp Centers, 2	160	8	21
Pecan Delights, 2, 1.83 oz	270	16	32
Sugar Free: Assort. Candies, 3, 1.55 oz	180	13	26
Pecan Delights, 2, 1.66 oz	210	17	27
Bags: Assorted Fruit, 3, 0.6 oz	40	0	17
Butter Cream Caramels, 3, 1.52 oz	150	10	25
Chocolate Peanuts, 25, 1.4 oz	190	14	20
Chocolate Truffles, 3, 1.52 oz	180	13	25
Peanut Butter Cups, 2, 1.2 oz	160	12	17
Salt Water Taffy (Brach's), 5	170	2.5	36
Seashells *(Guylian)*, 1 shell, 1.4 oz	210	13	21
See's Candies:			
Almond Royal, 5 pieces, 1.3 oz	190	13	18
Butterscotch Chews (5), 1.5 oz	210	12	27
Krispy's: Caffe Latte, 5 pcs 1.3 oz	180	8	27
Mint, 5 pieces, 1.3 oz	170	8	27
Little Pops:			
Butterscotch (4), 0.5 oz	70	2	13
Cafe Latte (4), 0.5 oz	70	2	12
Chocolate (4), 0.5 oz	70	3	11
Vanilla (4), 0.5 oz	50	2	9
Lollypops, average, 0.7 oz	90	3	17
Milk Molasses Chips, 6 pieces, 1.4 oz	180	8	27
Milk Peppermints, 2 pieces, 1.23 oz	150	4	28
Peanut Butter Bar, 1 oz	150	10	15
Peppermint Twists (3), 0.53 oz	60	0	15
Raisins, Dark/Light (28), 1.4 oz	170	7	29
Toffee-ettes, 3 pieces, 1.6 oz	270	21	18
Sugar Free: Dark Bar, 1.5 oz	180	16	24
Dark Walnut Clusters, 1.5 oz	220	20	18
Peanut Brittle, 1.5 oz	170	14	17
Skittles: Sour, 2 oz bag	230	2.5	52
Tropical/Wild Berry, 2.17 oz	250	2.5	56
Fun Size, 1 bag, 0.5 oz	60	1	14
Tear & Share, 4 oz bag	420	4.5	93
Skor Toffee Bar (1), 1.4 oz	200	12	25
Smarties:			
Candy Rolls (1), ¼ oz	25	0	6
Giant, 2 pieces, ¼ oz	25	0	6

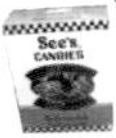

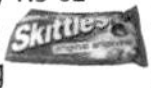

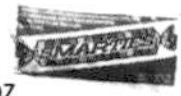

Brands & Generic (Cont)

Per Piece/Serving	C	F	Cb
Snack Barz *(Hershey's)*, 0.88 oz	120	5	16
Snickers: 2.07 oz bar	280	14	35
King Size, 3.29 oz 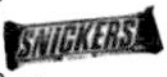	440	22	56
Fun Size, 2 bars, 1.2 oz	8	21	
Amond Bar, 1.76 oz	240	11	32
Creme Egg (1), 1 oz	150	8	17
Cruncher, 1.56 oz	230	13	25
Fudge, 1.78 oz 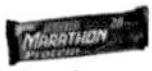	250	13	31
Marathon Bar, av., 1.9 oz bar	215	8	27
Miniatures, 4 pieces, 1.27 oz	170	9	22
Munch Bar, 1.4 oz bar	220	15	18
Sno Caps, ¼ cup, 1.4 oz	180	8	30
Soft 'N Chewy Butter Toffee, each	30	0.5	5
Sorbee: Choc., ½ bar, 1.4 oz	180	12	25
Crystal Light Hard Candy, 4 pieces	25	0	13
(Note: Carb figures include Isomalt which has fewer calories than sugar.)			
Sour Patch: All types, 1.5 oz 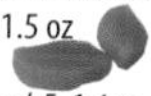	150	0	37
1 straw	20	0	5
Spearmint Leaves: *Jewel*, 5, 1.4 oz	140	0	35
Walgreens, 4 pieces, 1.62 oz	160	0	39
Spree Candies: Original, 15 pieces	50	0	13
Chewy Spree, 8 pieces	60	0	13
Starburst: Candy Canes, 0.5 oz	70	0	18
Fruit Chews, each	20	0.4	4
2 oz pkg 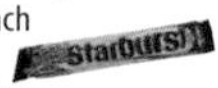	240	5	49
Jellybeans, 1.5 oz	150	0	37
Jellybean Egg, 2 oz	200	0	51
Tropical Fruit, 2.07 oz pack	240	5	49
Starlight Mints, 3 pieces, 0.56 oz	60	0	15
Suckers *(Walgreens)* (1), 0.39 oz	45	0	11
Sugar Babies, 1.4 oz	160	1.5	37
Sugar Coated Peanuts, 1 oz	120	8	10
Sunbursts Sunflowers *(Kimmie)*:			
Coffee Break Tube, 1.41 oz	200	11	22
Candy Bar Bag, 1.7 oz 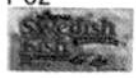	190	9	27
Swedish Fish (7), 1.48 oz	150	0	38
Sweet 'N Low: Chews (1)	20	0.5	5
Coffee Cremes (1)	40	3	6
Wafer Bars, average, 3 pieces	140	7	23
Mint Cremes, 3½ pieces	120	9	22
Mint Patteez, 4 pieces	100	2	29
Sweet Escapes: *See Hershey's*			
Symphony: 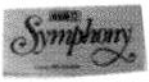			
Milk Choc: 1.5 oz bar	220	14	23
Large Block, 3 pieces, 1.27 oz	190	11	21
w. Almds & Toffee (1), 1.48 oz	220	13	21

Per Piece/Serving	C	F	Cb
Taffy, 1 piece, 1 oz	60	0	17
Take 5 *(Hershey's)*: 1.5 oz	200	11	25
King Size, 2.6 oz 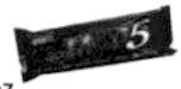	370	22	44
Snack Size, 2 pces	210	13	26
Marshmallow, 1.3 oz	180	9	22
3 Musketeers: Original, 2.13 oz	260	8	46
Fun Size, 3 pieces, 1.66 oz	190	6	34
Minis, 7 pieces, 1.4 oz	170	5	32
Mint Bar, 2 pieces, 1.24 oz	150	5	26
Pop'ables (15)	180	6	31
Tang-a-Roos, 1 roll	25	0	6
Terry's Choc Orange, (5), 1.5 oz	230	12	27
Tic Tac, all varieties, each	2	0	0
Toblerone: 1.8 oz bar	260	13	32
1 bar: 3.5 oz 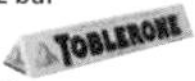	510	30	63
1.23 oz bar	180	9	23
Toffees, Regular, 1 oz	160	9	18
Toll House Milk Choc. Morsels, 1Tbsp	70	4	9
Tootsie Pops (1), 0.6 oz	60	0	15
Tootsie Roll: 2.25 oz roll	245	2	55
Mini Chews, 1.4 oz 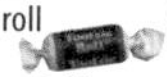	120	3.5	31
Truffles: Regular, 1 pce, 0.42 oz	60	4	6
Large *(Godiva)*, ¾ oz	110	6.5	12
Extra Large *(J.Schmidt)*, 1½ oz	220	13	24
Turtles *(Nestlé)*: Average, each	80	4.5	10
Sugar Free, 3 pieces, 1.34 oz	150	11	20
Twists (Sugar Free): Licorice; Strawberry, 7 twists, 1.4 oz	90	0	25
Twix: 2 cookies, 2 oz	280	14	37
Fun Size, 0.5 oz 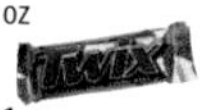	80	4	10
Twix 4 To Go	480	24	64
Minis, 3 pieces, 1 oz	150	8	20
Caramel, 0.85 oz	130	6	16
Peanut Butter 4 To Go	480	28	48
Peanut Butter, 1.8 oz	280	17	28
Twizzlers: Bites (17), 1.4 oz	140	0.5	32
Cherry Nibs, 2.3 oz package	220	2	50
Pull 'n' Peel Cherry, 1.16 oz	100	0	25
Sourz Assorted, 1.8 oz 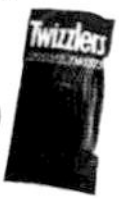	180	1.5	40
Strawz, 1 pkg., 1.6 oz	150	1	35
Sweet & Sour Filled (2)	140	2	30
Twists Strawberry, 1.6 oz	150	1	35
U-No Bar 1.5 oz	250	17	22
Weight Watchers *(Whitman's)*:			
Butter Cream Caramel (3)	150	8	23
Caramel Medallions (3)	160	9	24
English Toffee Squares (3)	150	9	21
Mint Patties (3) 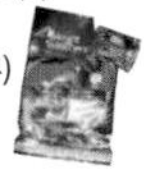	150	9	23
Peanut Butter Cups (4)	180	8	31
Pecan Crowns (3)	160	10	24

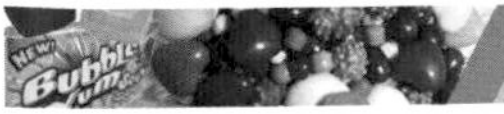

Brands & Generic (Cont)

Per Piece/Serving	C	F	Cb
Werther's: Original, 3 pce, 0.56 oz	70	1.5	14
Chewy Caramel (6), 1.31 oz	170	5	30
Caramelts (8), 1.4 oz	250	18	18
Sugar-Free, 5 pieces	40	1	14
Whatchamacallit Bar, 1.6 oz	230	12	28
King Size, 2.6 oz	370	20	45
Whitman's: Sampler (4), 1.75 oz	240	11	33
12 oz Box, 4 pieces, 1.59 oz	220	12	27
Sugar Free, 10 oz Box, 3 pcs, 1.42 oz	180	12	25
Reserve, 7 oz Box, 2 pcs, 1.16 oz	160	9	21
Whoppers, average all flav., 18 pcs	190	8	28
Wonka: Wonka Bar (1), 2.6 oz	360	19	49
Laffy Taffy: Orig., 5 bars, 1.5 oz	160	2	36
Stretchy & Tangy, 1½ oz	165	4	33
Nerds, 0.5 oz	60	0	14
Gobstopper, 9 pcs, 0.5 oz	60	0	14
Runts Fruit Box, 1.8 oz	210	0	49
Yogurt Candy,			
Coated Raisins, 27 pieces, 1.4 oz	180	8	28
York Peppermint Pattie:			
Regular, 1.4 oz	140	2.5	31
Fun Size, 0.6 oz	60	1	14
King Size, 1.45 oz	150	3	33
York Mints, (3)	10	0	3
Zachary Choc. Peanuts, 1.48 oz	240	15	21
Zagnut, 1.52 oz bar	200	8	31
Zero Bar: 1.8 oz bar	230	8	37
King Size, 3.4 oz	400	14	68
Zingos, 3 pieces, 0.07 oz	5	0	2

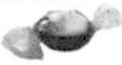
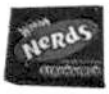

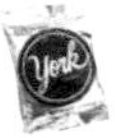

Gum ~ *Per Piece*

	C	F	Cb
Bazooka, each	15	0	4
Beechies	6	0	2
Big League Chew	10	0	2
Double Bubble Ball	20	0	5
Bubble Yum	25	0	6
Sugarless	10	0	3
Candilicious	30	0	2
Carefree (Sugarless/Regular)	5	0	2
Chiclets, 1 piece	5	0	1
Clorets, 1 stick	10	0	2
Dentyne	5	0	0.5
Estee, bubble/regular	5	0	2
Extra *(Wrigley's),*			
Sugar-Free	5	0	2
Freshen-Up	10	0	3
Hubba Bubba: Regular	20	0	5
Sugar-free, average	14	0	0.5
Ice Breakers	5	0	2
Jolt Gum, 2 pieces	10	0	3
Super Bubble	15	0	4
Trident, Original; White	5	0	1
Wrigley's, all flavors	10	0	2

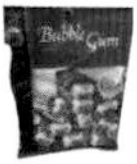

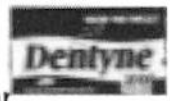

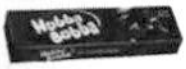

Updated Nutrition Data ~ www.CalorieKing.com
Persons with Diabetes ~ See Disclaimer (Page 24)

Carob Candy

Per Piece/Serving	C	F	Cb
Carob: Plain/Natural, 1 oz	155	9	15
Carob Coated: Raisins, 1 oz	130	8	15
Almonds/Peanuts, 1 oz	150	10	14
Malt Balls, 1 oz	135	8	15
Caramels, 1 oz	110	4	18
Dates, 1 oz	125	5	20
Soybeans	145	9	16
Trail/Party Mix, 1 oz	150	9	15
Carob Chips, unsweetened, 1 oz	155	9	15

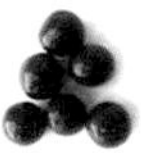

Cough Drops

	C	F	Cb
Beech Nut, 1 drop	10	0	2
CVS, Sour Lemon Throat Drops			
Diabetic Tussin, 1 drop	0	0	0
Halls Defense Vit. C, 1 drop	15	0	4
Sugar Free, 1 drop	5	0	3
Halls Fruit Breezers, 1 drop	15	0	4
Halls Menthol Drops, 1 drop	15	0	4
Sugar Free, 1 drop	5	0	4
Halls Plus, 1 drop	20	0	5
Listerine Lozenge (Amer. Chicle)	10	0	2
Luden's Throat Drops, all flavors, 1	10	0	2
Sugar Free, 1 drop	0	0	0
Pine Bros, 1 cough drop	10	0	2
Ricola: Cough Drops (1)	10	0	3
Sugar-Free Lemon Mint (2)	0	0	1
Rite Aid, Menthol Cough (1)	10	0	3
Robitussin: Regular, 1 drop	15	0	3
Honey Cough, 1 drop	40	0	10
Sugar Free Throat, 1 drop	10	0	3
Sunny Orange Vit. C, 1 drop	10	0	3
Rolaids Sodium Free, 1	5	0	1
Sathers Peppermint Lozenges, 1	15	0	3
Squibb Cough/Throat Loz.'s, 1	15	0	4
Sucrets *(Beecham)* Lozenges, 1	10	0	2
Wintergreen Loz. *(Walgreens),* 1	15	0	3

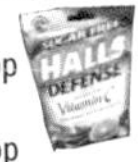

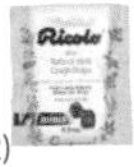

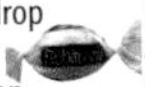

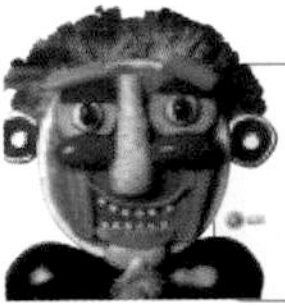

Eat at least 5 servings of fruit and vegetables every day . . . and Enjoy Better Health!

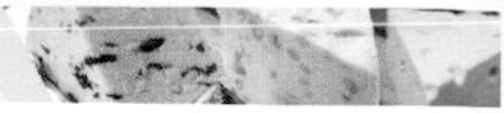

Quick Guide

Firm/Hard Cheeses	C	F	Cb
(American, Cheddar, Colby, Swiss)			
Regular Cheese:			
Thin Deli slice, ¾ oz	90	7	0
1 oz slice/piece	115	9	0.5
8 oz package	915	75	3
16 oz (1lb) package	1830	150	6
Cubes: 1" cube, ¾ oz	85	7	0.5
1¼" cube, 1 oz slice	115	9	0.5
Diced: 1 cup, 4½ oz	530	40	2
Grated: 1 Tbsp, ¼ oz	30	2.5	0
Shredded: Cheddar, ¼ cup, 1 oz	115	9	0.5
1 cup, 4 oz	455	37	1.5
Cheddar, Reduced-Fat, ¼ cup, 1 oz	80	6	1
Mozzarella: ¼ cup, 1 oz	85	6.5	0.5
Part-Skim, ¼ cup, 1 oz	70	5	1
Sliced: 1 thin (3½" square), ¾ oz	85	7	0.5
Rectangular (7"x 4"x ⅛"), 1½ oz	170	14	0.5
Round (3¼" diameter x ⅛"), ¾ oz	85	7	0.5
Semi-circular, 1¼ oz (5½" long, 3½" radius, ⅛" thick)	140	12	0.5
Fat-Free: Average all brands, 1 oz	40	0	2
Low-Fat: Average all brands, 1 oz	50	2	0.5
Reduced Fat: Average all brands, 1 oz	80	5	0.5

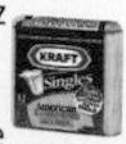

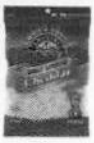

Cheese

Per 2 Tbsp, 1 oz Unless Indicated	C	F	Cb
American:			
Regular: 1 slice, 1 oz	105	9	0.5
Alpine Lace, 1 oz	90	7	2
Kraft, 0.7 oz slice	70	5	2
Shedded, ¼ cup, 1 oz	115	9	0.5
Land O'Lakes, 0.7 oz slice	70	5	2
Light: *Kraft* (2% Milk), 0.7 oz slice	50	3	1
Fat-Free: *Kraft,* 0.7 oz slice	30	0	2
Borden, Singles, 0.8 oz slice	80	0	2
Babybel, Mini *(Laughing Cow):*			
Original/Bonbel (1), ¾ oz	70	6	0
Light Original (1), ¾ oz	50	3	0
Gouda (1), ¾ oz	80	6	0
Blue/Bleu	100	8	0.5
Bonbel *(Laughing Cow),* 1 piece	70	6	0
Brick *(Land O'Lakes),* 1" cube, 1 oz	110	8	1
Camembert	85	7	0
Caraway	105	8	1
Castello *(Wegman's),* average, 1 oz	120	12	0

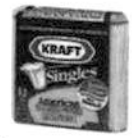

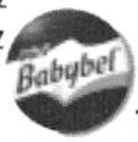

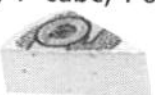

Cheese (Cont)

Per 2 Tbsp, 1 oz Unless Indicated	C	F	Cb
Cheddar: (Also see 'Quick Guide')			
Regular	115	9	0.5
Alpine Lace	90	7	0
Reduced-Fat/Low-Fat:			
Borden, Shredded, ¼ cup, 1 oz	80	6	1
Cabot Vermont, 50% Light, 1 oz	70	4.5	0.5
Fat-Free, Kraft, 0.7 oz slice	30	0	2
Cheese Balls *(Kaukauna),* average	100	7	0.5
Cheese Curds: Fresh, ¼ cup, 1 oz	110	9	0
Breaded & Fried ~ *See Page 80*			
Cheese Logs *(Kaukauna),* average	100	7	0.5
Cheshire	110	9	1.5
Colby: Regular	110	9	0.5
Reduced-Fat *(Kraft)*	80	6	0
Colby-Jack, regular	110	9	1
Cottage Cheese: ***Average All Brands***			
Creamed (4% milk fat): 2 Tbsp, 1 oz	30	1	1.5
½ cup, 4 oz	120	5	6
With fruit, ½ cup, 4 oz	130	4	15
Reduced-Fat (2%): 2 Tbsp, 1 oz	25	0.5	1
½ cup, 4 oz	100	2	4
Low-Fat (1%): 2 Tbsp, 1 oz	20	.5	1
½ cup, 4 oz	80	1	3
Fat-Free/Non-Fat: 2 Tbsp, 1 oz	20	0	1
(Jewel), ½ cup, 4 oz	80	0	5
Friendship: Low-Fat Pineapple, 4 oz	120	1	16
Non-Fat with Peach, ½ cup, 4 oz	110	0	15
Pot Style, ½ cup, 4 oz	90	2.5	3
Hood w. Chive/Onion, 4 oz	90	1	5
Knudsen:			
Free: Non-Fat, ½ cup, 4.oz	80	0	7
2% Milk Fat, ½ cup., 4 oz	100	2.5	6
Cottage Doubles, av., 5.5 oz carton	150	2.5	18
On the Go! Free, 4 oz carton	70	0	7
Low-Fat, 4 oz carton	90	2.5	6
Lactaid: Low-Fat, ½ cup, 4 oz	80	1	7
Light N' Lively: Fat-Free, 4.4 oz	80	0	8
Low-Fat, ½ cup, 4.4 oz	80	1.5	6
Live Active (Low-Fat 2%):			
Plain, 1/2 cup, 4 oz	90	2	10
Mixed Berry; Pineapple, av., 4 oz	120	1.5	18
Cream Cheese: *See Page 81*			
Edam, Regular	100	8	0.5
Farmer *(Friendship)*	50	2.5	0
Feta: Regular	75	6	1
Crumbled, ½ cup, 2½ oz	190	15	3
Red.-Fat *(Athenos)*	60	4	1
Fontina	110	9	0.5
Gjetost (Goat's Milk, fresh)	130	8	12

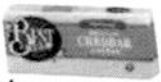

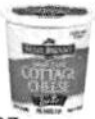

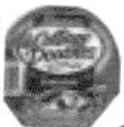

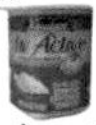

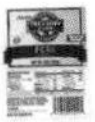

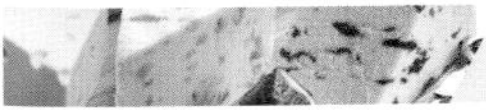

Cheese (Cont)

Per 2 Tbsp, 1 oz Unless Indicated

	C	F	Cb
Goat's Milk Cheese:			
Chevre, Soft	80	6	1
Chavril: Regular	60	4.5	0.5
Semi-Soft	100	8.5	1
Hard	130	10	0.5
Gorgonzola	100	8	0.5
Galbani Dolcelatte	95	8	1
Gouda	100	8	0.5
Gruyere	115	9	1
Havarti *(Land O'Lakes)*	110	8	1
Italian Blend *(Sargento)*	90	7	1
Jarlsberg *(Wegman's)*	100	8	0
Jarlsberg Reduced Fat, shredded	70	4	0
Kefir *(Alta Dena)*	70	6	2
Labneh (Lebanese Cream Cheese), 1.8 oz	70	4	4
Lactose Free Cheese *(Lifetime)*	40	0	1
Limburger	95	8	0
Mascarpone *(Wegman's)*	130	13	1
Mexican:			
Cacique: Cotija	110	9	0
Queso Fresco	80	6	0
Queso Quesadilla	70	5	2
Ranchero	80	6	0
Chi-Chi's: Con Quéso	90	7	4
Hot/Medium/Mild/Acante	10	0	2
Kraft, Taco, shredded	100	8	2
Sargento, Shredded	110	9	0.5
Supremo Chihuahua: Quéso Bianco	100	8	0
Quéso Fresco; Rancherito	80	6	0
Monterey	105	8.5	0
Monterey Jack: Regular	110	9	0
Kraft 2% Milk Reduced Fat	80	6	1
Alpine Lace, Co-Jack	90	7	0
Weight Watchers	90	6	1
Mozzarella:			
Regular	85	6.5	0.5
Land O'Lakes/Polly-O, average	90	6	1
Shredded	90	7	1
Light: *Polly-O Lite,* Shredded	60	2.5	1
Kraft 2% Milk Fat, Reduced Fat	70	4	1
Sargento Reduced Fat	80	4.5	1
Part Skim: *Alpine Lace*	70	5	1
Borden/Kraft, Shredded	80	5	1
Polly-O, String (2% milk), 1 stick	70	4.5	0.5
Fat-Free: *Polly-O*	35	0	1
Kraft, shredded	45	0	2
Muenster: Regular	105	9	0.5
Low-Fat	85	5	1
Myzithra, grated, 4 T. 1 oz	80	4	2
Neufchatel:	75	6	1
Philadelphia	70	6	1
Flavored: Fruit/Herbs	80	7	1
Chocolate *(Hickory Farms)*	110	8	1

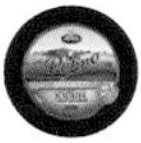

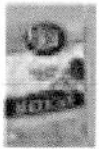

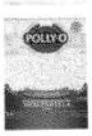

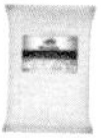

Cheese (Cont)

Per 2 Tbsp, 1 oz Unless Indicated

	C	F	Cb
Parmesan: Fresh/Block	110	7.5	1
Grated (Packaged): 1 Tbsp	20	1.5	0
1 oz quantity	120	8	1
½ cup, 1¾ oz	215	14	2
with Romano *(Frigo),* grated	110	7	0
Kraft Reduced-Fat Topping, 1 Tbsp	20	1	2
Pizza Cheese, shredded:			
Regular *(Kraft)* ¼ cup, 1 oz	90	7	1
Port de Salut	100	8	0
Port Wine (Kaukauna)	90	6	4
Pot *(Sargento)*	25	0	1
Provolone: Regular	100	7.5	0.5
Reduced-Fat: *Alpine Lace*	80	5	1
Sargento, 1 slice, ⅔ oz	50	3.5	0
Pub *(Rondele),* average	95	7	1
Quark: 40% fat	47	3	1
20% fat	32	1.5	1
Skim/Non-Fat	22	0	1.5
Queso: Anejo/Asadero/Blanco	105	9	1
Chichuahua/De Papa	110	9	2
Ricotta Cheese:			
Whole Milk	50	3.5	1
½ cup, 4½ oz	215	16	4
Part Skim,	40	2	1.5
½ cup, 4½ oz	170	10	6
Light/Low-Fat	25	1	1.5
½ cup, 4½ oz	125	5	6
Fat-Free, ½ cup, 4½ oz	100	0	10
Baked Ricotta, 2 oz portion	130	9	3
Romano: Block/Loaf	110	8	1
Grated (Package):	120	9	1
1 Tbsp, 0.2 oz	20	1.5	0
Roquefort	105	9	0.5
Sheep's Milk	45	3	1
Smoked: *Wegman's*	100	8	0
Tillamook, Smoked Cheddar	110	9	0
Stilton *(Wegman's)*	110	10	0
String *(Frigo/Kraft/Sargento)*	80	6	0.5
Light String-Ums *(Kraft)*	80	4.5	1
String Lite *(Frigo)*	60	2.5	0.5
Light *(Sargento),* 1 stick, 0.7 oz	50	2.5	0.5
Swiss: Regular	110	8	1.5
Reduced-Fat: *Alpine Lace,* 1.2 oz	110	7	1
Kraft, 2% Milk, 0.7 oz slice	50	2.5	2
Taco Cheese *(Kraft)* shredded, ¼ cup	120	10	1
Tilsit	100	7.5	0.5
Tybo	100	7	0.5
Vermont *(Cabot)*	110	9	0
Wensleydale	100	8	0.5
Whey Cheese	125	8	9

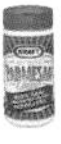

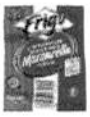

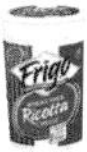

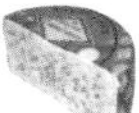

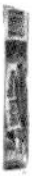

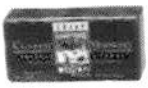

Cheese Products

	C	F	Cb
Cheese Food:			
Average all flavors: ¾ oz slice	70	5	2
1 oz slice	95	7	2.5
Alouette:			
Soft Spreadable: Per 2 Tbsp., 0.8 oz			
Berries & Cream	80	6	4
Light Garlic & Herbs	50	4	2
Peppercorn Parmesan	80	8	1
Cabot, 50% Red-Fat Ched., av., 1 oz	70	4.5	0
Cracker Barrel, Extra Sharp Ched., 1 oz	120	10	0
Handi-Snacks: *(Kraft)*			
Breadsticks 'n Cheez, 1.1 oz	110	4.5	14
Ritz Crackers 'n Cheez, 1 oz package	100	6	11
Kraft:			
American: Singles 1 slice, ¾ oz	45	2.5	2
Fat-Free, 1 slice, 0.67 oz	25	0	2
Snack Pack Cubes:			
Colby & Monteray Jack, 2%, 1.48 oz	160	13	1
Kraft Natural:			
Cheese Sticks: Cheddar (1), 1 oz	120	10	0
Mozzarella, 1 stick, 1 oz	80	5	0
Colby Jack, Red. Fat (1), 1 oz	90	6	0.5
2% Reduced Fat, 1 oz	90	6	1
Laughing Cow:			
Wedges: Original Creamy Swiss (1)	50	4	1
Light Varieties, 1 wedge	35	2	1
Gourmet Cheese Bites, Light, 5 pieces	35	2	1
Mini Babybel ~ See Page 78			
Lifetime:			
Cholest. Reducing, 1 Slice, 0.67 oz	30	1	2
Block, 1" cube, 1 oz	45	1.5	1
Lifeway Farmers Kefir, 2 Tbsp, 1 oz	25	1.5	4
Precious, Cheddar Chse Sticksters, 1 oz	110	9	1
Rondele:			
Spreadable: All Flavors, 2 Tbsp., 1 oz	70	7	1
Light, Garlic & Herb, 2 Tbsp., 1 oz	50	4	2
Sargento:			
Chef Style: Cheddar, shred., ¼ cup, 1 oz	110	9	1
Mozzarella, shredded, ¼ cup	80	6	1
Snack Bars, Mild Cheddar (1),	90	7	1
Sticks, Pepper Jack (1), 0.74 oz	80	6	0
Smart Balance:			
Creamy cheddar-flavor, 1 slice, ⅔ oz	40	2	2
Cheese Product Shreds, 1 oz	80	5	1
Smart Beat, Fat-Free, 0.6 oz slice	25	0	3
Velveeta: Regular, ¾ oz slice	60	4	2
Extra Thick, 1.2 oz	100	7	3
Shredded, ¼ cup, 1.3 oz	130	9	3
WisPride:			
Port Wine: Ball/Cup, 1.1 oz	90	7	4
Cup, Lite, 2 Tbsp, 1.1 oz	70	3.5	5

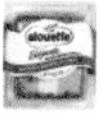

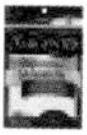
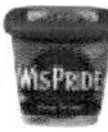

Cheese Whiz

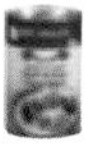

	C	F	Cb
Original, 2 Tbsp, 1.1 oz	90	7	4
Light, 2 Tbsp, 1.1 oz	80	3.5	6
Salsa Con Queso, 2 Tbsp, 1.1 oz	90	7	4

Cheese Curds

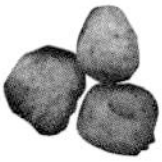

	C	F	Cb
Fresh: ¼ cup, 1 oz	110	9	0
1 cup, 4 oz	440	36	0
Breaded & Fried:			
A&W, 5 oz	570	40	27
Culver's, 6.7 oz	670	38	54

Cheese Substitutes

	C	F	Cb
Galaxy:			
Grated Parmesan Flavor, 2 tsp, 0.18 oz	15	0	0
Oat/Rice Slices, 1 slice, 0.7 oz	40	2	1
Veggy: American, 1 slice, ½ oz	40	2.5	0.5
Mozzarella Flavor, 1 slice, ½ oz	40	2.5	0.5
Lifetime, Swiss Rice Chunk, 1" cube	95	7	2
Lisanatti: Almond Cheese, average	50	1	3
Rice Cheese, average, 1 oz	60	3	2
Mori Nu:			
Tofu: Silken Soft, 1" slice, 3 oz	45	2.5	2
Firm, 1" slice, 3 oz	50	2.5	2
Soya Kaas: Cheddar, 1 oz	60	4	0
Fat-Free, all varieties, 1 oz	40	0	2
Soy-Sation, Shredded Cheese, av., 1 oz	70	4	2
Tofutti, Better Than Cream Cheese, 1 oz	85	5	9
Trader Joe's: *Per Slice*			
Soy Cheese:			
Cheddar Flavor, 0.7 oz	45	2	3
Mozzarella Flavor, 1 oz	70	4	3
Yogurt Cheese, 1 slice, 1 oz	100	8	0

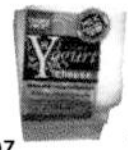

New Diet Aid
- The Refrigerator Air Bag!

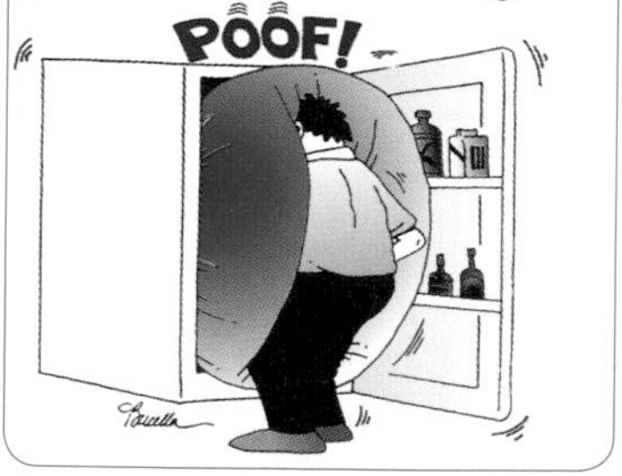

Cream Cheese

Cream Cheese	C	F	Cb
Regular/Soft, average all brands:			
2 Tbsp, 1 oz	90	9	2
8 oz package	720	72	13
with Chives; Herbs; Pimento, 1 oz	75	2.5	10
with Strawberry; Pineapple, 1 oz	90	8	4
Philadelphia *(Kraft): Per 2 Tbsp*			
Original, 1 oz	100	9	1
3 oz package	300	27	3
Regular, 1.1 oz	90	9	2
Flavored: Blueberry, 1 oz	90	7	5
Honey Nut; Strawberry, 1 oz	90	4.5	4
Garden Vegetable, 1 oz	90	8	2
Peaches 'N Creme Swirls, 1 oz	90	7	5
Light: Plain, 1.1 oz	70	5	2
Flavors, average, 0.7 oz	70	4	6
Fat-Free Varieties, 1 oz	40	0	6
Neufchatel, ⅓ Less Fat, 1 oz	70	6	1
Snacks: Bars, average (1), 1½ oz	180	11	20
Bagel & Crm Cheese To Go, 3.2 oz	240	8	34
Snack Bites, Turtle (1), 1 oz	130	7	15
Whipped: Regular, 0.7 oz	60	6	1
Mixed Berry, 0.7 oz	70	5	3

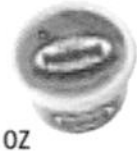

Dips/Spreads

Per 2 Tbsp, 1 oz, Unless Indicated

Dips/Spreads	C	F	Cb
Average All Brands			
Avocado/Guacamole	45	4	2
Baba Ghanoush *(Eggplant/Sesame)*	70	6	2
Cheese Fondue, ½ cup, 4 oz	260	15	4
French Onion Dip	60	4.5	3
Hummus: 2 Tbsp	50	1	5
½ cup, 4.5 oz	220	4.5	23
Tzatziki *(Cucumber/Yogurt)*	30	2.5	2
Clearman's: Original Spread	150	15	2
De La Casa, 5 Layer Party Dip	90	9	2
Frito: Chili Cheese	45	3	3
Bean; Hot Bean w/ Jalap.	35	1	5
Jalapeno Cheddar Chse	50	3.5	3
Guiltless Gourmet:			
Spicy Black Bean	40	0	7
Heluva Good Cheese: Fiesta Salsa	60	5	3
French Onion	60	5	2
Fat-Free	25	0	3
Fiesta Salsa	60	5	3
Average other flavors	60	5	3
Kaukauna: Parmesan Ranch	90	6	4
Smokey Cheddar	90	7	3

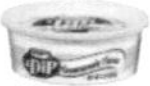

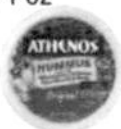

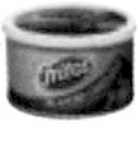

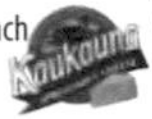

Dips/Spreads (Cont)

Per 2 Tbsp, 1 oz, Unless Indicated

Dips/Spreads (Cont)	C	F	Cb
Kemps			
Bacon & Onion	60	5	2
French Onion	60	5	2
Ranch Style	60	5	2
Top The Tater,			
Chive, Onion & Sour Cream	60	6	2
Kroger, all flavors	60	5	2
Kraft:			
Average all flavors	60	5	4
Cheez Whiz Dip:			
Original	90	7	4
Light	80	3.5	6
Marie's: *Per 2 Tbsp*			
Buttermilk Ranch	100	9	2
Creamy Dill	100	10	2
Guacamole	40	3	3
Marzetti: Choc Fruit	110	2	23
Caramel Apple	85	0	20
Veggie: Guacamole	130	13	2
Ranch	120	12	2
Fat-Free Ranch	30	0	6
Light Ranch	60	6	2
Nalley's,			
Ranch Chip Dip	100	10	2
Naturally Fresh: Chocolate Dip	70	0	14
Cream Cheese Strawberry	90	3.5	14
Caramel	100	4.5	16
Old Dutch, French Onion	50	3	5
Old El Paso:			
Cheese 'n Salsa: Mild; Medium	35	3	3
Thick N' Chunky	10	0	2
Prices: Pimiento Cheese Spread	85	7	3
Light Pimiento	55	3	3
Stop & Shop: Veggie Dip	110	10	3
Sour Cream French Onion	60	5	2
TGI Fridays:			
Spinach,Chse & Artichoke	45	3.5	2
Spinach Dip	50	3.5	2
Toby's: Tofu Pate	80	7	2
average other spreads	40	2.5	2
Tostitos Dip:			
Monterey Jack Queso	40	2.5	4
Salsa Con Quéso	40	2.5	5
Wise: French Onion	60	5	3
Nacho Cheese	50	4.5	3

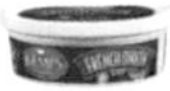

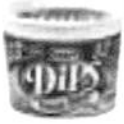

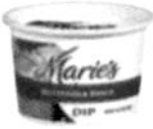

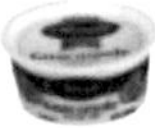

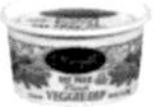

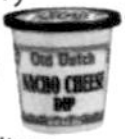

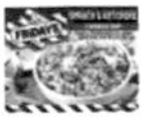

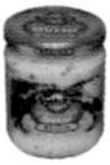

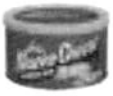

Condiments, Sauces

	C	F	Cb
Average of Brands & Homemade			
Apple Sauce: *Also see Page 104*			
Sweetened, ¼ cup, 2½ oz	55	0	13
Unsweetened, ¼ cup, 2 oz	25	0	7
Barbecue Sauce: Avg., 2 Tbsp, 1 oz	40	0	10
Bull's Eye, Original, 1 Tbsp, ½ oz	30	0	7
Bearnaise Sauce, ¼ cup, 2½ oz	190	19	5
Buffalo Wing Sce: Honey Mustard, 1 T.	40	3	3
Average other varieties, 1 Tbsp	25	2	2
Catsup (Ketchup), regular, 1 Tbsp	15	0	4
Cheese, h/made, ¼ cup, 2½ oz	150	10	12
Chef-Mate, Hot Dog, ¼ cup	70	2.5	9
Chili Sauce: *Heinz,* 1 T, ½ oz	20	0	4.5
Del Monte, 1 Tbsp, ½ oz	20	0	5
Cocktail Sauce, ¼ cup	110	0	15
Fat-Free *(Walden Farms)* 1 Tbsp	0	0	0
Cranberry, all types, ¼ c., 2½ oz	110	0	27
Demi Glaze Gold, 2 tsp	30	0.5	3
Honey Mustard *(French's)* 1 tsp	5	0	1
Horseradish: 1 tsp	2	0	0
Kraft, 1 tsp	20	1.5	1
Ketchup: Regular, 1 T., ½ oz	15	0	4
Heinz One-Carb, 1 Tbsp	5	0	1
Mole: *Doñg Maria,* 2 Tbsp, 1 oz	200	13	10
Rogelio Bueno 2 Tbsp, 1 oz	160	11	12
Mushroom Sauce, ½ cup, 2 oz	50	2	5
Mustard, average, 1 tsp	5	0	0.5
Pesto Sauce, ¼ cup, 2 oz	90	5	8
Pizza Sauce, cnd., ¼ cup, 2 oz	30	0	6
Seafood Cocktail Sce, ¼ c.	60	0	15
Soy Sauce: Avg., 1 Tbsp	10	0	1
Kikkoman Lite Soy, 1 Tbsp	10	0	1
Sour Cream Sce, ½ cup	250	15	22
Spaghetti Sce, ½ cup, 4½ oz	135	6	19
Steak Sauce: A1, 1 Tbsp, ½ oz	15	0	3
Lea & Perrins, 1 Tbsp, ½ oz	25	0	5
Carb Well *(A1)* 1 Tbsp, ½ oz	5	0	1
Strawb. Puree Sce, Unsweet., 2 T.	10	0	2
Sweet & Sour Sauce:			
Contadina, 1 Tbsp	40	1	8
Kraft, 1 Tbsp	60	0	13
La Choy, 2 Tbsp, 34g	60	0	14
Tabasco Sauce, 1 tsp	2	0	0
Taco Sauce, average, 2 Tbsp, 1 oz	10	0	1
Tartar Sauce: Heinz, 2 Tbsp, 1 oz	120	11	4
America's Choice, 2 Tbsp, 1 oz	160	17	1
Hellmann's, Regular, 2 Tbsp, 1 oz	80	7	4
McCormick, Fat-Free, 2 Tbsp, 1 oz	35	0	6
Teriyaki Sauce *(Kikkoman)* 1 T., ½ oz	15	0	3
Vinegar, White or Wine, 2 Tbsp	4	0	1
White Sauce, ½ cup, 5 oz	130	7	10
Worcestershire Sauce, 1 tsp	5	0	1

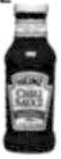
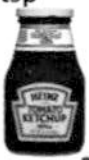
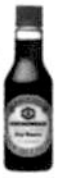
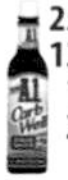
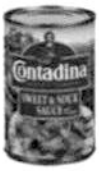

Pickles & Relish

	C	F	Cb
Average All Brands			
Bread & Butter Pickles, 4 sl., 1 oz	25	0	6
Chutney, 2 Tbsp, 1¼ oz	50	0	11
Dill Pickle:			
Slices, 4 slices, 1 oz	4	0	1
1 large, (3¾"x 1¼" diam.), 2¼ oz	12	0	3
Extra lrg (4"x 1¾" diam.), 5 oz	30	0	6
Halves: Small, 1 oz	3	0	0.5
Large, 2½ oz	8	0	2
Sweet, small, ½ oz	22	0	6
Gherkins, sweet, 1 med., 1 oz	30	0	7
Green Chiles, chopped, 2 Tbsp	5	0	1
Horseradish, 1 Tbsp	10	0	2
Jalapenos, pickled (2), 2 oz	10	0.5	2
Jalapeno Relish, 1 Tbsp, ½ oz	5	0	1
Mustard, avg. all brands, 1 tsp	5	0	0.5
Peppers, Hot/Mild (1), 1.6 oz	20	0	4
Pickled: Beets, ½ cup, 4 oz	75	0	19
Onions, 1 medium, ¾ oz	10	0	2
Cocktail Onion, 1 onion	2	0	0
Red Cabbage, ½ cup, 3 oz	65	0	15
Pickles: Sweet, 2 Tbsp, 1 oz	35	0	0
Large (3" x ¾ diam.), 1¼ oz	40	0	10
Pickle in a Pouch, 1 large	12	0	3
Relishes: Sandwich Spread, 1 tsp	20	1	5
Cranberry-Orange, 1 Tbsp	30	0	7
Hot Dog *(Heinz)*, 1 Tbsp, ½ oz	17	0	3
Sweet Pickle, 1 Tbsp, ½ oz	20	0	5
Sweet Cauliflower, 1 oz	35	0	8
Sauerkraut, Drained, 1 cup, 5 oz	25	0	6

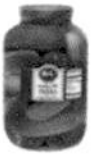
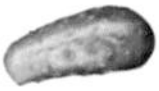
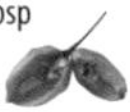
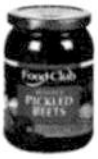

Salsa

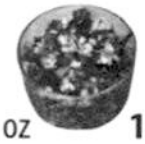

	C	F	Cb
Average all Types:			
Regular, no oil, 2 Tbsp, 1 oz	15	0	3.5
Made with oil, 2 Tbsp, 1 oz	40	3	8
Kaukauna, 2 Tbsp, 1 oz	15	0	3
La Victoria, 2 Tbsp, 1 oz	10	0	2
Old El Paso, 1 Tbsp, 1 oz	10	0	3
TGI Friday's, 1.2 oz	15	0	4

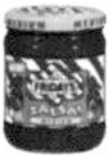

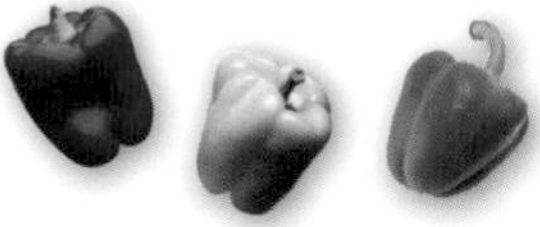

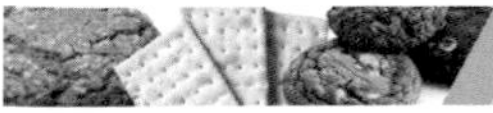

Quick Guide

	C	F	Cb
Cookies			
Average All Brands: *Per Cookie*			
Biscotti: Small, 0.5 oz	70	3	10
Regular, 1 oz	140	6.5	18
Chocolate Chip Cookies:			
Small/Thin 0.5 oz	70	3.5	9
Regular, 1 oz	140	7	18
Large, 2.5 oz *(Mrs Fields)*	330	16	46
Extra Large, 4 oz	555	28	73
Oatmeal/Oatmeal Raisin:			
Small/Thin 0.5 oz	65	2.5	10
Regular, 1 oz	130	5	20
Large, 2.5 oz *(Mrs Fields)*	330	14	44
Extra Large, 4 oz	510	20	78
Peanut Butter:			
Small/Thin 0.5 oz	70	3.5	9
Regular, 1 oz	135	7	17
Large, 2.5 oz *(Mrs Fields)*	330	17	41
Extra Large, 4 oz	540	27	67
Low-Fat Cookies			
Choc Chip (Low-Fat), (1), ½ oz	65	2	10
Oatmeal Raisin (Fat-Free), (1), 1 oz	95	0.5	22
Peanut Butter (Low-Fat), (1),1 oz	105	5	15

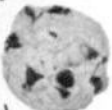
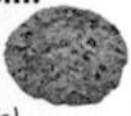
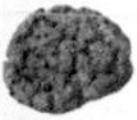

Quick Guide

	C	F	Cb
Crackers			
Average All Brands: *Per Cracker*			
Cheese Crackers: Plain, 1" square	5	0	0.5
Small, octagonal	10	0	1
Round (2" diam.)	15	0	1.5
Sandwich (Peanut Butter)	35	1.5	4
Graham, 2½" square	30	0.5	5
Melba Toast, plain, 1 piece	20	0	4
Oyster & Soup Crackers, ½ oz	60	2	10
(40 small oysters/20 lge hexagons)			
Rice Crackers: 1 small	9	0	1.5
Rice Snacks, Oriental-Style, 1 oz	130	2.5	23
Saltines, 5 crackers	65	2	11
Snack-type, 1 round cracker	15	0	2
Soda Crackers *(Saltine)*, 2	25	1	4.5
Water Cracker *(Carr's)*: Regular	30	0	7
Small, 1 cracker	15	0	3
Wheat, thin	9	0.5	1.5
Zweiback Toast, 1 piece	35	1	6

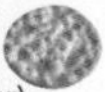
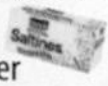
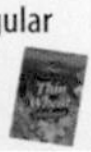

Brands

	C	F	Cb
Per Cookie/Cracker (Unless indicated)			
Albertsons			
Animal Crackers (6), 1 oz	130	3.5	22
Chocolate Chip:			
Original (3), 1 oz	150	7	20
Chewy (2), 1 oz	130	6	18
Chunky, 0.6 oz	80	3.5	10
Chocolate Sandwich Cremes (3) 1.1oz	150	6	23
Double Filled (2) 1 oz	130	6	20
Fudge Graham (3), 1 oz	140	7	19
Fudge Wafer (3), 1 oz	140	8	18
Graham Crackers: Cinnamon (2)	130	3	25
Honey (2), 1 oz	140	3	24
Low-Fat Honey (2), 1 oz	110	1	22
Marshmallow Ring, 1 oz	130	6	20
Milk Chocolate Chip, 2.5 oz	310	14	30
Striped Shortbread (3), 1.1 oz	160	7	21
Sugar, 2.5 oz	270	9	22
Triple Chocolate, 2.8 oz	310	12	33
White Chocolate Chip, 2.5 oz	280	11	37
Vanilla Wafers (9), 1.1 oz	160	4.5	24
Annie's			
Cheddar Bunnies			
Regular: 1 oz Snack Pack	150	7	19
7½ oz Box	1125	52	140
Sour Cream & Onion, 1 oz	140	6	18
White Cheddar, 1 oz	140	6	18
Whole Wheat, 1 oz	130	6	17
Bunny Classics: Buttery Rich, 1 oz	140	5	20
Cheddar, 1 oz	140	7	18
Saltine, 1 oz	140	3	22
Bunny Grahams: Friends, 1 oz	130	4.5	21
Chocolate, 1 oz	130	4.5	22
Austin			
Crackers: *Per Package*			
Cheese with Cheddar Cheese	190	10	23
Cheese with Peanut Butter	190	10	23
Sandwich:			
Chocolatey Peanut Butter Flavored	190	8	26
Grilled Cheese Flavored, 1.38 oz	190	9	24
PB & J Flavored, 1.38 oz	190	8	26
Toasty Crackers w/ P'nut Butter, 1.3 oz	190	9	23
Zoo Animal Crackers, 1 oz	120	1.5	23
Sandwich Cremes: *Per Package*			
Lemon OHs!; Vanilla Cremes, 1.2 oz	170	7	24

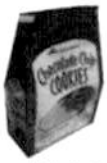
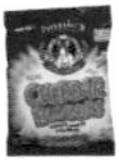

Updated Nutrition Data ~ www.CalorieKing.com
Persons with Diabetes ~ See Disclaimer (Page 24)

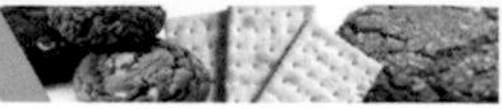

Per Cookie/Cracker, Unless Indicated

Barbara's Bakery:	C	F	Cb
Cookies: Fig Bars, average	**60**	0	14
Snackimals (10), average	**120**	4	19
Crackers: Rite Lite Rounds (5)	**60**	2	11
Wheatines (4)	**60**	1	11
Blue Diamond:			
Nut Thins:			
Almond: (16)	**130**	2.5	23
Cheddar Cheese (16)	**130**	4	23
Smokehouse (16)	**130**	3	23
Hazelnut (16)	**130**	3	23
Pecan (16)	**130**	3.5	23
Brent & Sam's:			
Chocolate Chip Pecan (2)	**110**	6	13
Key Lime White Chocolate (2)	**110**	5	14
Oatmeal Raisin with Pecans (2)	**110**	5	14
Triple Chocolate Bliss (2)	**110**	5	14
White Chocolate Macadamia (2)	**110**	6	14
Carr's:			
Crackers:			
Poppy & Sesame Seed (4)	**80**	5	9
Table Water (5)	**70**	1.5	13
Whole Wheat (2)	**80**	4	10
Cookies, Ginger Lemon Cremes (2)	**130**	5	20
Cheez•It ~ *See Sunshine (Page 89)*			
Chips Ahoy! ~ *See Nabisco (Page 87)*			
Country Choice			
Ginger Snaps (5)	**140**	5	22
Sandwich Cremes (2), average	**130**	5	19
Soft Baked, average all flavors	**100**	4	16
Vanilla Wafers (7)	**140**	5	22
Dr. Kracker:			
Crackers, Flatbread, average all flavors	**100**	4	11
Snacker: Klassic 3-Seed (8)	**120**	5	13
Seeded Spelt (8)	**120**	6	12
Spelt Sunflower Cheese (8)	**100**	6	12
Average other flavors (8)	**120**	5	15
Erin Baker's:			
Original Breakfast Cookies: *Per 3 oz*			
Mocha Cappuccino	**300**	6	53
Peanut Butter	**320**	11	47
Peanut Butter & Jelly	**320**	9	52
Vegan Peanut Butter Choc. Chunk	**330**	10	52
Minis: *Per 1 oz Cookie*			
Peanut Butter	**110**	3	16
Other flavors, average	**100**	2	18
Organic Brownie Bites, average	**95**	2	18

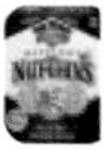

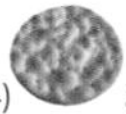

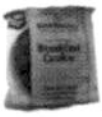

Per Cookie/Cracker, Unless Indicated

Famous Amos:	C	F	Cb
(Bite Size Cookies)			
Chocolate Chip: 4 cookies, 1 oz	**150**	7	20
1.4 oz Snack bag	**210**	10	28
3 oz (99cents) bag	**450**	21	60
12 oz bag	**1800**	84	240
15 oz box	**2250**	105	300
Chocolate Chip & Pecans (4)	**150**	8	18
Sandwich Creme:			
Chocolate; Vanilla, (3), 1 oz	**170**	7	25
Chocolate: 3 cookies, 1.2 oz	**170**	7	25
2.2 oz bag	**310**	9	33
14 oz package	**1980**	82	290
Fig Newtons ~ *See Nabisco, Page 87*			
Girl Scouts:			
Cookies: Caramel DeLites (2)	**140**	7	19
Do-si-dos (2)	**110**	5	16
Peanut Butter Sandwich (3)	**160**	6	26
Samoas (2)	**150**	8	19
Shortbreads (4)	**120**	4.5	19
Thanks-A-Lot (9)	**150**	6	22
Thin Mints (4)	**160**	8	22
Goldfish ~ *See Pepperidge Farm, Page 88*			
Grandma's:			
Homestyle Iced Lemon (1)	**190**	9	22
Peanut Butter Sandwich Creme (5)	**210**	10	28
Rich 'N Chewy, Choc Chip, 1 package	**270**	12	38
Vanilla Sandwich Creme (5)	**210**	9	30
Van./Choc. Mini Sandwich Creme (9)	**150**	7	22
Homestyle Big Cookies:			
Chocolate Chip	**190**	9	25
Fudge Choc. Chip	**170**	7	27
Oatmeal Raisin	**280**	6	30
Peanut Butter	**200**	9	29
Great American Cookies:			
Cookies: Original; Pecan	**230**	12	31
Chewy Pecan Supreme	**230**	12	31
Chewy Chocolate Supreme; Sugar	**200**	9	29
Double Fudge/ Reese's, average	**235**	11	32
Oatmeal	**230**	10	33
Original M&M/Reese's	**240**	12	32
Peanut Butter M&M	**250**	14	29
Snickerdoodles	**240**	11	33
White Chunk Macadamia	**250**	14	30
Double Doozies: Original	**690**	34	94
M&M Big Bite	**340**	17	46
Cookie Cakes: 16" Cookie	**460**	22	67
16" M&M Cookie	**500**	24	73
Heart Shaped	**440**	21	64
Sliced Cookie Cake, 1 slice	**580**	27	83

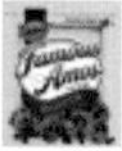

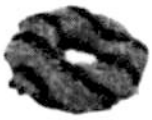

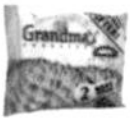

Per Cookie/Cracker, Unless Indicated

	C	F	Cb
Health Valley:			
Cookies:			
Cookie Cremes Sandwich (2), average	**125**	5	19
Oatmeal Raisin Cookie	**90**	3.5	14
Mini: Chocolate Chip (4)	**120**	5	16
Chocolate Chocolate Chip (4)	**130**	7	16
Crackers:			
Original Grahams: Amaranth Bran (6)	**120**	3	22
Oat Bran (6)	**120**	3	22
Rice Bran (6)	**110**	3	19
Organic: Bruschetta Vegetable (4)	**70**	3	10
Cracked Pepper; Sesame (4)	**70**	3	10
Stoned Wheat; Whole Wheat av., (4)	**70**	3	9
Hershey's:			
Cookies: York Cookies (2)	**130**	8	17
Almond Joy Cookies (2)	**140**	8	17
Hershey's Layered (2)	**130**	6	19
Reese's (2)	**150**	8	17
Reese's Layered (2)	**140**	7	18
Soft Baked (1)	**340**	16	50
Joseph's Cookies:			
Crispy Bite Size: *Sugar Free, Per 4 Cookies*			
Almond; Chocolate Peanut Butter	**95**	5	13
Chocolate Mint	**95**	5	14
Choc. Walnut; Pecan Chocolate Chip	**95**	5	13
Chocolate Chip	**100**	5	13
Lemon; Peanut Butter, average	**95**	4	15
Oatmeal Choc Chip w. Pecans	**100**	6	14
Oatmeal; Pecan Shortbread, average	**100**	5	15
Kashi TLC:			
Cookies: *Per Cookie*			
Happy Trail Mix, Chewy	**140**	5	21
Oatmeal: Dark Choc.	**130**	5	21
Raisin Flax	**130**	5	20
Crackers:			
Mini: Country Cheddar (18)	**130**	4.5	20
Fire Roasted Vegetables (15)	**130**	3.5	21
Honey Sesame (15)	**130**	3	22
Original 7 Grain (15)	**120**	3.5	21
Toasted Asiago (15)	**130**	4	21
Party: Mediterranean Bruschetta (4)	**120**	4	18
Roasted Garlic & Thyme (4)	**130**	4.5	18
Stoneground 7 Grain (4)	**130**	5	17
Snack Packs: Original 7 Grain (15)	**120**	3.5	21
Whole Grain: Original (7)	**120**	3.5	22
Roasted Garlic (7)	**120**	3.5	22

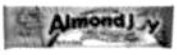
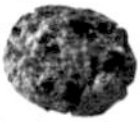

Per Cookie/Cracker (Unless indicated)

	C	F	Cb
Keebler:			
Crackers:			
Club: Original (4)	**70**	3	9
Reduced Fat (5)	**70**	2	12
Grahams: Original (8)	**120**	3.5	22
Cinnamon; Honey, average(8)	**135**	4	23
Low-Fat varieties (8)	**110**	1.5	23
Town House: Original (5)	**80**	4.5	10
Reduced Fat (6)	**60**	1.5	11
Wheatables:			
Crackers: Original (17)	**140**	6	20
Reduced Fat (19)	**140**	4	22
Honey Wheat; Multigrain, (17)	**140**	6	20
Nut Crisps, average all flavors (16)	**140**	6	20
Cookies:			
Chips Deluxe:			
Chocolate Lovers; Coconut	**80**	4.5	10
Original (2)	**170**	9	19
Rainbow	**80**	4	10
Rainbow Mini's 1.4 oz package	**200**	10	27
Soft & Chewy	**180**	3.5	11
Country Style Oatmeal (2)	**130**	6	19
Danish Wedding (4)	**130**	6	18
E.L. Fudge: Original	**90**	3.5	13
Double Stuffed (2)	**180**	9	24
Fudge Shoppe:			
Deluxe Grahams (3)	**140**	7	17
Fudge Sticks (3)	**150**	8	20
Fudge Stripes (3)	**150**	7	21
Mini's, 1 package	**200**	9	27
100 Calorie Package	**100**	3.5	16
Grasshopper (4)	**140**	7	19
Gripz, average, 1 pouch	**125**	5	17
Iced Animal (6)	**140**	5	22
Sandies Cookies:			
Choc Chip Pecan (2)	**170**	10	18
Pecan Shortbread (2)	**160**	10	18
Reduced-Fat (2)	**160**	7	21
100 Calorie Package	**100**	3	17
Soft Batch, Peanut Butter (2)	**160**	7	22
Vienna Fingers: Regular (2)	**150**	6	23
Reduced Fat (2)	**140**	4.5	24
Wafers: Vanilla (8)	**150**	6	21
Mini Vanilla (18)	**140**	6	21

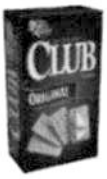
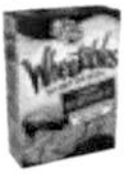
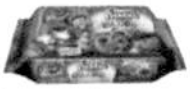

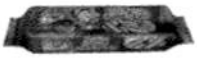
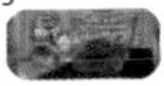
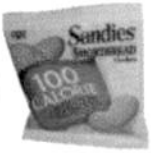
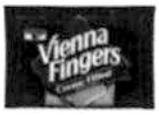

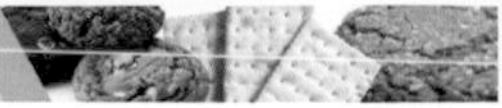

Per Cookie/Cracker, Unless Indicated

Kroger	C	F	Cb
Cookies: Chip Mates			
Original (3), 1.5 oz	160	8	22
Chewy (2), 1 oz	130	6	20
Chunky (2), 1 oz	130	6	18
Olde Southern Pecan Shortbread, 1 oz	150	9	15
Sugar Wafers (4), 1.1 oz	170	10	21
Vanilla Wafers (7), 1.1 oz	130	3.5	23
Crackers:			
Grahams, Original; Honey (4)	120	3	20
Saltines, Original, (5), 0.5 oz	60	1.5	10
Kid-O's			
Mint (2) 1 oz	140	6	22
Choc. Lovers Dbl Filled Choc, (2) 1 oz	140	6	21
Double Filled Sandwich (2) 1 oz	140	6	21
Chocolate Sandwich (3) 1.15 oz	150	6	25
Lance			
Nekot, Peanut Butter, 1 package	240	11	30
Strawberry Cookies (5)	230	10	33
Crackers: Toasty, 1 package	180	9	16
Nipchee, 1 package	190	9	23
Toastchee: Original, 1 package	220	11	23
Reduced-Fat, 1 package	190	8	23
Malt Crackers, 1 package	190	10	18
Little Debbie			
Fig Bar	160	3	31
Marshmallow Pie, average	180	7	28
Marshmallow Treat	160	4	31
Oatmeal Creme Pie , 1.34 oz	170	7	26
Nutty Bar (2), 2 oz	310	18	33
Crackers: Cheese w/ Peanut Butter (4)	130	6	15
Peanut Butter Toasty (4)	130	6	16
Lu			
Le Petit Beurre (4)	140	4	24
Le Petit Ecolier, average (2)	130	6	17
Pim's, Orange (2)	100	3	16
Macaroni & Cheese, *(Nabisco)*			
Average all flavors	150	7	18
Manischewitz			
Matzo Boards: *See Page 105*			
Chocolate Macaroon	45	2	8
Matzo Cracker, Miniatures (10)	110	0	25
Tam Tam Crackers: Everything (10)	130	5	19
Onion (10)	140	5	21

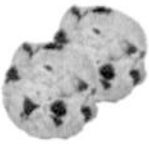

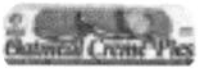

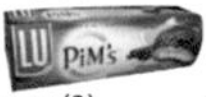

Per Cookie/Cracker, Unless Indicated

Miss Meringue	C	F	Cb
Chocolettes (10), average	130	3.5	24
Macaroons			
Traditional Recipe, 1.3 oz	180	10	20
Madeleines			
Chocolate (2), 1.2 oz	160	9	18
Traditional Recipe (2), 1.2 oz	160	9	19
Meringue Classiques			
Cappuccino (4), 1.1 oz	110	0	26
Mint Chocolate Chip (4), 1.1 oz	120	1.5	25
Triple Chocolate (4), 1.1 oz	120	1.5	25
Vanilla Rainbow/Van. (4), 1.1 oz	110	0	27
Meringue Minis			
Chocolate (13), 1.1 oz	110	0	26
Chocolate Chip (12), 1.1 oz	130	1.5	27
Mint Chocolate Chip (12), 1.1 oz	120	1.5	26
Orange Creamsicle (13), 1.1 oz	110	0	27
Vanilla; Rainbow Van. (13), 1.1 oz	110	0	27
Sugar-Free Chocolate (13), 0.5 oz	40	0	8
Sugar-Free Vanilla (13), 0.5 oz	35	0	9
Mother's			
Chocolate Chip (4), 1 oz	150	7	20
Circus Animal (6), 1 oz	150	7	20
Coconut Cocadas (5), 1.2 oz	160	8	21
Double Fudge (2), 1.3 oz	170	7	27
English Tea (2), 1.3 oz	180	7	27
Macaroons (2), 1 oz	170	11	17
Oatmeal (2), 1 oz	130	5	19
Taffy (2), 1.3 oz	180	8	27
Vanilla Creme (2), 1.3 oz	180	7	26
Iced: Lemonade (4), 1 oz	150	7	19
Oatmeal (1), 14 oz bag	150	6	23
Mrs Fields Cookies: *See Fast-Foods Section*			
Murray Sugar Free Cookies			
Fudge-Dipped: Grahams (4)	140	8	19
Mint Cookies (4)	130	7	17
Vanilla Wafers (4)	150	10	19
Creme Sandwiches:			
Lemon; Chocolate; average	130	6	20
Oatmeal (3)	140	7	21
Peanut Butter (3)	150	9	16
Shortbread (8)	130	5	21
Shortbread Pecan (3)	160	11	18
Vanilla Wafers (9)	130	5	24
Vanilla Creme Wafers (4)	130	8	19

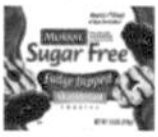

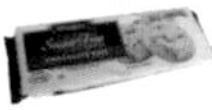

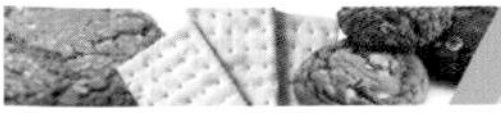

Per Cookie/Cracker (Unless Indicated)

Nabisco Cookies:	C	F	Cb
Chips Ahoy! : Chewy, 1 oz	120	6	18
Chocolate Chip, 1.13 oz	160	8	21
Chunky: Chocolate, 0.6 oz	80	4.5	11
Peanut Butter, 0.6 oz	90	5	10
Mini Choc. Chips Bite-Size (14)	150	7	20
Snak Saks (5)	150	8	21
Ginger Snaps (4)	120	2.5	23
Lorna Doone (4)	140	7	20
Mallomars	120	5	18
Newtons: Fig (2), 1.1 oz	110	2	22
Fig/Strawb. Minis, 1 pkg, 1.34 oz	130	3	26
100% Whole Grain (2)	110	2	21
Fat-Free (2)	90	0	22
Fruit Crisps, avg. (2)	100	2	20
Raspberry/Strawberry (2)	100	1.5	21
Nilla Wafers: (8), 1 oz	140	6	21
Reduced-Fat (8), 1 oz	120	2	24
Nutter Butter:			
Sandwich Cookies (2), 1 oz	130	5	20
Bites: 1.25 oz	170	7	24
Go-Paks (10), 1 oz	140	6	21
Snak-Saks (10), 1 oz	140	6	21
Wafers, Peanut Butter (5)	160	9	18
Oreo:			
Sandwich Cookies: Orig., White Creme	160	7	25
Reduced-Fat (3), 1.2 oz	150	4.5	27
Sugar Free (2), 0.8 oz	100	5	16
Chocolate Creme Filling (2)	150	7	21
Chocolate Fudge Covered, 0.7 oz	100	5	13
Double Stuff:			
Cool Mint (2), 1 oz	140	7	20
Peanut Butter (2), 1 oz	140	6	20
Golden: Original (3), 1.2 oz	170	7	25
Double Stuff (2), 1 oz	150	7	21
Uh-Oh with Chocolate Cream (3)	170	7	25
Fudge Rings (3), 1 oz	120	4.5	19
Fun Stix, Chocolate; Golden 1 packet	90	3.5	13
Go-Pak, Bite Size Choc (9), 1 oz	130	6	21
Snak-Saks: Bite Size Choc (9) 1 oz	130	6	21
Mini Golden Vanilla (9), 1 oz	140	6	21
Cakesters: Original (2), 2 oz	250	12	36
Peanut Butter Creme (2), 2 oz	210	9	31
Teddy Grahams:			
Snacks: Honey; Cinn. (24)	130	4	23
Chocolate, av., (24)	130	4.5	22
Snak Saks, Mini Choc Chip/Honey (47), av.,	130	4	22

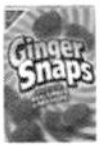

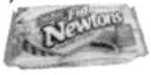

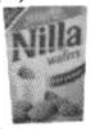

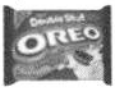

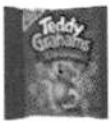

Updated Nutrition Data ~ www.CalorieKing.com
Persons with Diabetes ~ See Disclaimer (Page 24)

Per Cookie/Cracker (Unless Indicated)

Nabisco Cookies (Cont):	C	F	Cb
100 Calorie Packs: *Per Pack*			
Chips Ahoy! Thin Crisps	100	3	18
Barnum's Animals Choco Crackers	100	3	17
Honey Maid Thin Crisps	100	3	16
Lorna Doone Crisps	100	3	16
Milk Choc. Pretzels	100	3.5	16
Oreo Thin Crisps	100	3	16
Ritz Toasted Chips, Minis, 0.8 oz	100	3	17
Ritz Snack Mix Toasted, 0.8 oz	100	3	16
Nabisco Crackers: Per Serving			
Barnum's Animals (8)	120	3.5	22
Cheese Nips:			
Baked Cheddar, 1 oz	150	6	19
Four Cheese, 1 oz bag	150	7	18
Mini Go-Pak (53), 1 oz	150	6	19
Flavor Originals:			
Better Cheddars (22)	160	8	18
Chicken in a Biskit (12)	160	8	19
Sociables Baked Savory (7)	70	3.5	9
Vegetable Thins (11)	150	7	20
Honey Maid:			
Grahams: Average, (8)	130	3.5	24
Low-Fat (8), average	120	2	25
Mini S'Mores (8)	140	6	21
Premium Saltine: Fat-Free (5)	60	0	13
Hint of Salt (5)	60	1.5	12
Minis, Original (21)	70	2	11
Multigrain (5)	60	1.5	10
Original (5)	70	1.5	11
Soup & Oyster (22)	60	1.5	11
Unsalted Tops (5)	70	1.5	11
Wheat Thins: Big (11)	140	5	22
Multi-Grain (15)	140	4.5	22
Original (16), 1.1 oz	140	5	22
Parmesan Basil (15) 1 oz	140	5	21
Ranch (15), 1 oz	140	5	21
Reduced-Fat (16), 1 oz	130	3.5	22
Sundried Tomato & Basil (15) 1 oz	140	5	21
Wheatsworth, Stone Ground Wheat (5)	80	3.5	10
Zwieback, 0.28 oz	35	1	6

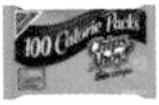

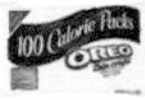

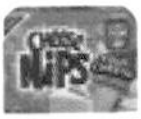

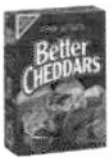

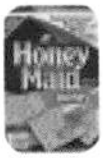

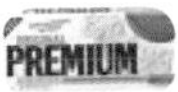

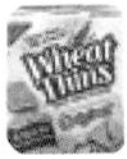

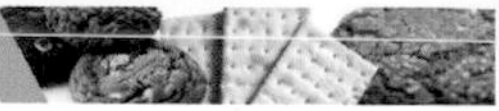

Per Cookie/Cracker (Unless Indicated)	C	F	Cb
Newman's Own Organics			
Alphabet Cookies (10) average	**120**	**3**	22
Champion Chip: Chocolate Chip (4)	**160**	**7**	21
Expresso Chocolate Chip (4)	**150**	**7**	21
Wheat-Free & Dairy-Free (4)	**160**	**8**	21
Other varieties, average	**160**	**8**	21
Fig Newman's: Fat-Free, 2 bars	**120**	**0**	28
Low-Fat, 2 bars	**140**	**2**	28
Wheat/Dairy-Free, 2 bars	**120**	**1.5**	26
Newman-O's: Original (2)	**130**	**4.5**	20
Choc. Creme (2); Mint Creme (2)	**130**	**4.5**	20
Ginger-O's (2)	**120**	**4.5**	19
Wheat-Free & Dairy-Free (2)	**130**	**4.5**	21
Oreo Cookies ~ *See Nabisco, Page 87*			
Peek Freans			
Assorted Creme (2)	**140**	**6**	19
Nice Biscuits (2)	**160**	**6**	25
Shortcake (2)	**140**	**7**	18
Pepperidge Farm			
Cookies			
Brussels (3)	**150**	**7**	20
Brussels Mint (3)	**190**	**10**	22
Chessmen (3)	**120**	**5**	18
Choc Chunk: Double	**140**	**7**	18
Dark Chocolate Chunk Nantucket	**140**	**7**	16
Dark Chocolate Pecan Chesapeake	**140**	**8**	15
Milk Chocolate, Macadamia Nut Sausalito	**140**	**8**	16
White Chocolate Macadamia	**130**	**6**	17
Average other varieties	**140**	**7**	18
Collection: Ginger Family (4)	**160**	**5**	26
Golden Orchard (3)	**140**	**6**	21
Geneva (3)	**160**	**9**	19
Homestyle: Ginger Man (4)	**130**	**4**	21
Shortbread (2)	**140**	**7**	16
Sugar (3)	**140**	**6**	20
Milano: Original (3)	**180**	**10**	21
Milk Chocolate (3)	**170**	**9**	21
Soft Baked Cookies: Oatmeal	**140**	**5**	22
Milk Chocolate Chunk	**150**	**7**	21
Snickerdoodle; Sugar	**140**	**5**	22
100 Calorie Pouches: *Per Packet*			
Chessmen	**100**	**3.5**	15
Dark Chocolate Chunk	**100**	**3.5**	15
Goldfish	**100**	**3.5**	14
Oatmeal Raisin	**100**	**3**	16

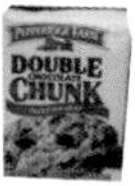

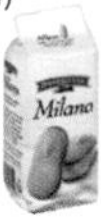

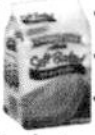

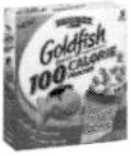

Per Cookie/Cracker (Unless Indicated)	C	F	Cb
Pepperidge Farm (Cont)			
Crackers			
Entertaining Quartet (4)	**70**	**2.5**	10
Golden Butter (4)	**70**	**2.5**	11
Harvest Wheat (3)	**80**	**3.5**	11
Wheat Crisps (17), 1 oz	**140**	**5**	21
Goldfish, average all flavors:			
1 oz (55)	**140**	**5**	20
1.5 oz pouch	**210**	**9**	27
2 oz carton	**280**	**10**	40
Pretzel Thins:			
Simply (11)	**110**	**0**	21
Snack Sticks:			
Artisan Cheese (11)	**130**	**4**	20
Toasted Sesame (12)	**140**	**5**	20
President's Choice			
Milk Choc Chunk Pecan (1), 0.8 oz	**120**	**7**	14
Peanut Butter (2), 1 oz	**140**	**8**	15
The Decadent: Choc Chip (2), 1.1 oz	**160**	**8**	21
Chocolate Chunk (2), 1.1 oz	**160**	**8**	21
Reverse White Choc. Chip (2), 1.1 oz	**160**	**8**	19
Ritz			
Crackers: Orig., ½ oz	**80**	**4.5**	10
Reduced-Fat, ½ oz	**70**	**2**	11
Honey Butter (5), 06 oz	**80**	**4**	10
Peanut Butter, 1.4 oz package	**190**	**9**	24
Real Cheese, 1.4 oz package	**200**	**11**	22
Whole Wheat, ½ oz	**70**	**2.5**	11
100 Calorie Snack Mix, 1 pkg, 0.8 oz	**100**	**3**	16
Ritz Bits Sandwiches: Cheese, 1 oz	**150**	**9**	17
Carry Me Pak , 2 oz	**290**	**17**	33
Cheddar Cheese, 1 oz packs	**130**	**7**	17
Cheese Go-Pak (12), 1 oz	**220**	**13**	24
Peanut Butter, 1.25 oz	**170**	**10**	20
Peanut Butter Go-Pak, 1 oz	**160**	**8**	18
Peanut Butter 2 Go, 1.38 oz	**190**	**9**	24
Single Serve, 1.5 oz	**220**	**13**	24
Ritz Chips: Toasted Original, 1 oz	**130**	**4.5**	21
Cheddar; Sour Crm & Onion, 1 oz	**130**	**6**	19
Safeway Select			
Homestyle: Choc. Chunk Brownie	**120**	**5**	19
Oatmeal Raisin, 1 oz	**130**	**6**	18
Indulgent: Double Choc Chunk, 1 oz	**130**	**7**	18
Milk Choc. Macadamia Nut, 1 oz	**140**	**8**	17
Pecan Choc Chunk, 1 oz	**140**	**9**	16
White Choc. Macadamia Nut, 1 oz	**140**	**8**	17
Tuxedos: Chocolate (3), 1.3 oz	**180**	**7**	26
Cinnamon Bun; Vanilla (3) 1.3 oz	**180**	**8**	26
Mint Chip Creme (2), 1 oz	**140**	**7**	20
Vanilla Creme Wafers (4)	**150**	**8**	20

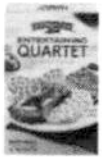

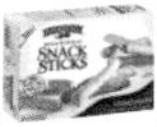

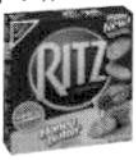

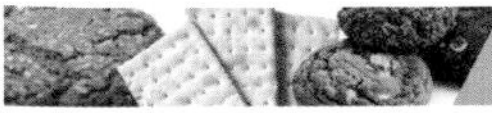

Snackwell's	C	F	Cb
Creme S'wich (2) 1 oz	**110**	3	20
Creme Sandwich, Packs To Go!, 1 pkg	**210**	5	38
Devil's Food Cake, Fat-Free, ½ oz	**50**	0	12
Lemon Creme Sandwich Sugar Free (3)	**130**	6	23
Shortbread Sugar Free (3) 1 oz	**130**	6	21
South Beach Living			
Cookies: *Per Package*			
Peanut Butter	**100**	5	15
Oatmeal Choc. Chip	**100**	5	16
Stella D'Oro			
Almond Toast (2)	**100**	2	20
Anginetti, 1 oz	**130**	3.5	22
Anisette Sponge Low-Fat (2)	**95**	1	19
Anisette Toast Low-Fat (3)	**125**	1	27
Biscotti, average, ¾ oz	**95**	4	13
Breakfast Treats: Chocolate Cookie	**90**	3	15
Original	**90**	3	15
Original Mini, 1 oz	**120**	3.5	21
Viennese Cinnamon	**90**	2.5	16
Coffee Treats: Almond Toast (2)	**100**	2	20
Angel Wings, 1 oz	**170**	12	14
Anisette Sponge (2)	**90**	1	18
Anisette Toast, 1.1 oz	**130**	1	27
Banana Walnut Toast, 1 oz	**100**	2	19
Blueberry; Cinnamon Toast, 1 oz	**100**	1	20
Roman Egg Biscuits, 1.1 oz	**130**	4	21
Continental Cookie Collection, 1 oz	**130**	4.5	20
Egg Jumbo, 1.1 oz	**120**	1.5	26
Lady Stella Assortment, 1 oz	**130**	4.5	20
Margherite (2)	**130**	5	20
Margherite Mini, 1.1 oz	**150**	5	24
Swiss Fudge (2) 1.1 oz	**170**	9	22
Streit's			
Wafers: Chocolate (3)	**160**	9	19
Vanilla (3)	**170**	11	18
Rolls, Chocolate (3)	**105**	6	12
Sunshine			
Krispy: Original; Whole Wheat (5)	**60**	1.5	11
Oyster & Soup, 16 crackers	**60**	1.5	11
Wheat (5)	**60**	1.5	11
Cheez-It: Original (27), 1 oz	**150**	8	17
Reduced-Fat (29), 1 oz	**130**	4.5	20

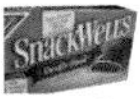

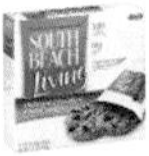

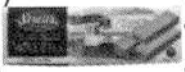

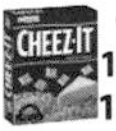

Also See Snacks ~ Page 154

Updated Nutrition Data ~ www.CalorieKing.com
Persons with Diabetes ~ See Disclaimer (Page 24)

Per Cookie/Cracker (Unless Indicated)	C	F	Cb
Trader Joe's			
100 Calorie Packs, average	**100**	2.5	18
Cherry Granola (2), 1 oz	**110**	4	18
Chocolate Almond Lacey's (2)	**170**	12	16
Chocolate Chip: Small (4), 1.1 oz	**140**	7	18
Large, Singles , 1.7 oz	**280**	14	35
Caramel Cashew (3), 1 oz	**140**	7	16
Dark Choc Chunks with Almonds (3)	**140**	7	17
Dunkers: Choc Chip (2), 1.2 oz	**160**	7	21
Choc Coated Choc. Chip (2), 1.3 oz	**190**	9	25
Ginger Snaps (5), 1 oz	**140**	6	21
Joe Joe's S'wich Cremes,			
Choc./Vanilla (2), 1 oz	**130**	5	20
Lemon Crisps (5)	**120**	4	19
Meringues: Low-Fat, Chocolate (4)	**120**	1.5	25
Fat-Free Vanilla (4)	**110**	0	27
Very Mini Meringues, Van. (100)	**100**	0	24
Oatmeal Raisin, 1.8 oz	**270**	12	35
Pecan Southern Style (4), 1 oz	**150**	9	15
Righteous Rounds Choc Chip (5), 1 oz	**130**	4	20
Thins: Meyer Lemon (9), 1 oz	**160**	5	25
Triple Ginger (9), 1 oz	**140**	4.5	24
Triple Choc Chunk, 1 oz	**140**	7	20
Ultimate Vanilla Wafers (5), 1 oz	**120**	6	15
Water Crackers (4)	**60**	1	12
Triscuit			
Baked Whole Wheat Crackers: *Per Serving*			
Original (15), 1 oz	**120**	4.5	19
Thin Crisps, Original, (15)	**130**	5	21
Roasted Garlic (8)	**120**	4.5	20
Voortman			
Shortbread Cookies (2), 1.3 oz	**180**	10	24
Sugar Free Cookies:			
Chocolate Chip (2), 1.4 oz	**160**	10	26
Lemon Wafers (3), 1 oz	**130**	8	17
Peanut Butter Wafers (4), 1 oz	**150**	7	17
Vanilla Wafers (3), 1 oz	**130**	8	17
Vanilla Wafers: Regular (3), 1.1 oz	**140**	7	20
***Zesta*:**			
Crackers: Whole Grain Wheat (5)	**60**	1.5	11
Fat Free (5)	**60**	0	13
Original (5)	**60**	1.5	11
365 *(Whole Foods):*			
Choc Chip (5), 1 oz	**130**	6	19
Classic Fig Bars (2), 1.3 oz	**140**	2.5	27
Lady Fingers (5), 1.1 oz	**120**	1.5	25
Lemon Wafers (5), 0.9 oz	**120**	5	17
Oatmeal (6), 1 oz	**130**	4.5	20
Sandwich Cremes (2), average	**130**	5	20
Sugar (5), 1.1 oz	**130**	4	22

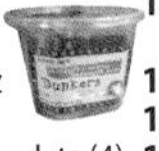

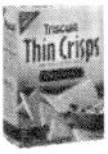

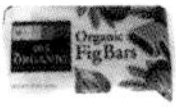

C Cookies ~ Refrigerated ◆ Crispbreads

Thaw, Bake & Serve

	C	F	Cb
Pillsbury Cookies: *Per Cookie Unless Indicated*			
Refrigerated Cookie Dough			
Big Deluxe Classics:			
Oatmeal Raisin	**150**	6	24
Peanut Butter Cup	**170**	8	22
White Chunk Macadamia Nut	**170**	9	22
Other varieties	**170**	8	23
Ready To Bake: Sugar Cookie (2)	**170**	8	23
Chocolate Chip with Walnuts (2)	**170**	9	22
Chocolate Chunk Chip (2)	**180**	9	22
Peanut Butter with Reese's Pieces (2)	**170**	8	21
S'mores (1); Chocolate Candy (2)	**160**	7	23
Create n Bake: Peanut Butter	**120**	6	16
Chocolate Chip	**130**	6	18
Oatmeal Choc. Chip; Sugar, average	**120**	5	18
Refrigerated Dough:			
Cinnamon Roll (1)	**140**	5	23
Flaky Cinnamon Twists with Icing (1)	**180**	9	22
Flaky Supreme with Icing (1)	**370**	19	48
Grands Cinnamon Rolls with Icing (1)	**310**	9	54
Simply Bake Bars:			
P.B. Choc.; Turtle Supreme, 1/12 pkg	**150**	8	19
Toll House *(Nestlé)*: *Per Cookie Unless Indicated*			
Refrigerated Dough:			
Chocolate Chunk (2)	**180**	9	23
Jumbo Chocolate Chip (1)	**180**	9	23
Mini Brownie Bites (3)	**160**	8	20
Mini Chocolate Chip (3)	**160**	8	21
Walnut Chocolate Chip (2)	**180**	9	22
Ultimates Refrigerated Dough			
Chocolate Chip Lovers	**180**	9	23
Choc. Chips & Chunks with Pecans	**190**	10	22
Peanut Butter Chips & Choc Chunks	**180**	9	23
Triple Chocolate Decadence	**170**	8	23
Turtle	**180**	9	23
White Chocolate Macadamia Nut	**190**	10	22

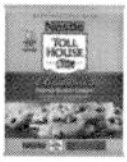

Crispbreads

	C	F	Cb
Per Crispbread Unless Indicated			
Finn Crisp: Original, Rye	**40**	0	10
Other types	**19**	0	3
Kavli Norwegian: Crispy Thin (3)	**50**	0	11
Hearty Thick (2)	**60**	0	12
Malsovit Meal Wafers	**75**	4	7
New York Flatbread Crisps	**35**	0	7
Ry-Krisp: Natural (2)	**50**	0	11
Seasoned (2)	**60**	1	11
Sesame (2)	**60**	2	10
Ryvita: Dark/Light (2)	**70**	0	16
WASA: Crisp'n Light 7 Grain (3)	**60**	0	13
Fiber	**30**	1	5
Hearty, 0.5 oz	**45**	0	11
Light Rye (2), 0.5 oz	**60**	0	14
Multi Grain, 0.5 oz	**45**	0	10
Whole Wheat, 0.5 oz	**50**	1	10

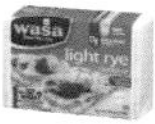

Matzos

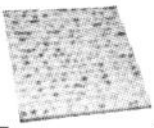

	C	F	Cb
Manischewitz			
Egg 'n Onion Matzo, 1 oz	**100**	1	23
Mandelin (9)	**35**	2	4
Matzo Meal, ¼ cup	**130**	0	28
Matzo Farfel, 1 cup, 2.7 oz	**180**	0.5	60
Passover Egg Matzos, 1.1 oz	**120**	0	28
Tam Tam Crackers, Onion (10)	**140**	5	21
Thin Salted; Thin Tea Matzos, 0.9 oz	**100**	0	22
Unsalted, 1 oz	**90**	0	20
Whole Wheat, 1 oz	**110**	0.5	23
Crackers: Miniatures (10)	**110**	0	25
Passover Egg Matzo (11)	**110**	0	20
Streit's			
Mediterranean Matzos, 1 Matzo, 1 oz	**90**	0.5	18
Unsalted Matzos, 1 Matzo, 1 oz	**100**	0	23

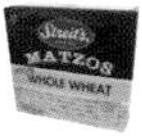

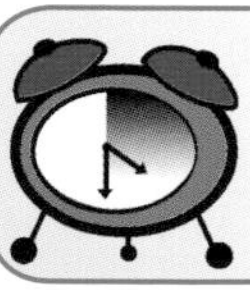

There are 1440 minutes in every day...

Schedule 30 of them for exercise!

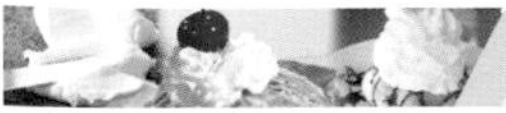

Quick Guide

Cream

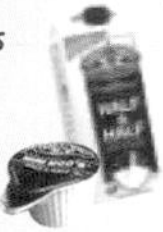

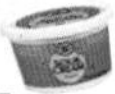

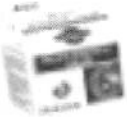

	C	F	Cb
Average All Brands			
Half & Half Cream:			
1 Tbsp, 0.5 oz	20	1.5	0.5
2 Tbsp, 1 oz	40	3	1
¼ cup, 2 oz	80	6	2
Single Serve Cup, ⅜ fl.oz	15	1.5	0.5
Light: Coffee/table (20% fat): 1 Tbsp	30	3	0.5
2 Tbsp, 1 oz	60	6	1
Sour Cream:			
Regular: 1 Tbsp, 0.5 oz	25	2.5	1
1 cup, 8 oz	490	48	10
Low-Fat/Light: 1 Tbsp, 0.5 oz	20	1.5	1
2 Tbsp, 1 oz	40	3	2
Fat-Free: Average, 2 Tbsp, 1 oz	25	0	4
Hood, 2 Tbsp, 1 oz	25	0	4
Kroger, 2 Tbsp, 1 oz	20	0	3
Naturally Yours; Oak Farm, 2 Tbsp	20	0	3
Knudsen, 2 Tbsp, 1 oz	30	0	5
Sour Cream Substitute:			
Albertson's, 2 Tbsp, 1 oz	60	5	2
Tofutti Sour Supreme, 2 Tbsp, 1 oz	85	7	9
Whipping Cream:			
Heavy (37% fat):			
1 T. fluid/2 T. whipped	50	5.5	0.5
¼ cup whipped	100	11	1
½ cup fluid/1 cup whipped	400	44	3.5
Light (30% fat):			
1 Tbsp fluid/2 Tbsp whipped	45	4.5	0.5
½ cup fluid/1 cup whipped	350	37	4

Coconut Cream/Milk

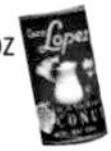

	C	F	Cb
Coconut Cream (Canned),			
Plain/unsweetened: 2 Tbsp, 1 oz	75	6.5	3
½ cup, 4 oz	285	26	12
Sweetened: *Coco Lopez,* 1 oz	130	5	21
½ cup, 4 oz	520	20	84
Coconut Milk (Canned):			
Natural Value: Reg., ¼ cup, 2 fl.oz	120	11	5
Lite, ¼ cup, 2 fl.oz	55	5	1
Thai Kitchen: Lite, ¼ cup, 2 fl.oz	45	4	1
Premium, 2 fl.oz	120	10	4
Coconut Water (Center), 1 cup	45	0.5	9

Updated Nutrition Data ~ www.CalorieKing.com
Persons with Diabetes ~ See Disclaimer (Page 24)

Whipped Toppings

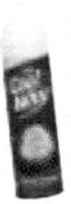

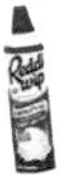

	C	F	Cb
Average All Brands			
Cream (Pressurized): 2 Tbsp	20	1	1
¼ cup	45	4	2
½ cup	90	8	4
Cream Topping: Lite, 2 Tbsp	20	1	3
Cool Whip: Extra Creamy, 2 Tbsp	25	2	2
Lite, 2 Tbsp, ¼ oz	15	1	2
Free, 2 Tbsp, 0.32 oz	15	0	3
Kraft: Dream Whip, 2 Tbsp	10	0	2
Reddi-Wip: Original, 2 Tbsp, 0.28 oz	15	1	0.5
Chocolate, 2 Tbsp, 0.28 oz	15	1	1
Extra Creamy, 2 Tbsp, 0.28 oz	20	1.5	0.5
Fat-Free, 2 Tbsp, 0.28 oz	5	0	1

Creamers (Non-Dairy)

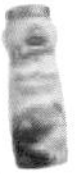

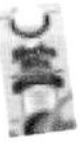

	C	F	Cb
Powder:			
Coffee-Mate/Cremora/N-Rich			
Original: 1 tsp	10	0.5	1
1 heaping tsp	25	2	2
Lite, 1 tsp	10	1.5	2
Flavors: 4 tsp	60	3	8
Fat-Free, Average, 4 tsp	50	0	11
Liquid/Refrigerated: *Per Tablespoon*			
Coffee-Mate			
Unflavored: Original, 1 Tbsp	20	1	2
Fat-Free, 1 Tbsp	10	0	2
Low-Fat, 1 Tbsp	10	0.5	1
Flavors: Average all flavors, 1 Tbsp	35	1.5	5
Fat-Free, all flavors, 1 Tbsp	25	0	5
Hood, Country Creamer, 1 Tbsp	20	1.5	2
International Delight:			
Average all flavors, 1 Tbsp	40	1.5	7
Fat-Free French Vanilla, 1 Tbsp	30	0	7
Kroger			
Coffee, Fat-Free & Lactose Free:			
French Vanilla, 1 Tbsp	30	0	6
Hazelnut, 1 Tbsp	35	1.5	6
Mocha Mix: Original, 1 Tbsp	20	1.5	2
Fat-Free, 1 Tbsp	10	0	1
Lite, 1 Tbsp	10	0.5	1
Silk: Original, 1Tbsp	15	1	1
French Vanilla; Hazelnut, 1 Tbsp	20	1	3

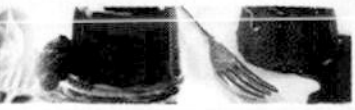

Ready-To-Serve

Ready-To-Serve	C	F	Cb
Instant Pudding, Regular, ½ cup	170	4	30
Reduced Calorie: *Estee*	70	0	12
Jell-O Snacks, sugar-free, ½ cup	60	1	13
Royal Flan,Vanilla sugar-free, ½ cup	80	0	21
Hunt's Snack Pack: *Per 3.5oz Cup*			
Puddings, average all flavors	120	3.5	21
Jell-O Puddings			
Pudding & Pie Filling: *Per ¼ Package*			
Cook & Serve, average, prepared	150	3	26
Instant, regular, average, dry	100	0	23
Fat & Sugar Free, average, dry	30	0	8
Pudding Snacks: Fat-Free, 4 oz	100	0	23
Cheesecake Snack, Strawb. 3½ oz	130	2	26
Mousse Temptations, average, 2.3 oz	60	3	10
Smoothie Snacks, 4 oz	100	2.5	18
Kozy Shack Puddings			
Regular Puddings:			
Chocolate, ½ cup, 4 oz	140	3.5	24
Key Lime, ½ cup, 4 oz	110	0	25
Low-Fat (1% Milk), 6-Pack,			
Average, 1 pudding cup	110	1	20
No Sugar Added, 4-Pack: *Per 1 Pudding Cup*			
Apple Pie A-la-Mode	70	3	10
Chocolate	60	1	10
Vanilla	90	3	10
Flans: Creme Caramel, 1 cup	150	3.5	27
Restaurant Style, 1 cup	190	6	28
Rice Pudding: *Per ½ Pudding Cup, 4 oz*			
Original	130	3	22
Cinnamon Raisin	140	3	24
European Style	130	3.5	22
No Sugar Added, 1 pudding cup	70	0.5	14
Rice, Country Peaches, ½ cup	140	4.5	23
Soy Puddings, average, 1 cup	115	2	22
Tapioca: All Natural, 1 pudding cup	130	3	23
No Sugar Added, 1 pudding cup	90	3	11
Frozen Desserts: Cream Puffs (6)	260	20	15
Chocolate Truffle Rolls (8)	240	13	27
Mini Eclairs (5)	250	16	23
Mini Napoleons (5)	280	14	35
Tiramisu, 1 cup	220	10	29
Kraft Handi Snacks: *Per Cup (3.5 oz)*			
"Doubles", average all flavors	100	1	22
Rice Pudding	140	6	19
Vanilla Pudding	90	1	20
Choc. Pudding, Fat-Free	90	0	21

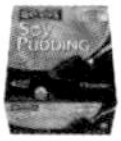

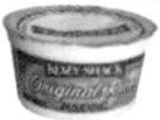

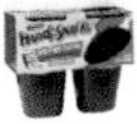

Ready-To-Serve (Cont)

Ready-To-Serve (Cont)	C	F	Cb
Kroger: *Per Container*			
Butterscotch, 3½ oz	110	2	22
Chocolate, 3½ oz	110	2.5	21
President's Choice			
Key Lime Pie (36 oz), ⅛ pie, 4.5 oz	440	20	59
Mississippi Mud Pie (36 oz), ⅛, 4.5 oz	405	22	49
Swiss Miss Pudding Snacks: *Per 4 oz Cup*			
Chocolate, Low-Fat	130	2	26
Chocolate Vanilla Swirl	140	3.5	27
Creamy Vanilla	140	3.5	24
Milk/Dark Chocolate	150	3.5	27
Old Fashioned Tapioca	140	3.5	24

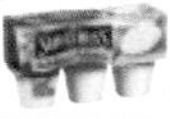

Homemade Puddings

Apple Tapioca, ½ cup	150	0	32
Bread Pudding, ½ cup	250	8	40
Blancmange, ½ cup	140	5	19
Chocolate, ½ cup	190	6	30
Crème Brûlée, ½ cup	400	35	16
Plum Pudding, 2 oz	170	3	32
Rice with Raisins, ½ cup	200	4	38
Sponge Pudding, 3½ oz	340	16	45
Tapioca Cream, ½ cup	110	4	15
Trifle, ½ cup	180	7	26

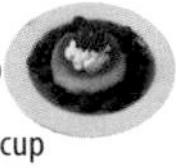

Custards

Custard Mix: Dry, ⅙ package	85	1	17
Prepared with 2% milk, ½ cup	140	3.5	21
Jello Flan, with 2% milk, ½ cup	140	2.5	20
Royal-Flan: Prep. with 2% milk, ½ cup	130	2.5	18
Homemade Custard			
Baked: Plain, ½ cup, 4½ oz	150	7	16
with skim milk, artif. sweetened	70	3	4
Boiled, ½ cup	165	7	18

Meringues

Meringue Swirl, ½ oz	50	0	8
Meringue Shell, 1 oz shell	100	0	16

Gelatin • Parfait • Jell-O

Gelatin Mix: *Jell-O, Royal ~ Made Up*			
Regular, all flavors, ½ cup	80	0	18
Sugar Free/Low Calorie, ½ cup	10	0	0
Creme Gelatin/Parfait: *Per ½ Cup*			
Ida Mae, ½ cup	60	2	10
Reser's, Dessert Parfait, 3.88 oz	100	2	19
Gel Snacks *(Jell-O):* Regular, 3.5 oz	90	0	22
X-Treme Snacks:			
Cherry/Raspb., 3½ oz	70	0	17
Watermelon/Apple, 3½ oz	100	0	24

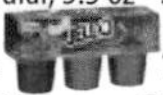

Chicken Eggs

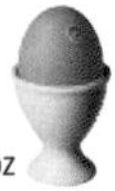

Fresh Eggs	C	F	Cb
Raw (weight with shell):			
Small, 1.4 oz	**65**	4	0
Medium, 1.55 oz	**70**	4	0
Large, 1.76 oz	**75**	4.5	0
Extra Large, 1.98 oz	**80**	5	0
Jumbo, 2.22 oz	**90**	5.5	0
Egg Yolk, 1 extra large	**63**	5	0
Egg White, 1 extra large	**16**	0	0
Dried Egg Powder			
Whole Egg: ¼ cup, 1 oz	**170**	12	0
1 Tbsp	**30**	2	0
Egg White, ¼ cup, 1 oz	**105**	0	0
Egg Yolk, ¼ cup, 1 oz	**195**	18	0

Egg Substitutes

¼ Cup (Equivalent to 1 Egg) ~ Zero Cholesterol.

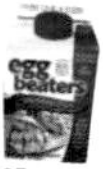

	C	F	Cb
Better 'n Eggs *(Papetti)*, ¼ cup, 2 oz	**30**	0	1
Egg Beaters *(Fleischmann's)* Frozen/Liquid, Regular/Flavors, ¼ cup, 2.2 oz	**30**	0	1
Ener-G, Egg Replacer, 1½ tsp, 4 g	**15**	0	4
Egg Substitute *(Albertson's)*, ¼ cup	**30**	0	1
Egg Whites, 4 Tbsp, ¼ cup, 2 oz	**30**	0	0
Nature Egg, Simply Egg White, ¼ cup, 2 oz	**25**	0	0
Second Nature, Fat-Free, ¼ cup, 2 fl.oz	**35**	0	1

Other Eggs

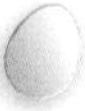

	C	F	Cb
Duck, 1 large, 2½ oz	**130**	9.5	0
Goose, 1 large, 5 oz	**280**	19	0
Quail, 3 eggs, 1 oz	**42**	3	0
Turkey, 1 large, 3 oz	**135**	9.5	0
Turtle, 1 egg, 1¾ oz	**75**	5	0

Omega-3 Fat Enriched

	C	F	Cb
Eggland's Best, 1 large	**70**	4	0
Eggs Plus *(Pilgrim's Pride)*, 1 large	**70**	4.5	1

Note: Cholesterol content same as regular eggs, but Omega-3 fats inhibit blood cholesterol increase.

(Extra Notes ~ *See Page 271*)

Cooked Eggs

	C	F	Cb
Boiled Egg: *Same as raw egg*			
Hard-Cooked *(Egg•Lands), Small,* Peeled	**65**	4	0
Fried Egg:			
With fat: 1 large egg	**105**	9	0.5
2 small eggs	**175**	13	1
No fat/nonstick pan, 1 large	**75**	5	0.5
Deviled Egg, 2 halves	**145**	13	0.5
Eggs Benedict (2) on toast or English muffin	**860**	56	25
Eggs Florentine (2) on toast or English muffin	**890**	59	25
Pickled Egg, 1 large	**80**	5.5	0
Poached Egg, 1 large	**65**	4	0
Quiche (Homemade, average):			
Egg & Bacon, 1 slice, 5.3 oz	**580**	43	27
Ham & Cheese, 1 slice, 5.3 oz	**475**	33	29
Scotch Egg, 1 egg	**300**	21	16
Scrambled Eggs: 1 large egg:			
With 1 Tbsp milk + 1 tsp fat	**120**	9	1
With 1 Tbsp skim milk/no fat	**85**	5.5	1
2 large eggs:			
With 2 Tbsp milk + 2 tsp fat	**260**	20	2
With 2 Tbsp skim milk, w/o fat	**180**	11	2

Omelets

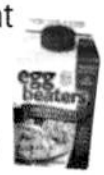

	C	F	Cb
1 Egg: Plain (with 1 tsp fat)	**125**	10	0.5
With ½ oz cheese	**175**	15	0.5
With ½ oz cheese + ½ oz ham	**200**	16	0.5
2 Eggs: Plain (with 2 tsp fat)	**250**	20	1
With 1 oz cheese	**360**	29	2
With 1 oz cheese+1 oz ham	**410**	32	2
3 Eggs: Plain (with 1 Tbsp fat)	**360**	29	1.5
With 2 oz cheese	**580**	47	2.5
With 2 oz cheese+2 oz ham	**680**	53	2.5
Extras: Tomato/Onion/Veggies	**20**	0	4.5
Egg Substitute *(EggBeaters)*:			
2 eggs (½ cup) + 1 tsp fat	**100**	4	2
3 eggs (¾ cup) + 2 tsp fat	**160**	8	3
Extras: 1 oz Cheese	**110**	9	1
1 oz Ham	**50**	3	1
Tomato/Onion/veggies	**20**	0	4.5

Egg Nog ~ *Per ½ Cup (4 fl.oz)*

	C	F	Cb
Average all Brands, ½ cup	**170**	9.5	17
Regular: *Borden*	**160**	9	17
Hood (Golden)	**180**	9	22
Light/Low-Fat: *Horizon; Hood*	**140**	4	22

Updated Nutrition Data ~ www.CalorieKing.com
Persons with Diabetes ~ See Disclaimer (Page 24)

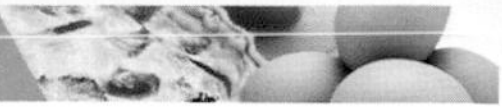

Breakfast Sides

	C	F	Cb
Toast: Plain, 1 thick slice	85	1	13
With 2 tsp butter/margarine	155	9	13
With 3 tsp/1 Tbsp fat	190	13	13
English Muffin: Plain, 2 oz	130	1	26
With 3 tsp fat	230	12	26
Bacon, 2 strips	70	5	0
Ham, Lean, 2 oz	100	3	0
Hash Browns:			
½ cup, 3 oz	125	6.5	14
1 cup serving, 6 oz	250	13	28
Sausages, 2 links (1 oz each)	180	16	1.5

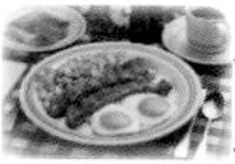

Frozen Egg Breakfasts

	C	F	Cb
Aunt Jemima Breakfast Sandwiches: *Per Package*			
Ham, Egg & Cheese Griddlecake	240	8	33
Sausage, Egg & Cheese Biscuit	340	21	27
Sausage, Egg & Cheese Croissant	350	23	22
Jimmy Dean			
Biscuit, Sausage, Egg & Cheese (1)	440	31	27
Croissant: Sausage, Egg & Cheese (1)	430	29	30
Muffin, Sausage, Egg & Cheese	350	21	28
Omelet: 3 Cheese (1)	290	23	4
Ham & Cheese (1)	250	19	4
Pillsbury: Toaster Scrambles,			
Cheese Sauce, Egg & Bacon	180	12	16
Cheese Sauce, Egg & Sausage	180	11	16
Red Baron			
Scrambles: Bacon (1), 5 oz	410	21	36
Sausage (1), 5 oz	370	19	36
Western (1), 5 oz	350	16	36
Swanson Great Starts			

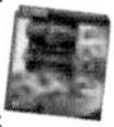

Frozen Pancake/Waffles: *See Page 122*

Frozen Egg Rolls

	C	F	Cb
Chun King/La Choy: ***Average All Brands***			
Pork & Shrimp Egg Rolls:			
Mini, 6 rolls, 3 oz	210	9	27
Shrimp Egg Rolls, Mini, 6 rolls	190	6	28
Lotus: Pork, 3.8 oz	180	7	18
Vegetable, 3.8 oz	70	1.5	13
Kahiki: Pork, 3 oz	140	3.5	20
Chicken, 3 oz	160	6	19
Vegetable Egg Roll, 3 oz	130	3.5	21

Fast-Foods/Restaurants

	C	F	Cb
Arby's: Bacon & Egg Croissant	335	22	23
Au Bon Pain: Scrambled Eggs, 6 oz	210	18	6
Bob Evans:			
Farmers Market Omelette	630	45	14
Ham & Cheddar Omelette	515	36	4
Three Cheese Omelette	530	40	5
Western Omelette	530	36	8
Bojangles: Egg Biscuit	400	30	26
Bacon, Egg & Cheese Biscuit	550	42	27
Bruegger's Bagels:			
Breakfast Sandwiches:			
Egg & Cheese	470	14	63
Egg, Cheese & Sausage	480	21	63
Burger King: Croissan'wich			
Bacon Egg & Cheese	340	19	26
Ham Egg & Cheese	330	16	27
Sausage & Cheese	380	24	26
Carl's Jr, Bacon & Egg Burrito	550	32	37
Chick-Fil-A			
Chicken, Egg & Cheese Bagel	500	20	49
Denny's: T-Bone Steak & Eggs	780	36	4
Omelette: Ham & Cheddar	590	44	4
Ultimate with Hash Browns	880	66	34
Veg.-Cheese with Hash Browns	700	49	30
Del Taco, Egg & Cheese Burrito	400	18	35
Dunkin Donuts			
Bacon, Egg & Cheese Croissant	510	31	39
Ham, Egg & Cheese Bagel	520	17	75
Eat 'N Park: Cheese Omelette	390	30	2
Western Omelette	345	21	7
Hardee's: Loaded Omelet Biscuit	640	44	37
Sausage & Egg Biscuit	590	42	36
IHOP: T-Bone Steak & Eggs	1160	n/a	70
Colorado Omelette	1890	n/a	130
Jack in the Box			
Bacon, Egg & Cheese Biscuit	440	26	37
McDonald's: Egg McMuffin	300	12	30
Bacon, Egg & Cheese Biscuit, regular	420	23	37
Scrambled Eggs (2)	170	11	1
Whataburger			
Breakfast Platter with Bacon , 2 slices	730	45	93

Quick Guide

Butter & Margarine

Average All Brands

	C	F	Cb
Regular: 1 tsp, 0.18 oz	35	4	0
1 Pat/Single Portion, 0.18 oz	35	4	0
1 Tbsp, approximately ½ oz	100	11	0
2 Tbsp, 1 oz	205	23	0
1 Stick, ½ cup, 4 oz	815	92	0
1 Pound, 2 cups, 16 oz	3260	368	0
Light (Regular) 40% Fat:			
1 tsp, 0.18 oz	25	3	0
1 Tbsp, ½ oz	75	8.5	0
2 Tbsp, 1 oz	150	16	0
Whipped Butter (Regular):			
1 tsp, 0.14 oz	30	3	0
1 Tbsp, 0.35 oz	70	7.5	0
1 Stick, ½ cup, 2 ⅔ oz	545	62	0
Whipped Light Butter (40% Fat):			
1 tsp, 0.18 oz	25	3	0.5
1 Tbsp, 0.32 oz	45	5	1
2 Tbsp, 0.63 oz	90	10	2
Unsalted: Same as Regular			

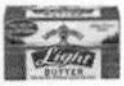

Flavored Butter/Spreads

Average All Brands

	C	F	Cb
Honey Butter (60% Fat):			
1 Tbsp, ½ oz	90	8	4
Downey's, 1 Tbsp, ½ oz	60	1	11
Garlic Butter (80% Fat):			
1 Tbsp, ½ oz	100	11	0
Sweet Cream Butter:			
Regular, 1 Tbsp	100	11	0
Stick *(Parkay)*, 70% Fat, 1 Tbsp	90	10	0
Tub *(Land O'Lakes)*, 50% Fat, 1 Tbsp	90	10	0

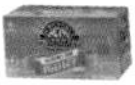

Ghee (Clarified Butter)

(Example: *Purity Farms*)
Note: Ghee is 100% fat compared to regular butter (80% fat + 20% water)

	C	F	Cb
1 tsp, 0.18 oz	45	5	0
1 Tbsp, ½ oz	120	14	0
2¼ Tbsp, 1 oz	250	28	0

Updated Nutrition Data ~ www.CalorieKing.com
Persons with Diabetes ~ See Disclaimer (Page 24)

Light & Reduced Fat Spreads

Per 1 Tbsp, ½ oz (Unless Stated)	C	F	Cb
Albertson's: Country (48%), 1Tbsp	60	7	0
Butter Blend, 1 Tbsp	80	9	0
Benecol: Spread, 1 T., ½ oz	70	8	0
Light, Spread, 1 T., ½ oz	50	5	0
Blue Bonnet, Homestyle (48% Veg Oil)	60	7	0
Brummel & Brown, Spread, 1 Tbsp	45	5	0
Country Crock *(Shedd's):* Regular	60	7	0
Light; Calcium & Vitamins	50	5	0
Spreadable Butter, 1 Tbsp	80	9	0
Downey's, Honey Butter, 1 Tbsp	60	1	11
Fleischmann's: Soft Spread	60	7	0
Original Stick, 1 Tbsp	80	9	0
Light Spread, 1 Tbsp	40	5	0
'I Can't Believe It's Not Butter': Reg.	70	8	0
Light Soft Spread	50	5	0
Imperial: Stick, 1 Tbsp	80	8	0
Tub, 1 Tbsp	50	5	0
Land O'Lakes: Butter, 1 Tbsp	100	11	0
Honey Butter, 1 Tbsp	90	8	4
Light Butter Whipped	45	5	0
Light Butter, 1 Tbsp	50	6	0
Parkay: Squeeze, 1 Tbsp	70	8	0
Light Spread, 1 Tbsp	45	5	0
Original Stick, 1 Tbsp	80	9	0
Promise: Buttery, 1 Tbsp	80	8	0
Fat-Free, 1 Tbsp	5	0	0
Light, 1 Tbsp	45	5	0
Smart Balance: 67% Buttery, 1 T.	80	9	0
Heart Right, 1 Tbsp	80	8	0
Light (37%), 1 Tbsp	45	5	0
Omega Plus, 1 Tbsp	80	9	0
Smart Beat, Fat-Free, 1 Tbsp	50	0	1
Smart Squeeze, 1 Tbsp	5	0	1

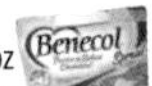

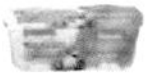

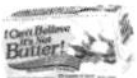

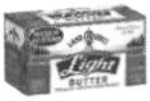

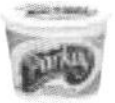

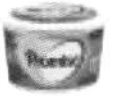

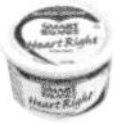

Butter Substitutes

	C	F	Cb
Butter Buds: 1 serving, ½ tsp	5	0	2
Sprinkles, 1 tsp	5	0	0
Earth Balance, Non GMO, 1 Tbsp	100	11	0
Molly McButter, ½ tsp	5	0	1
Shedd's Willow Run, Soy, 1 Tbsp	90	10	0
Sunsweet, Lighter Bake, 1 Tbsp, 0.67 oz (Butter/Oil Replacement)	35	0	9

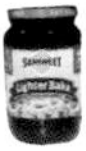

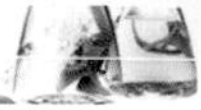

Spreads Comparison

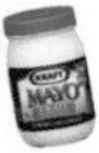
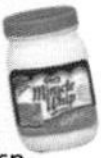
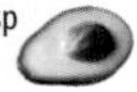

	C	F	Cb
Mayonnaise: Regular, 1 T.	90	10	0
Light, average, 1 Tbsp	45	0	2
Fat-Free, 1 Tbsp	10	0	2
Miracle Whip *(Kraft):*			
Regular, 1 Tbsp	40	3	2
Light, 1 Tbsp	25	1.5	3
Free, 1 Tbsp	15	0	3
Smart Beat Dressing: 1 Tbsp	10	0	3

Extra Listings for Mayonnaise & Dressings
~ See Page 89 ~

	C	F	Cb
Avocado, mashed, 1 Tbsp	45	4	2.5
Peanut Butter, 1 Tbsp	100	8	3.5
Nutella, 1 Tbsp	95	5.5	11

Animal Fats/Lards

Average All Types
Beef Tallow/Drippings, Lard (Pork), Chicken, Duck, Goose, Turkey.

	C	F	Cb
1 Tbsp (13g)	115	13	0
2¼ Tbsp, 1 oz	255	28	0
1 cup, 7¼ oz	1850	205	0
½ pound, 8 oz	2040	227	0
Ghee/Butter Oil: 1 Tbsp, ½ oz	120	14	0
2¼ Tbsp, 1 oz	250	28	0

Vegetable Shortening

Average All Types *(example: Crisco)*

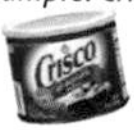

	C	F	Cb
1 Tbsp, 13g	115	13	0
2¼ Tbsp, 1 oz	250	28	0
1 cup, 7¼ oz	1810	205	0

Vegetable Oils

Includes almond, avocado, canola, corn, coconut, flaxseed, grapeseed, linseed, mustard, olive, palm, peanut, rice bran, safflower, sesame, sunflower, soybean, wheat germ. Note: Oil is 100% fat.

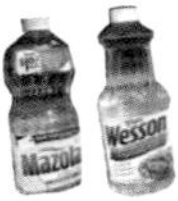

	C	F	Cb
1 tsp, 5g	45	5	0
1 Tbsp, ½ oz	120	14	0
2 Tbsp, 1 oz	250	28	0
1 cup, 7¾ oz	1930	205	0

Fish Oils

	C	F	Cb
Average All Types (Includes cod liver, herring, salmon, sardine): 1 Tbsp, ½ oz	125	14	0

Cooking Sprays/Squeezes

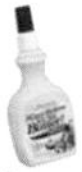

	C	F	Cb
Cooking Sprays *(PAM, Mazola, I Can't Believe It's Not Butter, Weight Watchers, Wesson):*			
Per serving	2	0	0
1-3 second spray	6	1	0
I Can't Believe It's Not Butter	0	0	0
Parkay Buttery Spray	0	0	0
Squeeze (Parkay), 1 Tbsp, ½ oz	70	8	0

Olestra (Olean)

	C	F	Cb
Olestra ***(Olean)***	0	0	0

Note: *Olean is Proctor & Gamble's* brand name for olestra – a no-calorie cooking oil that gives snacks (like potato chips, tortilla chips and crackers) taste and texture without adding fat or calories.

Examples:

- *Frito-Lay* Light Products *(Lays, Ruffles, Tostitos, Doritos)*
- *Pringles* Fat-Free Potato Crisps

Ruffles Light

Quick Guide

Mayonnaise

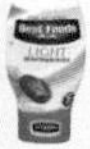
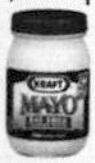

	C	F	Cb
Regular			
Average All Brands, 1 Tbsp	90	10	0
Best Foods, Kraft, 1 Tbsp	90	10	0
½ cup, 4 oz	720	80	0
Light/Reduced Fat			
Kraft, 1 Tbsp	45	4	2
Best Foods, 1 Tbsp	35	3.5	1
Hain, Safflower Oil, 1 Tbsp	100	11	0
Hellman's, 1 Tbsp	90	10	0
Smart Balance, Omega, 1 Tbsp	50	4.5	2
Spectrum: Canola Mayo, 1 Tbsp	100	11	0
Light Canola Mayo Eggless, 1 Tbsp	35	3.5	0
Fat Free			
Kraft: 1 Tbsp	10	0	2
½ cup, 4 oz	80	0	16
Smart Beat, 1 Tbsp	10	0	3
Sugar Free: *Dukes* Mayo, 1 Tbsp	100	12	0

Mayonnaise Style Dressing

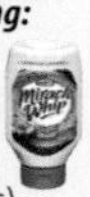

	C	F	Cb
Best Foods Sandwich Spread, 1 T.	60	5	2
Miracle Whip Salad Dressing:			
Regular, 1 Tbsp, ½ oz	35	3	2
Light, 1 Tbsp, ½ oz	25	1.5	3
Free, 1 Tbsp, ½ oz	15	0	3
Nayonaise *(Nasoya)* (Tofu Base/Dairy Free/Eggless)			
Regular, 1 Tbsp, ½ oz	35	3.5	1
Fat-Free, 1 Tbsp, ½ oz	10	0	2

Quick Guide

Fresh Fish	C	F	Cb
Low Oil (Less than 2.5% fat)			
White/Lightly-colored flesh. Examples: Cod, Flounder, Haddock, Halibut, Mahi Mahi, Perch, Pike, Pollock, Snapper, Sole, Whiting.			
Per 4 oz Edible Portion			
Raw, 4 oz (without bones)	90	1	0
Steamed, Broiled, Baked	130	1	0
Fried: Lightly Floured	210	8	3.5
Breaded	260	12	8
In Batter	320	16	27

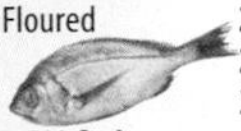

Medium Oil (2.5-5% fat)	C	F	Cb
Lightly-colored flesh. Examples: Bluefin Tuna, Catfish, Kingfish, Orange Roughy, Salmon (Pink), Swordfish, Rainbow Trout, Yellowtail.			
Raw, 4 oz (without bones)	140	5	0
Baked, Broiled, 4 oz	175	6	0
Fried, 4 oz	230	11	8

High Oil (Over 5% fat)	C	F	Cb
Darker-colored flesh. Examples: Albacore Tuna, Bluefish, Herring, Mackerel, Salmon (Atl./Chinook/Sockeye), Sardines, Trout, Whitefish.			
Raw, 4 oz (without bones)	230	16	0
Baked, Broiled, 4 oz	275	17	0
Fried, 4 oz	340	23	12

Cooking Yields (Fin Fish):
4 oz Raw wt. = 3½ oz Cooked weight
4 oz Cooked wt. = 5 oz Raw weight

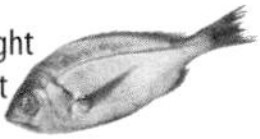

Calorie & Fat Variations
The amount of fat/oil in fish varies with the species, season and locality. Within the same fish, fat/oil content is generally higher towards the head.

Get Moving! Take a computer break every hour.

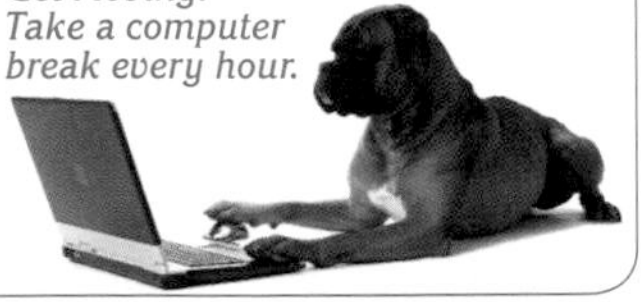

Fish & Shellfish

Edible Weights: (no bones/shell)	C	F	Cb
Abalone, Raw, 3 oz	90	0.5	5
Ahi Tuna, grilled, 6 oz fillet (w/o fat)	235	2	0
Anchovy: Paste, 1 Tbsp, ¼ oz	15	1	0.5
Canned in oil, drained, 5 only, ¾ oz	40	2	0
Pickled, 1 oz	50	3	0
Barracuda (Pacific), raw, 4 oz	130	3	0
Bass: Sea, raw, 4.6 oz fillet	125	2.5	0
Striped: Raw, 1 fillet, 5½ oz	150	3.5	0
Baked, 3 oz	105	3	0
Blue Fish: Raw, 1 fillet, 5¼ oz	185	6.5	0
Baked, 3 oz	130	5	0
Butterfish, raw, 3 oz	125	7	0
Cajun & Creole Dishes: *See Page 176*			
Calamari, breaded/fried, 7 oz	350	15	16
Carp, raw, 3 oz	110	5	0
Catfish (Wild): Raw, 4 oz	110	3	0
Fried, breaded, 1 fillet, 3 oz	200	12	7
Baked, 3 oz	90	2.5	0
Caviar, black/red, 1 Tbsp, 16g	40	3	0.5
Clams: Raw, 3 oz (4 large/9 small)	65	1	2
Fried, breaded, 6.6 oz (20 small)	380	21	20
Canned, drained, ½ cup, 2½ oz	120	1.5	4
Minced, ¼ cup, 2 oz	25	0	2
Clam Juice: (*Snow's*) 1 Tbsp	0	0	0
Cod, Atlantic/Pacific: Raw, 4 oz	95	1	0
Baked/Broiled, 1 fillet, 6¼ oz	190	2	0
Canned, 3 oz	90	1	0
Minced, ¼ cup, 2 oz	25	0	0
Smoked/Dry Heat, 3 oz	90	1	0
Crab: Alaska King, raw, 1 leg, 6 oz	145	1	0
1 leg, cooked, 4¾ oz	130	2	0
Blue: Raw, 1 crab			
(⅓ lb whole crab, ¾ oz flesh)	20	0.2	0
Steamed, 3 oz	85	1	0
Canned, drained, ½ cup, 2½ oz	65	1	0
Dungeness, 1 crab, 5¾ oz edible			
(from 1½ lb whole crab)	180	2	2
Imitation Crab Legs/Stix, 3oz	80	0.5	13
Crab Cakes (Low-fat), (1), 2 oz	95	4.5	0.5
Regular (1), 3 oz	130	6.5	0.5
Crab Legs, restaurant *(Red Lobster)*	260	4.5	0
Crayfish, raw, 4 oz (edible)	90	1	0
Croaker, raw, 3 oz	90	3	0
Cuttlefish, raw, 3 oz	70	1	1
Dolphinfish, raw, 1 fillet, 7 oz	175	1.5	0
Eel: Raw, 3 oz	155	10	0
Smoked/Dry Heat, 3 oz	200	13	0
Fish & Chips: *Arthur Treacher*	1540	101	132
Denny's, without condiments	960	54	83
Fish S'wich with Tartar Sauce, 5½ oz	430	23	41
Fish Sticks (1), frozen, breaded, 1 oz	70	3.5	6

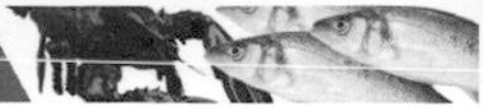

Fish & Shellfish (Cont)

Edible Weights: (no bones/shell)	C	F	Cb
Fish Oil, 1 Tbsp, ½ oz	125	14	0
Flounder/Sole: Raw, 4 oz	105	1.5	0
Baked, 1 fillet, 4½ oz	150	2	0
Frozen Fish & Entrees: *See Page 113-124*			
Gefilte Fish: *See Kosher/Deli Foods, Page 178*			
Grouper, raw, 4 oz	105	1	0
Haddock: Raw, 4 oz	100	1	0
Broiled, 1 fillet, 5¼ oz	170	1.5	0
Smoked, 3 oz	100	1	0
Baked, 3 oz	95	1	0
Halibut: Raw, 4 oz	125	3	0
Baked, ½ fillet, 2¾ oz	225	5	0
Herring: Atlantic, raw, 4 oz	180	10	0
Pickled, 2 pieces, 1 oz	80	5	3
In Sour Cream, 1 oz	55	3	5
Party Snacks, ¼ cup, dr., 2 oz	120	5	0
Rollmops, 1½ oz	110	8	6
Canned: Plain, drained, 3 oz	130	8	0
in Tomato Sauce, 3.5 oz	140	8	2
Smoked, kippered, 4 oz	245	14	0
Jellyfish: Raw, 4 oz	30	0	0
Dried, Salted, 1 cup, 2 oz	20	1	0
King Fish, raw, 4 oz	120	2.5	0
Ling, raw, 4 oz	100	0.5	0
Lobster, Northern: Raw, 4 oz	105	1	0.5
1 Lobster, 6¼ oz			
(from 1½ lb whole lobster)	160	1.5	1
Cooked, 1 cup, 5 oz	140	1	2
Lobster Newberg, avg. ¾ cup	360	20	9
Lobster Thermidor, avg. 1 serving	370	22	15
Lobster Salads, avg. ½ cup	220	13	5
Lobster Tail, restaurant *(Red Lobster)*	260	3	0
Lomi Salmon, ¼ cup, 4 oz	20	1	3
Lox, Regular/Nova, 2 oz	65	2.5	0
Mackerel: Atlantic, raw, 4 oz	230	16	0
Broiled, 3 oz fillet	230	16	0
Jack, canned, ½ c., 3⅓ oz	150	6	0
King, raw, 4 oz	120	2	0
Pacific/Jack: Raw, 4 oz	180	9	0
Broiled, 3 oz	170	9	0
Spanish, raw, 4 oz	160	7	0
Mahi-Mahi, raw, 4 oz	125	1	0
Milkfish, raw, 4 oz	170	7.5	0
Monkfish: Raw, 4 oz	85	1.5	0
Baked, 3 oz	80	2	0
Mullet, striped, raw, 4 oz	135	4.5	0
Mussels: Raw, 4 oz (edible wt.)	100	2.5	4
1 cup, 5¼ oz (edible wt.)	130	3.5	5
Cooked, moist heat, 3 oz	150	4	6

	C	F	Cb
Ocean Perch: Raw, 4 oz	105	2	0
Baked, 3 oz	105	2	0
Octopus, common, raw, 4 oz	95	1	2.5
Orange Roughy, raw, 4 oz	85	1	0
Oysters: Common, raw, 3 oz	70	2	4
Eastern raw: 6 medium, 3 oz	50	1.5	4.5
1 cup, 8¾ oz	150	4	14
Fried/breaded, 6 med., 3 oz	170	11	10
Pacific, raw, 1 med., 1¾ oz	40	1	2
Oysters Rockerfeller, 3 oysters	220	13	12
Perch, average, raw, 4 oz	105	1	0
Pike: Northern, raw, 4 oz	100	1	0
Walleye, raw, 4 oz	105	1.5	0
Pollock, raw, 4 oz	105	1	0
Pout (Ocean), raw, 4 oz	90	1	0
Pompano, Florida, raw, 4 oz	185	11	0
Porgy/Scup, raw, 4 oz	150	4	0
Quahogs ~ See Clams			
Red-Snapper, raw, 4 oz	115	1.5	0
Rockfish, Pacific, raw, 4 oz	110	2	0
Roe, raw, 2 Tbsp, 1 oz	40	2	0.5
Sablefish: Raw, 4 oz	220	17	0
Smoked, 3 oz	220	17	0
Salmon:			
Raw: Chinook, 4 oz	205	12	0
Atlantic; Coho/Silver, 4 oz	210	12	0
Chum; Pink, 4 oz	135	4	0
Red/Sockeye, 4 oz	190	10	0
Baked: Atlantic/Coho, 3 oz	160	5	0
Smoked Salmon: Chinook, 3 oz	100	4	0
Pacific Supreme, 2 oz	100	4	0
Canned Salmon: ***Average All Brands***			
Pink: 1 oz	40	2	0
¼ cup, 63g (2.2 oz)	90	5	0
3¾ oz can, whole	155	8.5	0
7½ oz can, whole	300	17	0
Skinless/boneless, ¼ c., 2 oz	70	2	0
Red Sockeye: 1 oz	50	3	0
¼ cup, 63g (2.2 oz)	110	7	0
3¾ oz can, whole	190	12	0
Atlantic, ½ cup, 3½ oz	230	14	0
Chinook/King, ½ cup	210	14	0
Chum, ½ cup, 3½ oz	140	5	0
Coho/Silver, ½ cup	155	5	0
Atlantic Steaks: Small, 8 oz	320	14	0
Medium, 12 oz	480	21	0
Large, 16 oz	640	28	0
Salmon Cake, take-out, 3 oz	240	15	6

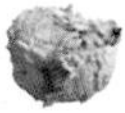

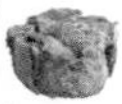

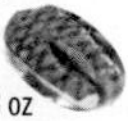

Fish (Cont)

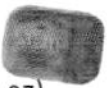

	C	F	Cb
Sardines (Canned): ***Average All Brands***			
In Oil, undrained, 1 oz	85	7	0
Drained of oil, 1 oz	60	3	0
3¾ oz can, drained, (3¼ oz)	190	11	0
1 large/2 med. ⅗" small, 0.8 oz	50	3	0
In Tomato/ Mustard Sauce, 1 oz	55	3	0
3¾ oz can (3 sardines)	210	12	1
Sashimi: *See Japanese Foods, Page 178*			
Scallop: Raw, 6 large/15 small, 3 oz	80	0.5	2
Breaded/fried, 6 pieces, 3½ oz	200	10	10
Sea Bass, raw, 4 oz	110	2	0
Seafood Salad, (Deli Style),			
½ cup, 3.5 oz	250	21	11
Shark: Raw, 4 oz	150	5	0
Batter-dipped, fried, 4 oz	220	13	6
Baked, 4 oz	185	7	0
Shark Fin, dried, 1 oz	30	0	0
Shrimp: Raw, in shell, ½ lb	140	2	1.5
Raw, shelled, 3 oz (12 large)	90	1.5	0.5
Breaded/fried, 3 oz (11 large)	210	11	10
Canned, 1 oz (10 shrimp)	30	0.5	0
Tiger, cooked, 1 shrimp, ½ oz	15	0.5	0
Battered, fried, 1 shrimp	60	4	3
Shrimp Cocktail, restaurant-style	140	2	1
Smelt, Rainbow, raw, 4 oz	110	3	0
Snapper: Raw, 3 oz	85	1	0
Cooked, 1 fillet, 6 oz	220	3	0
Sole, Raw, 4 oz	105	1.5	0
Squid: Raw, 4 oz	105	1.5	3.5
Fried, 3 oz	150	6	7
Surimi (Imitation Crab), 4 oz	110	0.5	17
Sweet & Sour Fish, ½ dish, 10 oz	580	29	53
Swordfish raw:			
Small Steak, 4 oz	135	4.5	0
Medium Steak, 6 oz	205	7	0
Tilapia, Rain Forest Fillets, 4 oz	110	2	0
Trout, Rainbow: Raw, 4 oz	135	4	0
Broiled, 3 oz	125	5	0
Smoked, 2 oz	110	6	0
Tuna: ***Average All Brands***			
Raw: Albacore, 4 oz	190	8	0
Bluefin, 4 oz	165	5.5	0
Skipjack, Yellowfin, 4 oz	125	1	0
Broiled, 3 oz	115	1	0
Canned:			
In Water, drained:			
Chunk/Solid: 2 oz can	75	1.5	0
3 oz can	110	2.5	0
6 oz can	220	5	0

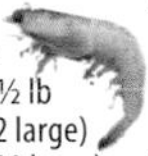

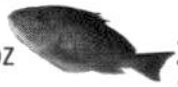

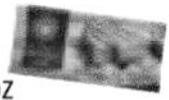

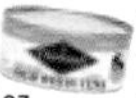

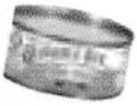

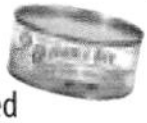

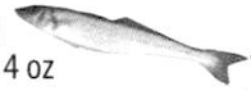

	C	F	Cb
Tuna (Cont)			
In Oil, drained:			
Chunk Light: 2 oz	110	5	0
6 oz can, drained	315	14	0
Solid White, 2 oz	105	4.5	0
6.3 oz can, drained	330	14	0
Tuna Salad: Deli Style, ½ cup, 4oz	300	24	15
Lower fat, 4 oz	210	10	11
Whitefish: Raw, 4 oz	150	6.5	0
Baked, 3 oz	145	6.5	1
Smoked, 3 oz	90	1	0
Whiting: Raw, 4 oz	100	1.5	0
Baked, 3 oz	100	1.5	0
Yellowtail: Raw, 4 oz	165	6	0
Grilled, 3 oz (from 4 oz raw)	160	6	0

Other Canned/Packaged Fish

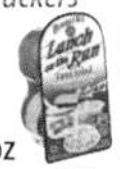

	C	F	Cb
Bumble Bee:			
Tuna Salad Kits: *With Crackers*			
Original, 3.5 oz	300	22	18
with Mayonnaise	420	23	24
Fat-Free, 3.5 oz	150	1.5	24
Lunch on the Run, 8.2 oz	560	31	59
Seafood Salad with Crackers, 3.3 oz	180	5.5	27
Sensations Bowls:			
Spicy Thai Chili, 3 oz	160	7	9
Lemon & Cracked Pepper, 3 oz	110	4	2
Chicken of the Sea			
Albacore Tuna in Water, 3 oz pouch	100	3	0
Light Tuna in Oil, 3 oz pouch	100	4	0
Pink Salmon, skinless/boneless, 2 oz	60	2	0
Shrimp, medium, 4 oz can	90	1	2
Starkist			
Pouch: *Per 3 oz Pouch, Drained*			
Albacore Tuna, in water, 2 oz	70	1.5	1
Tuna Chunk Light, in water, 2 oz	60	0.5	1
Lunch-To-Go Kit: Chunk Light Tuna			
with Mayo & Crackers, 4.5 oz	240	9	20
Tuna Creations, av. all varieties, 2 oz	70	1	0

Frozen Fish Products

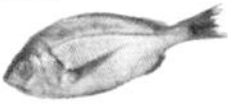

Gorton's: *Page 120*
Kroger: *Page 121*
Van De Kamp's: *Page 124*
Restaurant Chains: *Page 182*
Captain D's Seafood: *Page 94*
Long John Silver's: *Page 221*
Shoney's: *Page 249*
Southern Tsunami: *Page 253*
Wahoo's Fish Taco: *Page 265*

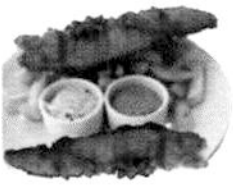

F Flours & Grains

Flours & Grains	C	F	Cb
Amaranth Flour, ½ cup, 3½ oz	365	6.5	65
Arrowroot Flour, ½ cup, 2¼ oz	230	0	56
Barley: Regular, ½ cup, 2.6 oz	255	1	55
Pearled, raw, 3½ oz	350	1	78
Buckwheat: Regular, ½ cup, 3 oz	290	3	61
Groats: Roasted, dry, ½ cup, 2.9 oz	285	2	62
Roasted, cooked, 3½ oz	80	0.5	17
Flour, whole-groat, ½ cup, 2 oz	200	2	42
Bulgur: Dry, ½ cup, 2½ oz	240	1	53
Cooked, ½ cup, 3.2 oz	75	0.5	17
Carob Flour, ½ cup, 1.8 oz	115	0.5	46
Corn Kernels av., ckd, ½ cup	80	0.5	18
Corn Bran, ½ cup, 1.3 oz	85	0.5	33
Corn Flour/Masa, ½ cup, 2 oz	215	2.5	43
Corn Grits: Dry, ½ cup, 2¾ oz	290	1	62
Cooked, ½ cup, 4¼ oz	70	0.5	15
Corn Germ, toasted, ½ cup, 4 oz	100	1.5	22
Cornmeal: Average all Types,			
3 Tbsp, 1 oz	105	0.5	22
½ cup, 2½ oz	255	1	54
Mixes: same as above	230	1	48
Made Up, ½ cup, 4.8 oz	95	0.5	20
Cornstarch: 1 Tbsp, 0.3 oz	30	0	8
½ cup, 2¼ oz	245	0	58
Couscous: Dry, 1 oz (3 oz cooked)	110	0	22
1 cup cooked, 5½ oz	175	0.5	37
Farina: Dry, ½ cup, 3.1 oz	325	0.5	69
Cooked, ½ cup, 4.1 oz	55	0	12
Flaxseed: Seeds, 1 Tbsp, 0.3 oz	45	3.5	2
Ground, 2 Tbsp, 0.3 oz	60	4.5	4
Garbanzo (Chick Pea), ½ cup, 1.6 oz	180	3	27
Kuzu Root Starch, 1 Tbsp, 0.35 oz	35	0	9
Matzo Meal, ½ cup, 2.2 oz	230	0.5	48
Millet: Raw, ½ cup, 3½ oz	380	4	73
Cooked, ½ cup, 3 oz	105	1	21
Oat Bran: Raw, ⅓ cup, 1.1 oz	75	2	21
Cooked, ½ cup, 3¾ oz	45	1	13
Oats, rolled/oatmeal:			
Dry/Groats, ½ cup, 1.5 oz	160	3	28
Cooked, ½ cup, 4.2 oz	75	1	13
Polenta: *See Cornmeal*			
Potato Flour, ½ cup, 2.8 oz	285	0.5	66
Psyllium Husks, 1 Tbsp, 0.15 oz	20	0	4
Quinoa: Dry ½ cup, 3 oz	320	5	59
Cooked, ½ cup, 3¾ oz	130	2	24
Rice Bran, ½ cup, 2 oz	180	12	28
Rice Flour, ½ cup, 2¾ oz	290	1	63

Flours & Grains (Cont)	C	F	Cb
Rice Polish, ½ cup, 3½ oz	360	0.5	80
Rye Flour: Dark, ½ cup, 2.3 oz	210	2	44
Medium, ½ cup, 1.8 oz	180	1	40
Light, ½ cup, 1.8 oz	190	1	41
Rye Grain: ½ cup, 3 oz	280	2	59
Flakes, ¼ cup, 1 oz	100	0.5	21
Semolina, ½ cup, 3 oz	300	1	61
Sorghum, ½ cup, 3.4 oz	325	3	72
Soy Flour:			
Defatted, 1 cup, 3½ oz	330	1	38
Low-Fat, 1 cup, 3 oz	325	6	33
Full-Fat, 1 cup, 3 oz	365	17	29
Soy Meal, defatted, 1 cup, 4.3 oz	415	3	49
Spelt Flour, ½ cup, 2 oz	190	1	41
Tapioca, Pearl:			
Dry, ½ cup, 2.7 oz	270	0	67
3 Tbsp, 1 oz	100	0	25
Teff (Seed) Flour, 2 oz	215	2	42
Tortilla Flour Mix, ½ cup, 2 oz	220	6	37
Triticale: ½ cup, 3.4 oz	325	2	70
Flour, whole-grain, ½ cup, 2.3 oz	220	1	48
Wheat Bran, unproc., ½ cup, 1 oz	65	1	19
Wheat Flakes, ½ cup, 1½ oz	160	1	35
Wheat Germ:			
Raw, ¼ cup, 1 oz	105	3	15
Toasted, ¼ cup, 1 oz	110	3	14
Wheat Flour:			
White, All Purpose/Self-Rising,			
1 level Tbsp, 0.28 oz	30	0	6
½ cup, 2.2 oz	230	0.5	48
1 cup, 4.4 oz	455	1.5	95
Whole Wheat, 1 cup, 4.2 oz	405	2	87

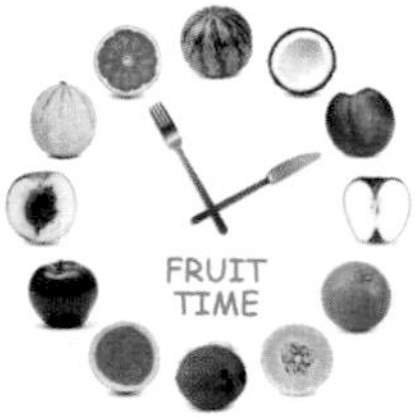

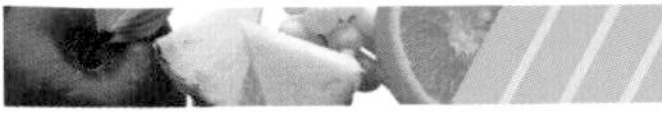

Weights As Purchased	C	F	Cb
Acerola, 1 cup, 20 pieces, 3½ oz	**30**	**0**	7.5
Apples: Whole, average all varieties,			
1 small (4 per lb), 4 oz	**55**	**0**	13
1 medium (3 per lb), 5½ oz	**70**	**0**	17
1 large (2 per lb), 8 oz	**110**	**0**	26
1 extra large, 11 oz	**150**	**0**	36
Without skin: 1 medium, 4½ oz	**60**	**0**	14
1 cup slices, 4 oz	**55**	**0**	13
Candy/Caramel Apple, 1 med., 6½ oz	**245**	**4**	54
Nut Coated, 1 medium, 7 oz	**325**	**11**	56
Chiquita Apple Bites, 10 slices, 3½ oz	**50**	**0**	12
Apricots: 1 small (12 per lb)	**17**	**0**	4
1 medium (8 per lb), 2 oz	**25**	**0**	6
1 large (5-6 per lb), 3 oz	**40**	**0**	10
Asian Pear (Nashi Fruit), 1 medium, 7 oz	**85**	**0**	21
Avocado (without seed/skin):			
Average, ½ medium, 3½ oz	**160**	**15**	8
1 salad slice, ½ oz	**25**	**2**	1
Mashed/Puree, 2 Tbsp, 1 oz	**50**	**4.5**	2
¼ cup, 2 oz	**90**	**9**	5
Californian, ½ medium, 3 oz	**160**	**14**	8
Mashed/Puree, ½ cup, 4 oz	**190**	**18**	10
Florida, ½ medium, 5½ oz	**180**	**15**	12
Mashed/Puree, ½ cup, 4 oz	**140**	**11**	9
½ cup cubed, 3 oz	**105**	**8**	7
Banana, (weight with skin):			
1 small (6", 4 per lb), 4 oz	**90**	**0**	23
1 medium (7", 3 per lb), 5 oz	**105**	**0**	27
1 large (8"), 7 oz	**120**	**0**	30
1 extra large (9"), 9 oz	**135**	**0**	35
without skin, 1 oz	**25**	**0**	6
Black Raspberries, 1 cup, 5 oz	**70**	**0**	16
Blackberries: 1 cup, 5 oz	**60**	**0.5**	14
Blueberries: Approx. 20, 1 oz	**15**	**0**	4
1 cup, 5 oz	**80**	**0.5**	20
1 pint, 14 oz	**225**	**1**	57
Boysenberries, 1 cup, 4.5 oz	**60**	**4.5**	14
Breadfruit, ½ cup, 4 oz	**115**	**0**	30
Cactus Pear, 1 fruit, 3½ oz	**40**	**0**	9
Cantaloupe: Flesh (without rind), 1 oz	**10**	**0**	2
1 cup pieces/balls, 5.5 oz	**55**	**0**	13
½ Circle Slices (no rind):			
1 thin (¼"), 1 oz	**10**	**0**	2
1 medium (½"), 2 oz	**20**	**0**	5
1 thick (¾"), 3 oz	**30**	**0**	7
Wedges (Length cut, w/o rind):			
1 thin, 1/16 medium, 2 oz	**20**	**0**	5
1 thick, ⅛ medium, 4 oz	**40**	**0**	9
Whole (Weights with seeds and rind):			
½ small, 20 oz	**195**	**1**	46
½ medium, 28 oz	**270**	**1.5**	65
½ large, 2½ lb	**370**	**2**	90
Carambola (Starfruit), 1 medium, 3 oz	**30**	**0**	6
Cassava, ⅓ cup, 2½ oz	**115**	**0**	27
Cherimoya, 1 cup, 5.5 oz	**115**	**1**	27

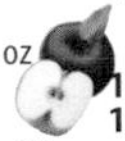

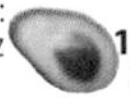
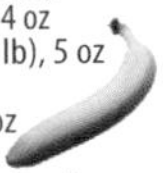
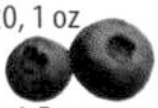
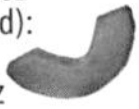
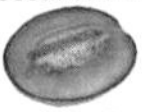

Weights As Purchased	C	F	Cb
Cherries: Sweet (Red/White), raw,			
8 cherries, 2 oz	**30**	**0**	8
1 cup, 4½ oz	**75**	**0**	19
½ lb (30 cherries)	**130**	**0.5**	32
Sour, red, raw, 1 cup, 4 oz	**50**	**0**	12
Clementine, 1 medium, 2.6 oz	**35**	**0**	9
Coconut: Fresh,			
1 piece, 2"x2"x ½", 1 oz	**100**	**10**	4.5
Shredded, fresh, ½ cup, 1.4 oz	**140**	**13**	6
Sweetened, dried, ½ cup, 1.6 oz	**235**	**16**	22
Crabapples, ½ cup slices, 2 oz	**40**	**0**	11
Cranberries, ¼ cup, 1 oz	**25**	**0**	6.5
Currants, raw, ½ cup, 2 oz	**35**	**0**	8
Custard Apple, 4 oz, edible	**115**	**1**	28
(from 7 oz with skin/seeds)			
Dates: *See Dried Fruits*			
Dragon Fruit (Pitahaya),			
1 medium, 11½ oz	**330**	**1.5**	76
Durian, flesh, 4 oz	**165**	**6**	31
Elderberries, ½ cup, 2½ oz	**55**	**0.5**	13
Feijoa (Pineapple Guava),			
1 medium, 2 oz	**30**	**0.5**	5.5
Figs, green/black:			
1 medium, 2 oz	**40**	**0**	10
1 large, 3 oz	**60**	**0**	15
Gooseberries, raw, ½ cup, 2½ oz	**35**	**0**	7
Grapefruit: Average all types,			
½ fruit, 10 oz (6 oz flesh)	**55**	**0**	13
1 cup sections w/ juice, 8 oz	**75**	**0**	18
Grapes: Average, 1 cup, 5½ oz	**105**	**0**	28
1 small bunch, 4 oz	**80**	**0**	20
1 medium bunch, 7 oz	**140**	**0**	36
1 large bunch, 16 oz	**315**	**0**	82
Granadilla, flesh, 3½ oz	**95**	**0**	23
Guava, 1 medium, 4 oz	**80**	**1**	16
Honeydew: 1 slice, ¾" thick, 3 oz	**30**	**0**	7
1 wedge (⅛ of 7" diam.),			
12 oz (with rind)	**80**	**0**	20
1 cup cubes/balls, 6 oz	**60**	**0**	14
½ small (4½ lb whole)	**180**	**0.5**	42
½ medium (6lb whole)	**230**	**1**	56
Honey Murcots, 1 only, 5 oz	**45**	**0**	11
Jaboticaba, flesh, 4 oz	**75**	**2**	15
Jackfruit, flesh, ⅛ average, 4 oz	**105**	**0**	27
Java-Plum, 4 plums, ½ oz	**10**	**0**	2
Jujube, 3 oz	**65**	**0**	17
Kiwifruit,: 1 Medium, 2.7 oz	**45**	**0**	11
1 Large, 3.2 oz	**55**	**0.5**	13
Kumquats, 5 medium, 3½ oz	**65**	**1**	15
Kiwano, ½ medium, 5 oz	**35**	**0**	8
Langsat, Duku, 1 medium, 2 oz	**25**	**0**	5
Lemon: 1 medium, 3 oz	**25**	**0**	8
1 wedge, 1 oz	**5**	**0**	1.5
Peel, grated, 1 Tbsp	**5**	**0**	1

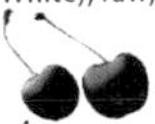
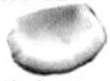
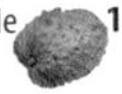
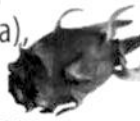
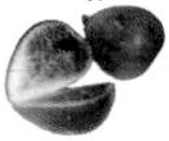
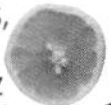
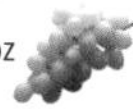
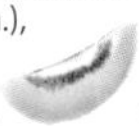

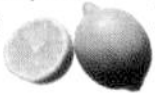

Weights As Purchased	C	F	Cb
Limes, 1 medium (2" diam.), 2.4 oz	20	0	7
Loganberries, frozen, ½ cup, 2½ oz	40	0	9
Longans, 5 fruit, ½ oz	10	0	2.5
Loquats, 4 fruit, 2¼ oz	30	0	8
Lychees, 4 fruit, 2¼ oz	30	0	7
Mamey Apple: ¼ fruit, 7 oz	100	1	25
Mandarin: 1 small, 3 oz	35	0	9
1 medium, 4 oz	45	0	11
1 large, 6 oz	50	0	13
Mango: Flesh, ½ cup slices, 3 oz	55	0	14
1 small mango, 7 oz	90	0.5	24
1 medium, 10 oz	130	0.5	34
1 cheek, 4 oz	60	0	14
1 large, 17 oz	220	1	58
1 extra large mango, 24 oz	310	1.5	82
Marionberries, 1 cup, 5 oz	75	1	15
Melon, average, 1 cup, cubes/balls, 6 oz	60	0	14
Monstera Deliciosa (Taxonia),			
Edible part, 4 oz	50	0	11
Mulberries, 20 fruit, 1 oz	15	0	3
Nashi Fruit (Asian Pear), 1 med. 7 oz	85	0	21
Nectarines: 1 medium, 4 oz	50	0	12
1 large, 5½ oz	70	0	16
Oheloberries, ½ cup, 2½ oz	20	0	5
Olives (Pickled): Green, 10 large, 1½ oz	60	6.5	1.5
Ripe, Greek Style, 10 medium, 1 oz	70	6	4
Ripe (Black) Californian:			
1 small/medium	5	0	0.2
1 large/extra large	6	0.5	0.5
1 jumbo	7	0.5	0.5
1 colossal	11	1	0.5
Oranges: Average all varieties (weights with skin)			
1 small, 5 oz	45	0	11
1 medium (3" diam.), 7 oz	85	0	21
1 large, 10 oz	130	0	33
Californian Valencia,			
1 medium (2¾" diam.), 6 oz	60	0	14
Calif. Navels (3" diameter), 7 oz	70	0	17
Sunkist Navel, large, 14 oz	130	0	30
Florida Orange, 1 med, 7 oz	70	0	17
Flesh only, 1 cup, 6 oz	85	0	21
Peel, 1 Tbsp	0	0	0
Papaya: ½ cup, cubed, 2½ oz	30	0	7
1 medium, (5"x3" diam.), 16 oz	120	0	30
Green (unripe), ½ cup, 3½ oz	20	0	5
Passionfruit,			
1 medium, 1¼ oz	35	0	8
PawPaw (see Papaya)			
Peaches: 1 small/donut, 3 oz	30	0	7.5
1 medium (4 per lb), 4 oz	45	0	11
1 large, 6 oz	65	0	16
1 extra large, 10 oz	110	0	27

Weights As Purchased	C	F	Cb
Pears, Average all types:			
1 mini, 2½ oz	35	0	8
1 small, 5 oz	75	0	18
1 medium, 7 oz	105	0	25
1 large, 9 oz	135	0	33
1 extra large, 12 oz	175	0	42
Pepino, ½ medium, 4 oz	20	0	4
Persimmons: Native, 1 oz	35	0	9
Japanese (2½"d. x 2½"h), 7 oz	120	0	30
Seedless (Maui), 1 medium, 5 oz	100	0	25
Pineapple (wts without skin):			
1 thin slice (½"), 2 oz	25	0	6
1 thick slice (¾"), 3 oz	40	0	10
1 cup, diced, 5½ oz	75	0	19
1 medium, 1½ lb (peeled)	325	0	86
Wedges *(Del Monte)*, 12 oz package	195	0	47
Canned: *See Page 104*			
Pitanga, (Surinam-Cherry) (5), 1.2 oz	10	0	2
Plaintains, ½ cup slices, 2½ oz	90	0	22
Plums: Average all types,			
Mini/Damson, (1" diameter), ½ oz	7	0	1.5
Small (2" diameter), 2¼ oz	30	0	7
Med. (2½" diam.), 3½ oz	45	0	10
Large (3" diameter), 5 oz	60	0	14
Pluot (plum-apricot), 1 medium, 5 oz	80	0	19
Pomegranate, 1 medium, 10 oz	105	0.5	25
Pummelo, flesh, ½ cup, 3½ oz	35	0	9
Prickly Pear, (Nopal):			
1 small, 2½ oz	20	0	5
1 medium, 5 oz	40	0	10
Quince, 1 medium, 3½ oz	55	0	14
Rambutan (Rambotang),			
Red/Yellow, 1 medium, 2 oz	15	0	4
Raspberries, ½ cup, 2 oz	30	0	7
10 Raspberries, ¾ oz	10	0	2
1 Cup, 4¼ oz	65	1	15
1 Pint, 11 oz	160	2	37
Sapodilla (Chico), 1 medium, 7½ oz	140	2	34
Sapote, ½ medium, 8 oz	150	0.5	38
Satsuma Tangerine, 1 medium, 3 oz	45	0	11
Soursop, 1 cup pulp, 8 oz	150	0.5	38
Starfruit, 1 medium, 3 oz	30	0	6
Strawberries: 1 cup, 5½ oz	50	0.5	12
6 medium/3 large, 2 oz	20	0	4
1 pint, 14 oz	115	1	27
Chocolate Dipped, 1 large	45	2.5	6
Sugar Apple (Custard Apple)			
½ cup pulp, 4 oz	120	0	30
Tamarillo, 1 med., 3 oz	20	0	3
Tamarind: 1 fruit (3"x1")	5	0	1.5
Pulp, ½ cup, 2 oz	140	0.5	37

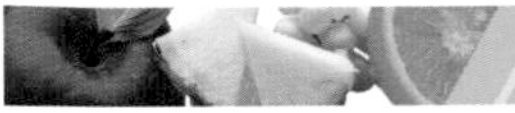

Weights as Purchased

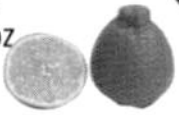
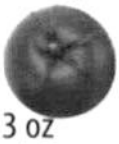
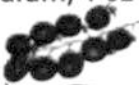

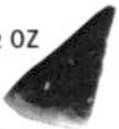
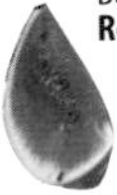
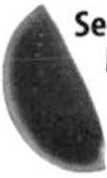

	C	F	Cb
Tangelo: 1 small, 4 oz	55	0	13
1 medium, 5 oz	70	0	17
1 large, 7 oz	95	0	23
Tangerine, 1 medium, (2½" diam.), 4 oz	50	0	13
Tangor, 1 medium, 4 oz	35	0	7
Tomatillos (3), 3½ oz	35	1	6
Tomatoes:			
1 small (2¼" diameter), 3 oz	15	0	3
1 medium (2¾" diameter), 5 oz	25	0	5
1 large (3½" diameter), 8 oz	40	0.5	9
1 extra large (3" diameter), 12 oz	60	0.5	14
Grape, 5 medium, 2 oz	10	0	2
Yellow Tear Drop, 3 medium, 1 oz	5	0	2
Cherry: 4 medium, 2 oz	10	0	2
1 cup, 5 oz	25	0	6
Slices (Medium Tomato):			
2 thin slices, 1 oz	5	0	1
2 thick (⅜"), 2 oz	10	0	2
Wedge, ¼ medium tomato, 1¼ oz	6	0	1
Chopped, 1 cup, 6½ oz	35	0.5	7
Fried Green Tomato, 2 slices, 2½ oz	140	11	9
Canned Tomatoes/Products: See Page 168			
Tree Tomato (Tamarillo), 3 oz	20	0	5
Ugli Fruit, Tangelo type, 5 oz	40	0	8
Watermelon: Flesh only, 1 oz	8	0	2
1 thin slice, (¼ circle, ⅜"), 2 oz	15	0	4
1 Extra			
1 cup cubes or balls, 5½ oz	45	0	11
10 balls, 4.3 oz	35	0	9
Buffet Slice, thin, 1 oz	8	0	2
Regular (Long Shape):			
1 thick (1") slice (¼ circle, 4½" radius)			
9 oz w. skin (5½ oz no rind)	50	0	12
1 thin (½") slice (¼ circle)	25	0	6
1 thick (1") slice (½ circle)			
18 oz with rind	100	1	22
1 whole melon (15" long, 7½"diameter)			
20 lb with rind, 10 lb w/o rind	1360	7	330
Seedless (Round Shape):			
Medium size (13 lb, 8¼" diameter)			
1 whole, 8½ lb without rind	1160	5	280
Wedge (⅛ whole melon),			
26 oz with rind	145	1	35
Flesh only, without rind, 8 oz	70	0.5	17
Mini size (6 lb, 6½" diameter),			
1 whole, 3½ lb without rind	480	2.5	110
Wedge (⅛ whole),			
1½ lb, with rind	60	0.5	14
Xoconostle: *see Prickly Pear*			

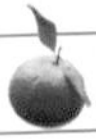

FRUIT & VEGETABLE JUICES
~ See Beverages Page 41

Dried Fruit

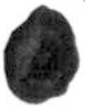
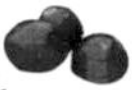

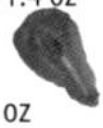

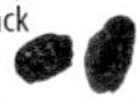

	C	F	Cb
Apples, 5 rings, 1 oz	80	0	19
Apricots, 8 halves, 1 oz	65	0	16
Banana Chips, ½ cup, 1½ oz	220	14	25
Banana Flakes, 4 Tbsp, 1 oz	80	0	20
Cranberries *(Craisins):*			
Sweetened, ¼ cup, 1 oz	100	0	24
Unsweetened, ¼ cup, 1 oz	80	0	19
Choc-coated, 1 oz	135	7.5	18
Currants, ¼ cup, 1¼ oz	100	0	25
Dates: 5 medium dates, 1½ oz	120	0	29
Large Calif.: 1 date, 0.7 oz	55	0	13
3 dates, 2 oz	170	0	39
½ cup, chopped, 3 oz	240	0	58
Pecan Date Rolls, 1 oz	100	2.5	19
Date Crumbles *(Bob's Redmill),*			
¼ cup, 1 oz	90	0	22
Figs, 3 medium figs, 1 oz	90	0	23
Goji Berries, 3 Tbsp, 1 oz	100	1	20
Longans; Lychees, 1 oz	80	0	20
Mango Slices, 5 pieces, 1.4 oz	25	0	6
Papaya Spears, 2 pieces, 1.4 oz	120	0	30
Peaches, 2 halves, 1 oz	60	0	15
Pears, 3 halves, 2 oz	140	0.5	34
Plums *(Sunsweet)* (5), 1.4 oz	100	0	24
Prunes (dried Plums): with pits, 1 oz	70	0	17
1 medium (60/lb)	16	0	4
1 large (50/lb)	22	0	5
1extra large (40/lb)	25	0	6
Without pits, 4 medium, 1 oz	70	0	17
Cooked: with sugar, ½ cup, 5 oz	155	0	38
without sugar, ½ cup, 4½ oz	135	0	33
Raisins: 2 Tbsp, 1 oz pack	85	0	20
½ cup, 2.8 oz	220	0.5	56

Candied/Glazed Fruit

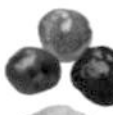

	C	F	Cb
Apricot, 1 medium, 1 oz	70	0	17
Cherry, (Maraschino) (1)	8	0	2
Citron/Fruit Peel, 1 oz	85	0	20
Ginger, 1 oz	90	0	21
Pineapple, 1 slice, 1¼ oz	120	0	29

Fruit Leather/Rolls

	C	F	Cb
Average All Brands, 1 oz	105	1	24
Fruit By The Foot, *(Betty Crocker)*			
1 roll, ¾ oz	80	0	17
Fruit Gushers, *(Betty Crocker),* 1 oz	90	1	20
Fruit Roll-Ups, *(Betty Crocker)* 1 roll	50	1	12
Stretch Island, Leathers, 2 pieces, 1 oz	90	0	24

Canned/Bottled Fruit

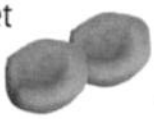
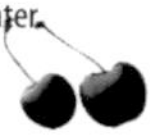
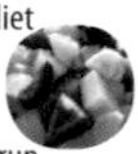
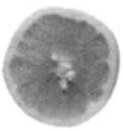
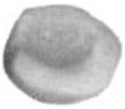
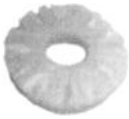

Solids & Liquids: *Per ½ Cup, 4½ oz*	C	F	Cb
Apricots: In water/diet	35	0	8
In juice/lite	60	0	15
In syrup	105	0	28
Black/Blueberries: Heavy syrup	120	0	30
In light syrup	110	0	26
Cherries, pitted: in water	55	0	15
In light syrup	85	0	22
In heavy syrup	105	0	27
In extra heavy syrup	135	0	34
Maraschino, 1 oz	50	0	12
Pie Cherries, ⅔ cup, 5 oz	90	0	23
Fruit Salad: In water/diet	35	0	10
In light juice	60	0	16
In heavy syrup	95	0	25
Gooseberries, Light syrup	90	0	24
Grapefruit: Juice pack	45	0	12
In light syrup	75	0	20
Lychees, ½ cup, 4.5 oz	105	0	26
Mixed Fruit: In water/diet	40	0	10
In fruit juices/light syrup	70	0	18
In heavy syrup	90	0	24
Peaches (halves/slices): In water/diet	30	0	7
In juice/light	55	0	14
In light syrup	70	0	18
Drained, ½ peach	55	0	14
In heavy syrup	100	0	26
Pears: In water/diet	35	0	10
In light juice	60	0	16
In heavy syrup	100	0	26
Pineapple: All types			
In own juice	75	0	20
In heavy syrup	100	0	26
1 slice (ring), drained, 1½ oz	15	0	4
Prunes: In heavy syrup	125	0	33
In Liqueur, ½ cup, 4.4 oz	280	0	70
Stewed in Water, ½ cup	135	0	35
Tropical Fruit Salad: In light syrup	80	0	21
In heavy syrup	110	0	29

Fruit Snack Cups

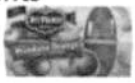
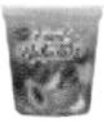
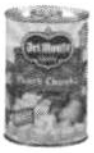
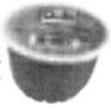

	C	F	Cb
Deli/Take-Out: Small, 6 oz	70	0	16
Large, 12 oz	140	0	32
Yogurt & Fruit Cup, 15 oz	380	4.5	75
Del Monte Fruit Cups			
Fruit Cups: *Per 4 oz Cup*			
Strawberry Banana Peaches	70	0	17
Mandarin Orange Segments	70	0	17
Pineapple Tidbits	70	0	18
Tropical Fruit	70	0	18
Fruit Naturals: *Per 8 oz Cup*			
Cherry Mixed Fruit	140	0	35
Peach Chunks	140	0	34
Pineapple Chunks	140	0	36
Red Grapefruit	120	0	32
Fruit-n-Gel Cups: *Per 4½ oz Cup*			
Mixed Fruit/Peaches in Fruit Gel	90	0	23
Lite varieties in Gel, average	60	0	14
Pull Top Cans: in 100% Juice, 4 oz	80	0	20
Lite varieties, 4 oz	60	0	15
Super Fruits: *Per ½ Cup*			
Mixed Fruit Chunks in Juice	60	0	15
Peaches in Pomeg. & Or. Juice	50	0	13
Dole Fruit Bowls			
4 oz Bowls: Diced Peaches	80	0	20
Mixed Fruit; Tropical Fruit	80	0	19
Pineapple	60	0	15
Fruit-n-Gel Bowls, Regular, 1 cup	60	0	14
Mott's: Healthy Harvest, 4 oz cup	50	0	13
Vons: Fruit Cocktail,			
In heavy syrup, ½ cup, 4.5 oz	90	0	25
In lite syrup, ½ cup	80	0	14

Apple & Fruit Sauces

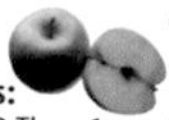
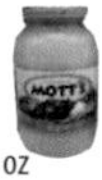
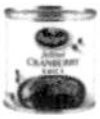

	C	F	Cb
Apple Sauce:			
Regular/sweetened, 2 Tbsp, 1 oz	20	0	6
4 oz package	85	0	22
¼ cup	50	0	13
Fruit Sauces & Purees:			
Average all fruit types, 2 Tbsp, 1 oz	25	0	6
½ cup, 4 oz	100	0	24
Mott's:			
Classics, average, 4 oz	100	0	24
Apple Sauce: Original, 4 oz	100	0	24
Fruit Flavored, average, 4 oz	90	0	23
No Sugar Added, 4 oz	50	0	12
Ocean Spray: *Per ¼ Cup*			
Jellied Cranberry Sauce	110	0	25
Whole Berry Cranberry Sauce	110	0	27

Pie Fillings ~ See Page 136

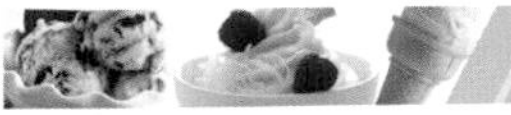

Quick Guide

Ice Cream

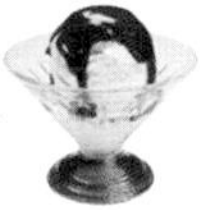

Vanilla: ***Average All Brands***
Other flavors ~ See Brand Listings.

	C	F	Cb
Regular Ice Cream (10% fat):			
Examples: *Borden/Hood*			
3 fl.oz scoop	105	5	12
½ cup, 4 fl.oz	140	7	17
1 Pint, 16 fl.oz	560	28	68
½ Gallon (4 Pints)	2240	112	272
Rich (16% fat):			
Example: *Hood (Red Sox)*			
3 fl.oz scoop	135	7.5	15
½ cup, 4 fl.oz	180	10	20
1 Pint	720	40	80
Super-Rich (20% fat): *Haagen-Dazs/Ben & Jerry's*			
3 fl.oz scoop	200	13	18
½ cup, 4 fl.oz	270	17	24
1 Pint	1080	68	96
Reduced-Fat/Light (6% fat):			
Breyer's Light/Hood Light			
3 fl.oz scoop	95	3	15
½ cup, 4 fl.oz	125	4	20
1 Pint	500	16	80
Fat-Free: *Baskin-Robbins FF/Borden FF/ Breyers FF/Dreyers FF/Hood FF*			
3 fl.oz scoop	70	0	16
½ cup, 4 fl.oz	90	0	21
1 Pint	360	0	84
Soft Serve: Regular, ½ cup	190	11	19
1 cup	380	22	38
Light, ½ cup	110	2	19
1 cup	220	4	38

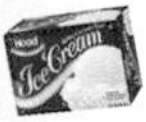

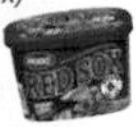

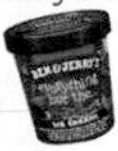

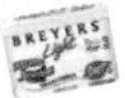

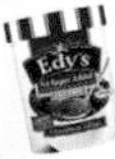

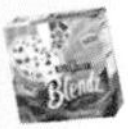

Quick Guide

Frozen Yogurt

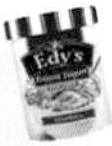

Average All Brands	C	F	Cb
Hard: Low-Fat, ½ cup	110	3	19
Non-Fat, ½ cup	110	0	24
Soft: Low-Fat, ½ cup	120	4	17
Non-Fat, ½ cup	100	0	30

Brands: *See Ice Cream & Ices Section*

Quick Guide

Gelato/Ices/Frozen Custard

	C	F	Cb
Gelato: *Per ½ Cup*			
Milk base: Vanilla	160	6	25
Chocolate Hazelnut	230	15	21
Water base, ½ cup	100	0	26
Frozen Custard: *Per ½ Cup*			
Chocolate	140	6	18
Orange Sherbet	105	2	21
Vanilla	130	6	16
Ice (Milk base): Average all flavors			
Hard (4% fat), ½ cup	100	3	15
Soft Serve (3% fat), ½ cup	110	2	19
Shaved Ice: Average, 12 fl. oz	160	0	40
Sherbet: Average, ½ cup	110	1.5	22
Sorbet: Fruit (without fat), ½ cup	70	0	19
Fruit Ice Pops	80	0	20
Tofu Frozen Desserts: *See Page 35*			

Sundaes

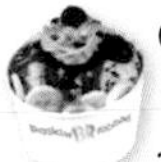

	C	F	Cb
Baskin Robbins:			
Banana Royale	620	28	87
Banana Split	1010	34	173
Brownie	920	47	119
Made With Snickers	1000	46	138
Oreo Outrageous	1130	55	158
Reeses Peanut Butter Cup	1220	80	109
Denny's: Banana Split	810	31	125
Oreo Blender Blaster	890	44	113
Oreo Sundae	760	37	103
Chocolate, Topping, 2 oz	135	0.5	34
Other Toppings ~ *See Page 203*			
McDonald's:			
Hot Caramel Sundae	340	8	60
Hot Fudge Sundae	330	10	54
Strawberry Sundae	280	6	49
Toppings: Peanuts, ¼ oz	45	3.5	2

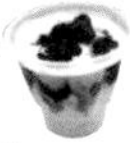

Ice Cream, Cones & Cups

Average All Brands	C	F	Cb
Wafer Cone/Cup, average	20	0	4
Sugar Cone, average	50	0	14
Waffle Cone:			
Small	50	1	10
Large	90	0.5	19
Brands:			
Oreo Chocolate Cone	50	1	10
Comet Sugar Cone	50	0	11
Keebler Sugar Cone	50	0	10

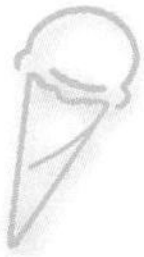

i Ice Cream & Frozen Yogurt

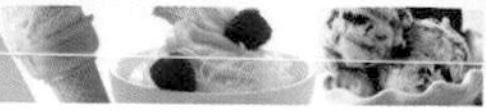

Brands

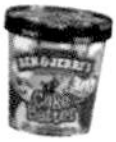
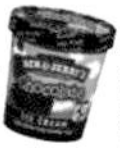
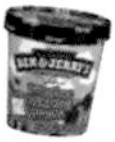
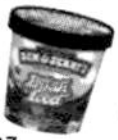
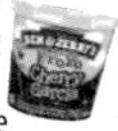

Item	C	F	Cb
Baskin-Robbins: *See Fast-Foods Section*			
Ben & Jerry's			
Hand Scoop: *Per ½ Cup*			
Butter Pecan, 3 oz	260	20	17
Cake Batter, 3 ¼ oz	240	14	24
Cherry Garcia, 3 oz	200	11	23
Chocolate, 3 oz	200	12	21
Chocolate Chip Cookie Dough, 3 oz	220	12	26
Chocolate Therapy, 3 oz	210	12	25
Cinnamon Buns, 3 oz	240	12	30
Coconut Seven Layer Bar, 3¼ oz	275	17	25
Coffee, Coffee BuzzBuzzBuzz, 3 oz	230	14	23
Half Baked, 3 oz	230	11	28
Imagine Whirled Peace, 3.2 oz	250	15	26
Mint Chocolate Chunk, 3 oz	230	14	23
New York Super Fudge Chunk, 3 oz	250	17	24
One Cheesecake Brownie, 3.2 oz	235	14	23
Phish Food, 3 oz	230	11	32
Strawberry Cheesecake, 3 oz	210	11	24
Sweet Cream & Cookies, 3 oz	240	13	24
Triple Caramel Chunk, 3 oz	230	12	38
Vanilla, 3 oz	190	12	18
Original: *Per ½ Cup*			
Banana Split, 3.9 oz	270	15	30
Boston Cream Pie, 3.65 oz	250	13	29
Cake Batter, 3.7 oz	280	17	28
Cherry Garcia, 3.7 oz	240	14	27
Chocolate Chip Cookie Dough, 3.7 oz	270	14	32
Everything But The... ,3.8 oz	300	19	31
Imagine Whirled Peace	270	16	28
Karamel Sutra, 3.77 oz	270	14	32
Milk & Cookies, 3.55 oz	270	15	30
Mission To Marzipan, 3.6 oz	260	13	32
New York Super Fudge Chunk, 3¾ oz	300	19	29
One Cheesecake Brownie, 3.65 oz	250	15	26
Peanut Britle, 3.65 oz	260	15	29
Peanut Butter Cup, 3.8 oz	340	24	28
Phish Food, 3.55 oz	270	12	37
Strawberry Banana, 3.35 oz	150	1.5	32
Triple Caramel Chunk, 3.77 oz	280	16	32
Turtle Soup, 3.65 oz	280	15	30
Frozen Yogurt: *Per ½ Cup*			
Fro Yo: Half Baked, 3.5 oz	180	3	35
Cherry Garcia, 3.5 oz	160	3	31
Chocolate Fudge Brownie	170	2.5	34
Strawberry Banana, 3.35 oz	150	1.5	32
Sorbet: Average all flavors	115	0	30

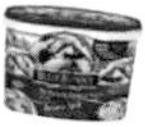
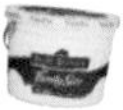
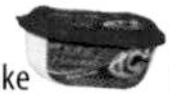
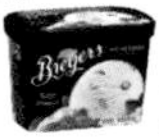
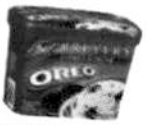
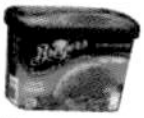

Item	C	F	Cb
Blue Bunny: *Per ½ Cup*			
Fat-Free, No Added Sugar:			
Brownie Sundae, 2.6 oz	90	0	23
Caramel Toffee Crunch, 2½ oz	90	0	24
Vanilla, 2½ oz	80	0	20
Reduced-Fat, No Added Sugar:			
Banana Split, 2½ oz	120	5	20
Butter Pecan, 2½ oz	130	6	16
Rocky Road, 2½ oz	130	6	21
Turtle Sundae, 2½ oz	140	7	20
Hi Lite: Chocolate, 2.3 oz	110	3	17
Fudge Nut Sundae, 2.3 oz	120	4	19
Homemade Vanilla, 2.35 oz	110	3.5	18
Personals (Light):			
Bunny Tracks, 2.4 oz	130	6	20
Choc. Raspb. Cheesecake	100	2.5	18
Super Fudge Brownie, 2.4 oz	120	3	23
Frozen Yogurt:			
Brownie Fudge Fantasy, 2.6 oz	110	0	24
Homemade Vanilla, 2.6 oz	100	0	19
Strawberry Cheesecake, 2 6 oz	100	0	21
Bars/Pops: See Page 110			
Breyers: *Per ½ Cup*			
All Natural:			
Original: Butter Pecan	150	10	14
Cherry Vanilla	130	6	18
Cookies & Cream; Rocky Road	150	7	19
Vanilla; Chocolate	130	6	15
Half The Fat: Butter Pecan	130	5	16
Chocolate Chocolate Chip	140	5	21
Cookies & Cream	130	4	20
Creamy, Chocolate/Vanilla, average	110	3.5	16
Mint Chocolate Chip	130	4.5	18
Strawberry Cheesecake	120	3.5	20
Vanilla Bean; Van. Choc. Strawberry	110	3	17
CarbSmart: Chocolate	90	6	13
Vanilla	90	6	13
Fun Flavors: Brownie Mud Pie	130	3.5	23
Heath English Toffee	160	6	25
Oreo	160	8	20
Snickers	170	8	20
Overload: Fried Ice Cream	140	4.5	23
Very Chocolate Cherry	120	3	21
Smooth & Dreamy:			
Fat Free: Chocolate Cookies & Cream	110	0	25
Chocolate Fudge Brownie	110	0	25
Creamy Vanilla	90	0	21
French Chocolate	90	0	22
Strawberry	90	0	22
No Added Sugar: Butter Pecan	110	6	14
Chocolate Fudge Brownie	90	1.5	20

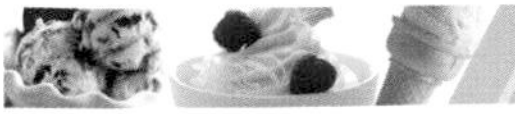

Brands (Cont)

	C	F	Cb
Brigham's: *Per ½ Cup, 4 fl.oz*			
Ice Cream: Big Dig	210	12	24
Chocolate	200	12	20
Coffee	190	12	17
Frozen Pudding	180	9	20
Just Jimmies	220	13	21
Mocha Almond; Pistachio	210	15	18
Vanilla	190	12	18
Elan Frozen Yogurt			
Average all flavors, ½ cup, 4 fl.oz	135	3	24
Bruster's			
Frozen Yogurt: *Per 3 fl.oz*			
Chocolate	150	4.5	24
Vanilla	150	4	24
Fat Free, No Added Sugar Ice Cream: *3 fl.oz*			
Chocolate	100	0	26
Chocolate Caramel Swirl	120	0	31
Cinnamon	100	0	23
Coffee	100	0	24
Fudge Ripple	110	0	30
Vanilla	100	0	23
Average other varieties	110	0	30
Carvel Ice Cream: *See Fast-Foods Section*			
Coldstone Creamery: *See Fast-Foods Section*			
CremaLita (Soft Serve)			
Calories will vary with density (air in product) and serving size. Best to weigh product and calculate on 25 cals per 1 oz weight.			
Vanilla: Small (4 fl.oz cup),			
If 4 oz weight*	100	0.5	23
If 6 oz weight*	150	1	35
(*) Most common weights			
Medium (8 fl.oz cup), 11 oz weight	275	1.5	63
Chocolate: Small, 6 oz weight	160	1	36
Dairy Queen/Brazier: *See Fast-Foods Section*			
Dippin' Dots			
Dots 'n Cream: *Per ½ Cup*			
Banana Split	170	10	6
Caramel Cappuccino	190	12	18
Mint Chocolate	165	10	15
Vanilla	170	10	16
Wild About Chocolate	240	14	26
Dove: *Per ½ Cup*			
Beyond Vanilla	240	15	23
Caramel Pecan Perfection	300	18	30
Chocolate & Brownie Affair	300	19	31
Chocolate & Cherry Courtship	270	16	27
Irresistibly Raspberry	240	12	30
Unconditional Chocolate	290	17	31
Vanilla with Chocolate Soul	300	18	30

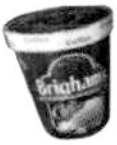

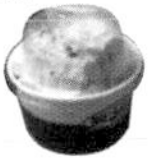

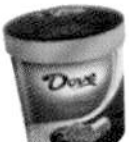

	C	F	Cb
Dreyers/Edys: *Per ½ Cup, 4 fl.oz*			
Grand: Chocolate	150	8	17
Fudge Swirl	150	7	19
Mint Chocolate Chip	160	9	18
Neapolitan; Vanilla Bean, average	140	8	15
Real Strawberry	130	6	16
Vanilla	140	8	15
Average other flavors	160	9	18
Loaded, Choc. Chip Cookie Dough	130	4	21
Slow Churned: Light, Neapolitan	100	3	15
Cookie Dough	130	4.5	20
Cups ½ Fat ⅓ Calories:			
Chocolate, 1 cup	170	6	25
Mint Chocolate Chip, 1 cup	210	8	29
Yogurt Blends: Cookies & Cream	120	4	20
Average other flavors	100	2	17
Friendly's: *Per Single Scoop*			
Ice Cream: Butter Crunch	130	6	16
Chocolate	110	6	10
Chocolate Almond Chip	120	7	11
Coffee	110	6	13
Hunka Chunka PB Fudge	180	11	17
Pistachio	130	7	14
Strawberry	110	5	14
Vanilla	120	6	14
Vienna Mocha Chunk	140	8	16
Frozen Yogurt: *Per ½ Cup*			
Raspberry Swirl, Non-Fat	90	0	19
Sundaes: *Per 3 Scoops*			
Royal Banana Split	880	35	132
Jim Dandy	1080	46	156
Reese's Peanut Butter Cup	870	51	90
Friend-Z's, Reese's P'nut Butter Cup	860	45	96
Gelati-da			
Gelato: *Per ½ Cup (4 oz)*			
Amaretto Chocolate	150	4.5	23
Choc Mint Milano	120	2.5	22
Coffee Fudge Latte	130	2	22
Limoncello	120	3	20
Red Raspberry	130	1.5	25
Vanilla Marsala	120	2	21
Haagen-Dazs			
Ice Cream, Sorbet, Frozen Yogurt: *See Fast-Foods Section*			
Bars: *See Page 111*			
Hola Fruta!: *Per ½ Cup, 3.35 oz*			
Pure Fruit Sherbet: Margarita	140	1	30
Peach	130	1	30
Pina Colada	140	1.5	31
Pomegranate; Raspberry	140	1	32
Pomegranate & Blueberry	150	1	31
Strawberry	130	1	31

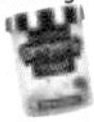

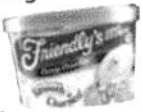

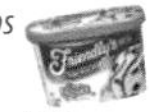

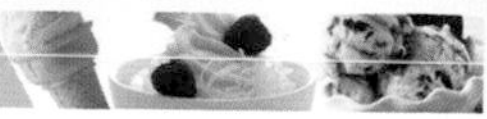

Brands (Cont)

	C	F	Cb
Hood: *Per ½ Cup*			
Frozen Fat-Free Yogurt:			
Maine Blueberry & Sweet Cream	**90**	**0**	19
Mocha Fudge	**100**	**0**	22
Strawberry	**80**	**0**	18
Strawberry Banana	**90**	**0**	20
Tangy, average all flavors	**110**	**1**	24
Vanilla	**90**	**0**	19
Ice Cream: *Per 2.33 oz*			
Birthday Party	**150**	**8**	19
Chocolate	**140**	**6**	18
Classic trio	**140**	**7**	17
Cookie Dough Delight	**160**	**8**	19
Cookies 'N Cream	**150**	**8**	19
Creamy Coffee	**140**	**7**	16
Fudge Twister	**140**	**6**	20
Golden Vanilla	**140**	**7**	17
Maple Walnut	**150**	**9**	17
Natural Vanilla Bean	**140**	**7**	17
Patchwork	**140**	**7**	17

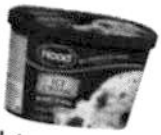

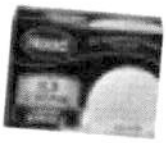

New England Creamery ~ *www.CalorieKing.com*

Bars: *See Page 111*

I Can't Believe It's Yogurt: *See Fast-Foods Section*

	C	F	Cb
Jerseymaid (Vons): *Per ½ Cup*			
Cookies & Cream	**160**	**8**	18
Choc Chip; Mint Choc Chip	**150**	**9**	16
Heavenly Hash; Nut Chunky Chocolate	**170**	**10**	17
Mocha Almd Fudge; Rocky Road	**160**	**10**	17
Neapolitan; Vanilla	**140**	**8**	15
Strawberry	**130**	**6**	17
Oberweis: *Per 6 oz Scoop*			
Super Premium:			
Chocolate	**480**	**31**	43
Chocolate Peanut Butter	**550**	**39**	42
Cookie Dough	**500**	**28**	56
Vanilla	**460**	**31**	40
Purely Decadent: *Per ½ Cup*			
Belgian Chocolate, 3.5 oz	**180**	**7**	30
Blueberry Cheesecake, 3.5 oz	**180**	**6**	33
Gluten Free: Key Lime Pie, 3.5 oz	**190**	**7**	34
Peanut Butter Zig Zag, 3.5 oz	**230**	**13**	32
With Coconut Milk: Chocolate, 3 oz	**150**	**9**	20
Coconut, 3 oz	**170**	**10**	19
Cookie Dough, 3 oz	**190**	**9**	24
Mint Chip, 3 oz	**170**	**9**	20
Vanilla Bean, 3 oz	**150**	**8**	19

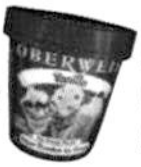

	C	F	Cb
Red Mango Frozen Yogurt: *No Toppings Included*			
Original/Tangomonium:			
Small	**90**	**0**	20
Regular	**160**	**0**	35
Large	**225**	**0**	50
Pomegranate: Small	**100**	**0**	22
Regular	**175**	**0**	39
Large	**250**	**0**	55
Rice Dream (Non-Dairy): *Per ½ Cup, 70g, Unless otherwise specified*			
All Natural: Carob Almond	**180**	**10**	26
Cocoa Marble Fudge	**160**	**7**	29
Cookies & Dream; Mint Carob Chip	**170**	**8**	27
Neapolitan	**160**	**6**	26
Orange Vanilla Swirl	**160**	**8**	26
Strawberry, 2.8 oz	**160**	**8**	25
Vanilla	**160**	**8**	26
Van. Hazelnut Fudge	**150**	**7**	22
Supreme: Chocolate Caramel Chai	**150**	**7**	22
Sweet Peach Pie	**150**	**6**	23

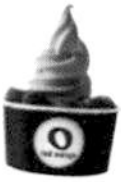

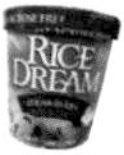

Bars: *See Page 112*

	C	F	Cb
So Delicious Organic: Butter Pecan	**160**	**7**	22
Chocolate Velvet, 2.85 oz	**130**	**3.5**	23
Cookies 'N Cream, 2.95 oz	**150**	**4**	26
Creamy Vanilla, 2.85 oz	**130**	**3**	24
Dulce de Leche, 2.95 oz	**140**	**3**	26
Mint marble Fudge, 3 oz	**140**	**3**	27
Mocha Fudge, 2.95 oz	**130**	**3**	26
Neapolitan; Strawberry, 2.85 oz	**120**	**3**	23
Soy Delicious: *Per ½ Cup*			
It's Soy Delicious: Choc Almond	**140**	**4.5**	23
Choc Peanut Butter	**135**	**3.5**	24
Pistachio Almond	**130**	**4.5**	23
Other flavors, average	**110**	**1.5**	25
Soy Dream (Non-Dairy): *Per ½ Cup, 70g*			
Butter Pecan	**150**	**9**	19
Chocolate	**120**	**6**	17
Choc. Fudge Brownie	**130**	**7**	18
French Vanilla; Vanilla	**140**	**8**	17
Green Tea	**140**	**8**	18
Mocha Fudge	**140**	**7**	21
Starbucks: *Per ½ Cup*			
Caramel Macchiato	**240**	**13**	27
Coffee	**210**	**13**	21
Java Chip Frappuccino	**250**	**15**	25
Mocha Frappuccino	**220**	**13**	23
Stonyfield Farm (Organic)			
Premium Ice Cream: *Per ½ Cup, 100g*			
Chocolate Raspberry Swirl	**230**	**13**	25
Cookies 'N Cream	**270**	**17**	27
Creme Caramel	**260**	**14**	28
Gotta Have Java	**250**	**16**	22
Gotta Have Vanilla	**250**	**16**	21
Vanilla Chai	**240**	**16**	21

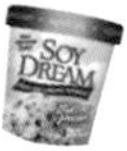

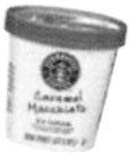

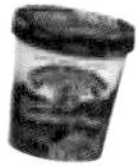

Brands (Cont)

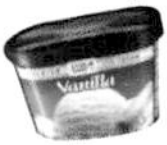

	C	F	Cb
Stop & Shop: *Per ½ Cup, 4 fl.oz*			
Butterscotch Ripple	140	6	20
Chocolate	150	8	18
Chocolate Chip, Regular/Chunky	150	8	18
Country Club	130	6	19
Heavenly Hash	170	8	22
Neapolitan; Vanilla	135	7	16
Vanilla Fudge Swirl	130	6	19
Tasti D-Lite (Soft Serve): *Per ½ Cup, 4 fl.oz*			
Calories will vary with density (air in product) and serving size			
Best to weigh product and calculate on 25 cals per 1 oz weight.			
Banana	70	1.5	11
Blueberry Cheesecake	90	1.5	14
Brownie Batter	90	2	14
Buttercrunch	100	3	13
Chocolate Marshmallow	90	1.5	16
Vanilla Cream; Vanilla Marshmallow	80	1.5	12
TCBY			
Soft Serve Frozen Yogurt: *Average all Flavors*			
98% Fat-Free:			
Kids, 2.68 oz	90	1.5	18
½ cup, 3.4 oz	110	2	23
Small, 6.7 oz	220	4	46
Regular, 8.7 oz	285	5	60
Large, 11 oz	365	6.5	76
Non-Fat: ½ cup, 3.4 oz	110	0	24
Small, 6.7 oz	220	0	48
Regular, 8.7 oz	285	0	62
Large, 11 oz	365	0	79
No Sugar Added/Fat-Free: ½ cup	90	0	24
Small, 6.7 oz	190	0	50
Regular, 8.7 oz	230	0	62
Large, 11 oz	300	0	79
Hand Scooped Frozen Yogurt			
Chocolate Chocolate: Child, 2 oz	90	2.5	15
Small, 4 oz	190	5	30
Medium, 6 oz	280	8	45
Large, 8 oz	380	10	60
No Added Sugar:			
Chocolate Swirl: Child, 2 oz	70	0	16
Small, 4 oz	130	0.5	32
Medium, 6 oz	200	1	49
Large, 8 oz	270	1.5	65
Tofutti, Non-Dairy Dessert: *Per ½ Cup*			
Premium Pints: Better Pecan	210	13	21
Chocolate Cookie Crunch	210	11	26
Chocolate Supreme	180	11	18
Vanilla	210	13	21
Vanilla Almond Bark	240	15	24
Vanilla Fudge; Wildberry, average	190	9	25

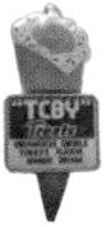

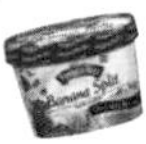

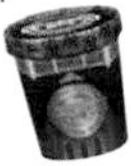

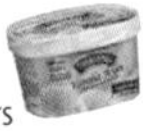

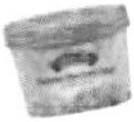

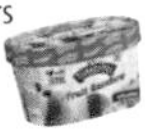

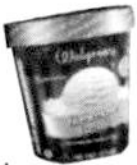

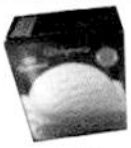

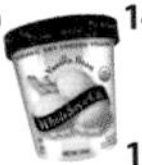

Per Serving	C	F	Cb
Turkey Hill: *Per ½ Cup, 4 fl.oz*			
Premium: Black Cherry	130	6	18
Butter Pecan	160	10	15
Choco Mint Chip	160	9	17
Choc. P'Nut Butter Cup	180	11	18
Cookies 'n Cream	150	8	19
Rocky Road	170	8	23
Tin Roof Sundae	150	8	19
Vanilla	140	7	16
Lite: Moose Tracks	130	6	19
Vanilla Bean	100	2.5	16
Average other flavors	130	4	19
All Natural: Average all flavors	150	8	17
No Sugar Added: *Per ½ Cup*			
Cherry Fudge Ripple	80	0	22
Dutch Chocolate; Vanilla	70	0	20
Moose Tracks	120	5	22
Frozen Yogurt:			
Choc. Chip Cookie Dough	120	2	23
Low-Fat, Skinny Minty	140	5	20
Fat-Free: Chocolate Marshmallow	110	0	24
Average other flavors	100	0	19
Sherbet	120	1	26
Walgreens			
Premium One Pint Container: *Per ½ Cup*			
Banana Split	150	6	22
Creme de Menthe	160	9	19
Homemade Vanilla	150	8	17
New York Cherry	130	6	17
Rocky Road	150	7	18
Strawberry Cheesecake	130	6	18
Toasted Butter Pecan	140	8	15
Waffle Cone	150	7	19
Premium 1.75 Quarts Container: *Per ½ Cup*			
Banana Split	150	6	22
Homemade Vanilla	150	8	17
New York Cherry	150	7	20
Old Fashioned 1.75 Quarts (Square)			
Average all flavors, ½ cup	140	7	16
Whole Soy Frozen Yogurt			
Average all flavors, ½ cup, 2½ oz	120	1	25

i Ice Cream Bars & Pops

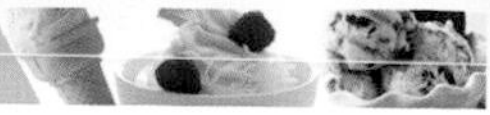

Bars & Pops

Per Bar/Serving Unless Indicated

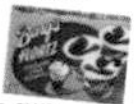
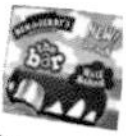
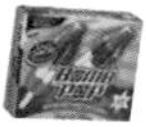

Item	C	F	Cb
Barq's			
Root Beer &			
Ice Cream Float, 4 fl.oz cup	120	3	22
Ben & Jerry's			
Bars: Cherry Garcia	270	19	28
Half Baked	360	18	46
Vanilla	310	21	26
The Cone: Cherry Garcia	310	16	41
Vanilla Almond	440	27	47
Big Bear: *See Klondike*			
Blue Bunny:			
Pops: Banana, 1.87 oz	35	0	9
Bomb Pops, average, 1.87 oz	50	0	12
Bars: Big Fudge, 2.22 oz	90	1	18
Big Star, 1.48 oz	110	7	11
Caramel Ice Cream Crunch, 1.69 oz	150	10	14
Choc. Ice Cream Sundae Crunch	170	9	21
Chocolate Raspberry, 2.82 oz	270	18	25
English Toffee, 1.38 oz	130	9	12
Milk Choc. with Almond, 3.14 oz	320	23	25
Orange Dream, 1.86 oz	70	1	15
Root Beer Float, 2 oz	80	2	14
King Size: Chocolate Eclair, 2.82 oz	220	12	27
Cookies 'n Cream, 2.47 oz	220	13	24
Crunch with Candy Center, 3 oz	340	28	24
Strawberry Shortcake, 2.78 oz	210	11	26
FrozFruit:			
Banana; Strawb. Cream, average	160	6	27
Creamy Pina Colada, 4.3 oz	190	3.5	37
Creamy Coconut	150	10	14
Champ Cones: Caramel Lovers, 3.5 oz	320	19	34
Caramel Nut	320	19	34
Chocolate Lovers	290	15	37
Fudge Nut	330	19	35
Vanilla	310	19	31
Sandwiches: Big Bopper, 5.01 oz	460	23	60
Big Double Strawberry, 3.84 oz	270	10	41
Mississippi Mud, 2.08 oz	150	4	25
Neapolitan, 2.18 oz	150	3.5	27
Chips Galore, 3.42 oz	310	16	40
Breyers			
Berry Swirls; Fruit Variety	40	0	10
Pomegranate Blends	40	0	10
Strawberry Tropical Raspb	25	0	5

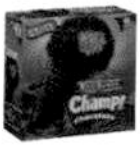

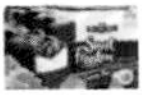

Per Bar/Serving Unless Indicated

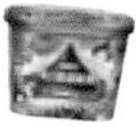
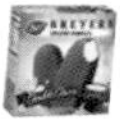

Item	C	F	Cb
Breyers (Cont)			
Ice Cream Poppers:			
Heath (27)	410	30	32
Hershey's Kisses:			
Chocolate (26)	470	31	31
Vanilla (26)	460	34	33
Oreo (27)	410	27	38
Reese's (27)	470	34	35
Double Churn Light Bars: Rocky Road	180	9	23
Creamy Vanilla	160	8	21
Vanilla & Almond	170	9	21
No Sugar Added: Creamy Vanilla	150	9	18
Krunch	150	9	18
Butterfinger *(Nestle)*: 1.9 oz bar	210	15	17
Loaded Bar, 2.8 oz	270	17	28
California Natural: Mango Sorbet	130	0	33
Lemon & Strawberry Sorbet Cups	120	0	31
Cool Classics:			
Arctic Blasters: Crispy Bar	160	11	15
Fudge Bar	80	0	20
Ice Cream Bar	150	10	13
Orange Cream	100	2.5	18
Icepix: Grape; Cherry; Orange	35	0	8
Honeydew; Watermelon Cantelope	35	0	9
Sugar-Free, Banana	15	0	3
Swirl Pops, Mango-Cherry	80	0	21
Creamsicles: Regular	100	2	20
Sugar-Free, all flavors	25	0	5
Crunch *(Nestle)*:			
Caramel	210	14	18
Vanilla Flavored	220	15	18
Reduced-Fat	140	8	15
Loaded, King Size, 2.68 oz	270	17	15
Dove: Milk Chocolate with Vanilla	330	21	31
Milk Chocolate with Almonds	340	23	28
Dark Chocolate with Vanilla	330	21	33
Dreyers/Edys			
Dibs: With Chocolaty Coating (26 Pieces)			
Chocolate	360	25	30
Crunch	340	24	30
Drumstick	350	25	30
Mint	340	24	30
Real Fruit Bars: Orange & Cream	80	1.5	16
Strawberry	80	0	21

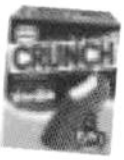

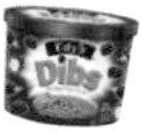

Bars & Pops (Cont)

Per Bar/Serving

	C	F	Cb
Drumstick *(Nestlé)*: Classic Vanilla	290	16	33
Vanilla Caramel	320	17	37
Vanilla Fudge	310	16	37
King Size, Triple Choc.	390	21	46
Simply Dipped: Vanilla	270	13	37
Cookies & Cream	300	14	39
Mint	290	14	38
Edy's, Fruit Bars:			
Creamy Coconut	120	3	21
Grape; Lemonade; Lime	80	0	20
Orange & Cream	80	1.5	16
Strawberry	80	0	21
Fat Boy:			
Sundae On A Stick:			
Casco Vanilla Nut, 3 oz	290	22	22
Chocolate	240	18	20
Peppermint, 3 oz	280	20	26
Sandwiches: Chocolate, 3 oz	210	9	31
Cookies n' Cream 3 oz	240	10	36
Raspberry Cheesecake, 2.8 oz	210	7	34
Strawberry, 3 oz	220	10	30
Vanilla, 3 oz	220	10	31
Fruit A Freeze:			
All Natural Creamy: Cappuccino	140	5	20
Coconut	160	7	20
Mango Cream	110	3.5	18
Strawberry	100	4	16
Choc. Covered Creamy: Banana	190	11	22
Coconut	190	7	22
Strawberry	190	12	20
Fudge Bar *(Nestlé)*: Polar	90	2	16
Mini's	80	2	14
Fudgesicle: *(The Original Brand)*			
Fudge Bar	100	2	17
Fat-Free	60	0	13
No Added Sugar	40	1	10
Good Humor: Oreo Bar	250	15	28
Candy Center Crunch	310	23	24
Chocolate Eclair	220	10	30
Premium Vanilla	260	17	24
Reese's Peanut Butter Cups	310	21	27
Toasted Almond	240	12	30
Cones: King	250	13	30
Premium Sundae	260	15	29
Triple Choc. Brownie	420	19	58
Vanilla & Chocolate	390	21	44
Sandwiches: Choc. Chip Cookie	270	10	44
Giant Neapolitan	250	9	38
Giant Vanilla	220	4	43
Snack Pops, average all flavors	210	13	23

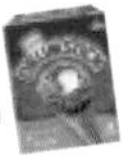
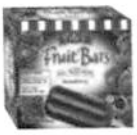
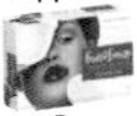

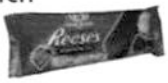

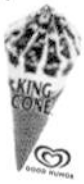

Per Bar/Serving

	C	F	Cb
Haagen-Dazs:			
Dark Chocolate: Chocolate	290	20	24
Vanilla	300	21	23
Milk Chocolate:			
Vanilla & Almonds	310	22	22
Vanilla	290	21	22
Snack Size: Coffee & Alm. Crunch	190	13	15
Vanilla & Almonds	190	14	14
Healthy Choice: Fudge Bar	80	1	13
Caramel Swirl S'wich	150	2	30
Mocha Swirl	90	1.5	17
Sorbet & Cream Bar	90	1	17
Vanilla Sandwich	130	2	25
Hood: Chocolate Eclair	150	10	14
Fudge Bar, Fudge Stix	70	0	14
Orange Cream	90	1.5	19
Rocket	120	5	16
Hoodsie Cups: Vanilla; Chocolate	100	5	12
Pops	60	0	16
Sundae	120	5	19
Sandwiches: Vanilla	180	6	29
Light	160	3	29
Ice Cream Sandwich *(Nestle)*: Mini	90	2.5	15
Super	260	11	39
Vanilla	160	4	29
Icee Freeze, 2.25 oz	70	0	17
Klondike			
Bars: Caramel Pretzel	260	15	29
Choco Taco	290	15	36
Dark Chocolate	250	14	29
Heath	230	15	24
Krunch	250	14	30
with Crispy Pieces	260	17	24
Neapolitan	250	14	29
Oreo	260	17	26
Original Vanilla, 3 oz	250	14	29
3.6 oz	330	23	28
Reese's	260	16	26
Triple Chocolate	230	14	26
Whitehouse Cherry	250	14	31
Cones: Nascar; Vanilla	280	14	35
Vanilla Caramel; Vanilla Fudge	290	14	37
Sandwiches			
Oreo	230	10	34
Vanilla	170	3	32
Slim-a-Bear Sandwich			
100 Calorie, Vanilla	100	1.5	21

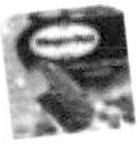
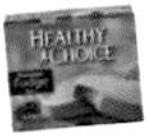

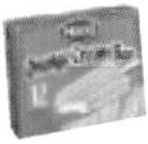
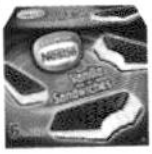
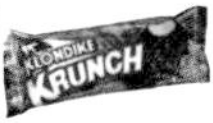

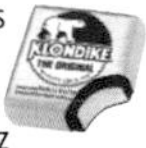

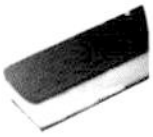
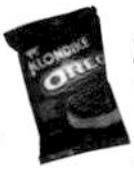

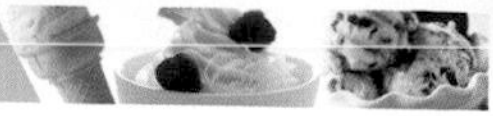

Bars & Pops (Cont)

Per Bar/Serving	C	F	Cb
Luigi's Real Italian Ice			
Squeeze Tubes	70	0	18
M&M's			
Cookie Ice Cream Sandwich:			
Single, 3 oz	260	12	34
6 pack, 1 sandwich, 2.3 oz	220	10	29
Cone, Single, 2.8 oz	250	12	33
Treats	190	15	13
Minute Maid: Juice Bars	60	0	15
Soft Frozen Lemonade	70	0	19
Molli Coolz!: *Per 2.5 oz Cup*			
Cookies N' Cream	140	10	10
Rocks: Cherry & Blue Raz & Lemon	80	1.5	15
Strawberry	50	0.5	12
Nestlé: Push Up Pop, average	70	1	16
Crunch Vanilla, 2.2 oz bar	220	15	18
Mini Sandwiches	90	3	14
Rolo Chocolate Cone	260	14	30
Rolo King Size, 4 oz	300	19	30
Vanilla Sandwich	160	4	29
Drumstick: Chocolate	310	17	34
Vanilla Fudge	310	16	37
Oreo: Sandwich	260	11	38
Popsicles			
Regular: Big Stick	70	0	17
Dora The Explorer; Scribblers	30	0	7
Firecracker	35	0	9
Rainbow	45	0	11
SpongeBob Pop-Ups	80	1	16
Super Heros	40	0	11
Sugar Free: Orange Cherry Grape	15	0	4
Tropicals	15	0	4
Slow Melts: Ice Age	40	0	10
Mighty Minis	40	0	10
Creamsicle:			
Low Fat, Orange & Raspberry	70	1	13
No Added Sugar, Orange; Cherry; Berry	25	0	5
Reese's Peanut Butter Ice Cream	270	18	24
Rice Dream Vanilla Nutty Bar, 95g	320	24	27
Safeway Select Coffee Almd Bar	270	17	26
Skinny Cow			
Ice Cream Cones, average	150	3	29
Fudge Bars, Low-Fat	100	0.5	22
Minis Fudge Pops (2)	100	2	19
Sandwiches, average all flavors	140	2	30
Truffle Bars, average all flavors	100	2	18

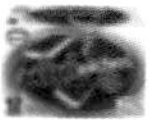

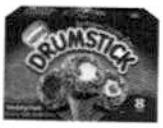

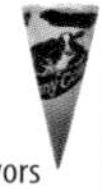

Slim A Bear ~ *See Klondike*

Per Bar/Serving	C	F	Cb
Snickers: Ice Cream Bar, 1.75 oz	180	11	18
Snack Size (1)	90	6	9
Cone, 2.9 oz	280	15	33
Snow Cone *(Wonder)*: 7 fl.oz Cone	60	0	15
So Delicious Sugar Free: Fudge Bar	80	5	12
Vanilla Bar	150	14	15
Soy Dream (Non-Dairy):			
Lil' Dreamers, all flavors	100	4.5	15
Sweet Nothings: Fudge Bar	100	0	23
Mango Raspberry	100	0	23
Tofutti (Non-Dairy):			
Cuties: Cookies 'N Cream	130	6	11
Peanut Butter	130	8	20
Vanilla	130	6	17
Sticks: Choc. Fudge Treats	30	1.5	6
Hooray! Hooray!	150	9	10
Marry Me Bar	170	8	22
Mint By Mintz	170	7	7
Totally Fudge Pops	95	1.5	19
Trader Joe's			
Fruit Floes: Cafe Latte	130	0	26
Caribbean	80	0	21
Lime Juice	60	0	16
Mango & Cream	60	2	10
Strawberry	100	0	24
Bars: Ice Cream Sandwich	440	21	60
Mini Mint Sandwich, 1.41 oz	120	6	18
Raspberry & Vanilla Cream	80	3.5	10
Turkey Hill: Double Decker	190	7	30
Vanilla Bean	190	7	29
Light S'wich, Van. Bean	160	3	32
Sundae Cone	320	18	33
Twix Bar, 2.65 oz	280	16	31
Walgreens			
Choc Nut Sundae Cones	200	11	24
Ice Cream Sandwiches, 2.2 oz	170	5	28
Turbo Tubes, 2.26 fl.oz	90	1	20
Weight Watchers			
Bars: Candy Bar	150	9	16
English Toffee Crunch	110	6	13
Giant: Chocolate Cookies & Cream	130	5	24
Chocolate Fudge Brownie	140	1.5	35
Cookies & Cream	130	5	23
Latte Bar	90	1	21
Cones, Average all flavors	140	4	30
Cups: Chocolate Chip Cookie Dough	140	2.5	31
Mint Chocolate Chip	140	3.5	29
Sandwiches: Vanilla	120	2	28
Round, Chocolate; Vanilla	140	1.5	31

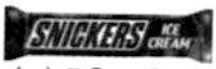

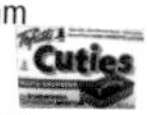

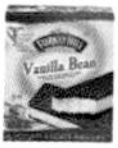

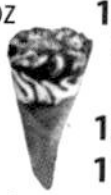

Canned & Packaged Meals

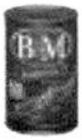

B & M: *Per ½ Cup (4½ oz)*	C	F	Cb
Baked Beans: Original	170	2	31
Barbeque	190	0.5	39
Vegetarian	160	1	28
Raisin Brown Bread, ½" slice, 2 oz	130	0.5	29
Banquet			
Homestyle Bakes: *Per Serving, Prepared*			
Asian Style Fried Rice	240	1.5	47
Chicken & Dumplings	230	4.5	33
Country Chicken, Mashed Potato & Bisc.	360	17	43
Creamy Cheesy Chicken Alfredo	400	22	36
Creamy Chicken & Biscuits	350	17	39
Lasagna	290	11	36
Pasta & Meatballs	310	10	41
Betty Crocker			
Complete Meals: *Per Serving, ⅕ Package*			
Cheesy Beef Taco	240	4.5	42
Chkn & Buttermilk Biscuits	280	11	37
Chkn Fettuccini Alfredo	230	6	34
Stroganoff	190	4	30
Three Cheese Chicken	240	7	36
Hamburger Helper: *Per Cup, Prepared*			
Beef Fried Rice	300	12	22
Beef Pasta	280	9	24
Cheeseburger Macaroni	310	10	26
Cheesy Hashbrown	400	19	39
Cheesy Jambalaya	320	13	28
Chili Macaroni	270	16	26
Crunchy Taco	340	13	33
Salisbury	280	9	24
Tuna Helper: *Per Serving*			
Creamy Parmesan	290	7	36
Average other varieties, average	310	12	37
Chicken Helper: *Per Cup, Prepared*			
Cheesy Chicken Enchilada	330	10	40
Chicken Fried Rice	250	7	22
Italian Fettuccini Alfredo	330	9	29
Side Dishes/Casseroles: *Per Serving, Prepared*			
Au Gratin, ⅔ cup	150	4	23
Cheddar & Bacon; Cheesy Scallops	140	4	25
Roasted Garlic	120	5	20
Scalloped Potatoes, ½ cup	130	5	25
Sour Cream and Chives, ⅔ cup	120	2.5	21
Deluxe Potatoes: *Per ½ Cup, Prepared*			
Cheesy Cheddar Au Gratin	180	8	25
Loaded Au Gratin	140	4	25
Three Cheese Mashed Potato Bake	190	9	24

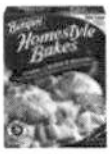

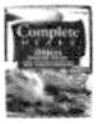

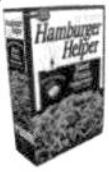

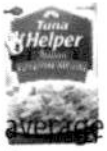

Betty Crocker (Cont)	C	F	Cb
Seasoned Skillets: *Prepared*			
Hash Brown, ½ cup	120	3	18
Roasted Garlic & Herb, ⅔ cup	170	7	21
Traditional, ½ cup	180	7	22
Bowl Appetit: *Per Bowl*			
Cheddar Broccoli Rice	290	6	52
Homestyle Chicken Pasta	250	5	44
Pasta Alfredo	350	9	55
Teriyaki Rice	250	1	57
Three-Cheese Rotini	340	7	59
Bush's Best: *Per ½ Cup*			
Black Beans	110	0.5	23
Chili Beans	120	1	20
Dark Red Kidney Beans	105	0	22
Garbanzo Beans	105	2	20
Refried Beans: Traditional	150	3	24
Fat Free	130	0	24
Baked Beans: Vegetarian	130	0	29
Average other flavors	150	1	32
Campbell's			
Beans: *Per ½ Cup*			
Baked Beans	160	2.5	30
Pork & Beans	140	1.5	25
Chunky Microwavable Bowls: *Per Cup*			
Firehouse; Roadhouse	230	8	25
Spaghetti O's: *Per Cup*			
Original	180	1	37
With Meat Sauce	180	2	32
With Meatballs	240	8	32
Chef Boyardee: *Per Cup*			
Beefaroni in Tomato Sauce	260	10	33
Beef Ravioli in Tomato & Meat Sauce	240	8	35
Cheesy Burger Macaroni	200	5	30
Cheesy Burger Ravioli	250	6	38
Pepperoni Pizzaroli	250	7	38
Spaghetti & Meatballs in Sauce	270	10	32
99% Fat-Free: Beef Ravioli in Sauce	170	1.5	33
Cheese Ravioli in Tomato Sauce	240	2.5	45
Forkables, Sports; Sealife:			
Pasta in Sauce with Meat	240	6	37
Microwaveable Big Bowls: *Per ½ Bowl*			
Beefaroni in Tomato Sauce	250	9	31
Lasagna	250	7	33
Mini Beef Ravioli in Sauce	240	8	33

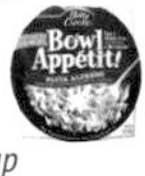

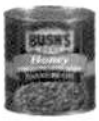

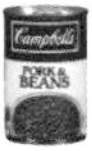

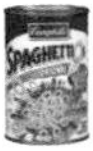

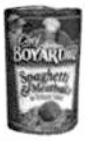

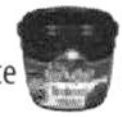

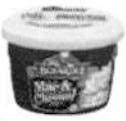
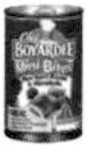
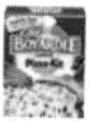
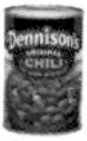
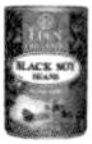

Chef Boyardee (Cont)	C	F	Cb
Microwaveable Cups: *Per Cup*			
Beefaroni	210	8	27
Beef Ravioli	190	5	29
Macaroni & Cheese	190	8	23
Spaghetti & Meatballs	200	8	23
Mini Bites: *Per Cup*			
Beef Ravioli with Meatballs	280	12	33
Pasta Shells with Meatballs	250	10	29
Spaghetti with Meatballs	250	10	30
Overstuffed: Beef Ravioli in Sauce	270	6	44
Italian Sausage Ravioli in Sauce	240	4.5	40
Twistaroni: Cheesy Nacho	220	7	32
Tomato & Beef	230	5	38
Dinner Kits: *Per Serving*			
Cheese Pizza	260	4.5	45
Lasagna	270	10	36
Dennison's Chili: *Per Cup*			
Chili Con Carne With Beans:			
Original	360	14	38
Chunky	300	10	32
99% Fat Free: Beef Chili with Beans	210	2	29
Turkey Chili with Beans	210	3	29
Dinty Moore *(Hormel Foods)*			
Beef Stew: 7½ oz cup	150	6	15
15 oz can, 1 cup, 8.3 oz	200	10	17
Microwave Cup: Beef Stew, 7.5 oz	150	6	15
Chicken & Dumplings, 7.5 oz	220	7	29
Noodles & Chicken, 7.5 oz	190	9	20
Average other varieties	180	8	17
Dr. McDougall's: *Per 10 oz*			
Ramen Noodles, Chicken flavor	200	1	40
Rice Pilaf, average	260	2	52
Eden Organics: *Per ½ Cup (4½ oz)*			
Baked Beans with Sorghum, Mustard	150	0	27
Black Eyed Peas	90	1	16
Black Soybeans	120	6	8
Refried: Black Beans	110	1.5	18
Pinto; Kidney Beans, av.	105	0.5	18
Farmhouse			
Pasta: *Unprepared*			
Herb & Butter, 4.7 oz	240	2	45
White Cheddar, 6.2 oz	260	2.5	47
Rice: *Unprepared*			
Chicken Flavor, 6 oz	200	1	43
Long Grain & Wild Herb & Butter	200	1.5	42
Mexican, 6 oz	190	0.5	42

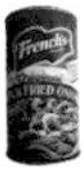
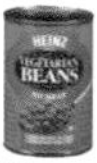
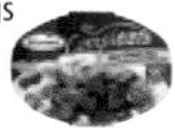
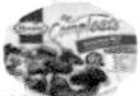
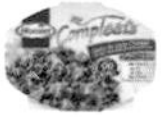
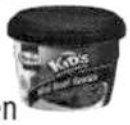
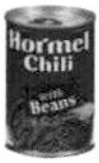

French's Fried Onions	C	F	Cb
Regular: 2 Tbsp, ¼ oz	45	3.5	3
¼ cup, ½ oz	90	7	6
1 cup, 2 oz	360	28	24
Cheddar: 2 Tbsp, ¼ oz	45	3.5	3
¼ cup, ½ oz	90	7	6
1 cup, 2 oz	360	28	24
Health Valley			
Chili, average all varieties, 1 cup	150	1	31
Microwavable Chili: *Per Cup*			
Vegetarian Spicy	120	1	25
Vegetarian Spicy 3 Bean	140	1	28
Heinz			
Vegetarian Beans, ½ cup	140	0.5	27
Hormel: *Per Cup*			
Compleats: *Per 10 oz Serving*			
Beef Pot Roast	270	6	29
Beef Steak Tips	270	9	29
Chicken & Dumplings	260	8	34
Chicken & Noodles	240	8	27
Chicken & Rice	280	11	34
Chicken Alfredo	330	18	28
Chicken Breast and Dressing	270	7	29
Chicken Breast & Gravy	200	3	24
Homestyle Beef	220	6	30
Lasagne with Meat Sauce	280	7	42
Meatloaf with Potato & Gravy	310	11	34
Salisbury Steak	280	11	30
Santa Fe Style Chicken	280	4	41
Sesame Chicken	320	8	41
Spaghetti	290	9	36
Teriyaki Chicken with Rices	270	1.5	50
Turkey & Hearty Vegetables	180	3.5	24
Turkey & Dressing	290	9	31
Kid's Kitchen: Beans & Wieners	310	13	37
Cheesy Mac'N Cheese	270	14	24
Mini Beef Ravioli	240	6	38
Noodle Rings & Chicken	140	4	18
Chili (15 oz Can):			
With Beans: *Per 8.7 oz*			
Regular; Hot; Chunky	260	7	33
99% Fat Free: Turkey	210	3	28
Vegetarian	190	1	35
Without Beans: *Per 8.3 oz*			
Regular; Hot Chili	220	9	18
Chunky	210	8	19
Turkey	190	3	16

	C	F	Cb
Hungry Jack Potatoes			
Instant Potato Flakes, ⅓ cup	80	0	19
Hunt's			
Manwich Sloppy Joe, Original, ¼ cup	30	0	7
Knorr:			
Sides: *Dry Mix Only*			
Note: Figures are only for package contents and not for extra ingredients added in preparation.			
Asian: Chicken Fried Rice, ½ cup, 2.3 oz	220	1.5	47
Teriyaki Noodles, ¾ cup, 2.3 oz	240	2	48
Teriyaki Rice, ½ cup, 2.1 oz	240	1.5	51
Cajun: Garlic Butter Rice, ½ cup, 2.4 oz	240	4	46
Red Beans & Rice, ½ cup, 2.8 oz	290	1	62
Fiesta: Mexican Rice, ½ cup, 2.4 oz	240	1	52
Spanish Rice, ½ cup, 2.3 oz	230	1	49
Taco Rice, ½ cup, 2.4 oz	230	1	48
Pasta: Alfredo, ⅔ cup, 2.2 oz	240	4.5	40
Alfredo Broccoli, ⅔ cup, 2.2 oz	240	4.5	41
Butter, ⅔ cup, 2.2 oz	240	4	43
Butter & Herb, ⅔ cup, 2.2 oz	230	3.5	44
Cheesy Cheddar, ¾ cup, 2.1 oz	220	2	41
Parmesan, ⅔ cup, 2.1 oz	220	4.5	37
Stroganoff, ⅔ cup, 2 oz	210	2	39
Rice: Cheddar Broccoli, ½ cup, 2.4 oz	240	1.5	49
Chicken Broccoli, ½ cup, 2.3 oz	210	1	46
Chicken Flavor, 2.3 oz	240	2.5	47
Sides Plus Veggies:			
Butter & Herb Rotini , 1 cup	260	3.5	49
Cheddar Rice, 2.4 oz	250	2	51
South Western Style Rice, 2.5 oz	250	1.5	51
Vegetable Fried Rice, ½ cup, 2.3 oz	240	1.5	50
Kraft			
Dinners: *Per Serving, Prepared*			
Macaroni & Cheese: Cheesy Alfredo	380	14	50
Pasta & Sauce	310	9	49
Scooby-Doo	290	6	50
Spirals	290	6.5	48
Thick 'N Creamy	380	15	50
Bistro Deluxe:			
Creamy Portobello Mushroom	310	11	40
Sundried Tomato Parmesan	300	11	40
Deluxe, Original; Sharp Cheddar	320	9	47
Easy Mac, average all varieties	220	5	39
Velveeta Shells & Cheese, Original	360	12	49

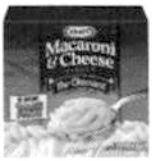

	C	F	Cb
Kraft (Cont)			
Velveeta Potatoes: *Per ½ Cup, Prepared*			
Cheesy: Au Gratin	190	6	26
Bacon Scalloped	200	7	26
Cheesy Mashed Potatoes	200	12	21
Kroger: *Prepared as Directed*			
Kitchen Creation Skillet Dinners: *Per Cup Prep'd*			
Cheeseburger	300	13	24
Cheesy Hashbrowns	400	20	39
Creamy Broccoli	300	12	33
Lasagna	280	12	26
Stroganoff	320	14	27
Noodles & Sauce: *Per Cup, Prepared*			
Alfredo	310	12	42
Butter	290	12	39
Chicken & Broccoli	290	8	42
Stroganoff	290	10	39
La Choy			
Beef Chow Mein, 1 cup	90	2	11
Chicken Chow Mein, 1 cup	100	3	10
Chop Suey Vegetables, ½ cup	15	0	3
Chow Mein Noodles, ½ cup	130	5	19
Lightlife			
Organic Tempeh:			
Flax; Soy, average, 4 oz	225	9	16
Garden Veggie, 4 oz	240	10	17
Three Grain; Wild Rice, 4 oz	230	9	21
Smart Tenders:			
Lemon Pepper (3)	130	3	8
Savory Chick'n (3), 3 oz	130	3.5	7
Tempehtations: Classic BBQ, 3 oz	160	6	16
Ginger Teriyaki, 3 oz	160	5	18
Zesty Lemon, 3 oz	160	8	10
Lunchables *(Oscar Mayer): Per Package*			
Cracker Stackers Ham & Cheddar	410	21	39
Mini Beef Taco Wrapz, 5.7 oz	400	10	61
Nachos Chse & Salsa, 4¾ oz	500	18	66
Maxed Out: Combo Ham & Cheddar	660	22	101
Combo Turkey & Cheddar, 5.4 oz	680	22	106
Pizza: Pepperoni, 7.1 oz	530	17	75
Extra Cheesy, 7.3 oz	510	12	77
Ultimate Nachos with Dip & Salsa	580	27	75
Lunchmakers *(Armour)*			
Loco Nachos	400	14	69
Cheese Pizza	360	9	53

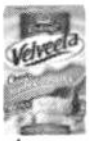

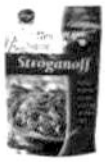

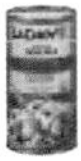
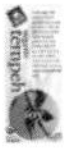

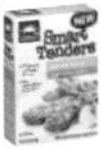

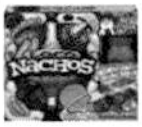

Maruchan	C	F	Cb
Ramen Noodles: Beef/Chicken/Shrimp Flavors, ½ block, 1½ oz	190	7	26
Noodles: Instant Lunch,			
Lime Chili with Shrimp Flavor	290	11	39
Roast Beef Flavor	290	12	38
Roast Chicken Flavor	290	12	38
Yakisoka: *Per ½ Package*			
Cheddar Cheese Flavor	280	14	33
Chicken Flavor	260	11	36
Teriyaki Beef Flavor	260	10	36
Minute Rice: *1 Cup, Prepared*			
Ready To Serve: *Per 4.4 oz Container, Prepared*			
Brown Rice	230	3.5	40
Chicken Rice Mix	230	5	41
White Rice	200	3	40
Yellow Rice Mix	190	4	35

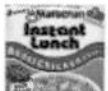
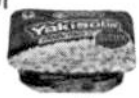
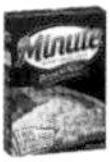

Nissin			
Chow Mein: Per ½ Package, 2 oz			
Chicken Flavor	240	9	35
Spicy Chicken Flavor	260	11	36
Teriyaki Beef; Thai P'nut	270	12	36
With Shrimp	280	14	32
Noodle Cups: *Per Cup*			
Beef/Shrimp Flavor	300	13	38
Beef Flavor Minestrone	270	11	37
Chicken Flavor	300	13	38
Top Ramen: *Per ½ Dry Noodle Block, w/ Seasoning*			
Beef/Chicken Flavor	190	7	27

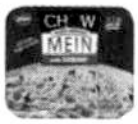
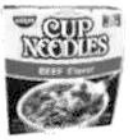

Old El Paso			
Dinner Kits: *Per Kit, Unprepared*			
Burrito	170	3.5	31
Soft Taco Bake	180	7	28
Side Dishes: *Prep'd*			
Spanish Rice, ⅓ packet	270	7	54
Cheesy Mexican Rice, ⅓ packet	280	7	55
Refried Beans: Traditional, ½ cup	90	0.5	16
with Green Chili, ½ cup, 4.3 oz	90	0.5	16
Vegetarian, ½ cup, 4.16 oz	90	0.5	16
Fat-Free varieties, ½ cup, 4.37 oz	100	0	18

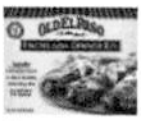

Pasta Roni: *Per Cup (Prepared)*			
Angel Hair Pasta varieties, average	310	13	41
Butter & Herb Italiano	300	12	40
Chicken & Broccoli	360	15	49
Chicken Flavor	300	12	39
Fettuccine Alfredo	450	25	47
Four Cheese Corkscrew	370	16	49
Shells & White Cheddar	290	12	38
Tomato Parmesan	270	9	40

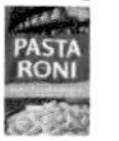
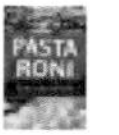

Pasta Roni (Cont): *Per Cup, Prep'd*	C	F	Cb
Nature's Way: Creamy Parmesano	280	9	41
Mushroom in Cream Sauce	280	10	39
Olive Oil & Italian Herb	250	8	38
Rice-A-Roni			
Classic Favorites: *Per Cup, Prepared*			
Beef; Herb & Butter; Rice Pilaf, av.	310	9	51
Broccoli Au Gratin	350	16	46
Chicken	300	9	50
Lower Sodium	270	5	51
Chicken & Broccoli	220	5	40
Chicken & Garlic	250	8	41
Fried Rice	310	10	50
Spanish Rice	260	8	44

(Reduced Fat Recipe: If only 1 Tbsp fat is used instead of 2 Tbsp, deduct 35 calories and 0.15 oz fat.)

Nature's Way: Parmesan & Romano	280	9	42
Italian Cheese & Herb	340	12	52
Long Grain & Wild Rice	250	7	43
Savory Whole Grains:			
Chicken & Herb Classico	260	8	41
Roasted Garlic Italiano	270	9	41
Spanish	250	8	42

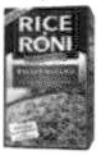
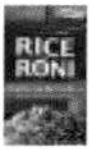
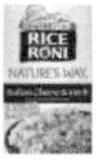

Rosarita			
Refried Beans: *Per ½ Cup*			
Traditional	120	2	18
Vegetarian; Spicy	120	2	19
Non-Fat: Black Bean	110	0	19
Traditional	100	0	19
S & W: *Per ½ Cup*			
Baked Beans: Original, 4.6 oz	160	1	32
With Maple Sugar, 4.6 oz	140	0.5	28
Black Beans, 4.5 oz	100	1	17
Chili Beans with Chipotle, 4.55 oz	110	1	23
Kidney Beans, 4.66 oz	120	1	20
White Beans, 4.48 oz	110	0.5	19

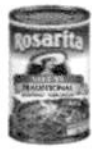
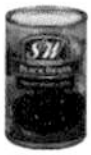
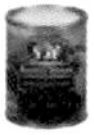

Shedd's			
Country Crock Side Dishes			
Garlic Mashed Potato, ⅔ cup, 5 oz	160	7	22
Homestyle Mashed Potato, ⅔ cup	180	9	23
Deluxe: Cheddar Broccoli Rice, 1 cup	270	11	35
Elbow Macaroni & Cheese, 1 cup	370	17	40
Four Cheese Pasta, 1 cup, 8.11 oz	380	17	41
Loaded Mashed Potatoes, ⅔ cup	200	11	23

Simply Asia

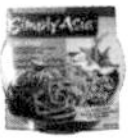

	C	F	Cb
Noodle Bowls: *Per 8.5oz Bowl*			
Roasted Peanut	510	14	78
Sesame Teriyaki	410	3.5	79
Soy Ginger	420	5	78
Spicy Mongoklian	450	6	86
Noodles & Sauce: *Per 1/3 package*			
Chili Garlic	320	4.5	62
Sesame Teriyaki	300	3	60
Soy Ginger	320	4.5	60
Spicy Kung Pao	310	4	58
Quick Noodles: *Per 8.8 oz Tray*			
Honey Teriyaki	430	3.5	85
Pad Thai	460	3	93
Szechwan Garlic Chow Mein	460	7	83
Average other varieties	430	3	86
Stir-Fry Meals: *Per ½ Cup*			
Honey Teriyaki	240	2	47
Mandarin Orange	230	1	49
Spicy Kung Pao	230	3	43

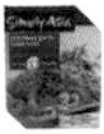

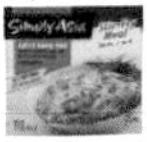

South Beach Living *(Kraft)*

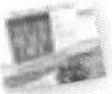

	C	F	Cb
Wraps/S'wiches: *Per Package*			
Deli Ham & Turkey	220	10	23
Grilled Chicken Caesar	230	11	22
Southwestern Style Chicken	240	11	26
Turkey & Bacon Club	240	12	24

Stagg Chili

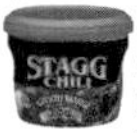

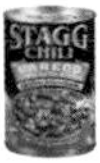

	C	F	Cb
14.3 oz Can: *Per Cup*			
Chili with Beans: Classic; Dynamite	335	17	29
Chunkero	320	16	28
Country Brand; Laredo	320	16	29
Fiesta Griller	250	10	25
Ranch House Chicken	240	8	26
Silverado Beef	250	7	30
White Chili	260	12	20
No Beans: Steakhouse	320	22	14
Low-Fat: Turkey Ranchero	260	5	34
Vegetable Garden 4 Bean	200	1	37

Taco Bell

	C	F	Cb
Home Originals: *Per Serving*			
Dinner Kits: Taco, ⅙ package	250	11	20
Cheesy Double Decker Taco, ⅙ pkg	350	16	30
Soft Taco, ⅕ package	370	13	40
Refried Beans:			
Fat-Free, 4.6 oz	100	0	18
Vegetarian Blend, 4.6 oz	120	1	20

Tasty Bite

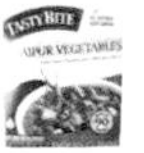

	C	F	Cb
Vegetarian Entrees: *Per ½ Package, 5 oz*			
Agra Peas & Greens	140	10	9
Bengal Lentils	160	8	16
Bombay Potatoes	100	4	13
Jaipur Vegetables	170	11	10
Jodhpur Lentils	100	4	12
Madras Lentils	120	5	14
Punjab Eggplant	140	9	13

Thai Kitchen

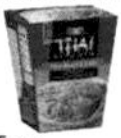

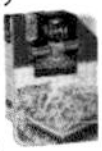

	C	F	Cb
Microwaveable Take-Out Meals: *Per ½ Package*			
Original Pad Thai	240	2	52
Thai Basil & Chili	230	5	43
Thai Peanut	220	4.5	42
Noodle Carts: *Per 2¼ oz Tray*			
Pad Thai	230	2.5	49
Thai Peanut	280	6	51
Rice Noodle Soup Bowls, average all flavors, 2.4 oz	250	3	49
Stir-Fry Rice Noodles: *Per ½ Package*			
Thai Curry	290	2	63
Thai Peanut	310	6	54

The Spice Hunter

	C	F	Cb
Meals In A Cup: *Per Meal*			
Stuffed Potato: Creamy Butter	140	3.5	25
Cheddar & Broccoli	170	3	31
Sour Cream & Chives	160	2	31
Risotto: 3 Cheese	260	3	47
Spinach & Garlic; Wild Mushroom	235	1	47

Tofurky

	C	F	Cb
Deli Slices, average 5 pieces, 1.83 oz	100	3	6
Holidays: Tofurky Roast, ⅕ package	250	6	13
Cranb.-Apple Potato Dumplings (2)	220	1	46
Jurky, 4 pieces	100	2	9
Sausages: Beer Brats (1), 3.5 oz	260	13	8
Kielbasa (1), 3.5 oz	240	12	12
Italian Sausage (1), 3.5 oz	270	13	12

Trader Joe's

	C	F	Cb
Chicken Chili with Beans, 1 cup	290	9	32
Pasta, Shells & White Cheddar, 1 cup	280	6	48
Organic Baked Beans, average, ½ cup	140	0	29
Turkey Chili with Beans, 1 cup	230	3	30
Black Beans: Regular, ½ cup	110	0	19
Cuban Style, ½ cup	100	0.5	19
Pasta Bowls: *Per 5 oz Bowl*			
Fusilli with Tomato Basil Sauce	380	5	72
Penne with Creamy Vodka Marinara Sce	400	8	72
Pesto Tortellini	470	23	58
Potatoes: Garlic Mashed, ½ cup	150	7	19
Cheddar Cheese Au Gratin, ½ cup	140	5	21

Uncle Ben's	C	F	Cb
Country Inn: *Per Cup, Prepared w/o Margarine*			
Broccoli Rice Au Gratin	200	2	43
Chicken & Vegetable Rice	200	1.5	41
Mexican Fiesta Rice	200	1	42
Oriental Fried Rice	200	1	42
Ready Rice: *Per 1 Cup, Prepared*			
Butter & Garlic Flavored Rice	220	4	41
Roasted Chicken	220	3.5	41
Teriyaki	220	3	42
Whole Grain Brown	240	3	39
Ready Whole Grain Medley: *Per 1 Cup, Prepared*			
Brown & Wild	220	3.5	42
Chicken Medley	210	3.5	41
Roasted Garlic	200	3	38
Santa Fe	220	3	42
Vegetable Harvest	220	3	34

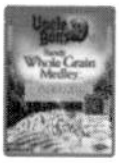

Valley Fresh	C	F	Cb
Chicken: *Per 2 oz*			
Premium White	80	3	0
White & Dark	80	3.5	0
Turkey, Premium White	80	3	0

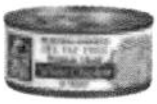

Van Camps	C	F	Cb
Pork & Beans, ½ cup	110	1	23
Original Baked Beans, ½ cup	140	1	30
Beanee Weenee Original, 10½ oz	340	11	39

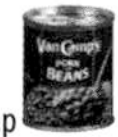

White Wave	C	F	Cb
Seitan: Chicken with Broth, 5 oz	110	2	4
Traditional, 3 oz	90	1	3

Soy Milks & Yogurts: *See Pages 48, 170*

Tofu: *See Page 162*

Worthington/Loma Linda	C	F	Cb
Big Franks: 1 link, 1.8 oz	110	6	3
Low-fat, 1 link, 1.8 oz	80	2.5	3
Chili, 1 cup, 8.10 oz	280	10	25
Choplets, 2 slices, 3.2 oz	90	1	4
Diced Chik, 2 oz	50	0	2
Linketts, (1), 1¼ oz	70	4	1
Little Links (2), 1.6 oz	90	5	3
Low-Fat Veja-Links (1), 1 oz	45	1.5	3
Multigrain Cutlets, 2 slices, 3¼ oz	100	1	5
Prime Stakes (1) 3¼ oz	120	6	7
Redi-Burger, ⅝" slice, 3 oz	120	2.5	7
Saucettes (1), 1 oz	90	6	1
Super Links (1), 1.7 oz	110	8	2
Tender Bits (6), 2.8 oz	120	4	7
Tender Rounds (6), 2.8 oz	120	4.5	6
Veja-Links (1), 1 oz	50	3	1
Vege-Burger, ¼ cup, 2 oz	60	0.5	2
Vegetable Skallops, ½ cup, 3 oz	90	1	4
Vegetarian Burger, ¼ cup, 1.9 oz	70	1.5	3

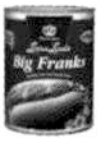
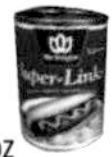
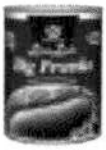

Yves Veggie Cuisine (*Vegetarian*)	C	F	Cb
Breakfast: Patties (2), 1.8 oz	80	2	4
Canadian Bacon, 3 slices	80	0.5	2
Burgers: Meatless Beef Burger (1)	110	4	8
Meatless Chicken (1)	100	3	5
Deli: Bologna, 4 slices	80	2.5	2
Ham, 4 slices	100	2	5
Pepperoni, 6 slices	60	1	4
Roast Beef, 4 slices	110	2.5	4
Salami, 4 slices	80	0	4
Smoked Chicken, 4 slices	100	1.5	5
Turkey, 4 slices	100	1.5	5
Hot Dogs & Brats:			
Jumbo Dog (1), 2.7 oz	110	3	5
Good Dog (1), 2 oz	70	3.5	1
Hot Dog (1), 1.6 oz	50	0.5	2
Tofu Dog (1), 1.3 oz	45	1	2
Brats: Veggie Classic (1), 3.3 oz	160	5	9
Zesty Italian (1), 3.3 oz	150	5	9
Skewers:			
Lemon Herb Chicken (1), 2.8 oz	100	1	7
Meatless:			
Ground: Turkey, ⅓ cup, 1.95 oz	60	1	4
Taco Stuffers, ⅓ cup, 1.95 oz	90	2.5	5
Rounds: Original, ⅓ cup, 1.95 oz	60	0.5	5
Asian Lettuce Wrap, ⅓ cup, 1.95 oz	60	0.5	8
Strips: Beef, 3 oz	120	1	4
Chicken, 3 oz	110	1	3

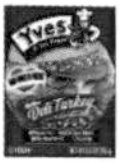

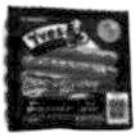

Zatarain's	C	F	Cb
Beans & Rice Mix: *Per ⅓ Cup Dry Mix Only*			
Black Beans & Rice	220	0.5	47
Blackeyed Peas & Rice	220	0.5	46
Caribbean Rice	160	1.5	34
Chicken Creole Rice	130	0.5	28
Chicken Flavor Rice	210	1	44
Fire Roasted Vegetables & Rice	170	0	38
Garlic & Herb & Rice	150	0	33
Gravy & Rice	200	0.5	45
Rice Pilaf	200	0	45
Smothered Chicken Rice	130	0	28
Yellow Rice	190	0	43

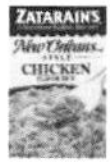

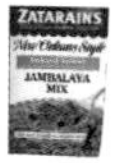

Amy's (Vegetarian)

Per Serving

	C	F	Cb
Asian Meals: Thai Stir Fry, 9.5 oz	310	11	45
Asian Noodle Stir Fry, 10 oz	290	7	50
Bowls: Brown Rice & Veges, 10 oz	260	9	36
Santa Fe Enchilada, 10 oz	350	11	47
Burritos: Bean & Cheese, 6 oz	300	9	43
Bean & Rice, 6 oz	300	8	48
Breakfast Burrito, 6 oz	250	7	38
Entrees: Cheese Enchilada, 4.9 oz	240	14	18
Cheese Lasagna, 10.3 oz	380	14	44
Macaroni & Cheese, 9 oz	410	16	47
Macaroni & Soy Cheeze, 9 oz	370	15	42
Roasted Vegetable Lasagna, 9.8 oz	350	11	47
Tofu Vegetable Lasagna, 9.5 oz	330	11	41
Whole Meals: Cheese Enchilada, 9 oz	350	15	38
Black Bean Enchilada, 10 oz	330	8	53
Bl. Bean Tamale Verde, 10.3 oz	330	10	55
Enchilada Verde, 10 oz	390	13	54
Veggie Loaf, 10 oz	290	8	47
Pot Pies: Broccoli	430	22	46
Mex. Tamale; Shepherd's Pie	155	4	27
Vegetable, 7½ oz	420	19	54
Snacks: Nacho, 5-6 pieces	210	8	26
Cheese Pizza, 5-6 pieces	190	7	22
Veggie Burgers,			
Californian Veggie (1), 2½ oz	140	5	19
Wraps: Breakfast Scramble, 5.5 oz	380	19	30
Indian Samosa, 5 oz	250	9	34
Indian Spinach Tofu, 5.5 oz	310	14	35
Teriyaki, 5,5 oz	310	7	51

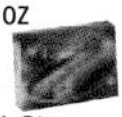

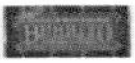

Extra Product Listings ~ www.CalorieKing.com

Bagel Bites

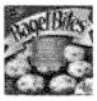

	C	F	Cb
Three Cheese, 4 pieces, 3 oz	210	6	30
Cheese Sausage & Pepperoni, 4 pieces	210	7	30

Banquet

	C	F	Cb
Breaded Chicken: Breast Patties (1)	160	9	11
Chicken Breast Nuggets (6), 3 oz	240	16	12
Crispy Chicken, Skinless, 4.2 oz	360	23	13
Popcorn Chicken, 11 pieces	180	9	18
Wings: Hot & Spicy, 3 oz	270	18	11
Honey Barbecue, 3 oz	270	18	11
Crock Pot Classics			
Chicken & Dumplings, ⅔ cup	200	8	21
Hearty Beef & Veggies, ⅔ cup	140	6	15
Meatballs in Stroganoff Sauce, ⅔ cup	300	14	29

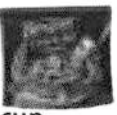

Updated Nutrition Data ~ www.CalorieKing.com
Persons with Diabetes ~ See Disclaimer (Page 24)

Banquet (Cont)

	C	F	Cb
Dinners:			
Boneless Pork Rib, 10 oz	320	11	42
Chicken Fingers, 7.1 oz	480	21	56
Fettuccine Alfredo, 8 oz	290	12	34
Lasagna with Meat Sauce, 8 oz	270	8	35
Mac & Cheese, 8 oz	260	6	39
Macaroni & Beef, 8 oz	210	4.5	32
Meatloaf Meal, 9.5 oz	280	13	28
Pepperoni Pizza, 5.75	340	12	47
Salisbury Steak Meal, 9.5 oz	290	16	25
Spaghetti & Meatballs, 9 oz	380	16	42
Swedish Meatballs, 10.25 oz	440	18	51
Turkey , 9.25 oz	250	7	32
Hearty One Dinners:			
Chicken Fried Beef Steak	750	42	66
Chicken Fried Chicken	660	40	48
Select Recipe: Chicken Parmesan	360	16	37
Corn Dog Meal, 7.5 oz	460	16	68
Fried Chicken Meal, 9 oz	440	26	30
Homestyle Pot Roast, 9.6 oz	170	5	19
Pot Pies: Beef, 7 oz	390	22	36
Chicken; Turkey, average, 7 oz	3880	21	36

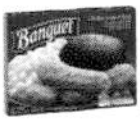

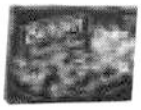

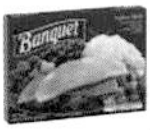

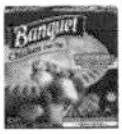

Birds Eye – Voila!

Per 1 Cup, Cooked

	C	F	Cb
Voila!: Beef & Broccoli Stir Fry	210	6	27
Chicken Parmesan	240	8	31
Creamy Tomato Penne with Chicken	210	4.5	29
Garlic Chicken	240	8	29
Garlic Shrimp	230	9	27
Shrimp Scampi	190	2.5	31
Sweet & Sour Chicken	200	1	38
Family Skillets: Alfredo Chicken	280	12	27
Cheesy Chicken	250	6	35
Garlic Chicken	240	8	29
Three Cheese Chicken	210	8	21

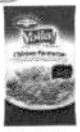

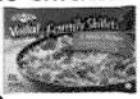

Boca (Vegetarian)

	C	F	Cb
Burger: Cheeseburger, 2.5 oz	100	4.5	6
All American Classic, 2.5 oz	140	5	9
Vegan, Original, 2.5 oz	70	0.5	6
Organic Burgers: Vegan, Original	100	2.5	9
Grilled Vegetables, 2.5 oz	80	1	7
Chik'n: Orig Nuggets (4)	180	7	17
Patties (1), 2.5 oz	160	6	15
Veggie Patties, Bruschetta	90	1.5	9

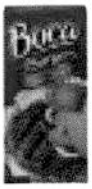

Boston Market

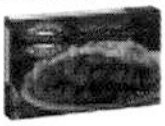

	C	F	Cb
Dinners: Beef Steak & Noodles, 14 oz	460	12	58
Chicken Parmesan	620	24	69
Salisbury Steak	710	40	53
Swedish Meatballs	760	43	57
Turkey Breast Medallions with Potato	360	14	35
Entrees: Chicken Pot Pie, 8 oz	560	36	43
Honey Roasted Chicken, 9.2 oz	410	17	46

Claim Jumper

	C	F	Cb
Beef Pot Roast, 8 oz	270	11	27
Chicken Alfredo, 8 oz	320	13	33
Chicken Fried Beef Steak, 16¼ oz	720	39	71
Country Fried Chicken, 17¼ oz	700	34	75
Creamy Fettuccine Bake, 8 oz	320	16	28
Lasagna with Meat Sauce, 8 oz	310	14	30
Meatloaf Dinner, 15¼ oz	520	31	36
Roased Turkey Breast with Brocc., 14 oz	430	17	49
Salisbury Steak, 16 oz	640	35	48
Family Meal, Chicken & Noodle, 8 oz	300	15	34
Pot Pies: Beef, 1 cup, 8 oz	590	42	39
Chicken, 1 cup	550	37	39

Contessa

	C	F	Cb
On The Stove: *Per Serving, Unprepared*			
Beef/Chicken Stir Fry, average, 7 oz	180	2	24
Cashew Chicken with Sauce, 1½ cups	260	5	39
Jambalaya with Sauce, 1½ cups	240	7	29
Mongolian Beef with Sauce, 1¾ cups	310	7	47
Shrimp Stir-Fry with Sauce, 2 cups	180	0.5	29
Microsteam: *Per 1 Cup Prepared*			
Chicken Alfredo	270	13	27
Italian Sausage Rigatoni	310	11	43
Spaghetti Bolognese	250	11	27

GardenBurger

	C	F	Cb
Veggie Burgers: *Per Patty*			
Portabella	100	2.5	17
Sun-Dried Tomato Basil	100	2.5	17
The Original	100	3	18

Gorton's

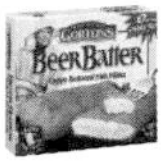

	C	F	Cb
Fish Fillets:			
Battered:			
Beer Battered (2), 3.63 oz	250	18	16
Crispy Battered (2), 3.81	230	12	22
Lemon Peppered Battered (2), 2.7 oz	270	18	20

Gorton's (Cont)

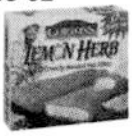

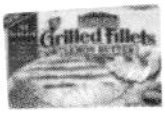

	C	F	Cb
Fish Fillets:			
Breaded: Classic Crunchy Golden (2)	240	12	23
Crunchy Tilapia (2), 3.8 oz	250	12	23
Garlic & Herb (2)	230	12	22
Lemon Herb (2)	240	13	21
Potato Crunch (2)	240	14	20
Grilled: Garlic Lemon Butter (1)	100	3	1
Salmon (1), 3.15 oz	100	3	2
Tilapia (1), 3.15 oz	80	2.5	1
Shrimp:			
Butterfly (5)	250	11	27
Shrimp Scampi, 4 oz	120	6	8
Grilled: Classic, 4 oz	110	1.5	5
Shrimp Scampi, 4oz	130	4.5	3

Healthy Choice

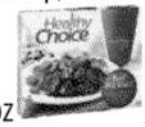

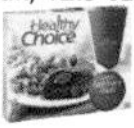

	C	F	Cb
All Natural Entrees:			
Portabella Spinach Parmesan, 9.4 oz	270	7	40
Ravioli: Lobster Cheese, 9 oz	250	6	37
Pumpkin Squash, 9.2 oz	300	6	52
Sweet Asian Potstickers, 10 oz	380	4.5	75
Tortellini Primavera Parmesan, 9 oz	220	4.5	35
Asian/Cafe/Mediterranean Steamers:			
5-Spice Veef & Vegetables, 10.2 oz	290	4.5	48
Chicken Margherita, 10 oz	320	7	45
Chicken Pad Thai, 10 oz	270	3.5	40
Chicken Pesto Classico, 10.6 oz	320	9	39
Grilled Whiskey Steak	250	4	34
Lemon Garlic Chicken & Shrimp, 10 oz	260	6	35
Complete Meals:			
Beef Pot Roast, 11 oz	260	5	40
Chicken Parmigiana, 11½ oz	340	9	49
Homestyle Salisbury Steak, 12.5 oz	290	6	42
Lemon Pepper Fish	310	4.5	53
Sweet & Sour Chicken	400	10	61
Select Entrees:			
Bacon & Smokey Cheddar Chicken	260	6	32
Ravioli Florentine, 8.5 oz	240	4	38
Spicy Caribbean Chicken, 8.5 oz	310	2	56

Hot Pockets

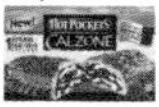

	C	F	Cb
Calzones: *Per ½ Calzone, 4.2 oz*			
4 Meat & 4 Cheese	290	12	33
Pepperoni & 3 Cheese	330	16	34
Supreme	280	12	33

Hot Pockets (Cont)

	C	F	Cb
Mexican Style: *Per Sandwich*			
Beef Taco	290	12	34
Three Cheese & Chicken Quesadilla	280	11	34
Paninis: *Per ½ Panini*			
Bruschetta Chicken	220	7	28
Deli Style Ham & Swiss	220	8	26
Steak & Cheddar	220	8	25
Pizzeria: Four Cheese Pizza	330	13	39
Sausage & Pepperoni Pizza	340	16	39
SideShots, Cheeseburger, Mini, (2)	300	10	40
Soft Baked Subs: *Per Sub*			
Ham & Three Cheese	260	9	34
Meatballs & Mozzarella	330	16	34
Philly Steak & Cheese	310	13	33
Spicy Pepperoni Pizza	360	18	34
Stuffed Sandwiches: *Per 4 oz Sandwich*			
Barbecue Recipe Beef	340	14	44
Cheeseburger	310	12	38
Meatballs & Mozzarella	340	16	36
Philly Steak & Cheese	310	13	37

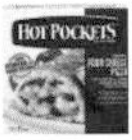

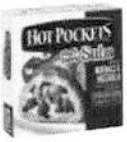

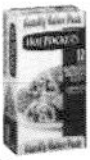

Hungry-Man

	C	F	Cb
Hungry-Man Dinners:			
Boneless Fried Chkn	860	39	85
Boneless Pork Rib	840	36	105
Buffalo Chicken Strips	860	50	57
Classic Fried Chicken	1050	65	62
Meatloaf	690	29	74
Mexican Style Fiesta	590	22	87
Roasted Carved Turkey	570	18	80
Rotisserie Chicken	460	36	31
Salisbury Steak	580	31	50
Hungry-Man XXL Dinners: *Per ½ Package*			
Backyard BBQ, 12 oz	570	28	52
Carved Turkey Breast	430	18	47
Gr. Beef Steak Strips	620	14	94
Meatloaf	690	27	86
Roasted Carved Turkey Dinner	1360	70	114
Southern Fried Boneless Chicken	500	26	44
XXL Sandwiches: *Per 8 oz Sandwich*			
Angus Beef Charbroil	700	41	55
Buffalo Fried Chicken	660	27	70
BBQ Pork Ribs	750	45	60
Country Fried Pork	660	33	70
Chili Cheese Dogs	300	15	31
Crispy Fried Chicken	670	30	68

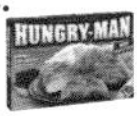

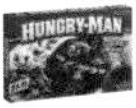

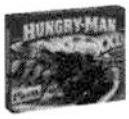

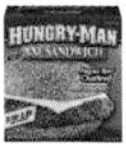

José Olé

	C	F	Cb
Breakfast Burrito			
Egg & Bacon, 4 oz	250	9	32
Egg & Ham, 4 oz	250	8	34
Egg & Sausage, 4 oz	270	10	34
Burrito: Steak & Cheese (1)	310	10	40
Chicken Monterey (1)	270	7	41
Chimichangas:			
Premium: Chicken & Cheese (1), 5 oz	330	11	45
Steak & Cheese (1), 5 oz	350	14	41
Snacks:			
Chimichangas, Steak & Ched. Mini (3)	370	20	37
Empanadas, Chicken & Cheddar (2)	320	14	37
Quesadillas: Grilled Chkn & 3 Cheese (1)	270	9	31
Grilled Steak & 3 Cheese (1)	260	9	32
Tacos, Beef & Cheese Mini, (4)	230	12	23
Taquitos: Chicken, Corn Tortillas, (3)	200	8	26
Steak & Cheese, Flour Tortillas, (2)	250	12	26

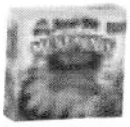
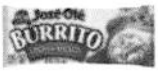

Kid Cuisine

	C	F	Cb
All American Fried Chicken	470	20	48
All Star Chicken Breast Nuggets	400	15	51
Cheese Blaster Mac & Cheese Meal	410	9	69
Magical Cheese Stuffed Crust Pizza	410	10	63
Popstar Popcorn Chicken	420	13	62
Twist & Twirl Spaghetti with Meatballs	430	13	61

Kroger

	C	F	Cb
Meals Made Simple			
Chicken Alfredo, 1¾ cups, 7.4 oz	410	16	47
Chicken Florentine, 2¼ cups, 6.9 oz	330	19	25
Shrimp Fried Rice, 1¼ cups, 8 oz	190	0.5	36
Shrimp Linguini, 1⅓ cups, 8 oz	340	8	51
Oven Ready			
Breaded Calamari Rings (13), 3 oz	230	14	18
Coconut Shrimp with Dipping Sauce	310	18	24
Shrimp Scampi, 1 cup, 4 oz	80	2.5	2
Pot Pies: Beef, (1), 7 oz	450	27	36
Chicken (1), 7 oz	380	22	36
Turkey (1), 7 oz	370	20	38

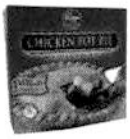

Lean Cuisine

	C	F	Cb
Entrees: *Per Complete Meal*			
Cafe Cuisine:			
Beef & Broccoli	260	5	39
Beef Chow Fun	320	5	54
Beef Portabello	220	6	25
Chicken with Almonds	250	4	38
Sun Dried Tomato Pesto Chicken	290	9	34
Thai Style Chicken	220	4	28
Comfort Cuisine:			
Baked Chicken	240	5	32
Beef Pot Roast	210	6	26
Roasted Turkey & Vegetables	150	5	12
Dinnertime Selects:			
Chicken Fettuccini	400	8	48
Lemon Garlic Shrimp	350	7	54
Salisbury Steak	270	8	27
Simple Favorites:			
Asian Style Pot Stickers	260	4	47
Cheese Ravioli	220	5	33
Macaroni and Cheese	290	7	41
Spa Cuisine:			
Butternut Squash Ravioli	280	7	43
Lemongrass Chicken	260	6	33
Salmon with Basil	220	6	26

Pizzas ~ *See Page 138*

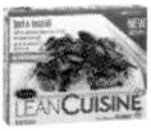

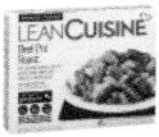

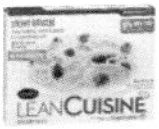

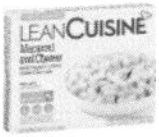

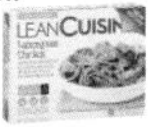

Lean Pockets

	C	F	Cb
Sandwiches: *Per Single Pocket*			
Original: Cheeseburger	290	8	41
Meatballs & Mozzarella	290	9	40
Philly Steak & Cheese	270	8	39
Mexican Style, average all flavors	250	7	35
Pizzeria: Four Cheese	280	6	41
Pepperoni	280	8	40
Quesadillas: Average	360	9	48
Breakfast	240	7	33
Whole Grain: Chicken Brocc. & Chedd.	250	6	39
Garlic Chicken White Pizza, 4.48 oz	260	8	38
Grilled Chicken Mushroom & Spinach	250	6	37
Ham & Cheddar	270	8	39
Meatball & Mozzarella	240	7	22
Supreme Pizza	220	6	33
Turkey, Broccoli & Cheese	260	8	38
Soft Baked Subs, average	250	7	36

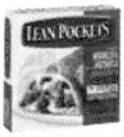

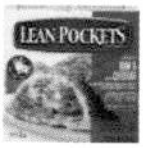

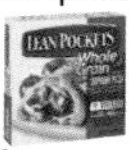

Marie Callender's

	C	F	Cb
Complete Dinners: *Per Meal*			
Country Fried Chicken & Gravy	560	26	61
Golden Battered Fish Fillet	410	12	60
Grilled Chicken Breast	400	17	32
Honey Roasted Chicken	340	12	37
Honey Roasted Turkey	320	10	31
Meatloaf & Gravy with Potatoes	450	18	41
Old Fashioned Beef Pot Roast	260	6	31
Salisbury Steak & Gravy	370	15	35
Spaghetti with Meat Sauce	490	14	67
Swedish Meatballs	540	28	48
Pasta Al Dente:			
Cavatappi Genovese, 11 oz	400	16	40
Fettuccine Chicken Balsamic, 10.5 oz	440	18	46
Penne Chicken Piccata, 10 oz	360	14	35
Rigatoni: Con Pesce, 10.5 oz	340	12	44
Marinara Classico, 10.5 oz	460	24	41
Tortellini Romano, 10 oz	430	14	59
Pot Pies: Chicken	640	38	56
Grilled Chicken Alfredo	680	39	58
Savory Herb Turkey, 10 oz	660	36	64

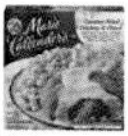
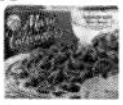
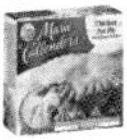

Michael Angelo's *Per Single Serve Package*

	C	F	Cb
Baked Ziti & Meatballs, 12 oz	480	15	60
Chicken Alfredo, 12 oz	470	14	57
Chicken Cacciatore, 10 oz	260	8	26
Chicken w/ Creamy Garlic, 10 oz	310	9	31
Chicken Piccata, 10 oz	510	24	52
Chicken Toscana, 12 oz	490	15	58
Eggplant & Chkn, 12 oz	360	16	28
Eggplant Parmesan, 12 oz	480	28	16
Four Cheese Lasagna, 12 oz	600	33	42
Lasagna with Meat Sauce, 12 oz	450	16	45
Manicotti with Sauce, 12 oz	460	24	22
Shrimp Scampi, 10 oz	570	30	53
Vegetable Lasagna, 12 oz	345	11	35

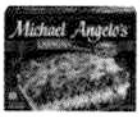

Morningstar Farms

	C	F	Cb
Burgers: *Made with Organic Soy*			
Mushroom Lovers (1)	110	6	8
Spicy Black Bean (1)	120	4	13
Grillers: Original Veggie Burger (1)	130	6	5
Prime Veggie Burger (1)	170	9	4
Vegan Burger (1)	100	2.5	7

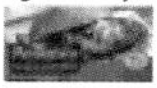

Morningstar (Cont)

	C	F	Cb
Chik'n: Buffalo Wings (5)	200	8	20
Chik'n Nuggets (4)	190	9	19
Patties: Breakfast Pattie (1)	80	3	4
Chik Patties, Original (1)	140	5	16
Garden Veggie Pattie (1)	110	3.5	9
Italian Herb Chik Pattie (1)	170	5	22

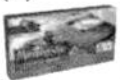

Safeway Select

	C	F	Cb
Beef Salisbury Steak, 9.35 oz	400	25	23
Bow Tie Pasta Pepperoni, 9.5 oz	340	14	36
Chicken Parmesan, 9.25 oz	350	11	48
Classic Lasagna, 11 oz	280	9	35
Fettucini Alfredo, 11.5 oz	480	15	75
Five Vegetable Lasagna, 10.6 oz	330	7	58
Orange Chicken, 9 oz	450	15	64
Pasta Primavera, 9 oz	300	11	41
Penne Pasta, 8 oz	340	12	53
Pot Roast, 9 oz	280	14	26
Spaghetti with Meat Sauce, 12 oz	450	16	61
Swedish Meat Balls, 11.5 oz	470	24	43
Triple Rich Macaroni & Cheese, 7.95 oz	360	18	37

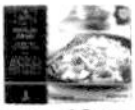

Stouffer's

	C	F	Cb
Corner Bistro: *Per Single Serve Packet*			
Flatbread Melts:			
Chicken Quesadilla, 6 oz	370	15	41
Steak, Mushroom & Cheddar	390	17	40
Stromboli: Italian-Style Supreme	430	19	45
Pepperoni & Provolone, 6 oz	430	17	45
Toasted Subs: Meatball Italiano, 7 oz	400	18	42
Philly-Style Steak & Cheese, 6 oz	370	16	39
Craveable Classics: *Per Serving*			
Creamed Chipped Beef, 4.4 oz	140	7	11
Macaroni & Cheese, 8 oz	340	16	36
Easy Express Skillets: *Per Serving*			
Broccoli & Beef, 12.5 oz	350	6	57
Chicken & Pasta Parmesan, 12.5 oz	480	15	60
Teriyaki Chicken, 12.5 oz	310	4.5	44
Yankee Pot Roast, 12 oz	300	8	39
Homestyle Classics: *Per Per Single Serve Packet*			
Beef Pot Roast	240	8	27
Fish Fillet	400	16	36
Meatloaf	340	19	20
Roast Turkey Breast	290	12	30
Homestyle Recipe: *Per Package*			
Chicken Pot Pie	660	37	62
Turkey Pot Pie	710	41	61
Homestyle Selects: *Per Serving*			
Five Cheese Lasagna, 9 oz	330	14	33
Meatloaf, 8 oz	600	31	45
Salisbury Steak, 8 oz	710	39	48

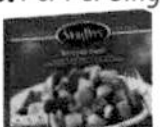

Updated Nutrition Data ~ www.CalorieKing.com
Persons with Diabetes ~ See Disclaimer (Page 24)

Stouffer's (Cont)

	C	F	Cb
Restaurant Classics: *Per Package*			
Cheese Ravioli	380	13	47
Chicken Parmigiana	410	14	47
Green Pepper Steak	240	4	32
Veal Parmigiana	460	22	46
Restaurant Selects: *Per Package*			
Bourbon Steak Tips	490	17	61
Chicken Fettuccini Alfredo	840	38	94
Monterey Chicken	530	21	54
Sesame Chicken	590	16	87
Shrimp Scampi	400	12	56

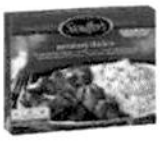

Swanson

	C	F	Cb
Classics: *Per Complete Meal*			
Breaded Fish Fillet, 7.3 oz	370	14	45
Boneless Fried Chicken, 7.5 oz	240	13	21
Fried Chicken Strips 6¾ oz	290	14	28
Macaroni & Cheese, 10.25oz	450	17	61
Meatloaf, 9.5 oz	230	9	22
Mexican Style Fiesta	380	15	51
Roasted Carved Turkey	250	11	29
Salisbury Steak, 9.5 oz	230	12	19
Pot Pies: Beef (1), 7 oz	390	24	33
Chicken/Turkey (1), 7 oz	380	22	34

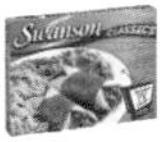

TGI Friday's

	C	F	Cb
Beer Battered Onion Rings (3)	180	8	26
Buffalo Wings (3)	180	11	4
Chicken Quesadilla	260	11	28
Honey BBQ Wings (3)	150	9	6
Mozzarella Sticks & Sauce, 1 oz	80	4.5	7
Popcorn Chicken, 3 pieces, 2.6 oz	250	8	29
Potato Skins, Cheddar & Bacon, 3 pieces	210	12	17

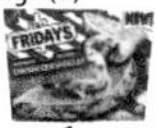

Trader Joe's

	C	F	Cb
Meals: *Per Serving*			
Asian Style Chkn Stir Fry w/ Sauce, 8 oz	190	1	30
Chicken Chow Mein, ⅓ package, 6.35 oz	210	2	35
Chicken Fried Rice, 1 cup, 5 oz	200	3.5	33
Chicken Quesadilla (1), 6 oz	320	16	26
Citrus Glazed Chicken with rice, 8 oz	270	5	40
Macaroni & Cheese, 1 cup, 6.98 oz	360	15	42
Rice Bowls, average, 11 oz bowl	390	3.5	55
Shrimp Stir Fry, 8 oz	220	1	29
Sweet & Sour Shrimp with Rice, ⅓ pkg	190	0	39
Turkey Sausage Stromboli, ¼ loaf, 4.5 oz	250	7	31
Pies: Chicken Pot Pie, ½ Pie, 8 oz	360	22	28
Spinach Pie, ¼ pie, 6 oz	240	4	37

Tyson

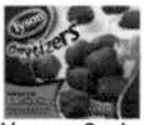

	C	F	Cb
Any'tizers:			
Buffalo Style: Chicken Wyngs, 3 pieces	**150**	7	8
Hot Wings (Bagged), 3 pieces	**230**	15	1
Stuffed Chicken Peperoni Minis (3)	**200**	11	10
Stuffed Chicken Cordon Bleu Minis (3)	**180**	10	9
Popcorn Chicken (Boxed), 6 pieces	**220**	10	19
Popcorn Chicken Bites (Bag), 7 pces	**180**	9	11
Fully Cooked Chicken: *Per Serving*			
Buffalo Style Chicken Strips (2)	**230**	10	21
Fajita Chicken Strips, 3 oz	**110**	4	1
Grilled Chicken Breast Strips, 3 oz	**100**	2	1
Honey BBQ Chicken Strips (1)	**180**	8	18
Southwestern Style Chkn Brst Strips	**120**	3	3
100% All Natural Breaded Chicken			
Breast: Fillets (1), 4.5 oz	**240**	9	20
Patties (1), 2.57 oz	**180**	11	12
Southern Style Tenderloins (1)	**150**	7	9
Tenders (5)	**240**	14	15
Crispy Strips (2)	**200**	10	13
Nuggets (5), 3.2 oz	**270**	17	15
Skillet Creations: *Per Serving*			
Asian Style Orange Chicken, ½ package	**340**	5	50
Chicken Tuscany & Penne, ½ package	**320**	6	44
Grilled Chicken Fajitas (2)	**250**	7	32

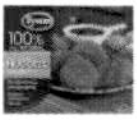

Van De Kamp's

	C	F	Cb
Crispy Battered Halibut (3), 4 oz	**280**	13	24
Crunchy Fish Sticks (6), 4 oz	**240**	11	22
Fish Shaped Nuggets (4), 4.25 oz	**280**	13	25
Fried: Beer Battered Fillets (2)	**240**	13	18
Breaded: Butterfly Shrimp, 7 pieces	**330**	16	31
Popcorn Fish, 8 pieces, 4.13 oz	**270**	13	25

Weight Watchers

	C	F	Cb
Smart Ones			
Anytime Selection:: *Per Meal*			
Calzone Italiano, 10 oz	**290**	6	47
Chicken & Cheese Quesadilla, 8 oz	**220**	7	26
Entrees: *Per Meal*			
Angel Hair Marinara	**230**	4	40
Broccoli & Cheddar Roasted Potato	**240**	7	35
Chicken Carbonara	**250**	4.5	32
Chicken Enchiladas Suiza	**290**	5	49
Chicken Fettuccini	**340**	6	47
Chicken Parmesan	**290**	5	35
Cranberry Turkey Medallions	**250**	2	43
Honey Mango BBQ Chicken	**240**	3.5	34
Lasagna Bake with Meat Sauce	**270**	4	43

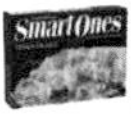

Weight Watchers (Cont)

	C	F	Cb
Entrees cont: *Per Meal*			
Lemon Herb Chicken Piccata	**230**	1.5	41
Macaroni & Cheese	**270**	2	52
Meatloaf with Mashed Potatoes	**250**	8	23
Orange Sesame Chicken	**320**	8	48
Pasta Primavera	**280**	6	44
Picate Chicken & Pasta	**260**	4	32
Pineapple Beef Teriyaki	**260**	4.5	38
Roasted Chicken with Potato	**180**	4	20
Roast Turkey Medallions	**220**	1.5	38
Salisbury Steak, 9.5 oz	**280**	3.5	33
Shrimp Marinara	**180**	1.5	31
Sirloin Beef Asian Vegetables	**220**	1.5	27
Spaghetti with Meat Sauce	**310**	6	48
Spicy Szechuan Style Vege. & Chicken	**240**	5	36
Stuffed Turkey Breast	**290**	6	42
Swedish Meatballs	**270**	5	35
Sweet & Sour Chicken	**210**	2	31
Teriyaki Chicken & Vegetables	**230**	2.5	39
Thai Style Chicken & Rice Noodles	**26**	4	43
Three Cheese Mcaroni	**300**	6	48
Traditional Lasagna with Meat Sauce	**300**	6	43
Tuna Noodle Gratin	**240**	4.5	37
Morning Express: *Per Meal*			
Breakfast Quesadilla	**220**	6	28
Canadian Style Bacon English Muffin	**210**	6	27
English Muffin Sandwich	**210**	5	27
Stuffed Breakfast Sandwich	**240**	7	28

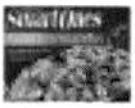

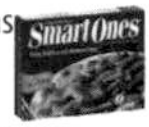

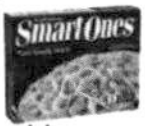

Worthington/Loma Linda

	C	F	Cb
Chic-ketts, 2 slices	**110**	5	3
Dinner Roast, ¾" slice	**180**	11	6
Fried Chik'n with Gravy, 2 pieces	**150**	10	5
FriPats, 1 pattie, 2¼ oz	**130**	6	5
Leanies, 1 link, 1.4 oz	**100**	7	2
Meatless: Chicken Style Roll, ⅜" slice	**90**	4.5	2
Smoked Turkey Roll, ⅜" slice	**130**	8	4
Prosage Links (2), 1.6 oz	**80**	3	3
Stakelets, 2.5 oz piece	**150**	7	7
Stripples, 2 slices	**60**	4.5	2
Swiss Stake, 1 piece	**130**	6	9

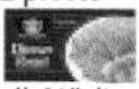

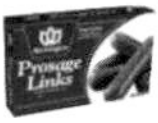

Zatarains

Per 12oz Package Unless Indicated

	C	F	Cb
Blackened Chicken Alfredo, 10.5 oz	**500**	25	46
Jambalaya seasoned with Chicken	**400**	5	69
Jambalaya seasoned with Sausage	**480**	14	77
Red Beans & Rice with Sausage	**510**	20	68

Note: Cooking reduces weight of meat by 20-45% due to water and fat losses. Average weight loss is 30%. Actual loss depends on cooking method and cooking time. Examples:

4 oz raw weight = approx. 3 oz cooked weight
4 oz cooked weight = approx. 5½ oz raw weight

What 3 oz Cooked Meat Looks Like

- Half the size of this book (4¼" x 3" x ⅜" thick)
- Rectangular piece (4" x 2½" x ½" thick)
- Deck of cards (3½" x 2½" x ⅝" thick)

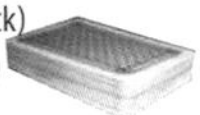

STEAK QUICK GUIDE

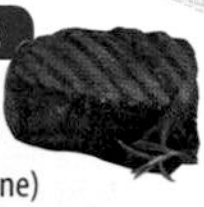

Sirloin (Choice Grade)
External fat trimmed to ¼"
Broiled, Edible Portion (no bone)

	C	F	Cb
Small/Regular Serving, 3 oz (cooked)			
(from 4-4½ oz raw)			
Lean + external fat (¼"), 3 oz	**225**	13	0
Lean + marbling, 3 oz	**195**	10	0
Lean only, 3 oz	**160**	6	0
(No external fat or marbling)			
Medium Serving, 5 oz (cooked wt)			
(from approximately 7 oz raw)			
Lean + external fat (¼"), 5 oz	**350**	21	0
Lean + marbling, 5 oz	**325**	17	0
Lean only, 5 oz	**265**	10	0
Large Serving, 8 oz (cooked wt)			
(from 11-12 oz raw)			
Lean + external fat, 8 oz	**600**	36	0
Lean + marbling, 8 oz	**520**	27	0
Lean only, 8 oz	**425**	15	0
Extra Large Serving, 12 oz (cooked wt)			
(from approximately 16-17 oz raw)			
Lean + external fat (¼"), 12 oz	**900**	52	0
Lean + marbling, 12 oz	**740**	40	0
Lean only, 12 oz	**640**	23	0
Pan Fried			
Sirloin (choice), medium serving:			
Lean + external fat (¼"), 5 oz	**460**	33	0
Lean only, 5 oz	**340**	16	0

Other Steaks

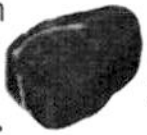

	C	F	Cb
Filet Mignon (Tenderloin):			
1 Medium steak (6 oz raw weight)			
Broiled, with ¼" fat trim			
Lean + fat (¼"), 4 oz	**360**	27	0
Lean only, 3½ oz	**230**	12	0
New York/Club Steak:			
Top Loin/Short Loin			
1 steak, regular (9¼ oz raw, ¼" fat)			
Broiled: Lean + fat (¼"), 6¼ oz	**580**	43	0
Lean + marbling, 5½ oz	**400**	25	0
Lean only, 5¼ oz	**360**	20	0
Porterhouse Steak:			
1 Medium, 6 oz raw weight (no bone), broiled			
Lean + fat (¼"), 4¼ oz	**410**	33	0
Lean only, 3½ oz	**210**	11	0
1 Large ,12 oz raw weight (no bone), broiled			
Lean + fat (¼") 8½ oz cooked	**820**	66	0
Lean only, 7 oz cooked	**420**	22	0
T-Bone Steak: *Broiled or Grilled*			
Medium Size: *8 oz raw weight*			
(Approximately 6 oz cooked)			
Lean + Fat (¼"), 5 oz (no bone)	**400**	28	0
Lean only, 4 oz (no bone)	**265**	12	0
Large Size: *12 oz raw weight*			
(Approximately 9 oz cooked)			
Lean + fat (¼"), 7 oz (no bone)	**560**	39	0
Lean only, 6 oz (no bone)	**400**	18	0
Extra Large Size: *20 oz raw weight*			
(Approximately 16 oz cooked)			
Lean + Fat (¼"), 12 oz (no bone)	**960**	66	0
Lean Only, 10 oz (no bone)	**660**	30	0

Also See Fast-Foods & Restaurants Section ~
Lone Star Steakhouse
Outback Steakhouse

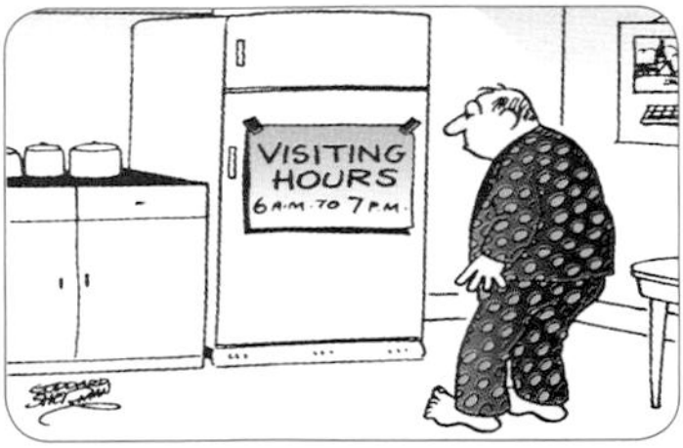

Beef – Individual Cuts

Average All Grades Edible Weight (no bone)	C	F	Cb
Brisket, whole, braised:			
Lean + fat (¼″ trim), 3 oz	330	27	0
Lean + marbling, 3 oz	250	17	0
Lean only, 3 oz	185	9	0
Chuck blade, braised:			
Lean + fat (¼″), 3 oz	310	24	0
Lean + marbling, 3 oz	295	22	0
Lean only, 3 oz	245	13	0
Flank: Raw, 4 oz	175	8	0
Braised, 3 oz	225	14	0
Broiled, 3 oz	155	6	0
Round, bottom, braised:			
Lean + marbling, 3 oz	190	7.5	0
Lean only, 3 oz	185	6.5	0
Round, eye/tip, roasted:			
Lean + fat (¼″), 3 oz	205	11	0
Lean (with marbling), 3 oz	150	5	0
Round, top: *Per 3 oz (cooked wt)*			
Braised, Lean + fat	210	10	0
Lean only	170	4	0
Broiled, Lean + fat	180	8	0
Lean only	160	5	0
Pan-fried, Lean + fat	235	13	0
Lean only	195	7	0

Beef Ribs

	C	F	Cb
Back Ribs (7″ long, visible fat trimmed to ¼″) 10.3 oz raw (with bone) or 3½ oz cooked (braised, no bone)			
1 average rib	410	34	0
3 ribs	1230	102	0
Short Ribs (2½″ long, visible fat trimmed to ¼″) 6 oz raw (with bone) or 2½ oz cooked (braised, no bone)			
1 average rib	320	28	0
3 ribs	960	85	0

Ground Beef

	C	F	Cb
Ground Beef, Raw: *Per 4 oz*			
70% lean (30% fat)	380	34	0
75% lean (25% fat)	335	29	0
80% lean (20% fat)	290	23	0
85% lean (15% fat)	245	17	0
90% lean (10% fat)	200	12	0
95% lean (5% fat)	155	6	0
Baked/Broiled: Reg. (70%), 3 oz	230	16	0
Lean (80%), 3 oz	215	14	0
Extra lean (90%), 3 oz	185	10	0
Pan-Broiled: Reg. (70%), 3 oz	230	15	0
Lean (80%), 3 oz	210	14	0
Extra lean (90%), 3 oz	195	10	0
Ground Beef Patties: Average (23% Fat)			
Raw, 4 oz	330	25	0
Broiled, 3 oz (from 4 oz raw)	250	19	0

Quick Guide

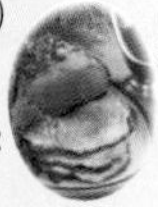

Roast Beef (Roasted)	C	F	Cb
Round (Eye/Tip, average) Average All Cuts			
Small/Regular Serving, 3 oz (2 thin slices/1 thick slice)			
Lean + fat (¼″)	200	11	0
Lean only	150	5	0
Medium Serving, 5 oz (3-4 thin slices)			
Lean + fat	330	19	0
Lean only	245	9	0
Large Serving, 8 oz (3 thick slices)			
Lean + fat	525	30	0
Lean only	390	14	0

Roast Dinner Extras

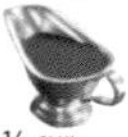

	C	F	Cb
Gravy: Thin, 2 Tbsp	20	0.5	3.5
Thick, 2 Tbsp	50	2	0.5
1 Ladle/4 Tbsp	100	4	1
Veggies: Beans, green, ½ cup	20	0	5
Cauliflower with cheese sauce, 4 oz	135	9	15
Corn, kernels, ¼ cup	35	0	9
Carrots, ¼ cup	20	0	3
Peas, ¼ cup	35	0	6
Potato: Roasted with fat, 1 small	155	8	30
Baked in Jacket, 1 large	280	0	63
with 1 Tbsp whipped butter	350	8	63
with Sour Cream, 2 Tbsp	270	5	64
Sweet Potato/Yam, 1 medium	105	1	24
Beef Kebob (Cooked):			
Beef & Veggies, 2 oz	160	10	4
If very lean meat	100	4	4

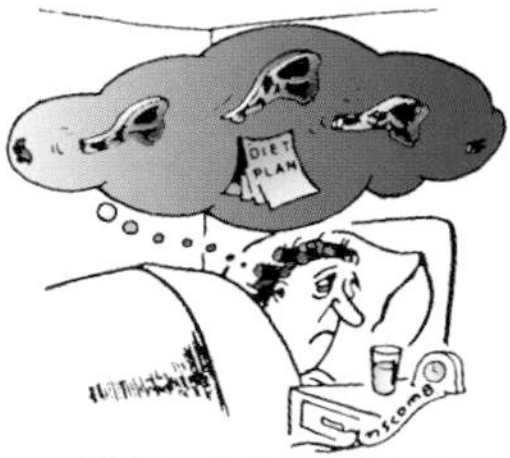

"347 ~ 348 ~ 349..."

Updated Nutrition Data ~ www.CalorieKing.com
Persons with Diabetes ~ See Disclaimer (Page 24)

Lamb

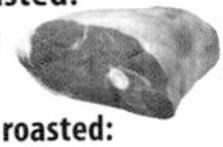
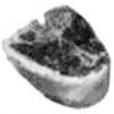
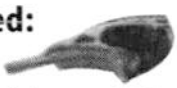

	C	F	Cb
Choice Grade			
Leg (Whole), roasted:			
Lean + fat, 3 oz	220	14	0
Lean only, 3 oz	160	7	0
Leg (Sirloin Half), roasted:			
Lean + fat, 3 oz	250	18	0
Lean only, 3 oz	175	8	0
Leg (Shank Half), roasted:			
Lean + fat, 3 oz	190	11	0
Lean only, 3 oz	155	6	0
Loin Chop, broiled:			
1 chop (raw weight, 4¼ oz):	250	17	0
Lean + fat (2¼ oz edible)	180	12	0
Lean only (1.6 oz edible)	85	3.5	0
Rib Chop, broiled/roasted:			
1 chop (raw wt., 3½ oz)			
Lean + fat (2½ oz edible)	255	21	0
Lean only (1¾ oz edible)	105	6	0
Shoulder (Arm/Blade):			
Braised: Lean + fat, 3 oz	295	21	0
Lean only, 3 oz	240	12	0
Broiled: Lean + fat, 3 oz	240	17	0
Lean only, 3 oz	170	8	0
Roasted: Similar to Broiled			
Cubed Lamb (Leg/Shoulder):			
For stew or kabob			
Braised, lean only, 3 oz	190	8	0
Broiled, lean only, 3 oz	160	6	0

Veal

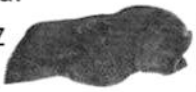

	C	F	Cb
Edible Weights			
Leg (Top Round):			
Braised: Lean + fat, 3 oz	180	6	0
Lean only, 3 oz	175	5	0
Pan-fried, breaded:			
Lean + fat, 3 oz	195	8	9
Lean only, 3 oz	185	6	9
Pan-fried, not breaded:			
Lean + fat, 3 oz	180	7	0
Lean only, 3 oz	155	4	0
Roasted: Lean + fat, 3 oz	135	4	0
Lean only, 3 oz	130	3	0

Veal (Cont)

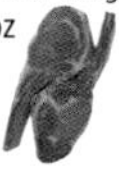
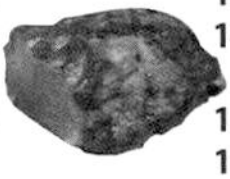

	C	F	Cb
Loin Chop: 1 chop, (7 oz raw weight)			
Braised: Lean + fat, 3 oz	240	15	0
Lean only, 3 oz	190	8	0
Roasted: Lean + fat, 3 oz	185	11	0
Lean only, 3 oz	150	6	0
Rib, roasted: Lean + fat, 3 oz	195	12	0
Lean only, 3 oz	150	7	0
Shoulder, Arm/Blade, roasted:			
Lean + fat, 3 oz	155	7	0
Lean only, 3 oz	140	5	0
Sirloin, roasted:			
Lean + fat, 3 oz	170	9	0
Lean only, 3 oz	145	6	0
Cubed for Stew, braised:			
Leg/Shoulder, lean only, 3 oz	160	4	0

(1 lb raw yields approx. 9¼ oz cooked)

Pork

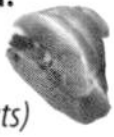
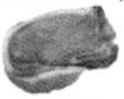
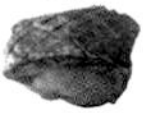

	C	F	Cb
Fresh Pork (Cooked Weight, no bone)			
(4 oz raw weight = approx. 3 oz cooked weight)			
Blade Steak, broiled:			
Lean + fat, 3 oz	220	15	0
Lean only, 3 oz	190	11	0
Country Style Ribs, broiled/roasted:			
Lean + fat, 3 oz	280	22	0
Lean only, 3 oz	210	13	0
Spareribs, braised: lean & fat, 6 oz			
(from 1 lb raw weight)	675	52	0
Leg (Ham),whole, roasted:			
Lean + fat, 3 oz	230	15	0
Lean only, 3 oz	180	8	0
(Ham, cured ~ See Cold Meats)			
Loin Chops, broiled: Average			
(From 1 chop: 5 oz raw weight with bone or 4 oz raw weight, without bone)			
Lean + fat, 3 oz	200	11	0
Lean only, 3 oz	165	7	0
Loin Roast, roasted:			
Lean + fat, 3 oz	210	13	0
Lean only, 3 oz	180	8	0
Rib Chops, (Boneless), broiled:			
Lean + fat, 3 oz	220	14	0
Lean only, 3 oz	185	9	0
Rib Roast, roasted:			
Lean + fat, 3 oz	215	13	0
Lean only, 3 oz	180	9	0

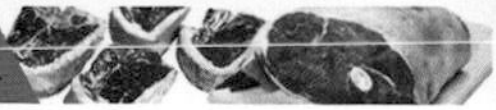

Pork (Cont)

	C	F	Cb
Sirloin Chop, broiled:			
Lean + fat, 3 oz	180	8	0
Lean only, 3 oz	165	6	0
Sirloin Roast, roasted:			
Lean + fat, 3 oz	175	8	0
Lean only, 3 oz	170	7	0
Tenderloin (Boneless), roasted:			
Lean + fat, 3 oz	125	4	0
Lean only, 3 oz	120	3	0
Ground Pork			
Raw: Average, ¼ lb, 4 oz	300	24	0
Broiled, 3 oz	250	18	0
Pan-fried, drained, 3 oz	260	19	0

Bacon

	C	F	Cb
Raw: 1 medium slice (20 lb), ¾ oz	95	9	0
1 thick slice (12 lb), 1⅓ oz	175	17	0
(1 lb raw yields approximately 5 oz cooked)			
Broiled/Pan-Fried:			
1 medium slice., 0.3 oz	40	3	0
3 medium slices, 0.8	125	10	0
2 thin slices, ½ oz	75	6	0
1 thick slice, 0.85 oz	65	5	0
Canadian Bacon: Cooked, 1 slice, 1 oz	45	2	0.5
Packaged, 3 slices, 2 oz	90	4	1
Bacon Bits, 1 Tbsp, ¼ oz	35	2	0
Breakfast Strips, Broiled, 1 sl.,, 0.42 oz	50	4	0

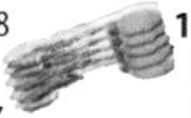

Ham

	C	F	Cb
Boneless Ham, cooked:			
Regular, (approximately 13% fat):			
Roasted, 3 oz	150	8	0
Extra Lean (5% fat), Roasted, 3 oz	125	5	0
Whole Ham, cooked:			
Lean + fat (as purchased)			
Roasted, 3 oz	210	15	0
Lean only, Roasted, 3 oz	135	5	0
Canned Ham: Similar to boneless ham			
Chopped, canned, 3 oz	200	16	0
Ham Patties, cooked, 1 pattie, 2¼ oz	220	20	1
Ham Steak, extra lean, 2 oz	70	2.5	0

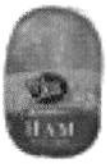

Lunch Slices: *See Deli Meats, Page 131*

Game & Other Meats

	C	F	Cb
Bison Steak,			
lean, 6 oz (raw)	205	4	0
Boar (wild), roasted, 3 oz	140	4	0
Buffalo Steak: *New West Foods,* 4 oz	70	3	0
Trader Joe's, 1 pattie	430	30	1
Caribou, roasted, 3 oz	140	4	0
Deer/Venison, roasted 3 oz	135	3	0
Goat (Capretto): Raw, 3 oz	95	2	0
Roasted, 3 oz	120	2.5	0
Ostrich: *Blackwing Ostrich Meats,*			
Sport Jerky, ½ oz piece	25	0	0
Sausage Patties (2) 2 oz	60	0.5	0
New West Foods:			
Ground Ostrich, 4 oz	165	7	0
Ostrich Steak, 4 oz steak	130	2.5	0
Rabbit: Roasted, 3 oz	165	7	0
Stewed, 1 cup, diced, 5 oz	290	12	0

Variety & Organ Meats

	C	F	Cb
Brain (Lamb): Braised, 3 oz	125	9	0
Pan-fried, 3 oz	230	19	0
Chitterlings, pork, simmered, 3 oz	260	25	0
Ears, pork, simmered, 1 ear, 4 oz	185	12	0
Feet, pork: Simmered, 3 oz	200	14	0
Cured, pickled, 3 oz	170	14	0
Hormel, 2 oz	80	6	0
Head Cheese (Pork Snouts/Ears/Vinegar/Spices):			
1 oz slice	50	4	0
Heart, Beef, braised, 3 oz	140	4	24
Jowl, pork, raw, 4 oz	750	80	0
Kidneys, braised, 3 oz	140	5	0
Liver (beef): Raw, 4 oz	150	4	4
Braised, 3 oz	140	4	3
Pan-fried, 3 oz	185	7	7
Pancreas, pork, braised, 3 oz	185	8	0
Pork Cracklins, 0.5 oz	80	6	0
Pork Hocks, 1 piece, 6 oz	340	23	0
Scrapple, pork, 2 oz	120	8	8
Spleen, pork, braised, 3 oz	130	3	0
Stomach, pork, raw, 4 oz	185	12	0
Sweetbreads: Beef, cooked, 3 oz	125	9	0
Lamb, cooked, 3 oz	125	9	0
Tail, pork, simmered, 3 oz	340	31	0
Tongue, braised: Veal, 3 oz	170	9	0
Beef/Lamb/Pork, average, 3 oz	235	17	0
Tripe, beef, raw, 3 oz	85	3.5	0

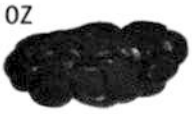

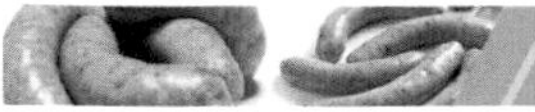

Quick Guide

Franks & Weiners

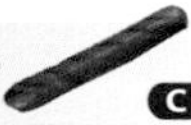

Average All Brands	C	F	Cb
Regular/Smoked: *Per Frank*			
Regular, 1.5oz (10/16 oz package)	**140**	13	1
Jumbo, 2 oz (8/16 oz package)	**170**	16	0
Bun Length, 2 oz	**180**	17	2
Extra Long, 2.75 oz	**240**	21	2
Small/Cocktail (50/lb) each	**30**	3	0.5
Beef Franks: *Per Frank*			
Regular, 1.6 oz (10/16 oz package)	**140**	13	2
Jumbo, 2 oz (8/16 oz package)	**170**	15	2
Bun Length, 2 oz	**180**	16	2
¼ lb Dog, 4 oz	**300**	24	4

Franks & Weiners

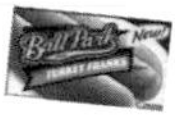

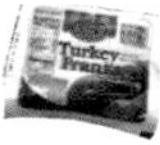

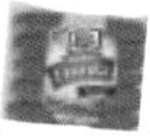

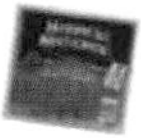

	C	F	Cb
Ball Park			
Franks & Wieners: *Per Frank*			
Angus Beef Franks	**170**	15	3
Cheese	**180**	15	4
Turkey Franks	**110**	7	6
GrillMaster: Deli Style Beef; Beef	**250**	21	3
Lite Franks, Beef	**100**	7	3
Foster Farms			
Chicken/Turkey Franks (1), 2 oz	**140**	12	1
Hebrew National			
Beef: 1.72 oz link	**150**	14	1
¼ Pound	**360**	33	3
Jumbo, 3 oz link	**270**	25	2
97% Fat-Free, 1.6 oz link	**40**	1	3
Jennie-O			
Turkey Franks:			
1.2 oz link	**70**	5	1
Jumbo, 2 oz link	**120**	9	2
Oscar Mayer			
Beef, Light, 1.6 oz	**90**	7	2
Cheese Dogs, 1.6 oz	**140**	13	1
Turkey Frank: 1.6 oz	**100**	8	2
Bun Length, 2 oz link	**120**	10	3
Shelton's			
Chicken Franks, 1.2 oz link	**70**	6	0
Turkey Franks, 1.2 oz link	**70**	6	0
Zacky Farms			
Turkey Franks, 2 oz link	**160**	12	1

Quick Guide

Fresh Sausages

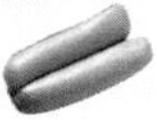

Pork/Beef: *Average All Types*	C	F	Cb
Small: Raw, 4" link, 1 oz	**85**	7.5	0
Broiled/Pan-fried	**80**	7	0
Medium: Raw, 2 oz	**170**	15	0
Broiled/Pan-fried	**165**	14	0
Large: Raw, 3 oz	**255**	22	0
Broiled/Pan-fried	**245**	21	0
Italian: Raw, 3.2 oz	**315**	28	0.5
Cooked, 2.4 oz	**230**	18	3
Chorizo: Beef Chorizo, 2.5 oz piece	**250**	23	5
Pork Chorizo, 2 oz piece	**250**	23	5

Note: Fat is lost in broiling/pan frying.
(Cooked weight = approx. 60-70% raw weight)

Smoked Sausage

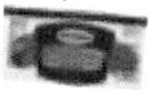

	C	F	Cb
Average All Brands: 2 oz link	**170**	15	0
3 oz link	**255**	22	0
Ball Park, Turkey, Bun Size, 1.75 oz	**45**	0	5
Butterball			
Turkey, 1.8 oz	**100**	6	4
Eckrich, Grillers, 2 oz	**180**	16	2
Hillshire Farm, Beef/Pork/Trky, 2 oz	**190**	16	3
Hardwood Smoked Chicken, 2 oz	**90**	5	3
Italian, 2 oz	**190**	16	4
Turkey, 2 oz	**90**	5	3

Breakfast Sausages/Patties

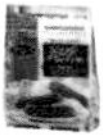

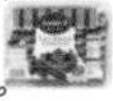

	C	F	Cb
Armour, Sizzle 'n Serve			
Beef Sausage, 3 links, 2 oz	**230**	22	1
Pork/Turkey, 3 links, 2.1 oz	**210**	19	2
Lite Original, 3 links, 1.8 oz	**90**	7	1
Butterball: Turkey Burger Pattie (1)	**150**	8	0
Turkey Breakfast Links (3)	**130**	7	0
Jennie-O:			
Fully Cooked: Sausage Links, 2 oz	**110**	7	0
Sausage Patties, 1 oz	**65**	4	0
Maple Turkey Sausage (1)	**140**	11	3
Jimmy Dean, *Heat 'N Serve*			
Sausage Links (3)	**210**	19	1
Sausage Patties (2)	**200**	17	1
Maple Sausage Links (3)	**170**	14	2
Breakfast Sandwiches: *See Page 94*			
Jones *Golden Brown:*			
All Natural:			
Beef Sausage Links (3)	**200**	18	2
Maple Sausage (3)	**240**	22	2
Sausage Patties, Maple Pork (1)	**130**	12	1

Vegetarian Patties:
Boca: *See Page 119*
Garden Burger: *See Page 120*

Bagel, Corn & Hot Dogs

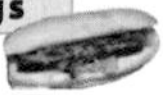

Hot Dogs, Ready-To-Go (Includes Ketchup/Relish; w/o Mayo)	C	F	Cb
Regular (1.5 oz frank, 1.5 oz bun)	260	15	22
Bun Length (2 oz frank, 1.5 oz bun)	290	18	21
Jumbo Dog (2 oz frank, 2 oz bun)	360	20	36
¼ lb Beef Dog (¼ lb dog, 2 oz bun)	480	15	36
Mile Long Dog (2.6 oz dog, 1.5 oz bun)	360	24	23
Weinerschnitzel: *See Fast-Foods*			
Corn Dogs			
Beef/Pork Frank: Average, 2.6 oz	170	10	16
Foster Farms			
Chili Cheese Dog (1), 2.7 oz	200	9	24
Honey Crunchy Dog (1), 2.7 oz	180	10	15
Mini (4), 2.7 oz	210	12	18
State Fair with Ball Park Franks,			
Beef Corn Dogs (1), 2.7 oz	220	10	25
Mini Beef Corn Dogs (6)	260	15	24
Bagel Dogs			
Vienna Beef: Bageldog (1), 5 oz	420	17	33
Mini (1), 2.8 oz	150	4	20

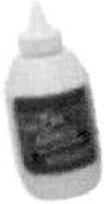

Hot Dog Toppings/Extras:	C	F	Cb
American Cheese, 1 slice, 1 oz	110	9	1
Catsup, 1 Tbsp	16	0	4
Chili (w. Beans), ¼ cup	70	3.5	9
Ketchup, 1 Tbsp	15	0	4
Mustard, 1 Tbsp	20	0	1
Onions, Chopped, 1 Tbsp	5	0	1
Pickle Relish, 1 Tbsp	20	0	5
Sauerkraut, ½ cup	20	0	5

Deli & Lunch Meats

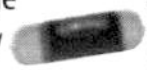

Beef Jerky/Meat Snacks:	C	F	Cb
Bridgford: Beef Jerky, 1 oz	100	0.5	5
Beef Stick (5.5 oz stick), 1 oz	150	13	2
Beef Steak, 1 oz	70	0.5	2
Beef & Cheese (Giant Size), ½ package, 1.5 oz	170	14	1
Pepperoni Sticks (2), 1 oz	160	13	2
Pepperoni (1" diameter), 1 oz	130	12	0
Teriyaki, 1 oz package	80	0.5	4
Original; Hot 'n Spicy	70	1	5
Berliner (pork/beef), 1 oz	65	5	1
Beerwurst (Beef):			
Small (2.75"diam), $\frac{1}{16}$" slice	20	2	0
Large (4"diam), ⅛" slice	75	7	0.5

Deli & Lunch Meats

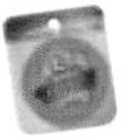

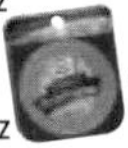

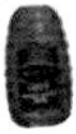

Beerwurst (Pork):	C	F	Cb
Small (2.75"diameter), $\frac{1}{16}$" slice	15	1	0
Large (4"diameter), ⅛" Slice	55	4	0.5
Bologna: 1 Slice, 1 oz	65	6	1
Fat-Free, 1 slice, 1 oz	20	0	2
Beef Bologna: 1 slice, 1 oz	90	8	1
Light, 1 slice, 1 oz	60	4	2
Light *(Oscar Mayer)*, 1 slice, 1 oz	60	4	2
98% Fat Free *(Oscar Mayer)*, 1 oz	25	0.5	3
Ring *(Boar's Head)*, 2 oz	150	13	1
Turkey, average, 1 oz	60	5	0.5
Blood Sausage, 1 oz	100	9	0.5
Bratwurst: Average, 1 oz	80	7	1
Boar's Head, cooked, 1 wurst, 4 oz	300	25	0
Bob Evan's, Beer, 2.6 oz link	270	21	1
Braunschweiger (Pork/Liver/Sausage),			
Oscar Mayer, 1 oz slice	110	10	1
Chicken, *Average All Brands*			
1 thick or 2 thin slices, 1 oz	30	1	1
Hillshire Farm, Rstd/Smkd, av.,2 oz	60	1	2
Corned Beef: Average, full fat, 1 oz	60	5	0.5
Hillshire Farm, 2 oz	60	1	0.5
Ham, Sliced:			
Baked/Boiled, sliced, 1 oz	30	1	0.5
Chopped, *Eckrich* (97% FF), 1 oz	25	1	1
Armour: Canned, 1 oz	35	1.5	0.5
97% Fat Free, 1 oz	25	1	1.5
Oscar Mayer, 1 oz slice	60	2	0.5
Honey/Brown Sugar, Average, 1 oz	30	1	1
Prosciutto, average, 1 oz	70	5	0
Ham & Cheese Loaf, average, 1 oz	70	5	1
Italian Sausage, 2.6 oz	250	20	3
Kielbasa (Polish Sausage), 2 oz	65	5	1
Beef, 2 oz link	190	17	1
Boar's Head, 1 oz	60	5	0
Hillshire Farm, 2.68 oz	250	22	4
Knockwurst, 1 oz	90	8	0.5
Linguica *(Gaspar's)*, 2 oz	180	8	1
Liverwurst, 1 oz	65	5	2
Liver Pate, fresh, average, 1 oz	90	8	1
Luncheon Loaf *(Foods Co)*, 1 oz	65	5	2
Mortadella, 1 oz	105	9	0
Olive Loaf: Average, 1 oz	70	5	3
Oscar Mayer, 1 oz	75	6	2

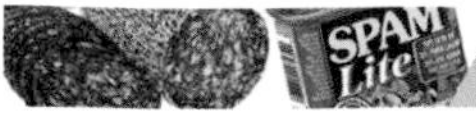

Deli & Lunch Meats (Cont)

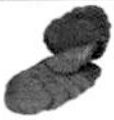
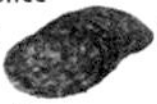
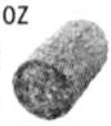

	C	F	Cb
Pastrami (Beef):			
Healthy Deli, 2 oz	70	2	1
Hillshire (DeliSelect), 6 slice, 2 oz	60	1	0
Boar's Head, Round, 2 oz	80	3.5	1
Peppered Beef, 1 oz slice	40	2	1
Pepperoni, 5 slices, 1 oz	140	13	0
Pickle Loaf, av., 1 oz	70	5	5
Pickle & Pimento Loaf			
Oscar Mayer, 1 oz	75	6	3
Proscuitto/Proscuitti: Average, 1 oz	70	5	1
Hormel, 1 oz	90	7	1
Roast Beef: Lean, 1 oz	40	2	0
Healthy Choice, all types, 2 oz	60	1.5	1
Salami: Beef, average, 1 oz	80	7	1
Beer Salami, average, 1 oz	50	4	0.5
Cotto: *Oscar Mayer*, 1 slice, 1 oz	70	6	1
Dry: Hard, average, 4 slices, 1 oz	110	10	3
Oscar Mayer, 2 slices, 1.6 oz	100	8	1
Genoa: Average, 1 oz	120	9	1
Stick *(Best's Kosher)*, 2, 1.75 oz	180	15	2
Italian *(Bridgeford)*, 1 oz	120	11	0
Turkey, average, 1 oz	55	4	1
SPAM *(Hormel): Per 2 oz Serving*			
Classic: 2 oz serving	180	16	2
7 oz can	630	56	3
12 oz can	1030	96	6
Spam Lite: 2 oz	110	8	1
12 oz can	660	48	6
Other Spam Products:			
Hickory Smoked, 2 oz	170	15	2
Hot & Spicy, 2 oz	180	16	2
Oven Roastd Turkey, 2 oz	80	4	2
Spam with Bacon, 2 oz	180	16	1
Spam with Cheese, 2 oz	170	15	1
Spam Spread, 2 oz	140	12	1
25% Less Sodium	180	16	1
Spam Singles:			
Classic, 3 oz package	250	22	2
Lite, 3 oz package	160	11	2
Summer Sausage:			
Bridgford, 1 oz	100	9	1
Hillshire Farm, 2 oz	190	16	0.5
Oscar Mayer, 1 slice, 1 oz	90	7	1

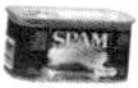

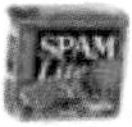

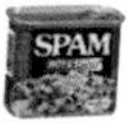

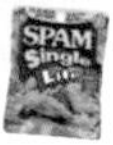

Deli & Lunch Meats (Cont)

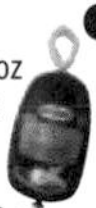
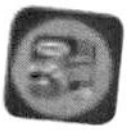

	C	F	Cb
Treet *(Armour)*, canned, 2 oz	140	3.5	4
Turkey: Average, 1 oz slice	30	1	0.5
¾ oz slice	22	0.5	0.5
Turkey Breast:			
Butterball Fat Free, 3 slice, 2 oz	60	0	4
Hillshire Deli Select, 6 slice, 2 oz	50	0.5	3
Healthy Choice: Deli Thin: *Per 4 Slices, (1.8 oz)*			
Oven-Roasted	60	1.5	2
Smoked/Rotisserie Seasoned	60	1.5	3
Honey Roasted & Smoked	60	1.5	4
Hearty Deli Sliced,			
Oven Rsted Turkey Breast, 1 sl., 1 oz	30	1	1
Turkey Ham, 1 slice, 1 oz	35	1.5	0.5
Turkey Pastrami, 1 oz	35	1.5	1
Turkey Roll, 1 oz	40	2	0.5
Turkey Loaf, 1 oz	30	1	0.5

Vegetarian Deli *(Worthington, Yves): See Page 76*

Meat Spreads

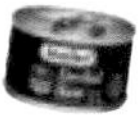
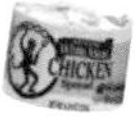

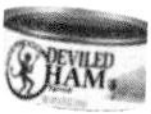

	C	F	Cb
Average All Brands: *Per ¼ Cup (2 oz)*			
Chicken	90	10	2
Ham, Deviled	140	11	0
Liverwurst	190	16	2
Roast Beef	130	10	2
Sandwich Spread	140	10	9
Turkey	110	7	2
Underwood: *Per 2 oz*			
BBQ Chicken	130	8	2
Chicken, White Meat	130	8	2
Deviled Ham	180	15	1
Liverwurst	160	13	4
Roast Beef	130	10	2
Turkey, White Meat	140	9	2

Paté

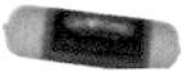

	C	F	Cb
Boar's Head Liverwurst Pate, 2 oz	145	12	0
Les Trois Petit Cochons: *Per 2 oz*			
Black Peppercorn	240	24	1
Chicken Livers & Black Truffle	140	11	2
Country Pate	220	25	1
Duck Liver with Port Wine	130	11	2
Smoked Salmon	110	9	2
Marcel Henri			
Pate de Champagne	210	19	1
Chicken Liver with Port Wine, 2 oz	200	19	1
Duck Truffle with Port Wine, 2 oz	240	24	1
Old Wisconsin Pate			
All types, 2 oz	210	18	3

Nuts

Per 1 oz Unless Indicated

	C	F	Cb
Acorns, raw 1 oz	**110**	7	12
Almonds, dried/dry roasted:			
Whole, 24-28 medium, 1 oz	**170**	15	5.5
½ cup, 2½ oz	**420**	37	13
Chopped,½ cup, 2¼ oz	**380**	34	12
Sliced, ½ cup, 1⅔ oz	**280**	25	9
Choc. coated (5-6), 1 oz	**150**	10	15
Oil Roastd *(Blue Diamond)*, 1 oz	**170**	16	5
Honey Roasted, 1 oz	**170**	14	8
Almond Meal (partially defattened)			
1 cup (not packed), 2¼ oz	**260**	11	11
Brazil Nuts, 8 medium, 1 oz	**185**	19	3.5
Cashews, dry or oil roasted:			
14 large/18 medium/26 small, 1 oz	**165**	14	9
½ cup, 2.4 oz	**375**	31	20
Honey Roasted, 1 oz	**165**	13	10
Chestnuts, av. all: Dried, 1 oz	**105**	1	22
Raw/Fresh, 5-6 nuts, 1 oz	**60**	0	13
Canned, water chestnuts,			
sliced/whole/drained, 1 oz	**30**	0	7
Coconut, fresh:			
1 piece, 2"x2"x ½", 1 oz	**100**	10	4.5
Shredded, fresh, ½ cup, 1.4 oz	**140**	13	6
Dried (Desiccated):			
Unsweetened, 1 oz	**185**	18	7
Sweetened: Shredded, 1 oz	**140**	10	13
Grated, ½ cup, 1.3 oz	**185**	12	18
Cream (canned), ½ cup, 5.2 oz	**285**	26	12
Milk (canned), ½ cup, 4 oz	**225**	24	3
Water (center liquid), ½ cup, 4¼ oz	**25**	0	4.5
Filberts or Hazelnuts:			
Shelled, 18-20 nuts	**180**	17	4.5
Chopped, ¼ cup, 1 oz	**180**	18	5
Ground, ¼ cup, 0.6 oz	**120**	12	3
Ginkgo Nuts, canned, 14 medium, 1 oz	**32**	0.5	6.5
Hickory, 30 small nuts, 1 oz	**200**	18	5
Macadamia Nuts, shelled:			
Raw, 7 medium/14 small, 1 oz	**200**	21	4
½ cup, 2.3 oz	**480**	51	10
Dry Roasted, 1 oz	**205**	22	4
½ cup, 2.4 oz	**480**	51	9
Choc. coated, 2-3 pieces, 1 oz	**170**	12	14
Mixed Nuts: 18-22 nuts, 1 oz	**170**	15	7
Planters: Dry Roasted/Honey	**160**	12	9
Oil Roasted, all types	**170**	16	6
Sweet Roasts, 26 pieces, 1 oz	**160**	12	10
Nut Toppings, chopped, 1 Tbsp, ¼ oz	**40**	4	1.5

Per 1 oz Unless Indicated	C	F	Cb
Peanuts:			
Raw/Dried:			
In shell, 1 oz	**117**	10	3
Shelled, 1 oz	**160**	14	4.5
Boiled, shelled, ½ cup, 3.1 oz	**285**	20	19
Roasted: 30 large/60 small, 1 oz	**165**	14	6
1 cup, 5.1 oz	**860**	76	22
Chopped, 3 Tbsp, 1 oz	**165**	14	6
Planters: Cocktail, 1 oz	**170**	14	6
Rich Roasted in Chocolate, 2½ oz	**220**	14	19
Roasted in Shell, Salted, 1 oz	**160**	14	5
Dry Roasted, 1oz	**160**	13	6
Honey/ & Dry Roasted, 1 oz	**160**	13	8
Spanish Raw, 1 oz	**150**	13	6
Spanish Redskin, 1 oz	**180**	14	5
Sweet N' Crunchy, 1 oz	**140**	7	16
Pecans: Kernel halves, 1 oz	**195**	20	4
(20 jumbo or 31 large halves)			
1 cup halves, 3.8 oz	**755**	78	15
Chopped, ½ cup, 2 oz	**380**	39	7.5
Oil Roasted, 15 halves, 1 oz	**205**	20	4
Honey Roasted, 1 oz	**200**	21	4
Pilinuts, dried, ¼ cup, 1 oz	**215**	24	1
Pine Nuts, dried, 1 Tbsp, 0.3 oz	**70**	7	1.5
Pistachios: Unshelled, ½ cup, 2 oz	**165**	14	7
Shelled, ¼ cup, 45 nuts, 1 oz	**170**	14	8.5
Lance, 1.1 oz package	**95**	7	4
Sesame Nut Mix: *Planters*, 1 oz	**160**	13	9
Soy Nuts: Dry Roasted, 1 oz	**130**	6	9
½ cup, 3 oz	**390**	18	28
Dr Soy: Chocolate coated, 1 oz pkg	**140**	7	13
Average other flavors, 1 oz	**150**	8	8
Trail Mix *(Planters)*: Fruit & Nut, 1 oz	**140**	9	14
Golden Nut Crunch, 1 oz	**160**	11	12
Honey Nut & Caramel, 1 oz	**160**	10	16
Mixed Nuts & Raisins, 1 oz	**150**	11	10
Nut & Chocolate, 1 oz	**160**	10	16
Nuts, Seeds & Raisins, 1 oz	**160**	12	11
Spicy Nuts & Cajun Sticks, 1 oz	**150**	10	13
Sweet & Nutty, 1 oz	**150**	10	14
Walnuts:			
Black: 15-20 halves, 1 oz	**175**	17	3
Chopped, ¼ cup, 1.1 oz	**195**	18	3
English/Persian:			
14 halves, 1 oz	**185**	18	4
Chopped, ¼ cup, 1 oz	**190**	19	4
Ground, ¼ cup, 0.7 oz	**130**	13	3

Quick Guide

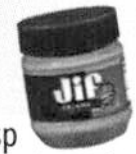

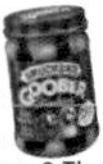

	C	F	Cb
Peanut Butter: *Average All Brands*			
1 level tsp, 0.2 oz	35	3	1.5
1 level Tbsp, 0.6 oz	105	8.5	3.5
2 level Tbsp, 1.2 oz	210	17	7
1 oz Quantity	170	14	6
½ cup, 5 oz	850	70	30
Jif: Reduced Fat, 2 Tbsp	190	12	15
Creamy; Crunchy; Simply, 2 Tbsp	190	16	7
Peanut Butter & Honey, 2 Tbsp	180	14	10
Laura Scudder's:			
Smooth; Crunchy, 2 Tbsp	210	16	6
Reduced-Fat, 2 Tbsp, 1¼ oz	200	12	12
Peanut Wonder, Original, 2 Tbsp	100	2	13
Peter Pan: Creamy; Crunch, 2 Tbsp	200	16	6
Whipped, 2 Tbsp	150	12	5
Smucker's Goober,			
Grape/Strawberry 3 Tbsp	240	13	24
Skippy: Reduced Fat, 2 Tbsp	180	12	15
Roasted Honey Nut Creamy, 2 Tbsp	190	16	7

Peanut Butter & Jelly Sandwich

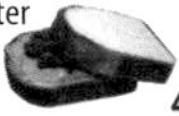

	C	F	Cb
1 sandwich, with 2 oz Bread:			
Light Spread: (1 Tbsp Peanut Butter + 1 Tbsp Jelly)	310	10	48
Thick Spread: (2 Tbsp Peanut Butter + 2 Tbsp Jelly)	480	19	67
With **Goober Grape,** 3 Tbsp, 2 oz	380	15	52

Nutella

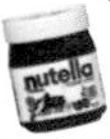

	C	F	Cb
Nut & Chocolate Spread			
1 Tbsp, 0.7 oz	100	5.5	11
2 Tbsp, 1.3 oz	200	11	22

Note: *Nutella* contains approximately 50% sugar and only 13% hazelnuts

Other Nut & Seed Butters

	C	F	Cb
Almond Butter, 1 Tbsp, ½ oz	100	10	3.5
Almond Butter Honey Roasted, 1 Tbsp	90	7	5.5
Beanut Butter, 1 Tbsp, ½ oz	90	5.5	7
Cashew Butter, 1 Tbsp, ½ oz	95	8	4.5
Hazelnut Butter, 1 Tbsp, ½ oz	105	10	2.5
Pecan Butter, 1 Tbsp, ½ oz	110	10	2
Pistachio Butter, 1 Tbsp, ½ oz	90	6.5	4.5
Sesame Butter (Tahini), 1 Tbsp, ½ oz	90	8	3
Soy Nut Butter, 1 Tbsp, ½ oz	75	5	4

Tahini ~ *See Sesame Butter*

Seeds

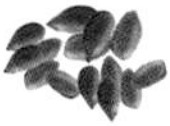

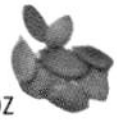

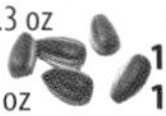

	C	F	Cb
Alfalfa Seeds, sprouted, ½ cup, ½ oz	5	0	1
Caraway, Fennel, 1 tsp	7	0.5	1
Cottonseed Kernels, roasted, 1 Tbsp	50	3.5	2
Flax Seeds, 3 Tbsp, 1 oz	140	9	9
Lotus Seeds, dried, ½ cup, ½ oz	55	0.5	10
Poppy Seeds, 1 tsp	15	1	1
Pumpkin & Squash Seeds, whole:			
Roasted/Tamari, 1 oz	150	12	4
½ cup, 4 oz	590	48	15
Dried, (hulled), ¼ cup, 1 oz	155	13	5
Safflower Kernels, dried, 1 oz	150	11	10
Sesame Seeds:			
Dried, 1 Tbsp, 0.3 oz	50	4.5	2
Roasted/Toasted, 1 oz	160	14	7.5
Sunflower Kernels/Seed:			
Dried, ¼ cup without hulls, ¼ oz	200	18	7
Dry Roasted, 1 Tbsp, 0.3 oz	45	4	2
¼ cup, 1 oz	165	14	7
Oil Roasted, ⅕ cup, 1 oz	170	14	6.5
Watermelon Seeds, dried, ¼ cup, 1 oz	150	13	4

Nut eaters are healthier and live longer, say scientists.

Nuts are a nutritious source of protein, vitamins, minerals, fiber, healthy fats, and antioxidants.

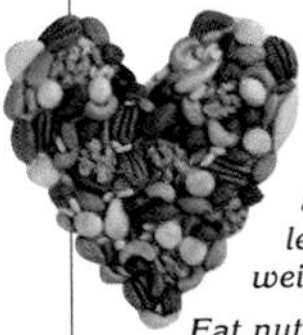

The fat and fiber of nuts can help reduce blood cholesterol. Their protein and fiber also promotes meal satiety (fullness) and reduces hunger levels – of benefit in weight control.

Eat nuts instead of high-sugar snacks, candy and soft drinks. Add chopped nuts to breakfast cereals.

P Pancakes & Waffles

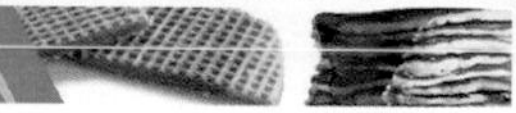

Quick Guide

	C	F	Cb
Pancakes			
Plain: *Average All Types*			
Small (3" diameter), ¾ oz	50	2	6
Medium (4" diameter), 1¼ oz	85	3.5	11
Large (5" diameter), 2½ oz	175	7.5	22
Add Extra for Syrups/Butter			
Pancake Syrup: Regular, 1 Tbsp	50	0	13
¼ cup, 4 Tbsp	210	0	52
Lite, 1 Tbsp	25	0	6
¼ cup, 4 Tbsp	100	0	26
Butter/Margarine: Regular, 1 Tbsp	100	11	0
Whipped, 1 Tbsp	70	7.5	0
Waffles			
Homemade: 7" waffle, 2½ oz	245	13	26
From Mix: 7" waffle, 2½ oz	205	8	28

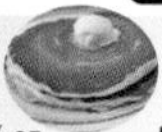

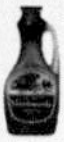

Frozen Breakfasts

	C	F	Cb
Aunt Jemima			
Pancakes: Buttermilk (3)	240	6	41
Homestyle (3)	240	6	41
Low-Fat (3)	200	3	39
Whole Grain (3)	240	6	42
Mini Pancakes (11)	240	4.5	44
Frozen Breakfasts:			
French Toast: Cinnamon, 2 slices	220	4.5	37
Homestyle, 2 slices	220	4.5	37
Sticks (5)	360	12	58
Eggo *(Kellogg's)*			
Bake Shop Swirlz, Cinnamon (1), 2.2 oz	150	3	28
French Toast: Toaster Swirlz, (4)	120	3	20
French Toaster Sticks, average, (2)	225	6	37
Stuffed French Toaster Sticks (2)	300	7	54
Pancakes: Buttermilk (3)	280	9	44
Minis (11)	260	8	31
Krusteaz			
Pancakes: Mini (8)	160	2	30
Buttermilk (3)	270	4	52
French Toast: Homestyle; Thick, 1 sl.	170	3.5	28
Sticks, Griddled (4)	230	5	41
Pillsbury			
Pancakes: Buttermilk (3)	240	4	47
Mini (11)	240	4	45
Chocolate Burst (3)	280	7	51
Toaster Strudel, av. all flavors (1)	190	9	26

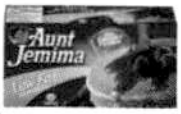

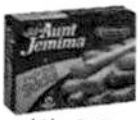

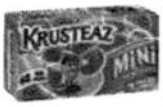

Pancake Brands

	C	F	Cb
Aunt Jemima Mixes: *Prepared as Directed*			
Buttermilk, 4 x 4"	180	5	23
Original Complete, 2 x 4"	160	1.5	32
Original, 4 x 4"	250	6	33
Whole Wheat Blend, 3 x 4"	200	5	30
Betty Crocker Pancake Mixes			
Complete Orig./Buttermilk (3)	200	2.5	40
Bisquick (Shake 'N Pour), (3)	220	3	42
Hungry Jack Pancakes			
Mixes: *Per ⅓ Cup, Prepared as Directed*			
Complete: Buttermilk, 3 x 4"	150	1.5	31
Extra Light & Fluffy, 3 x 4"	150	2	30
Original, with 2% Milk, Oil, Egg	250	8	37
With Skim Milk, Oil, Egg Whites	180	1	37
Easy Packs: *Per ⅓ Cup Dry Mix, Prepared*			
Blueberry Wheat	160	2.5	32
Buttermilk	150	1.5	31
Northern Pines: (3), 3 x 4", 3.5 oz	200	3.5	38

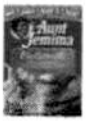

Frozen Waffles

	C	F	Cb
Aunt Jemima: Buttermilk (2)	200	6	33
Homestyle; Blueberry (2)	190	6	32
Low-Fat (2)	160	3	31
Eggo *(Kellogg's)*: Blueberry (2)	190	6	29
Chocolate Chip (2)	210	7	32
French Toast (1)	140	6	19
Homestyle	190	7	27
Nutri-Grain: (2), av.	170	4.5	27
Low-Fat (2)	140	2.5	27
GO-LEAN *(Kashi)*: Average (1)	170	3	33
Nature's Path: Flax Plus (2), average	185	7	24
Homestyle (2)	270	10	44
Mesa Sunrise (2)	200	7	34
Van's: Belgian Homestyle (2)	220	9	31
Hearty Oats: Berry Boost (2)	190	8	26
Maple Fusion (2)	190	9	26
Mini: Chocolate Chip (12)	240	9	35
Homestyle (12)	210	8	32
Wheat Free Minis (12)	210	7	35
97% Fat Free, Original (2)	140	2	26

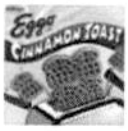

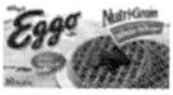

Updated Nutrition Data ~ www.CalorieKing.com
Persons with Diabetes ~ See Disclaimer (Page 24)

- Pasta includes all shapes and sizes; (e.g. spaghetti, fettuccini, elbows, shells, twists, sheets, cannelloni, tubes, ziti).
- All regular pasta products have the same cals/fat/carbs on a weight basis.
- 1 oz Dry = approximately 2½ -3 oz cooked.

Dry Spaghetti/Pasta

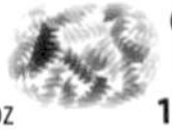

	C	F	Cb
1 oz quantity	105	0.5	21
1lb box/package, 16 oz	1685	7	339
Elbows, 1 cup, 3¾ oz	380	2	80
Shells, small, 1 cup, 3¼ oz	330	1.5	69
Spirals, 1 cup, 3 oz	305	1.5	64

Cooked Spaghetti/Pasta

	C	F	Cb
Plain, All Types (no added fat):			
Firm/Al Dente (8-10 minutes), 1 oz	42	0.5	8.5
Medium (11-13 minutes), 1 oz	37	0.5	7.5
Tender (14-20 minutes), 1 oz	32	0.5	7
(Longer cooking increases water absorbed)			
Spaghetti, ½ cup, 2 ½ oz	90	0.5	18
Medium serving, 1 cup, 5 oz	225	1.5	44
Large Serving, 2 cups, 10 oz	450	3	88
Extra Large, 3 cups, 15 oz	675	5	132
Elbows/Spirals, 1 cup, 5 oz	220	1.5	43
Small Shells, 1 cup, 4 oz	180	1	36
Protein-fortified: Dry, 1 cup, 3⅓ oz	350	2	63
Cooked, 1 cup, 5 oz	230	0.5	45
Spinach/Vegetable: Dry, 1 cup, 3 oz	310	1	61
Cooked, 1 cup, 5 oz	180	0.5	38
Whole-wheat: Dry, 1 cup, 3¾ oz	365	1.5	79
Cooked, 1 cup, 5 oz	175	1	37

Fresh Pasta (Refrigerated)

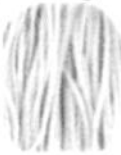

	C	F	Cb
Plain/Spinach/Tomato, average:			
As purchased, 4.5 oz	370	3	70
Cooked, 1 cup, 5 oz	185	1.5	35
Home-made, without egg:			
Cooked, 1 cup, 5 oz	175	1	35
Buitoni			
Cut Pasta: *Per ⅓ of 9 oz Pkg*			
Angel Hair	230	2.5	43
Fettuccine	260	3	46
Linguine	240	2.5	45
Whole Wheat Linguine	240	3	41
Ravioletti, Three Cheese, 1 cup, 3.2 oz	270	5	43

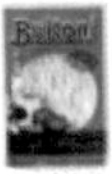

	C	F	Cb
Buitoni (Cont):			
Ravioli: Four Cheese, 1¼ cups	330	10	45
Light Four Cheese, 1¼ cups	260	4.5	41
Whole Wheat Four Chse, 1¼ cups	320	11	40
Tortellini: Herb Chicken, 1 c., 4 oz	350	10	52
Spinach Cheese, 1 cup, 3.7 oz	320	7	49
Three Cheese, 1 cup, 3.7 oz	320	7	50
Tortelloni: Cheese & Rstd Garlic, 1 c.	270	8	37
Other varieties, average, 1 cup	330	10	47

Pasta Sauces: *See Page 148*

Macaroni & Cheese

Packaged: *Kraft/Hormel* ~ *See Page 114-115*

	C	F	Cb
Restaurant, average: Side, 6 oz	265	13	26
Medium serving, 1 cup, 9 oz	350	17	34
Large serving, 2 cups, 18 oz	700	34	68

Noodles

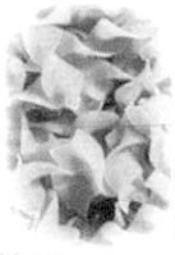

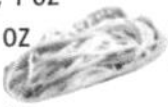

	C	F	Cb
Plain/Egg: Dry, 1 oz	110	1.5	20
1 cup, 1⅓ oz	145	1.5	27
Cooked: 1 oz	40	0.5	7
½ cup, 2¾ oz	110	1.5	20
1 cup, 5½ oz	220	3.5	40
Stir-Fried: 1 cup, 5½ oz	270	9	40
2 cup serving, 11 oz	540	18	80
Yolk Free (Cooked): *Per Cup*			
'No Yolks' *(Foulds)*, 2 oz	210	0.5	41
Passover Gold *(Manischewitz)*	200	0	41
Chinese: Cellophane/Rice, dry, 1 oz	100	0	25
Chow Mein/hard, dry, 1 oz	150	9	16
Japanese: Soba, dry, 1 oz	95	0.5	21
Cooked, 1 cup, 4 oz	115	0.5	24
Somen, dry, 1 oz	100	0.5	21
Cooked, 1 cup, 6 oz	230	0.5	49
Japanese Style Pan Fried:			
Maruchan's Yaki-Sobu, 5.6 oz cup	260	3	50
Ramen Noodles(*Maruchan/Nissin*): *See Page 116*			
Rice Noodles: Dry, 3.5 oz	365	0.5	83
Cooked, 1 cup, 6.2 oz	190	0.5	44
Stir Fry (*Yakisoba)*, 3.5 oz serving	430	6	52
Tofu Shirataki *(House Foods)*, 4 oz	20	0.5	3
Udon (*Chikara)*, average, 7.5 oz pkt	250	1	52

Simply Asia/Thai Kitchen ~ *Page 117*

Egg Roll/Won Ton Wrappers

	C	F	Cb
Egg/Spring Roll (1), 0.8 oz	65	0	15
Won Ton Wrapper (1), ¼ oz	20	0	4

Quick Guide

Fruit Pies: *Average All Brands (9")*

Apple; Blueberry; Cherry:	C	F	Cb
Small, ⅛ pie, 4¾ oz	320	15	46
Medium, ⅙ pie, 6⅓ oz	425	20	61
Large, ¼ pie, 9½ oz	640	30	92
Whole Pie (9"), 38oz	2560	120	368
Other Pies: *Per Serving (⅙ of 8" Pie)*			
Chocolate Cream Pie	345	22	38
Custard; Coconut Custard	270	14	31
Lemon Chiffon Pie	360	14	50
Lemon Meringue	360	13	57
Pecan Pie	440	23	57
Pumpkin Pie	300	12	42
Strawberry Pie	230	9	37

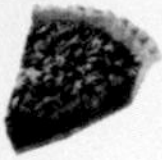

Brands ~ *Per Serving*

	C	F	Cb
Denny's: Apple Pie, 7 oz	510	23	72
French Silk Pie, 7 oz	770	57	59
Hostess: Fruit; Cherry Pie, 4.5 oz	480	20	68
Lemon Pie, 4.5 oz	490	22	69
Long John Silver's:			
Chocolate Cream Pie	280	17	28
Pineapple Cream Pie	300	17	35
Turtle Pie	290	16	34
Marie Callender's			
Cobbler, ⅛ pie, average	330	17	44
Mrs Smith's:			
Classsic Pies: Apple, ⅙ pie	320	14	47
Dutch Apple Crumb, ⅙ pie	340	14	52
Peach, ⅙ pie	310	14	42
Deep Dish, Apple, ⅒ pie	290	13	41
Peach Cobbler, ⅛ cobbler	210	6	39
Sara Lee			
Pies: Choc Dream Pie, ⅛ pie	420	24	47
Choc Mint Creme Pie, ⅛ pie	420	27	44
Key West Lime Pie, ⅛ pie	380	18	50
Peach Pie, ⅛ pie	310	15	42
Southern Pecan Pie, ⅛ pie	470	23	62
Oven Fresh Pies (9", 37 oz Box): *Per Slice (4.6 oz)*			
Apple Pie, ⅛	340	16	47
Cherry Pie, ⅛	340	16	45
Mince Pie; Blueberry Pie, av., ⅛	380	17	53
Pumpkin Pie, ⅛	260	10	39
Southern Sweet Potato Pie, ⅛	280	9	45
Simple Sweets: Apple Pie, ¼ pie	290	15	37
Cherry Pie, ¼ pie	330	16	45
Tastykake: Apple Pie	270	11	40
Coconut Cream Pie	370	20	42
Lemon Pie	300	14	44
Strawberry Pie	340	12	55

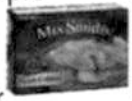

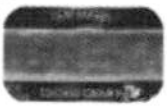

Croissants

Average all Brands	C	F	Cb
Plain/Butter/Cheese: Mini, 1 oz	115	6	13
Small, 1½ oz	170	9	19
Medium, 2 oz	230	12	26
Large, 2½ oz	290	15	32
Extra Large, 3 oz	330	19	37
Sweet Croissants:			
Almond Filled, 3 oz	330	18	39
Chocolate Filled, 3 oz	360	19	43
Dunkin' Donuts: Plain Croissant	310	16	35
Sara Lee: French Style Petite, 2 oz	230	11	26
French Style Original, 1½ oz	170	8	20

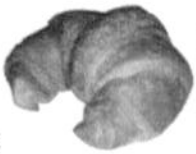

Croissant Sandwiches: *See Page 172*

Pastry & Pie Crust

	C	F	Cb
Pie Crust: Baked, 9" diameter shell			
1 Pie Shell, 6½ oz	970	64	87
2-crust Pie, 9", 11¼ oz	1660	109	150
Filo Pastry: 4 sheets, 2½ oz	210	2.5	40
Athens, 14"x18", 2½ sheets, 2 oz	180	1.5	37
Puff *(Pepp.Farm)*, ½ sheet, 4.5 oz	510	33	42
Bake & Fill Shell, 1.7 oz	190	13	16
Arrowhead Mills, Pie Crust, ⅛ of 9"	110	5	14
Bisquick: Baking Mix,			
Original, ⅓ cup, 1½ oz	160	4.5	26
Heart Smart, ⅓ cup, 1½ oz	140	2.5	27
Keebler:			
Ready Crust: *Per ⅛ of 9" Crust*			
Chocolate	100	4.5	14
Graham	110	5	14
Reduced Fat	100	3.5	15
Shortbread Crust	110	5	14
Graham Crackers Minis (1), 0.8 oz	110	5	15
Marie Callenders, Deep Dish Pie Shell, ⅛ pie, 1 oz	140	10	11
Mrs Smith's, Homestyle			
Deep Dish, 9", ⅛	130	7	15
Nabisco:			
Honey Maid Graham, ⅙ of 9", 1 oz	150	8	18
Nilla Pie Crust, ⅙ of 9", 1 oz	140	8	18
Pillsbury (All Ready Rolled), ⅛,1 oz	110	6	12
Trader Joe's, Pie Crust, ⅛ pie, 1.2 oz	170	12	12

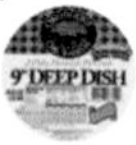

Pie Fillings (Canned)

Fruit: *Average all Fruits* (Apple/Blueberry/Cherry/Strawberry)	C	F	Cb
Sweetened: ⅓ cup, 3.2oz	90	0	22
1 cup, 9½ oz	270	0	66
1 can, 21 oz	600	0	150
Light/Lite, ⅓ cup, 3.2 oz	60	0	15
Unsweetened, ⅓ cup, 3.2 oz	35	0	8
Lemon Cream/Creme, ⅓ cup, 3.2 oz	130	1.5	28

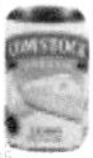

Pizzas ~ Ready-To-Eat

Average All Retail Outlets/Restaurants

Cheese Pizza

Medium Size (12"):

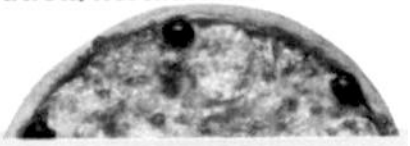

	C	F	Cb
Thin Crust:			
⅛ Pizza (1 slice)	**200**	8	22
½ Pizza (4 slices)	**800**	32	88
Whole Pizza (8 slices)	**1600**	64	172
Deep Dish/Pan:			
⅛ Pizza (1 slice)	**270**	13	27
½ Pizza (4 slices)	**1080**	52	108
Whole Pizza (8 slices)	**2160**	104	216

Pepperoni

Medium Size (12"):

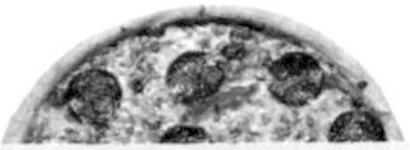

	C	F	Cb
Thin Crust:			
⅛ Pizza (1 slice)	**210**	10	23
½ Pizza (4 slices)	**840**	40	84
Whole Pizza (8 slices)	**1680**	80	168
Deep Dish/Pan:			
⅛ Pizza (1 slice)	**280**	15	27
½ Pizza (4 slices)	**1120**	60	108
Whole Pizza (8 slices)	**2240**	120	216

Supreme:

Medium Size (12"):

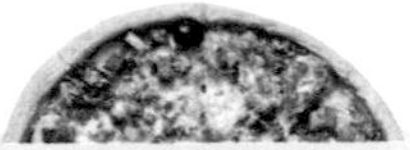

	C	F	Cb
Thin Crust:			
⅛ Pizza (1 slice)	**240**	11	23
½ Pizza (4 slices)	**960**	44	92
Whole Pizza (8 slices)	**1920**	88	184
Deep Dish/Pan:			
⅛ Pizza (1 slice)	**310**	16	28
½ Pizza (4 slices)	**1240**	64	112
Whole Pizza (8 slices)	**2480**	128	224

Meat Deluxe

Medium Size (12"):

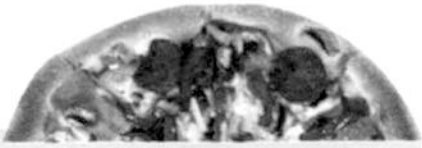

	C	F	Cb
Thin Crust:			
⅛ Pizza (1 slice)	**310**	18	23
½ Pizza (4 slices)	**1240**	72	92
Whole Pizza (8 slices)	**2480**	144	184
Deep Dish/Pan:			
⅛ Pizza (1 slice)	**380**	22	28
½ Pizza (4 slices)	**1520**	88	112
Whole Pizza (8 slices)	**3040**	176	224

Hawaiian *(Ham & Pineapple)*

Medium Size (12"):

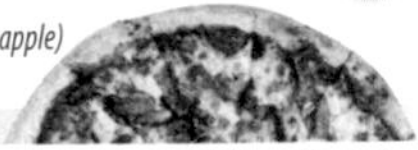

	C	F	Cb
Thin Crust:			
⅛ Pizza (1 slice)	**190**	7	23
½ Pizza (4 slices)	**760**	28	92
Whole Pizza (8 slices)	**1520**	56	184
Deep Dish/Pan:			
⅛ Pizza (1 slice)	**250**	11	28
½ Pizza (4 slices)	**1000**	44	112
Whole Pizza (8 slices)	**2000**	88	224

Veggie:

Similar to Hawaiian

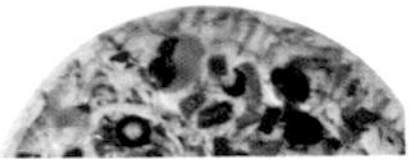

Single Slices

(Extra Large):
(Example: Sbarro's)

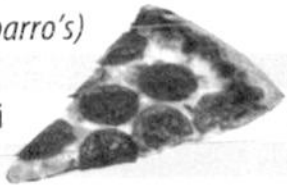

	C	F	Cb
Cheese	**460**	13	60
Pepperoni	**730**	37	61
Sausage	**670**	31	60
Supreme	**630**	27	63

Individual Pizza (6")

Deep Dish/Pan
(Approx. 9 oz weight):

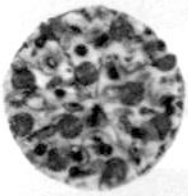

	C	F	Cb
Cheese	**600**	24	69
Hawaiian	**570**	21	70
Meat Deluxe	**900**	50	70
Pepperoni	**650**	30	67
Veggie	**560**	22	70

Large (14") Thin Crust

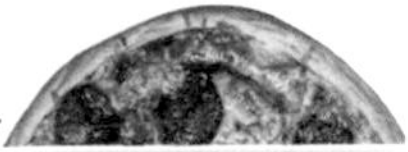

	C	F	Cb
Cheese: ⅛ Pizza	**290**	12	30
½ Pizza	**1160**	48	120
Hawaiian: ⅛ pizza	**260**	9	33
½ Pizza	**1040**	36	132
Pepperoni: ⅛ Pizza	**310**	15	30
½ Pizza	**1240**	60	120
Supreme: ⅛ Pizza	**340**	17	32
½ Pizza	**1360**	68	128
Meat Deluxe: ⅛ Pizza	**440**	26	31
½ Pizza	**1760**	104	124
Veggie: ⅛ Pizza	**260**	10	32
½ Pizza	**1040**	40	128

Frozen Pizzas

Food	C	F	Cb
Amy's: *Per ⅓ Pizza*			
Cheese Pesto	360	18	37
Cheese Pizza	290	12	33
Mushroom & Olive	250	9	33
Pesto	310	12	39
Roasted Vegetable	270	9	42
California Pizza Kitchen			
Crispy Thin Crust: *Per ⅓ Pizza*			
Margherita	290	13	31
Sicilian Recipe	310	14	30
White	290	12	31
For One:			
Four Cheese, 6.9 oz	510	17	69
Margherita, 6 oz	420	18	45
Sicilian, 5.5 oz	450	22	42
Self Rising Crust: *Per ⅓ Pizza*			
BBQ Chicken, 4.3 oz	270	9	33
Five Cheese & Tomato, 4.3 oz	330	11	41
Garlic Chicken, 4.3 oz	260	9	31
Celeste			
Pizza For One: Original, 1 pizza	350	16	39
Deluxe; Pepperoni; Cheeseburger	410	21	42
Meatball	420	22	40
Sausage & Pepperoni; Suprema	420	23	39
Zesty 4 Cheese	350	16	38
DiGiorno			
Crispy Flatbread Pizza: *Per Slice*			
Italian Sausage & Onion, 5.5 oz	400	26	27
Mushroom Medley, 4.3 oz	320	19	26
Pepperoni & Roasted Peppers, 4.5 oz	340	20	26
Tuscan Style Chicken, 4.7 oz	280	14	25
For One: *Per Pizza*			
Garlic Bread Crust:			
Pepperoni	840	44	81
Thin Crust Supreme	590	24	63
Classic Crust: Pepperoni	770	35	83
Supreme	790	36	85
Microwave: *Per ½ Pizza*			
Rising Crust: Four Cheese	370	15	44
Supreme	410	18	45
Three Meat	420	19	44
Thin Crispy Crust, Four Cheese	320	12	38
Rising Crust: Per ⅙ Pizza			
Four Cheese	310	11	40
Pepperoni	330	13	40
Thin Crispy Crust: *Per ⅕ Pizza*			
Four Meat	320	14	32
Grilled Chicken Tomato & Spinach	260	8	33

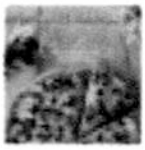
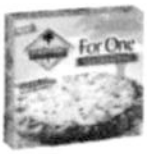
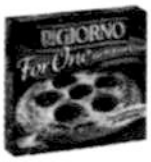
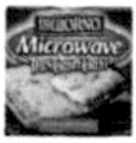

DiGiorno (Cont)	C	F	Cb
Ultimate Thin Crust: *Per ⅕ Pizza*			
Four Cheese	330	14	33
Four Meat; Pepperoni, average	390	20	33
Ultimate Toppings: *Per ⅕ Pizza*			
Cheese	320	13	34
Pepperoni; Supreme, average	365	19	33
Four Meat; Pepperoni, average	390	20	33
Freschetta			
Naturally Rising: *Per ⅕ of Large Pizza*			
4 Cheese	360	13	43
4 Meat	380	14	44
Can. Bacon P'apple	310	9	44
Pepperoni	360	14	44
Supreme	320	13	37
PizzAmore:			
6 Cheese, ¼ pizza	380	14	47
Meat Medley, ⅕ pizza	340	14	38
Pepperoni Duo, ¼ pizza	340	15	38
Supreme, ⅕ pizza	340	14	38
Stuffed Breadsticks: Garlic (1)	110	3	19
Cinnamon with Cream Cheese (1)	140	4	23
Healthy Choice: *Per Pizza, 6 oz*			
French Bread Pizza	345	4.5	54
Jeno's: *Per Pizza , 7 oz*			
Crispy 'N Tasty: Cheese	450	21	51
Sausage; Pepperoni, average	485	25	50
Home Run Inn (Chicago): *Per ⅙ Pizza*			
Classic Large 12": Cheese, 4.5 oz	340	18	30
Sausage, 5 oz	360	19	29
Sausage & Pepperoni, 5.15 oz	380	20	30
Signature, Sausage Supreme, 5½ oz	360	18	31
Kashi, Original Crust, av., ⅓ pizza	290	9	38
Lean Cuisine:			
Casual Eating: *Per Pizza, 6 oz*			
Deep Dish: Roasted Vegetable	320	5	52
Spinach & Mushroom	340	7	52
French Bread: Cheese	340	7	53
Deluxe	340	10	46
Traditional: Four Cheese	340	6	51
Pepperoni	350	8	50
Wood Fired: Margherita	300	7	43
Roast Garlic Chicken	330	8	42
Private Selection			
Flat Bread: *Per Pizza*			
Chicken	550	16	77
Margherita	600	22	70
Thin Crust: BBQ Chicken, ⅓ pizza	360	15	36
Extra Pepperoni, ⅓ pizza	440	24	32
Grilled Chicken Caesar, ⅓ pizza	350	15	35
Margherita, ⅓ pizza	310	13	32

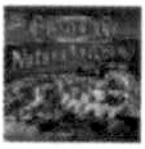
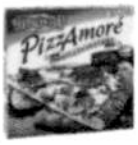
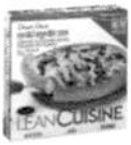

Persons with Diabetes ~ See Disclaimer (Page 24)

Frozen Pizzas (Cont)

Red Baron

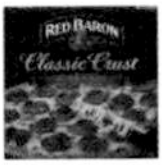

	C	F	Cb
Classic (Large):			
4 Cheese, ¼ pizza	380	16	40
Pepperoni, ¼ pizza	370	16	40
Supreme, ⅕ pizza	310	14	33
Sausage & Pepperoni, ¼ pizza	400	19	41
Special Deluxe, ¼ pizza	380	18	41
Fire Baked Singles: *Per Pizza*			
4-Cheese	550	22	67
Pepperoni	570	24	67
Thin & Crispy Tuscan Style: *Per ⅓ Pizza*			
5 Cheese	360	16	39
Pepperoni	410	20	40
Singles: *Per Pizza*			
Deep Dish: 4 Cheese	410	18	45
Meat Trio	400	18	45
Pepperoni	420	19	45
Supreme	420	19	45
Deep Dish Mini Pizza: *Per 4 Pizza's*			
Cheese	420	20	44
Pepperoni	460	25	44
French Bread: *Per Single Serve*			
Pepperoni	360	15	42
Supreme	310	10	42
5 Cheese & Garlic	410	22	39

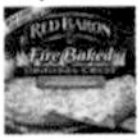

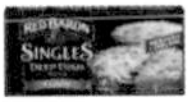

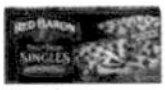

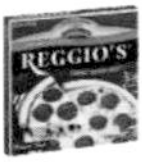

	C	F	Cb
Reggio's			
Deep Dish: Cheese, ⅙ pizza	350	16	39
Sausage, ⅙ pizza	410	20	39
Dinner Size: Cheese, ¼ pizza	330	12	41
Pepperoni & Sausage, ¼ pizza	400	18	41
Sausage; Supreme, av., ¼ pizza	380	16	41
Safeway Select			
Thin and Crispy:			
Four Cheese, ⅙ pizza	310	11	37
Pepperoni, ⅕ pizza	350	16	37
Ultra Thin Crust: *Per ⅓ Pizza Unless Indicated*			
BBQ Chicken ¼ pizza	250	10	23
Margherita	330	17	28
Primo Italiano Meat	330	17	28
Stouffer's: *Per ½ Pizza*			
French Bread Pizzas: Deluxe	430	21	45
Extra Cheese	400	18	44
Pepperoni	430	21	44
Sausage & Pepperoni	460	24	43

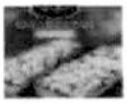

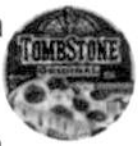

	C	F	Cb
Tombstone			
Original: *Per ⅕ of Large 12" Pizza Unless Indicated*			
4 Meat	310	14	30
Canadian Style Bacon, ¼ pizza	320	12	37
Deluxe	290	12	31
Extra Cheese, ¼ pizza	350	15	37
Pepperoni, ⅓ pizza	280	14	28
Pepperoni & Sausage	370	17	37
Sausage & Mushroom	290	13	30
Supreme	300	14	31
Double Top: Sausage, ⅙ pizza	310	16	27
Sausage & Pepperoni, ⅙ pizza	330	18	26
Harvest Wheat Thin Crust:			
Cheese, ⅓ pizza	300	10	37
Pepperoni, ¼ pizza	260	10	29
Supreme, ¼ pizza	260	10	29
Light Vegetable	230	6	31
Thin Crust: Three Cheese, ¼ pizza	310	15	28
Pepperoni; Sausage, av., ¼ pizza	325	18	29
Brick Oven Style, Cheese, ⅓ pizza	350	15	38
Pepperoni; Supreme, av., ¼ pizza	315	16	29
Tony's			
Original Crust: Cheese, ⅓ pizza	290	12	37
Pepperoni, ⅓ pizza	310	14	36
Ssg & Pepperoni; Supreme, av., ⅓	340	17	37
Deep Dish (Individual):			
Cheese (1)	400	16	47
Pepperoni (1)	470	24	49

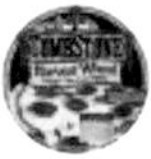

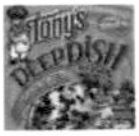

	C	F	Cb
Totino's			
Crisp Crust Party Pizza: *Per ½ Pizza*			
Cheese	320	15	34
Classic Pepperoni	370	20	35
Pizza Rolls: Cheese (6), 3 oz	180	5	26
Pepperoni (6), 3 oz	210	10	24
Trader Joe's:			
3 Cheese, ⅓ pizza	310	9	42
Parlanno, ¼ pizza	340	16	34
Spinach, ⅓ pizza	300	12	38
Weight Watchers (Smart Ones): *Per Pizza*			
Fajita Chicken	380	7	58
Four Cheese	370	7	57
Pepperoni	390	8	58
Wolfgang Puck			
All Natural Pizzas: *Per ⅓ Pizza*			
4 Cheese Tomato & Pesto	330	17	30
BBQ Chicken	360	15	40
Cheese	340	16	33
Margherita	330	16	33
Uncured Pepperoni	360	19	32

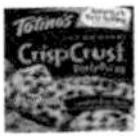

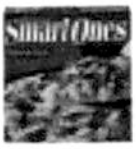

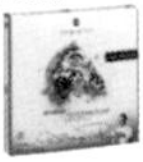

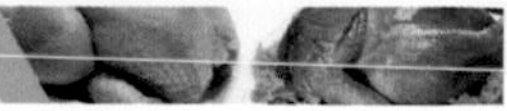

Quick Guide

Chicken	C	F	Cb
From 3lb ready-to-cook chicken			
Breast/Wing Quarter			
Roasted: With skin	300	15	0
Without skin	185	5	0
Fried, batter dipped	530	30	17
Leg Quarter:			
Thigh & Drumstick			
Roasted: With skin, 4 oz	265	15	0
Without skin, 3.35 oz	180	8	0
Fried, batter dipped	430	25	14
(**KFC:** *See Fast-Foods Section)*			

Per 4 oz Edible Portion

Average of Light Meat: *Per 4 oz (no bone)*			
Roasted: With skin	250	12	0
Without skin	175	4.5	0
Stewed: With skin	230	12	0
Without skin	180	4.5	0
Fried: Batter-dipped, 4 oz	315	17	11
Flour-coated, 4 oz	280	14	2
Average of Dark Meat: *Per 4 oz (no bone)*			
Roasted: With skin	290	18	0
Without skin	235	11	0
Stewed: With skin	265	17	0
Without skin	220	10	0
Fried: Batter-dipped, 4 oz	340	21	11
Flour-coated, 4 oz	325	19	5

Chicken Parts

Broilers or Fryers: Edible Weights (no bone)			
Breast: *Per ½ Breast*			
Raw: With skin, 5 oz	250	14	0
Without skin, 4¼ oz	130	1.5	0
Roasted: With skin, 3½ oz	195	8	0
Without skin, 3 oz	140	3	0
Stewed: With skin, 4 oz	200	8	0
Without skin, 3¼ oz	145	3	0
Fried: Batter-dipped, 5 oz	365	19	13
Flour-coated, with skin, 3½ oz	220	9	2
Drumstick: *Per Drumstick*			
Roasted: With skin, 2 oz	115	6	0
Without skin, 1½ oz	75	2.5	0
Fried: Batter-dipped, 2½ oz	195	11	6
Flour-coated, 1¾ oz	120	7	1
Stewed: With skin, 2 oz	115	6	0
Without skin, 1½ oz	80	3	0

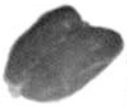

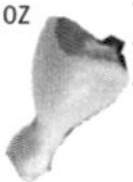

Chicken Parts (Cont)

	C	F	Cb
Thigh Portion: Edible Weight (no bone)			
Raw: With skin, 3.3 oz (4¼ oz with bone)	200	14	0
Without skin, 2.4 oz	80	3	0
Roasted: With skin, 2¼ oz	155	10	0
Without skin, 2 oz	110	6	0
Stewed: With skin, 2½ oz	160	10	0
Without skin, 2 oz	105	5	0
Fried: Batter-dipped, 3 oz	240	14	8
Flour-coated, 2¼ oz	165	9	2
Wing: *Per Wing*			
Raw Weight 3.2 oz (with bone)			
Raw: With skin	110	8	0
Without skin	35	1	0
Roasted: With skin	100	7	0
Without skin	45	2	0
Fried: Batter-dipped	160	11	5
Flour-coated	105	7	1
Stewed: With skin, 4 oz	100	7	0
Buffalo Wings: *See Fast-Foods Section*			
Neck: Simmered, with skin	95	7	0
Without skin	30	2	0
Skin Only: *Skin from ½ Chicken*			
Raw skin, 2¾ oz	275	26	0
Roasted skin, 2 oz	255	23	0
Stewed skin, 2½ oz	260	24	0
Fried, Flour-coated, 2 oz	280	24	5
Fried, Batter-dipped, 6¾ oz	750	55	44
Roasters			
Average of Light & Dark Meat:			
Roasted: With skin, 4 oz	250	15	0
Without skin, 4 oz	190	8	0
Light Meat: Without skin, roasted	175	5	0
Dark Meat: Without skin, roasted	200	10	0
Stewing Chicken			
Average of Light & Dark Meat: *Per 4 oz Stewed*			
With skin	325	22	0
Without skin	270	14	0
Light Meat: Without skin	240	9	0
Dark Meat: Without skin	290	17	0
Capon Chicken			
Roasted: With skin, 4 oz	260	13	0
½ Chicken, with skin	1460	74	0
Chicken Offal & Stuffing			
Giblets: Simmered, 1 cup	230	7	0.5
Fried, flour-coated, 1 cup	400	20	6
Gizzard, simmered, 1 cup	210	4	0
Heart, simmered, 1 cup	270	12	0.2
Liver: Raw, 4 oz	130	5.5	0
Simmered, 1 cup	215	8.5	1
Liver Pate Fresh, 1 Tbsp, ½ oz	30	2	1
Stuffing: Average, ½ cup	180	9	22

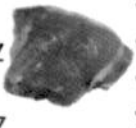

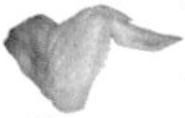

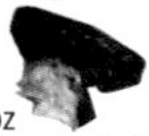

Updated Nutrition Data ~ www.CalorieKing.com
Persons with Diabetes ~ See Disclaimer (Page 24)

Chicken Products

Chicken Products	C	F	Cb
Bumble Bee: *Per 4oz Pouch*			
Chicken Breast, Skinless fillet:			
Garlic & Herb	110	1.5	1
With Barbeque Sauce	170	1.5	10
With Southwest Seasoning	120	1	0
Foster Farms			
Grilled Chicken Breast Strips, 3 oz	100	1.5	2
Wings: Chipotle, 4 wings, 2.9 oz	190	14	1
Honey BBQ, 4 wings, 2.9 oz	170	10	5
Hot & Spicy, 4 wings, 2.9 oz	170	13	1
Tyson:			
Any'tizers:			
BBQ Style Wings (3)	200	13	7
Buffalo Style Hot Wings (3)	230	15	1
Breaded Nuggets (5)	270	17	15
Breast Nuggets (5)	220	13	15
Southern Style Nuggets (6)	270	21	11
Breast Patties: Southern Style (1)	260	20	11

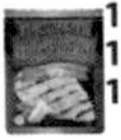
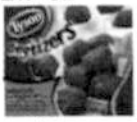

Duck, Goose, Quail

Duck: Roasted,			
With skin, 3 oz	290	24	0
Without skin, 3 oz	170	10	0
½ whole duck, with skin	1290	108	0
Goose: Roast, with skin, 3 oz	260	19	0
Without skin, 3 oz	200	11	0
Pheasant, cooked, 3 oz	210	10	0
Quail, cooked, 1 whole, 6 oz	400	24	0

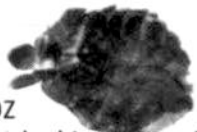

Turkey

Fryer-Roasters: *Per 3 oz Serving*			
Roasted: Light Meat, with skin	140	4	0
Without skin	120	1	0
Dark Meat: With skin	155	6	0
Without skin	140	4	0
½ of Whole Turkey: (Approx. 3¼ lbs raw weight Without neck and giblets; 1.8 lbs cooked weight)			
Roasted: With skin	1650	74	0
Without skin	1125	31	0
Ground Turkey, Raw: (4 oz raw wt. = 3 oz ckd wt.)			
Regular (85% lean), 4 oz	170	10	0
Lean (93% lean), average, 4 oz	160	8	0
Foster Farms (94% lean), 4 oz	150	7	0
Jennie-O (93% lean), 4 oz	170	8	0
Trader Joe's (93% lean), 4 oz	150	8	0
Breast, no skin, 4 oz	115	1	0
Patties: Small, 3 oz	130	7	0
Medium, 4 oz	170	10	0
Large, 5.3 oz	225	13	0

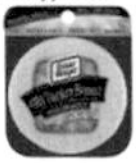

Turkey Parts

Turkey Parts	C	F	Cb
Roasted, Edible Weights (no bone)			
Breast (½): (from 17¼ oz raw weight with bone)			
With skin, 12 oz (no bone)	525	11	0
Without skin, 10¾ oz	415	2	0
Back (½): With skin, 4½ oz	265	13	0
Without skin, 3½ oz	165	6	0
Leg (Thigh & Drumstick): (from 1 lb raw weight with bone)			
With skin, 8½ oz (without bone)	410	13	0
Without skin, 7¾ oz	355	8.5	0
Wing: (from 7¼ oz raw weight)			
With skin, 3 oz (without bone)	185	9	0
Without skin, 2 oz (with bone)	100	2	0
Neck: Simmered, 1 neck, (9 oz with bone)	275	11	0
Giblets, simmered, 1 cup, 5 oz	240	7	3

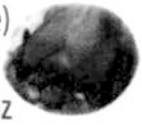

Young Hens (Roasted)

Light Meat: With skin, 3 oz	175	8	0
Without skin, 3 oz	135	3	0
Dark Meat: With skin, 3 oz	200	11	0
Without skin, 3 oz	165	7	0
Young Toms – Similar to Young Hens			

Turkey Products

Banquet: *See Frozen Meals, Page 119*			
Foster Farms:			
Homestyle Meatballs (3)	160	9	3
Hormel: Turkey Chunks (canned), cooked:			
Chunk Turkey, 2 oz	70	2.5	0
White & Dark Turkey, 2 oz	60	1.5	0
Jennie-O:			
All Natural: Lean Meatloaf, 4 oz	250	20	1
White Burgers, 5.25 oz	180	7	0
Fully Cooked: Italian Meatballs, 3 oz	170	11	1
Home Style Meatballs, 3 oz	180	12	2
Turkey Bacon, 1 slice	35	3	1
Turkey Bratwurst, lean, 4 oz	170	10	2
John Morrell: Off the Bone,			
Oven Roasted Turkey Strips, 4 oz	140	5	10
Spam, Oven Roasted Turkey, 2 oz	80	4	2
Swanson: *Frozen Meals, Page 123*			
Trader Joe's, Ital. Turkey Meatloaf, 3 oz	140	8	5

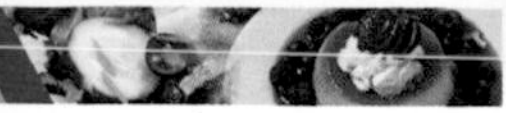

See CalorieKing.com for All Recipes & Serving Sizes

Starters/Appetizers:			
Cheesy Grape Balls (1)	**20**	1.5	1
Shiitake Summer Rolls (1)	**120**	1	24
Spring Rolls (1)	**135**	4.5	15
Soups:			
Beef Stew	**435**	8	35
Cheesy Broccoli Potato Soup	**150**	5	16
Chicken Soup with Rice Dumplings	**155**	0.5	31
Chili Con Carne	**360**	15	25
Creamy Butternut Squash Soup	**115**	3	22
Spicy Pumpkin Soup	**205**	5	29
Sweet Potato Soup	**130**	3	22
Salads:			
Apple Raspberry Salad	**95**	2.5	11
Cherry and Smoked Turkey Salad	**265**	9	31
Citrus Fruit Salad	**125**	0.5	30
Green Bean Potato Salad	**185**	5	32
Hot Rosemary Potato Salad	**180**	2	37
Watermelon Salad	**40**	0	10
Meat Entrees:			
Beef and Mushroom Burgers (2)	**450**	14	51
Grilled Marinated Lamb Filet, 3½ oz	**150**	7	1
Lamb and Rosemary Kebobs (1)	**220**	9	3
Mustard Steak with Tuscan Salad	**235**	8	8
Veal and Mushrooms	**235**	7	11

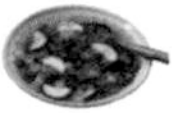

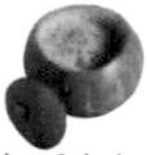

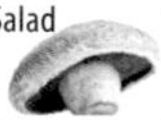

CALORIE KING TIPS
TO REDUCE CALORIES:

- **Use non-fat milk** in place of whole or 2% milk
- **Use low-fat yogurt** in place of sour cream
- **Skim fat** from surface of soups and casseroles after cooling
- **Add extra vegetables** to soups and hot entrees
- **Cakes/cookies/muffins:** Replace most or all the fat/oil with applesauce and/or prune puree (Example: *Sunsweet Lighter Bake*)
- **Drinks:** Replace sugar with no-calorie sweeteners such as *Equal, Stevia, Splenda and Sweet 'N Low*

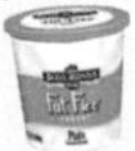

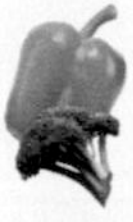

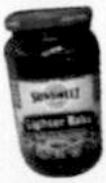

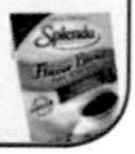

Chicken Entrees:			
Baked Chicken with Mushrooms	**155**	2	4
Baked Rosemary Drumsticks	**320**	11	22
Basil & Lemon Chicken Thighs	**150**	9.5	3
Chicken Cacciatore	**345**	7	40
Chicken Kiev	**315**	8	26
Easy Chicken Pot Pie	**275**	12	23
Lemon Chicken with Olives	**200**	9	8
Mushroom & Chicken Coq au Vin	**360**	9	9
Fish Entrees:			
Fish Cutlets in Herb Tomato Coulis	**300**	4.5	5
Grilled Fish with Corn & Leek, 4 oz	**245**	10	12
Stir-Fry Mixed Seafood & Noodles	**250**	4	28
Thai Fish Cakes	**260**	4	36
Tuna-Mayo Wrap	**250**	3.5	26
Vegetarian:			
Avocado Tacos	**100**	3	17
Coconut Vegetable Curry	**200**	11	12
Eggplant Stuffed with Tofu	**215**	5	40
Fettuccini w/Tomato & Basil Sauce	**340**	8	56
Gourmet Vegetable Pizza	**170**	5	24
Nutty Soy 'n Rice Burgers	**140**	3.5	23
Slow Cooker Veggie Lasagna	**185**	8.5	14
Vegetable Burgers	**185**	6.5	18
Zucchini Moussaka	**260**	5	36
Desserts:			
Angel Food Cake	**85**	0	18
Apple and Rice Pudding	**110**	0.5	25
Brandy Pumpkin Flan	**145**	5	17
Fruit Salad Dessert Cake	**175**	8.5	23
Low-Fat Carrot Cake	**185**	2	39
Melon Sorbet	**100**	2	21
Non-Fat Brownies	**115**	0	26
Non-Fat Chocolate Cupcakes	**105**	0	22
Non-Fat Vanilla Ice Cream	**60**	0	11
Watermelon Blueberry Banana Split	**175**	1	42
Drinks: *Per 1 Cup, 8 fl.oz*			
Apple and Fruit Frappe	**135**	0	33
Banana Daiquiri	**190**	2	44
Fruity Iced Tea	**50**	0	12
Mocha Shake	**95**	0	14
Pineapple Float	**180**	0	44
Watermelon Coconut Margarita	**235**	6	34
Watermelon Kiwi Smoothie	**115**	0	24

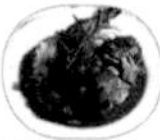

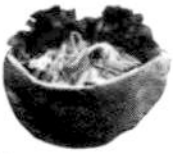

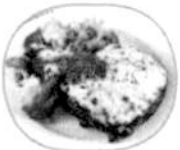

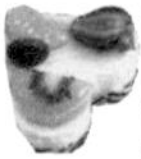

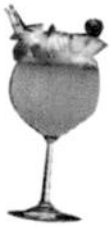

Updated Nutrition Data ~ www.CalorieKing.com
Persons with Diabetes ~ See Disclaimer (Page 24)

White Rice

	C	F	Cb
Raw: Short/Med. Grain, 1 cup, 7 oz	715	1	158
Long Grain, 1 cup, 6½ oz	675	1	148
Glutinous, 1 cup, 6½ oz	685	1	151
Cooked Rice (Boiled/Steamed):			
Short/Medium Grain:			
½ cup, 3¼ oz	135	0	30
1 cup (½ Pint), 7.2 oz	270	0.5	59
2 cups (1 Pint), 13 oz	480	1	106
Long Grain: ½ cup, 2¾ oz	105	0	22
1 cup, 5½ oz	205	0.5	44
Glutinous/Sticky, cooked, 1 c., 6 oz	170	0.5	37
Parboiled, cooked, ½ cup, 3 oz	105	0.5	22
Precook./Instant: Dry, ½ cup, 3½ oz	370	0	80
Cooked, ½ cup, 3 oz	90	0	20
Wild Rice: Raw, 1 cup, 5½ oz	570	2	120
Cooked, 1 cup, 5¾ oz	165	0.5	35

Brown Rice

	C	F	Cb
Average of Short or Long Grain			
Raw/Dry: ½ cup, 3¼ oz	340	2.5	71
1 cup, 6½ oz	685	5.5	143
Cooked: ½ cup, 3½ oz	110	1	22
1 cup, 7 oz	220	2	46

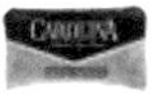

Rice Dishes

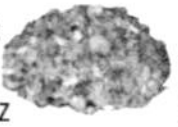

	C	F	Cb
Chinese Fried Rice:			
½ cup, 2½ oz	140	4.5	21
1 cup, (½ Pint), 5 oz	280	9	42
2 cups, (1 Pint), 10 oz	565	18	84
Mexican Rice: 1 cup	500	12	90
Taco John's, 1 serving (6 oz)	250	5	45
Taco Time, 1 serving (4 oz)	160	2	30
Rice-A-Roni: *See Page 116*			
Rice with Raisins/Pinenuts, 1 cup	400	11	60
Rice Pilaf: Restaurant, 1 cup	275	7.5	46
O'Charley's, 1 order	190	5	30
Rice Pudding *(Kozy Shack),*			
Original, ½ cup	130	3	22
Risotto, 1 cup	420	12	70
Saffron Rice, 4 oz	175	7	25
Spanish Rice: 1 cup	390	9	72
El Pollo Loco, small, 5 oz	160	1	35
Taco Cabana, 4 oz	180	5	30
Sticky Rice, 5 oz	155	0.5	34
Sushi Rice: 1 Tbsp	25	0	5
1 cup, 5.2 oz	390	0	77

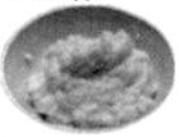

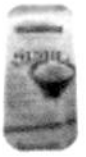

Other Packaged Rice Products:

Rice-A-Roni: See Page 116
Uncle Ben's / Zatarain's: See Page 118

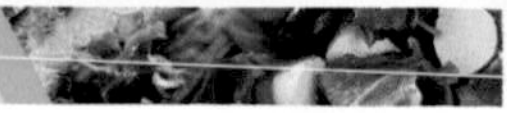

Deli Salads

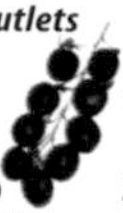
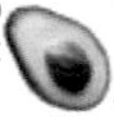
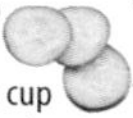
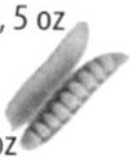
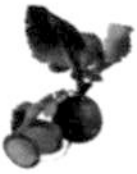
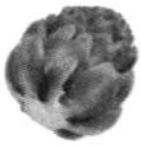

	C	F	Cb
General Average, All Outlets			
Antipasto Salad, ½ cup	135	8	13
3-Bean Salad, ½ cup	110	4	17
Bulgur Salad, ½ cup	70	2	12
Caesar Salad, Classic, 1 cup	200	14	15
Side Salad, without Dressing	25	0	6
Carrot Raisin: Without Dressing, ½ cup	20	0	5
With Dressing, ½ cup	135	12	6
Chef's Salad: Regular, without Dress.	620	37	8
With 2 oz 1000 Island	860	61	8
Chicken Salad, ½ cup/scoop, 4 oz	280	21	2
Coleslaw: Traditional, ½ cup	150	8	18
With Low Cal Dressing, ½ c	50	2	8
Corn, Mexican, ½ cup	240	12	33
Cucumber: Non-Oil Dressing, ½ cup	60	0	14
With Oil Dressing, ½ cup	140	12	8
Eggplant Salad, ½ cup	75	5	7
Fettucini with veges, ½ cup	135	6	16
Garden Salad, without Dressing, 1 cup	10	0	2
Greek Salad, 1 cup	105	8	7
Greek Vegetables, 1 cup	110	8	6
Lettuce, hearts, ½ head	15	0	2.5
Lobster Salad, ½ cup, 4 oz	250	21	11
Macaroni Salad, ½ cup, 5 oz	360	26	26
Nicoise, 1 cup	450	32	18
Pasta Salad, ½ cup	200	11	19
Potato Salad: Dijon, 3 oz	120	7	13
With Mayonnaise, ½ cup, 4 oz	215	15	17
Lowfat, ½ cup	110	1.5	21
Rice Salad, ½ cup	150	10	13
Saffron Rice, 4 oz	175	7	25
Spinach Salad, 1 cup	180	13	13
Tabouli, ½ cup	125	7	13
Three Bean Salad, ½ cup	90	4.5	12
Tomato & Mozzarella, ½ cup	180	14	10
Tortellini with Basil Pesto, ½ cup	150	9	15
Waldorf with Mayo, ½ cup	110	7	12
Signature Salads: *Per 6 oz Serving*			
(Supplied to Deli's and Institutions)			
Antipasto Salad, 6 oz	510	50	4
Artichoke Salad, marinated	400	41	8
California Medley	120	7	15
Cheese Agnolotti	250	8	23
Chicken Salad	420	33	11
Crabmeat Flavored	450	38	20

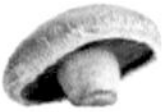
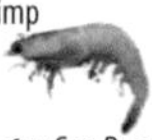

	C	F	Cb
Signature Salads (Cont): *Per 6 oz Serving*			
Egg Salad	300	23	14
Fresh Button Mushroom	190	16	6
Garden Olive	630	67	3
Ham Salad	400	32	14
Prima Pasta Salad	360	30	18
Seafood Pasta Del Mar	170	10	21
Seafood with Crab & Shrimp	420	34	20
Shrimp Salad	360	32	8
Tuna Salad	450	36	14

Fast-Food Restaurants: *See Page 182*

Fresh Salad Packs

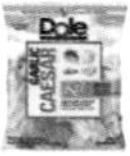

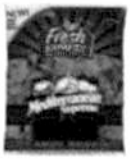

	C	F	Cb
Pre-Packaged (Supermarkets)			
Dole:			
Kits: *Per 3½ oz, Includes Dressing*			
Asian Island Crunch	140	7	17
Caesar	140	11	8
Hearty Italians	180	13	10
Perfect Harvest	160	12	11
Southwest Salad	150	11	10
Salad Blends: *Without Dressing*			
American; Mediterranean, 3 oz	15	0	3
Baby Arugula with Spinach, 3 oz	40	1	8
Fresh Express			
Complete Salad Kits: *Per Serving, Prepared*			
Asian Supreme, ¼ bag	120	5	17
B.L.T. Caesar, ⅓ bag	170	14	8
Caesar: Classic, ⅓ bag	150	13	8
Lite, ⅓ bag	100	7	8
Supreme, ⅓ bag	140	12	7
Mediterranean Supreme, ⅓ bag	150	10	16
Pacifica! Veggie Supreme, ½ bag	220	15	18
Salsa! Ensalada Supreme, ¼ bag	120	8	10

Salad Toppings

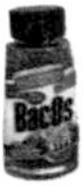

	C	F	Cb
Bacon Bits: Bacos, 1 Tbsp	30	1.5	2
Hormel, 1 Tbsp	25	1.5	0
Chow Mein Noodles, dry, ½ cup	120	7	13
Croutons, 2 Tbsp, 0.3 oz	40	1	7
Olives, 5 medium	25	2	0
Sunflower Seeds, 1 Tbsp, 0.3 oz	45	4	1.5
Toasted sliced Almonds, 2 Tbsp, ½ oz	85	7	3
Tortilla Chips, 12 chips, 1 oz	140	7	19

Updated Nutrition Data ~ www.CalorieKing.com
Persons with Diabetes ~ See Disclaimer (Page 24)

Quick Guide

Salad Dressings

Average All Brands Per 2 Tbsp (Approx 1 fl.oz)	C	F	Cb
Balsamic Vinaigrette: Regular	**90**	**9**	3
Light, 2 Tbsp	**45**	**4**	2
Fat Free, 2 Tbsp	**25**	**0**	6
Blue Cheese: Regular, 2 Tbsp	**150**	**16**	2
Regular, ¼ cup, 2 oz	**300**	**32**	4
Light, 2 Tbsp	**30**	**1**	4
Caesar: Regular, 2 Tbsp	**155**	**17**	1
Regular, ¼ cup, 2 oz	**310**	**34**	2
Light, 2 Tbsp	**70**	**8**	5
Coleslaw: Regular, 2 Tbsp	**125**	**11**	8
Regular, ¼ cup, 2 oz	**245**	**21**	15
Light, 2 Tbsp	**110**	**7**	14
French/Italian: Regular	**150**	**14**	5
Regular, ¼ cup, 2 oz	**290**	**28**	10
Light, 2 Tbsp	**65**	**4**	9
Fat/Oil-Free, 2 Tbsp	**40**	**0**	10
Ranch: Regular, 2 Tbsp	**145**	**16**	2
Regular, ¼ cup, 2 oz	**290**	**31**	4
Light, 2 Tbsp	**80**	**3**	7
Fat-Free, 2 Tbsp	**50**	**0.5**	11
Thousand Island: Regular	**120**	**11**	5
Regular, ¼ cup, 2 oz	**230**	**22**	9
Light, 2 Tbsp	**60**	**4**	7
Fat-Free, 2 Tbsp	**40**	**0.5**	10

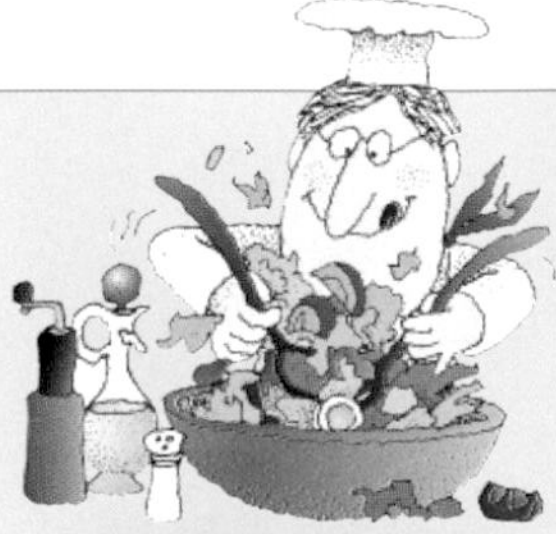

Enjoy a healthy salad but don't drown it in high-fat salad dressings.

Use 'light' dressings to halve the fat and calories.

Brands ~ Salad Dressings

Annie's Naturals: *Per 2 Tbsp*	C	F	Cb
Artichoke Parmesan	**130**	**13**	1
Goddess	**120**	**12**	2
Lemon & Chive	**150**	**16**	1
Shiitake & Sesame	**130**	**14**	1
Tuscany Italian	**80**	**7**	5
Vinaigrette: Balsamic	**110**	**11**	2
Roasted Red Pepper	**70**	**6**	3
Lite, Honey Mustard	**40**	**3**	5
Organic: Buttermilk	**60**	**6**	1
Creamy Asiago Cheese	**80**	**9**	0
Green Goddess	**130**	**13**	2
Thousand Island	**80**	**7**	4
Vinaigrette, Red Wine & Olive Oil	**140**	**15**	0
Bernstein's: *Per 2 Tbsp*			
Creamy Caesar	**120**	**13**	1
Herb Garden French	**130**	**12**	6
Italian	**110**	**12**	1
Restaurant Recipe Italian	**120**	**12**	1
Sweet Herb Italian	**130**	**11**	8
Fat-Free Cheese & Garlic Italian	**10**	**0**	2
Light Fantastic: Cheese Fantastico	**25**	**1.5**	3
Roasted Garlic Balsamic	**45**	**3.5**	3
Best Foods:			
Dijonnaise, 1 tsp	**5**	**0**	1
Mayonnaise: *Per 1 Tbsp*			
Canola	**45**	**4.5**	0
Low-Fat	**15**	**1**	2
Light	**35**	**3.5**	1
Real Mayonnaise	**90**	**10**	0
Tartar Sauce, 2 Tbsp	**80**	**7**	4
Bob's Famous: *Per 2 Tbsp*			
Bleu Cheese	**140**	**15**	1
Lite	**80**	**8**	1
Ranch Country	**150**	**16**	1
Roquefort	**140**	**15**	1
Thousand Island	**90**	**5.5**	4
Bolthouse Farms:			
Creamy Yogurt Dressings: *Per 2 Tbsp*			
Chunky Blue Cheese	**70**	**6.5**	2
Classic Ranch	**80**	**7.5**	3
Thousand Island	**140**	**14**	4
Brianna's: *Per 2 Tbsp*			
Blue Cheese	**120**	**11**	5
Blush Wine Vinaigrette	**120**	**7**	14
Chipotle Cheddar	**110**	**11**	4
French Vinaigrette	**130**	**14**	0
New American	**160**	**17**	6
Rich Santa Fe Blend	**25**	**0**	5
Zesty French	**150**	**15**	4

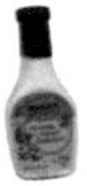
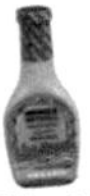
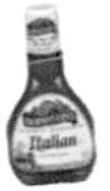
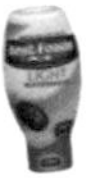
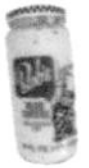
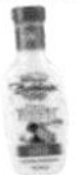
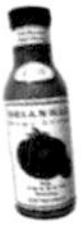

Brands ~ Salad Dressings (Cont)

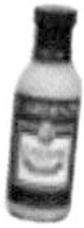
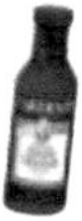
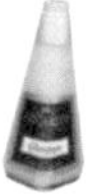
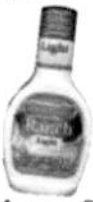
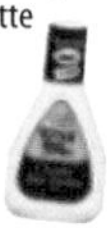

Per 2 Tbsp (Approx 1 fl.oz)	C	F	Cb
Cardini's			
Caesar, 2 Tbsp	160	17	1
Fat-Free Caesar	40	0	9
Light Caesar	80	7	5
Honey Mustard	140	13	5
Italian	100	8	7
Parmesan Ranch	150	16	1
Roasted Asian Sesame	120	10	7
Vinaigrette Dressing:			
Balsamic	100	8	5
Lite: Balsamic	50	3	5
Caesar	80	7	5
Greek	50	4.5	2
El Torito: Cilantro Pepita Caesar	140	14	1
Emeril's: *Per 2 Tbsp*			
House Herb Vinaigrette	100	10	1
Kicked Up French	80	5	8
Girard's: *Per 2 Tbsp*			
Apple Poppyseed	110	9	8
Caesar	140	15	1
Light Caesar	90	8	5
Champagne	150	16	1
Light Champagne	60	5	2
Creamy Balsamic Vinaigrette	100	9	6
Olde Venice Italian	130	13	2
Fat-Free: Balsamic; Red Wine, av.	25	0	6
Caesar	40	0	9
Raspberry	60	0	14
Vinaigrette: Blue Cheese	100	10	3
Hidden Valley: *Per 2 Tbsp*			
Regular Ranch: Italian Ranch	140	14	2
Old-Fashioned Buttermilk Ranch	140	14	2
Bacon Ranch	140	14	1
Cracked Peppercorn Ranch	120	12	2
Cole Slaw	150	15	5
Light, Original Ranch	80	7	3
Fat-Free, Original Ranch	30	0	6
Ken's Steak House Dressings: *Per 2 Tbsp*			
Balsamic & Basil Vinaigrette	110	12	2
Caesar	170	18	1
Chunky Blue Cheese	150	16	1
Country French	150	12	10
Peppercorn Ranch	180	19	1
Ranch	140	15	2
Italian with Aged Romano	120	12	2
Thousand Island	140	13	4
Lite: Caesar; Olive Oil Vinaigrette, av.	65	6	3
Ranch	90	7	5

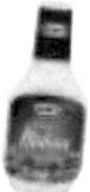
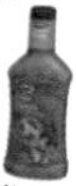
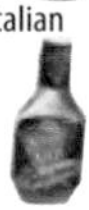
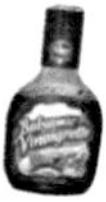
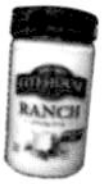

Kraft	C	F	Cb
Regular Dressings: *Per 2 Tbsp*			
Caesar Vinaigrette with Parmesan	70	5	3
Coleslaw Maker	110	9	7
Creamy Italian	100	11	2
Greek Vinaigrette	110	12	2
Honey Dijon	100	9	6
Light Raspb. Vinaigrette	60	4	5
Ranch	120	12	3
Roka Blue Cheese	120	13	1
Sundried Tomato Vinaigrette	60	5	4
Sweet Honey Catalina	130	10	8
Tangy Tomato Bacon	100	6	10
Thousand Island with Bacon	100	8	7
Tuscan House Italian	130	13	3
Kraft Free (Fat-Free): Italian	20	0	4
Classic Caesar	50	0	11
Honey Dijon	50	0	12
Light Done Right!:			
Red Wine Vinaigrette	45	4	3
Seven Seas: Viva Robust Italian	90	9	2
Red Wine Vinegar & Oil	90	9	2
Special Collection:			
Parmesan Romano	140	14	2
Kroger: *Per 2 Tbsp*			
3 Cheese Ranch; Creamy Ranch	130	14	2
Balsamic Vinaigrette	90	9	2
California Honey French	140	12	9
Chunky Bleu Cheese; Creamy Cucumber	150	16	3
Creamy Italian	120	13	3
Peppercorn Ranch	110	12	2
Poppy Seed	160	14	8
Thousand Island	70	5	5
Zesty Italian	90	9	3
Fat-Free: Creamy Ranch	30	0	7
Zesty Italian	20	0	4
Lite: Creamy Caesar	80	8	3
Creamy Ranch	70	6	3
Zesty Italian	35	2	4
Litehouse: Caesar	130	13	2
Chunky Bleu Cheese	150	16	1
Coleslaw	100	8	8
Jalapeno Ranch	120	12	2
Lite Bleu Cheese	70	6	2
Tangy Orange Citrus	50	0	13
Thai Peanut	60	3	6

Updated Nutrition Data ~ www.CalorieKing.com
Persons with Diabetes ~ See Disclaimer (Page 24)

Brands ~ Salad Dressings (Cont)

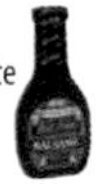

Maple Grove: *Per 2 Tbsp, 1 fl.oz*	C	F	Cb
Regular: Honey Mustard	100	8	8
Sweet-N-Sour	90	6	10
Fat Free: Balsamic Vinaigrette	5	0	1
Caesar	10	0	3
Greek	15	0	3
Honey Dijon; Poppyseed Vin., av.	40	0	10
Average other varieties	25	0	6
Lite: Caesar	60	4.5	4
Honey Mustard	70	4	8

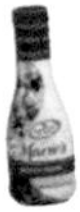

Marie's: *Per 2 Tbsp*	C	F	Cb
Caesar	170	19	1
Chunky Blue Cheese	160	17	0
Creamy Ranch	170	19	1
Honey Dijon	130	12	5
Poppy Seed	150	13	8
Sesame Ginger	100	8	7
Thousand Island	150	15	4
Premium, Spinach Salad	70	1.5	13

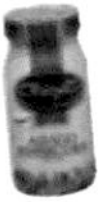

Marzetti's	C	F	Cb
Asiago Peppercorn	160	16	1
Asian Ginger	120	12	4
Bistro Blue Cheese	180	19	1
Chunky Blue Cheese	150	15	1
Honey Balsamic	120	11	4
Original Slaw	160	15	6
Ranch	160	17	1

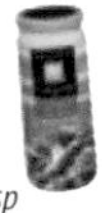

Nasoya: *Per 2 Tbsp*	C	F	Cb
Vegi-Dressing (Tofu Base/Dairy Free):			
Thousand Island	60	5	2
Other flavors	60	7	1
Nayonaise: Original	70	7	2
Fat-Free	20	0	4

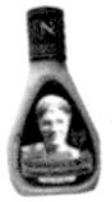

Newman's Own: *Per 2 Tbsp*	C	F	Cb
Balsamic Vinaigrette	90	9	3
Creamy Caesar	170	18	1
Family Recipe Italian	120	13	1
Olive Oil & Vinegar	150	16	1
Parmesan Roasted Garlic	110	11	2
Ranch	150	16	2
Lighten Up: Light Italian	60	6	0
Light Raspberry & Walnut	70	5	7
Light Balsamic Vinaigrette	45	4	2

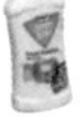

San-J: *Per 2 Tbsp*	C	F	Cb
Tamari Peanut	70	2	9
Tamari Sesame	40	2	5
Fat-Free, Tamari Ginger	25	0	5
Seven Seas:			
Green Goddess	130	13	2
Viva Robust Italian	90	9	2

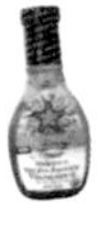

Spectrum: *Per 2 Tbsp*	C	F	Cb
Organic Omega-3:			
Asian Ginger	140	14	3
Creamy Garlic Ranch	120	13	1
Golden Balsamic Vin.	110	11	3
Pomegranate Chipotle	130	13	2
Vegan Caesar	90	9	2

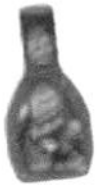

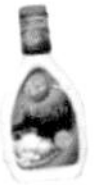

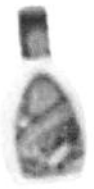

Wishbone	C	F	Cb
Creamy: Chunky Blue Cheese	150	15	2
Creamy Caesar	170	18	1
Creamy Italian	110	10	4
Deluxe French	120	11	5
Garlic Ranch	140	15	2
Ranch	120	13	2
Russian	120	6	14
Sweet 'n Spicy	130	12	6
Thousand Island	130	12	6
Light: Blue Cheese	50	2	6
Creamy Caesar	50	2	7
Country Italian	30	1.5	3
Honey Dijon	50	2	8
Italian	35	2	4
Parmesan Peppercorn Ranch	50	2	7
Ranch	40	2	5
Thousand Island	50	2	9
Fat-Free:			
Chunky Blue Cheese	35	0	7
Italian	20	0	4
Ranch	30	0	7
Oil & Vinegar: Balsamic Vinaigrette	50	5	3
House Italian	100	10	3
Red Wine Vinaigrette	80	5	9
Robusto Italian	80	7	4
Light Vinaigrette: Balsamic & Basil	60	5	3
Asian with Sesame & Ginger	70	5	6
Raspberry Walnut	80	5	7
Salad Spritzers: Average all flavors, 10 sprays (¼ fl.oz) for 1 cup salad	10	1	1

Gravy

	C	F	Cb
Homemade Gravy, average:			
Thin, little fat, 2 Tbsp, 1 oz	20	1	3
Thick, 2 Tbsp, 1¼ oz	50	2	9
¼ cup, 2½ oz	100	4	18
Pillsbury (Gravy Mixes): *Prepared*			
Brown; Homestyle, ¼ cup, 2 oz	15	0	3
Chicken, ¼ cup, 2 oz	20	0	4

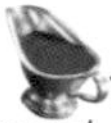

Gravy-In-Jars-Homestyle

	C	F	Cb
Boston Market, ¼ cup, 2 oz	40	2	3
Franco-American (In Jars):			
99% Fat Free, ¼ cup, 2 oz	25	0.5	3
Heinz, Regular, all flavors, ¼ cup, 2 oz	25	0	4
Fat Free Roast Turkey, ¼ cup, 2 oz	20	0	4
Vons, all flavors, ¼ cup, 2 oz	20	0.5	4

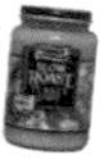

Tomato Products

	C	F	Cb
Whole/Chopped/Crushed/Diced			
1 cup, 8½ oz	50	0	10
In Aspic, ½ cup	50	0	12
With Green Chili, 1 cup, 8½ oz	60	0	16
Stewed, ½ cup, 1.7 oz	40	1.5	6.5
Wedges in Tomato Juice, 1 cup	70	0.5	18
Salsa, average, 1 Tbsp	15	0	3.5
Tomato Ketchup:			
Regular: 1 Tbsp, ½ oz	15	0	4
Single Serve, 1 packet	10	0	3
One-Carb *(Heinz)*, 1 Tbsp, ½ oz	5	0	1
Tomato Paste, 2 Tbsp, 1 oz	25	0	6
Regular, ¾ cup, 6 oz	140	1	32
Tomato Puree, ½ cup, 4½ oz	50	0	10
Tomato Sauce:			
Regular, ½ cup, 4.4 oz	50	0	11
Spanish Style, ½ cup, 4.3 oz	40	0	9
With Mushr., ½ cup, 4.3 oz	45	0	10
With Onions, ½ cup, 4.3 oz	50	0	12
Tomato Seasoning, 3 tsp	20	0	4
Sundried Tomatoes:			
Natural, 5-6 pieces, 0.4 oz	22	0	5
In Oil, drained, 6 pieces, ½ oz	40	2.5	4

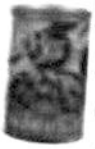

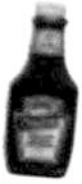

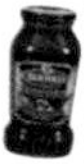

Sauces ~ Brands

	C	F	Cb
A-1			
Steak & Marinades Sauce: *Per Tablespoon (½ oz)*			
Bold & Spicy; Teriyaki; New York	20	0	5
Carb Well Steak Sauce	5	0	1
Chicago	20	1	3
Jamaican Jerk	25	0.5	5
New Orleans Cajun	25	0	5
Steak Sauce	15	0	3
Barilla: *Per ½ Cup*			
Green & Black Olives	80	3	10
Roasted Garlic	60	1	12
Average other varieties	70	2.5	12
Bertolli: *Per ½ Cup*			
Italian Sausage	100	3	15
Olive Oil & Garlic	90	3	14
Marinara; Roast Pepper, av.	80	2	13
Portobello with Merlot	80	2.5	12
Tomato & Basil	80	2	13
Vineyard Selection, Marinara	80	2	14
Best Foods/Hellmann's: *Per 2 Tbsp*			
Tartar Sauce	80	7	4
Buitoni			
Pasta Sauces: *Per ½ Cup Serving, 4½ oz*			
Alfredo	130	11	4
Light Alfredo	90	6	5
Marinara	70	3	10
With Roasted Garlic	60	1.5	10
Pesto: With Basil	300	28	6
Reduced Fat	240	14	9
Tomato Herb Parmesan	130	8	10
Vodka	100	7	7
Bull's Eye: *Per 2 Tbsp*			
Original BBQ Sauce	50	0	13
Sweet & Tangy	60	0	13
Catelli			
Garden Select Pizza Sauce, av., 1 fl.oz	65	0.5	1
Meat Sauce, ½ cup, 4 oz	85	2.5	11
Garden Select 6 Vege Recipe Sauce: *Per ½ Cup*			
Parmesan & Romano	80	2.5	12
Thick & Chunky, Diced Tomato & Basil	70	1.5	12
Other varieties, average	80	1.5	13

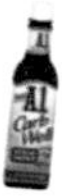

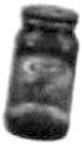

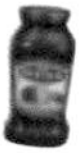

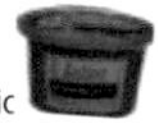

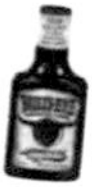

Updated Nutrition Data ~ www.CalorieKing.com
Persons with Diabetes ~ See Disclaimer (Page 24)

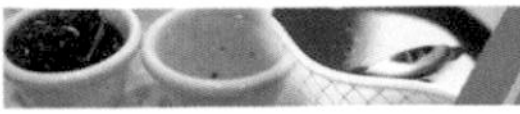

Sauces (Cont)

	C	F	Cb
Cento: *Per ½ Cup*			
Sauces: Passata Tomatoes	30	0	5
All Natural: Pasta	50	3	3
Pizza	40	1.5	6
Tomato: Arrabbiata	140	9	12
Marinara	120	9	9
Puttanesca	140	9	12
White Clam	170	15	4
Classico: *Per ½ Cup Unless Indicated*			
Organic Spinach & Garlic	70	2	11
Rsted Red Pepper Alfredo, ¼ cup	60	5	3
Spicy Tomato & Basil	90	3.5	12
Signature Recipes Sauce:			
Basil Pesto, ¼ cup	230	21	6
Cabernet Marinara with Herbs	70	2	11
Caramelized Onion & Roasted Garlic	85	3	13
Creamy Alfredo, ¼ cup	100	9	3
Fire Roasted Tomato & Garlic	50	1	8
Florentine Spinach & Cheese	80	4	9
Mushrooms & Ripe Olives	60	2	10
Spicy Red Pepper	60	2.5	8
Spicy Tomato & Pesto	90	5	10
Sun-Dried Tomato	80	4	11
Traditional Favorites Sauce: *Per ½ Cup*			
Four Cheese	80	3	12
Italian Sausage with Peppers & Onions	80	3	10
Roasted Garlic	50	1	9
Colgin, Liquid Smoke	0	0	0
Contadina: *Per ¼ Cup*			
Pizza Sauce: Flavored w/ Pepperoni	35	1	5
Original; Four Cheese, average	30	0.5	6
Cooking Sauce: Sweet & Sour, 1 Tbsp	40	1	8
Tomato Sauce, average, ¼ cup	20	0	4
Crosse & Blackwell: *Per 1 Tbsp*			
Ham Glaze	25	0	7
Mint Sauce	5	0	1
Del Monte			
Spaghetti Sauces: *Per ½ Cup*			
with Four Cheeses	70	1.5	15
with Meat/Mushrooms, av.	60	1	14
Other varieties, average	75	1	16
Chunky Sauce: Garlic & Herb	60	1.5	11
Italian Herb	60	1	12
Sloppy Joe Sauce, Original, ¼ cup	50	0	11

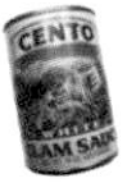
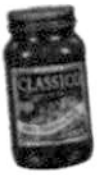
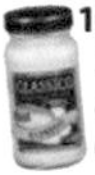
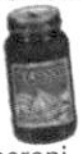
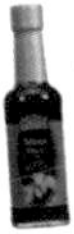
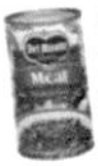

Sauces (Cont)

	C	F	Cb
Emiril's			
Pasta Sauces: *Per ½ Cup*			
Homestyle Marinara	90	3	14
Kicked Up Tomato	80	3.5	11
Puttanesca	80	5	9
Roasted Gaaahlic	80	3.5	12
Roasted Red Pepper	70	3.5	9
Vodka Sauce	110	7	12
Francesco Rinaldi: *Per ½ Cup*			
Traditional: Original	80	3.5	12
Meat/Mushroom	80	3	12
Average other varieties	70	2.5	12
French's			
Worcestershire Sauce, 1 tsp	60	0	1
Heinz: *Per 1 Tbsp, Approx. ½ oz*			
57	20	0	4
Barbecue Sauces, all flavors	35	0	9
Chili Sauce	20	0	5
Horseradish Sauce	75	6	2
Tomato Ketchup: Regular	15	0	4
Reduced Sugar	5	0	1
Worcestershire Sauce, 1 Tbsp	10	0	1
Original Cocktail Sauce, ¼ cup, 2.2 oz	60	0	15
House of Tsang: *Per 1 Tbsp (Approx. ½ oz)*			
Bangkok Peanut	45	2.5	4
Classic Stir Fry	25	1	4
Ginger Soy	20	0	4
General Tsao	45	0.5	10
Hibachi Grill: Kobe Steak	50	4	3
Hunan Smokehut	40	1	8
Sweet Ginger Sesame	40	1	8
Thai Peanut	50	3	5
Tokyo Teriyaki	40	0	10
Hoisin, 1 tsp	15	0	4
Imperial Citrus Stir-Fry	25	0	5
Korean Teriyaki Stir-Fry	35	1.5	5
Mandarin Marinade	25	0	6
Oyster	30	0	7
Saigon Sizzle Stir-Fry	45	2	7
Spicy Brown Bean	15	0	3
Sweet & Sour Stir-Fry	35	0	9
Szechuan Spicy Stir-Fry	25	1	4

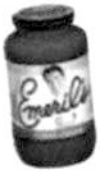
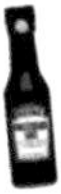
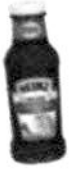
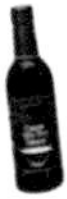

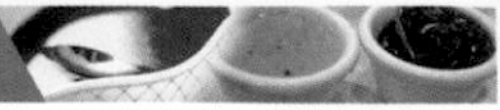

Brands (Cont)

	C	F	Cb
Hunt's			
BBQ Sauce: Original, 2 Tbsp	60	0	15
Hickory & Brown Sugar, 2 Tbsp	70	0	18
Manwich Sloppy Joe Sauce, ¼ cup	40	0	9
Spaghetti Sauce: Per ½ Cup			
Classic Italian: Four Cheese	50	1	10
Garlic & Herb	40	1	8
Zesty & Spicy	60	2	10
Original Style: Traditional	50	1	10
Meat Flavor	60	1	11

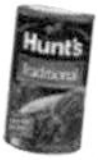

	C	F	Cb
Jack Daniel's			
Original No. 7 BBQ Sauce, 2 Tbsp	50	0	12
Hickory Brown Sugar, 2 Tbsp	50	0	13
Honey Smokehouse, 2 Tbsp	50	0	12
Jim Beam			
Hot Wing Sauce, 2 Tbsp	20	2	0
KC Masterpiece: *Per Tbsp.*			
Marinades: Garlic & Herb	30	1	5
Honey & Teriyaki with Sesame	40	0.5	9
Steakhouse	40	1.5	7

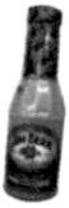

	C	F	Cb
Kikkoman Marinades			
Black Bean Sauce, 2 Tbsp	50	1	6
Hoisin Sauce, 2 Tbsp	80	1.5	17
Honey Mustard, 1Tbsp	30	0	6
Roasted Garlic & Herbs, 1 Tbsp	20	0	4
Teriyaki, 1 Tbsp	15	0	2
Teriyaki Roasted Garlic, 1 Tbsp	25	0	4

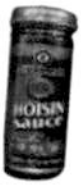

	C	F	Cb
Knorr			
Classic Sauce: *Per 2 Tbsp*			
Bernaise:			
Prepared with Whole Milk	65	5.5	3
Prepared with Non-Fat Milk	60	4.5	3
Hollandaise:			
Prepared with Whole Milk	65	5.5	3
Prepared with Non-Fat Milk	60	4.5	3
Classic Brown Gravy, av., ¼ cup	20	0.5	3

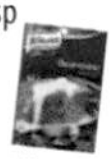

	C	F	Cb
Kraft			
Specialty Sauce: Cocktail, 2 Tbsp	60	0.5	11
Coleslaw Maker, 1 oz	110	9	7
Horseradish, 1 tsp	15	1.5	1
Sandwich Spread, 1 Tbsp	35	2.5	3
Sweet 'n Sour, 2 Tbsp	60	0	13
Tartar: Original, 1 Tbsp	60	4.5	4
Fat-Free, 1 Tbsp	25	0	5
Hot & Spicy, 1 Tbsp	70	6	4
Barbecue Sauces, average, 2 Tbsp	50	0.5	12

	C	F	Cb
Las Palmas			
Red Chile Sauce, ¼ cup, 2 oz	15	0.5	2
Enchilada Sauce: Green Chile	25	1.5	3
Hot Red Original, ¼ cup, 2 oz	15	0.5	2
Lawry's 30 Minute Marinade: *Per Tbsp*			
Caribbean Jerk; Teriyaki, av.	25	0	5
Herb & Garlic	10	0	2
Lemon Pepper	10	0	2
Mesquite	5	0	1
Sesame Ginger	30	0	7
Steak & Chop	5	0	1
Packet Seasonings: *Per 2 teaspoons (Dry)*			
Fajitas; Taco, average	10	0	3
Average other flavors	20	0	4

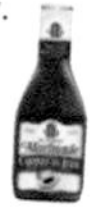

	C	F	Cb
Lea & Perrins			
Worcestershire Sauce: 1 tsp	5	0	1
Thick, 2 Tbsp	30	0	8
Mom's, Garlic & Basil	70	3	7
Monterey			
Pesto Sauce, ¼ cup, 2 oz	300	30	3
Mr Yoshida's			
Original Gourmet Sweet Teriyaki, 2 T.	90	0	20
Hawaiian Sweet & Sour, 2 Tbsp	70	0	18

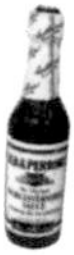

	C	F	Cb
Mrs. Dash Marinades (Salt-Free)			
Garlic Lime, 1 Tbsp	30	1.5	4
Lemon Herb Peppercorn, 1 Tbsp	25	2	2
Southwestern Chipotle, 1 Tbsp	20	1.5	2
Spicy Teriyaki, 1 Tbsp	25	1	5
Muir Glen: *Per ½ Cup*			
Organic Pasta Sauce:			
Portobello Mushroom	50	0	10
Other varieties, average	50	1	11

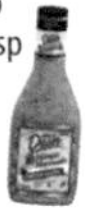

	C	F	Cb
Newman's Own: *Per ½ Cup*			
Bombolina (Tomato & Basil)	90	4.5	13
Five Cheese	80	3	10
Fra Diavolo	70	3	10
Marinara; Sockarooni	70	2	12
Roasted Garlic & Peppers	70	2.5	11
Vodka	110	5	11
O Organics			
Mild Salsa, 2 Tbsp	15	0	2

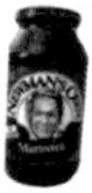

	C	F	Cb
Old El Paso			
Enchilada Sauce:			
Green Chile, ¼ cup	25	1.5	4
Other varieties, ¼ cup	25	1	3
Sauce Mixes, 2 tsp	10	0	2
Picante Sauce, 2 Tbsp	10	0	2
Taco Sauce, 1 Tbsp	5	0	1

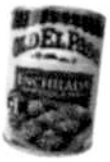

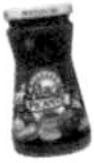
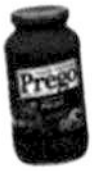
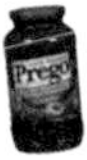
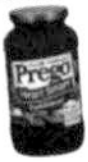
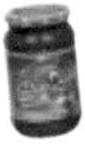
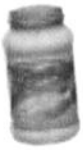
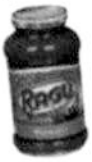

Brands (Cont)	C	F	Cb
Old El Paso (Cont)			
Salsas, Thick & Chunky:			
Medium, 2 Tbsp	10	0	2
Mild, 2 Tbsp	10	0	2
Pace: *Per 2 Tbsp*			
Chunky Salsa	10	0	2
Picante Sauce	10	0	2
Mexican Four Cheese, Salsa Con Queso	90	7	5
Prego: *Per ½ Cup*			
Classic Italian Sauce: Marinara	80	3	10
Flavored with Meat	80	2.5	13
Fresh Mushroom	70	1.5	13
Italian Sausage & Garlic	90	3	13
Mini Meatball	100	3	13
Mushroom & Garlic	80	2.5	13
Roasted Garlic Parmesan	70	1	13
Three Cheese; Tom. Basil & Garlic, av.	80	2	13
Traditional	70	1.5	13
Chunky Garden:			
Combo	70	1.5	13
Mushroom Supreme	90	3	13
Other varieties, average	90	3	13
Heart Smart: Traditional Italian	70	1.5	13
Mushroom Italian	70	1.5	13
Premier Japan			
Hoisin	15	0	3
Tamari; Ginger; Wasabi	5	0	1
Ragu: *Per ½ cup Unless Indicated*			
Pizza Quick Sauce, *Per ¼ Cup*			
Traditional	40	2	6
Pizza Sauce, Homemade Style, ¼ cup	30	1	5
Cheesy: *Per ¼ Cup*			
Classic Alfredo	110	10	2
Light Parmesan	70	5	3
Roasted Garlic Parmesan	110	10	3
Chunky:			
Mushroom & Green Pepper	80	2.5	12
Average other varieties	80	2.5	12
Light varieties, average	50	0	10
Old World Style: Margherita	70	2	10
Meat Flavor	70	3	9
Mushroom; Traditional	70	2.5	10
Organic: Garden Veggie	80	2.5	12
Traditional	80	3	11

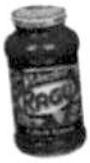
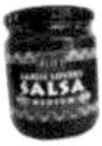
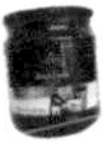

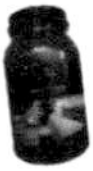
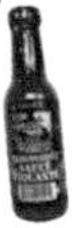
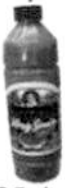
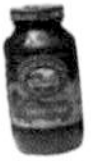

Ragu (Cont): *Per ½ Cup (Unless Indicated)*	C	F	Cb
Robusto!: 7-Herb Tomato	80	3	12
Chopped Tomato, Olive Oil & Garlic	95	5	10
Roasted Garlic	80	2.5	13
Sauteed Onion & Garlic	90	3.5	12
Six Cheese	90	3	12
Safeway Select			
Salsa: *Per 2 Tbsp*			
Chipotle	15	0	3
Garlic Lover's	10	0	3
Peach Pineapple	20	0	4
Salsa Verde	20	0	5
Southwest	10	0	2
Sauces:			
Fiesta Fajita, 2 Tbsp	15	0	2
Enchilada, ¼ cup, 2.2oz	20	0	4
Green Taco; Red Taco, 2 Tbsp	10	0	2
Roasted Tomato, 2 Tbsp	15	0	2
Select Sauces: *Per ½ Cup*			
Arrabbiata	110	8	10
Artichoke Pesto	60	2	9
Four Cheese	70	3	10
Garlic Basil	70	4	6
Marinara	60	2	10
Spicy Red Bell Pepper	50	1	9
Sundried Tomato & Olive	70	0	12
Tomato Alfredo	130	10	9
Vodka	130	10	9
Seeds of Change: *Per ½ Cup*			
Tomato Basil Genovese	60	3.5	9
Marinara di Venezia	60	3.5	6
Vodka Americana	120	10	8
The Wizard's			
Hot Stuff, 1 Teaspoon	0	0	0
Vegetarian Worcestershire, 1 tsp	0	0	1
Tony Roma's			
Wing Sauce, 1 Tbsp	15	1	0
Trader Joe's, BBQ Sauce, Kansas City Style, 2 Tbsp	60	0	15
Walnut Acres: *Per ½ Cup (125g)*			
Marinara & Zinfandel	50	1	9
Tomato & Basil	50	1	9
Low Sodium	40	0	9
Tomato & Mushroom	50	1	9

Home-Popped Popcorn

	C	F	Cb
Popping Corn Kernels:			
2 Tbsp, 1 oz	**110**	1	26
(makes approximately 5 cups)			
Air-popped (without oil), plain, 1 oz	**110**	1	22
1 cup, 0.2 oz	**20**	0	5
Oil-popped, plain, 1 oz	**145**	8	16
1 cup, 0.4 oz	**55**	3	6
Popcorn Oil, 1 Tbsp	**120**	14	0

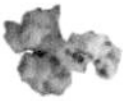

Microwave Popcorn

	C	F	Cb
Average all Brands: *Per 1 Cup Popped, Unless Indicated*			
Butter: Regular	**35**	2	4
Light	**25**	1	4
Act II Popcorn:			
Butter, 0.3 oz	**30**	2	4
5 cups, 1 oz	**160**	10	18
Light Butter, 0.2 oz	**25**	1	4
5 cups, 1 oz	**110**	4.5	19
Butter Lovers,0.3 oz	**35**	2.5	4
4½ cups, 1 oz	**170**	12	16
94% Fat-Free Butter	**30**	1.5	4.5
4½ cups, 1 oz	**130**	2.5	28
American Fare (K-Mart):			
Butter, 0.3 oz	**40**	2	5
3 cups, 1 oz	**120**	2	23
Theater Butter, 1 cup	**40**	2	5
3½ cups	**140**	8	15
Jolly Time:			
America's Best	**20**	0	4
Blast O Butter: Reg.	**45**	3	5
Light	**30**	1.5	4
Healthy Pop: Butter Flavor	**20**	0	4
Caramel Apple	**20**	0	5
Newman's Own: Butter Flavor, 3½ c.	**130**	5	18
Light Butter Flavor, 3½ cups	**140**	4.5	22
Orville Redenbacher's:			
Movie Theater Butter	**35**	2	3
4½ cups, popped	**170**	12	16
Smart Pop!:			
Butter, 6½ cups	**110**	2	24
100 Calorie Mini Bags (1)	**100**	2	24
Tender White	**40**	3	3
Pop Secret:			
1-Step, Cheddar	**40**	2.5	3
100 Calorie Pop, Butter	**15**	0.5	3
Butter	**40**	2.5	3
Extra Butter	**40**	2.5	3
Homestyle	**20**	1	3
Light Butter	**20**	1	3
Movie Theater Butter	**40**	2.5	4
94% Fat-Free: Butter	**20**	0	4
Kettle Corn	**15**	0	4
Smart Balance, Light Butter,1 cup	**25**	1	3

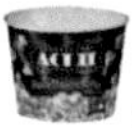

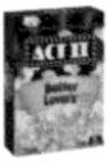

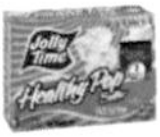

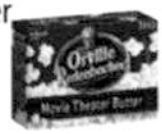

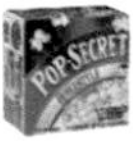

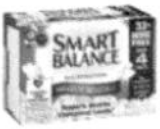

Bagged Popcorn

	C	F	Cb
Average All Brands (Ready-to-Eat)			
Regular/Plain: ½ oz package	**80**	5	8
1 oz package	**160**	10	16
4 oz package	**640**	40	64
2 oz Box (store/airport)	**320**	16	32
3 oz Bag (9" high x 5" wide)	**480**	24	48
Caramel Popcorn,			
without nuts, 1 cup, 2 oz	**240**	4	46

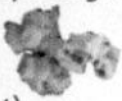

Brands ~ Bagged Popcorn

	C	F	Cb
7-Select (7-11): Popcorn, 1.5 oz pkg	**230**	16	21
Boston's: Lite, 3½ cups, 1 oz	**130**	4.5	20
Homestyle, 2½ cups, 1 oz	**160**	9	18
Cracker Jack: Original,			
½ cup, 1 oz	**120**	2	23
1 cup, 2 oz	**240**	4	46
99-Cents Package, 3⅜ oz	**410**	7	78
Crunch 'N Munch			
Caramel			
⅔ cup, 1 oz	**85**	4	11
1 cup, 2 oz	**170**	8	22
4 oz box	**335**	17	42
7.5 oz box	**630**	32	70
10 oz box	**840**	42	105
Fiddle Faddle:			
Butter Toffee/Caramel			
1 oz	**120**	3.5	22
1 cup, 2 oz	**240**	7	44
8 oz box	**960**	28	176
Jay's: Fat Free Caramel Corn, ¾ cup	**110**	0	26
Korn Krunch: *(Kornfections & Treasures):*			
Almond Pecan (Sugar Free), 1 oz	**150**	8	19
Orville Redenbacher's:			
Popcorn Cakes, Minis, average, (8)	**60**	1	12
Poppycock: Pecan Delight, ½ cup	**150**	8	20
Original Clusters, ½ cup, 1 oz	**160**	8	20

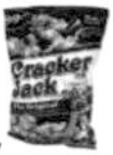

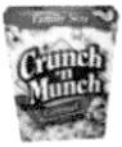

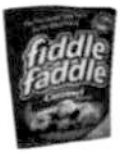

Movie Theater Popcorn

	C	F	Cb
Small (7 cups): Plain	**385**	21	44
With Butter (3 pumps, ¾ oz)	**570**	42	44
Medium (15 cups): Plain	**825**	45	94
With Butter (4 pumps, 1 oz)	**1075**	73	94
Large (20 cups): Plain	**1100**	60	124
With Butter (6 pumps, 1½ oz)	**1485**	102	124
Butter: 1 Pump, ¼ oz	**65**	7	0
4 Pumps (2 Tbsp), 1 oz	**250**	28	0

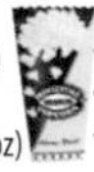

Updated Nutrition Data ~ www.CalorieKing.com
Persons with Diabetes ~ See Disclaimer (Page 24)

Corn & Tortilla Chips

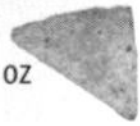

Average All Brands	C	F	Cb
Corn Chips:			
Average all types, 1 oz	**150**	8	18
8 oz bag	**1200**	64	144
Fritos, Original, 32 chips, 1 oz	**160**	10	15
Tortilla Chips: Average, 1 oz	**140**	7	18
(1 oz = approx. 12 chips or 13 strips)			
Doritos: 13 chips, 1 oz	**140**	7	18
White Nacho Cheese, 1 oz	**150**	8	17
Reduced Fat (13), 1 oz	**130**	5	19
Baked! Nacho Cheese (15), 1 oz	**120**	3.5	21
Snyder's, Multigrain, 1 oz	**130**	5	20
Stacy's,			
Simply Naked Pita Chips (14), 1 oz	**130**	5	19
Utz Reduced-Fat Baked,			
10 chips, 1 oz	**140**	7	18
Tostitos:			
Crispy Rounds, 1 oz	**140**	7	19
Multigrain, 1 oz	**140**	7	19

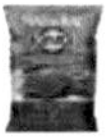

Potato Chips/Crisps

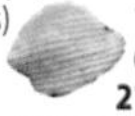

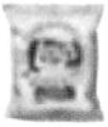

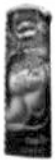

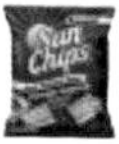

Average All Brands	C	F	Cb
Regular:			
Plain or flavored, (2 chips)	**15**	1	1.5
1 oz package (20 chips)	**150**	10	15
4 oz quantity	**600**	40	60
14 oz package	**2100**	140	210
Brands:			
Lay's Classic, 1 oz	**150**	10	15
Lay's Stax, av. all, 1 oz	**150**	10	15
Pringles: Original (16)	**150**	9	15
Large, 6.41 oz can	**960**	58	96
Minis, 1 bag, 0.8 oz	**140**	9	16
Snack Stack, 0.8 oz tub	**120**	8	12
Extreme, av., (15), 1 oz	**150**	9	15
Ruffles, 12 chips, 1 oz	**160**	10	14
Reduced Fat:			
Pringles, 16 Chips, 1 oz	**140**	7	17
Sun Chips, Original			
16 chips, 1 oz	**140**	6	18
Low-Fat/Baked:			
Lay's Baked!, Original (15), 1 oz	**120**	2	23
Ruffles Baked!: Original (9),1 oz	**120**	3	21
Cheddar Sour Cream (10), 1 oz	**120**	3	22
Baked! Tostitos Scoops (15) 1 oz	**120**	3	22
Fat Free: *Lay's Light*, Original, 1 oz	**75**	0	17
Pringles (Fat-Free) (15). 1 oz	**70**	0	15

Pretzels

Average All Brands	C	F	Cb
Hard-Baked Pretzels: *Each*			
1 oz quantity	**100**	0	22
Sticks, thin, 2¼" (9/oz)	**12**	0	3
Twists, thin, ¼" thick, (5/oz)	**25**	0	5
Dutch (2¾"x 2⅝") ½ oz	**55**	1	11
Sourdough *(Snyder's)*, ¾ oz	**100**	0	22
Soft Pretzels (Twists) average: *Each*			
Plain: Regular, 2.2 oz	**210**	2	43
King Size, 5.1 oz	**485**	4.5	99
New York Street Vendors, 7 oz	**660**	6	135
Big Cheese, 1.76 oz	**130**	3	22
Peanut Butter filled *(Tr. Joe's)* 1 oz	**150**	8	14
Choc-Coated *(Snyders)*, 1 oz	**140**	6	18
White Choc covered, 7 pieces, 1 oz	**140**	6	19

Brands ~ Pretzels

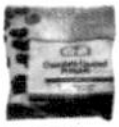

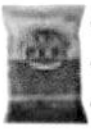

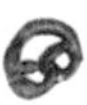

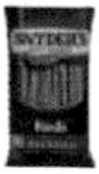

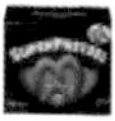

	C	F	Cb
7-Select:			
Choc Covered Pretzels			
10 pieces, 2 oz	**265**	13	35
1 pkg (4 oz), actual weight, 4.75 oz	**630**	30	84
Rold Gold *(Frito-Lay)*			
Braided Twists,			
Honey Wheat (8), 1 oz	**110**	1	23
Classic: Pretzel Sticks, 1 oz	**100**	0	23
Rods; Tiny Twists, 1 oz	**110**	1	23
Fat-Free, Tiny Twists, 1 oz	**100**	0	23
Snyder's of Hanover Pretzels			
100 Calorie Pack, Snaps, 0.9 oz	**100**	0.5	22
Multigrain:			
Pretzel Sticks, 1 oz	**120**	2	23
Pretzel Nibblers,			
Honey Mustard, 1 oz	**130**	3	23
Homestyle (15), 1 oz	**120**	1	25
Mini (20), 1 oz	**110**	0	25
Nibblers, all flavors (16), 1 oz	**130**	3	24
Rods (3), 1 oz	**120**	1	24
Thins, 1 oz	**110**	0	23
SuperPretzel: Soft Pretzels (1)	**160**	1	34
Softstix (2)	**130**	3	22
Soft Pretzel Bites (5)	**150**	0.5	32
Pretzelfils: Pizza (2)	**120**	2	20
Pepperjack; Mozzarella, (2)	**130**	4.5	19
Utz: Pretzels, average, 1 oz	**110**	1	21
Real Choc-covered Pretzels (2)	**120**	8	17

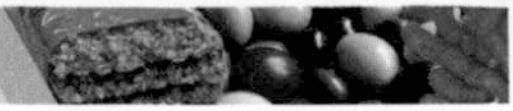

Snacks

Note: Actual weight of packaged snacks is usually 5-10% more than label Net Wt. For accuracy, weigh snack and allow extra calories, fat and carbs for any extra weight.

Snacks	C	F	Cb
Apple Chips *(Seneca)*, 1 oz	150	9	18
Bagel Crisps *(N.Y. Style)* 6 crisps, 1 oz	130	5	17
Banana Chips, ¼ cup, 13 chips, 1 oz	150	7	21
Beef Jerky *(Lance)*, average, 1 oz	70	1	4
Beef Sticks *(Lance)* 1 oz	130	10	4
Bugles, Original, 1⅓ cup, 1 oz	160	9	18
Cheese Balls *(Utz)*, 1 oz package	130	7	16
Cheese Crackers *(Lance)* (6), 1.4 oz	190	9	25
Cheese Curls: 1 cup, 1 oz	150	8	16
Cheese Nips, 1.25 oz package	170	7	22
Cheese Puffs: Average, 1 oz	160	10	15
American Fare, 1½ cup, 1 oz	160	11	13
Snyder's Multigrain, 1 oz	130	6	19
Cheese Twists (Snyders),1 oz	140	8	15
Cheerios, Snack Mix,			
average, ⅔ cup, 1.1 oz	125	3.5	22
Cheetos: Average all flavors, 1 oz	160	10	15
4 oz package	640	40	60
Baked!, 1 oz	130	5	19
Cheez Balls, 27 balls, 1 oz	150	9	11
Cheez-It Crackers:			
Average all flavors, 1 oz	150	7	18
1.25 oz package	190	9	24
3 oz package	420	21	57
Reduced Fat, 1 oz	130	4.5	20
Party Mix, ½ cup, 1 oz	130	4.5	20
Chex *(General Mills)*:			
100 Calorie Pouch, average	100	3	18
Mix: Bold Party Blend, ½ cup, 1 oz	120	4	18
Traditional, ½ cup, 1 oz	120	4	20
Chips Ahoy! Choc Chip Cookies,			
1.4 oz package	190	9	27
Mini: 3 oz package	410	20	57
Go-Pak!, 4 oz cup	550	27	77
Snak-Saks, 8 oz pkg	1100	51	154
Churros *(Mex. Pastry)* 10", 1 oz	100	5	12
Combos *(Oven Baked)*:			
Crackers, ⅓ cup, 1 oz	140	6	18
1 cup, 3 oz	420	18	54
Pretzels, ⅓ cup, 1 oz	130	4.5	19
1 cup, 3 oz	390	14	57
Cookies: *See Pages 83-89*			
Cool Cuts, Carrot & Ranch, 2.3 oz	70	5	5
Corn Chips: *See Page 153*			
Corn Crunchies/Spirals, 1 oz	95	0	22
Corn Nuts: ⅓ cup, 1 oz	130	4.5	20
1.7 oz bag	220	7.5	34
Corn Puffs: *(Pirate's Booty)*, 1 oz	130	5	18
Wotsits *(Walker)*, ¾ oz package	105	6.5	11
Dunkin Stixs *(Hostess)*, 3, 4oz	490	25	63

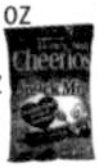

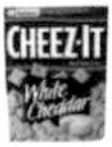

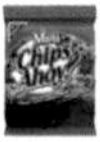

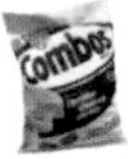

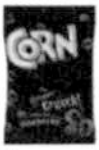

Snacks (Cont)

Snacks (Cont)	C	F	Cb
Fig Newtons: Regular, 2 oz package	200	4	39
Fat-Free, 2.1 oz package	180	0	44
Minis, Fig/Strawb., av., 1.34 oz pkg	130	3	27
Flavor Twists *(Fritos)*, 1 oz	160	10	16
French's Potato Sticks ¾ cup, 1 oz	180	12	16
Funyuns, Onion flavor (13), 1 oz	140	7	18
Genisoy Soy Crisps, average, 1 oz	120	3	17
Garden Harvest Tst'd Chips, av., 1 oz	120	3.5	20
Goldfish *(Pepperidge Farm)* 1 oz	140	5	20
Gold-N-Chees *(Lance)*, 1 oz	150	8	17
Hot Peanuts *(Lays)*, 3½ oz	310	25	10
Jerky (Beef), 1 oz stick	70	1	4
Lance S'wich Crackers, av., 1.4 oz	180	9	23
Munchies Snack Mix *(Frito-Lay)*:			
Cheese Fix, ¾ cup	140	7	18
Flaming; Totally Ranch, ¾ c.	140	6	19
Munchos, 16 pieces, 1 oz	160	10	16
Nibblers: Garlic Bread (13), 1 oz	130	3	24
Fat Free, Sourdough (16), 1 oz	120	0	25
Nutter Butter: Sandwich Cookies			
Singles, 1.9 oz package	250	10	37
Bites: 1.25 oz package	170	7	24
Milk Choc-Covered, 2.54 oz pkg	350	17	48
Onion Rings *(T.G.I. Friday)*, 1 oz	130	6	19
Oreo: 100 Calorie Pack, 0.84 oz	100	3	16
2 Go! (4 cookies), 2 oz	270	11	41
Double Stuf, 1.5 oz package	210	10	30
Mini Bite Size: (9 cookies), 1.25 oz	170	7	25
Go-Pak, 4 oz cup	530	22	81
Snak-Saks, 8 oz package	1040	48	168
Oreo Cakesters, 2 oz pkg	250	12	36
Oriental Mix *(Rice Snacks)*, 1 oz	125	3.5	21
Oyster Crackers *(Sunshine)*, 1 oz	60	1.5	11
Peanut Butter Nuggets (10), 1 oz	140	6	15
Pirate's Booty:			
1 oz bag	130	5	19
4 oz bag	520	20	76
With Caramel, 2.75 oz bag	330	5.5	63
Pirate's Cannon Balls: 1 oz	130	5	18
5 oz bag	715	27	99
Pita Chips, average, (9) 1 oz	130	4	18
Popcorn: *See Page 152*			
Pork Cracklins, 1 oz	180	14	0
Pork Skins/Rinds, 1 oz	160	10	0
Baken-ets, 99c package, 1.87 oz	300	19	0
Potato Chips: *See Page 153*			
Potato Skins *(TGI Friday)* (16), 1 oz	130	9	24
Pretzels *(Snyder's)*,			
Honey Mustard Onion Pieces, 2 oz	280	14	36

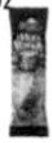

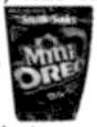

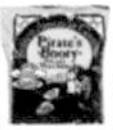

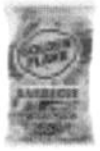

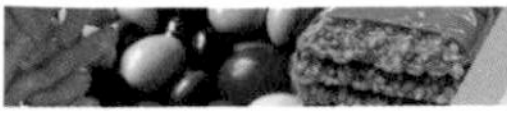

Snacks (Cont)

	C	F	Cb
Quakes Rice Snacks, average, 1 oz	130	4	26
Quaker Mini Delights, av.,1 bag, 0.7 oz	90	3.5	16
Rice Chips, Bar-B-Q/Onion, 1 oz	140	7	18
Ritz Bits S'wiches:			
Cheese: 1.5 oz package	220	13	24
Carry Me Pack, 2 oz	290	17	33
Go-Pak, 1 oz	150	9	17
P'nut Butter: 1.25 oz package	170	10	20
Big Bag (99cents), 3 oz	420	23	48
Sandwich Crackers *(Austin): Per Pkg*			
Cheese Cracker w/ Cheddar, 1.38 oz	190	10	23
Cheese Cracker w/ Pnut Butter, 1.3 oz	190	10	23
PB & J Flavored, 1.38 oz	190	8	26
Sesame Sticks *(Cityfarm)*, 1 oz	160	9	13
Smart Puffs *(Pirates Booty)*, 1.37 oz	180	8	23
Snack Mix *(Quaker)*:			
Baked Cheddar, 1 oz	130	4.5	19
Kids Mix, 1 oz	130	4.5	20
Snackwells Cookies, Pack 2 Go!, 1.7oz	210	5	38
Soy Crisps, average,1 oz	120	3	17
Soy Nuts: Dry Roasted, ¼ cup, 1 oz	130	6	9
Choc-coated, 1 oz	140	7	13
Sunflower Chips: *(Snyders)*			
100 Calorie Snack Pack (1)	100	4.5	14
Multigrain, all flavors, 1 oz	140	6	20
Takis Fajitas (12), 1 oz	140	7	17
4 oz package	560	28	68
TastyKake:			
Koffee Kake Jr., 2½ oz	280	10	45
Chocolate Jr., 3.3 oz	340	12	65
Creme Filled Koffee Kakes (2)	230	10	25
Tings *(Robert's)*, 2 oz bag	300	14	36
Toasted Cheese Crackers, 1 package	220	11	23
Tortilla Chips: *Page 153*			
Tostitos:			
Blue; Yellow; Scoops, average, 1 oz	140	7	19
Multigrain, 1 oz	150	8	18
Trader Joe's, Cheese Crunchies, 1 oz	130	6	19
7 oz package	910	42	133
Trail Mix (Nuts/Seeds/Dried Fruit):			
Regular, 3 Tbsp, 1 oz	140	9	13
Tropical, 3 Tbsp, 1 oz	130	7	16
with Chocolate Chips, 1 oz	180	12	16
Turkey Jerky: Teriyaki *(Oberto)*, 1 oz	70	1	8
BBQ Beef; Hot & Spicy, average, 1 oz	90	1	6
Veggie Crisps, *(Snyder's)*, 1 oz	140	7	20
Wasabi Peas, ¼ cup, 1 oz	120	3	19
Yogurt Pretzels (7), 1.5 oz	190	7	30
Yogurt Raisins *(Sun-Maid)*, 1 oz	120	4.5	20

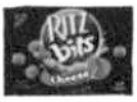

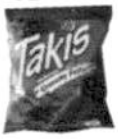

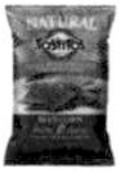

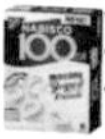

Fruit Snacks

	C	F	Cb
Betty Crocker: Fruit Gushers, 0.9 oz	90	1	20
Fruit by the Foot, 1 roll, 0.75 oz	80	1	17
Fruit Roll Ups: 1 roll, ½ oz	50	1	12
Scooby Doo; G-Force, 0.9 oz	90	0	21
General Mills:			
Dora the Explora , 0.9 oz	90	0	21
Other varieties	90	0	21
Kellogg's: Disney Fruit Snacks, 0.9 oz	80	0	19
Fruit Streamers, 1 Roll	80	1	17
Rolls,1 pouch, 0.63 oz	70	1.5	14
Yogos Bits, av., 0.7 oz	80	1.5	16
Sunkist: Fruit Snacks, 1 pouch	90	0	21
Fruit Smoothie Blitz, 1.3 oz	140	1	32

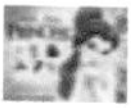

Vending Machines

	C	F	Cb
Cheese Balls *(Utz)*, 1 oz	130	7	16
Chips Ahoy, Choc Chip Cookies 1.4 oz	190	9	27
Choc Milk, 8 fl.oz	260	9	36
Coca-Cola Classic, 12 fl.oz	145	0	40
Diet Coke, 12 fl.oz	0	0	0
Corn Chips, 1 oz	160	10	16
Hostess Sweet Roll, 4¼ oz	400	12	69
Donut, plain, 1.4 oz	160	9	18
Fruit Pie *(Hostess)*, 4½ oz	480	20	68
Granola/Cereal Bars	140	3	26
***Hershey's,* 1.55 oz bar**	210	13	26
Hot Fries *(Andy Capp)*, 1 oz	150	7	17
Rice Krispies Treat	90	2.5	17
Lance Captain's Wafers, 1 package	200	9	27
M & M's: Milk Chocolate, 1.7 oz	240	10	34
Peanuts, 1.7 oz	250	13	30
Milk: Whole, 8 fl.oz	160	9	13
Reduced Fat, 2%, 8 fl.oz	140	5	14
Milky Way, 2 oz	260	10	41
Orange Juice, 8 fl.oz	190	14	6
Popcorn, plain, 1 oz	160	10	16
Pork Skins, 1 oz	160	10	0
Potato Chips: 1 oz	150	10	15
Reduced Fat, 1 oz	120	3	21
Pretzels, 1 oz	110	1	23
Raisins, ½ oz package	45	0	11
Reese's Peanut Butter Cups, 1½ oz	230	13	23
Snickers, 2.1 oz bar	280	14	35
Tortilla Chips, 1 oz	140	7	18

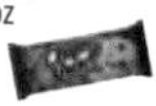

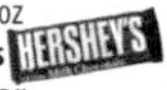

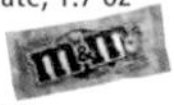

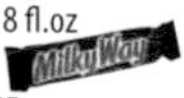

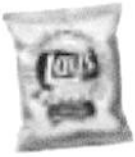

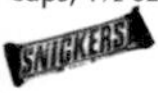

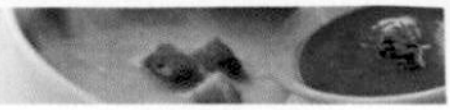

Homemade & Restaurant

Restaurant & Take-Out
Average All Preparations, Per 8 fl.oz

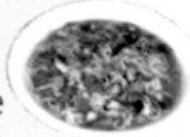
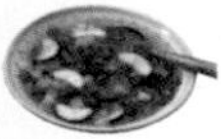
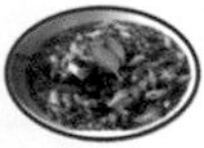
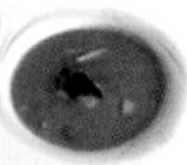

	C	F	Cb
Bean Medley	**200**	3	34
Beef Consomme	**30**	0	2
Borscht (with Sour Cream)	**130**	8	14
Bouillabaisse	**400**	15	10
Chicken & Corn	**290**	14	20
Chicken & Wild Rice	**80**	4	9
Chicken Consomme	**50**	0	2
Chicken Curry	**180**	8	18
Chicken Jambalaya	**160**	7	8
Chicken Noodle	**80**	2	12
with Chicken	**160**	4	12
Chicken Soup	**80**	2	6
Chili with Beans	**250**	12	25
Clam Chowder	**240**	15	17
Corn & Crab	**120**	3	18
Corn Chowder	**150**	8	16
Cream of Broccoli	**200**	12	20
Cream of Potato	**150**	6.5	17
Cream of Mushroom	**200**	13	15
Fish Chowder	**220**	15	6
French Onion	**420**	15	25
Gazpacho	**50**	0	5
Lentil Soup	**250**	9	28
Lobster Bisque	**320**	15	10
Matzo Ball (with 1 large ball)	**180**	7	24
Minestrone	**125**	2.5	20
Mulligatawny	**300**	15	8
Pea & Ham	**240**	10	25
Potato & Bacon	**170**	7	19
Pumpkin, Creamy	**210**	10	26
Shark Fin Soup	**100**	4	8
Spicy Shrimp Soup, 1 bowl	**160**	7	10
Split Pea Soup	**180**	2.5	30
Vegetable (Fat Free)	**75**	0	18
Vegetable Beef	**80**	2	10
Vichyssoise	**200**	9	15
Watercress	**90**	4	13

Other Soups: *See International & Fast-Foods Sections (Arby's, Au Bon Pain, Boston Market, Dunkin' Donuts, Denny's, Schlotzsky's, Sizzler, Souplantation, Sweet Tomatoes, Zoup!)*

Homemade Soups: Calculate calories, fat and carbohydrates from recipe ingredients.

Bouillon Cubes & Powders

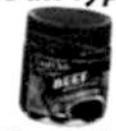

	C	F	Cb
Bouillon Cubes: ***Average all Types***			
Regular, 1 cube	**5**	0	1
Low Sodium (LiteLine)	**12**	0	1
Powders: Average, 1 tsp	**10**	0	1
Herb-Ox: Instant Broth & Seasoning,			
Beef, 1 envelope	**5**	0	1
Chicken; Vegetarian	**5**	0	1
Herbs, Spices: 1 tsp	**5**	0	1
Soup Oyster Crackers:			
10 small, 1 oz	**130**	3.5	21
4 large, ½ oz	**170**	4.5	28

Amy's (Organic)

Per ½ Can, 1 Cup, Unless Indicated

	C	F	Cb
Alphabet, Fat-Free	**80**	0	16
Black Bean Vegetable	**140**	1.5	26
Chunky Vegetable	**60**	0	13
Cream of Mushroom, ¾ cup	**150**	9	13
Cream of Tomato	**100**	2	17
Curried Lentil	**230**	8	30
Fire Roasted Southwestern Vegetable	**140**	4	21
Lentil Vegetable	**150**	4	23
Minestrone	**90**	1.5	17
No Chicken Noodle	**100**	3	13
Pasta & 3 Bean	**150**	4	22
Roasted Southwestern Vegetable	**140**	4	21
Spanish Rice	**140**	2.5	24
Split Pea	**100**	0	19
Summer Corn & Vegetable	**150**	6	23
Thai Coconut	**140**	10	9
Tuscan Bean & Rice	**160**	4.5	25
Vegetable Barley	**70**	1	13

'Light in Sodium' Range *(50% less sodium),* (Calories/Fat/Carb ~ Same as Regular Range)

Andersen's

~ Per Cup

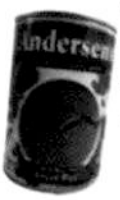

	C	F	Cb
Lentil	**110**	2	19
Split Pea	**130**	0	24
Split Pea with Bacon	**140**	1	23
Tomato	**130**	3.5	22

Baxters

Per ½ Can

	C	F	Cb
Luxury: Cream of Asparagus	**120**	6.5	13
Lobster Bisque	**140**	9	10
Mushroom Pottage	**165**	10	14
Slow Cooked Oxtail with Red Wine	**120**	4.5	14

Updated Nutrition Data ~ www.CalorieKing.com
Persons with Diabetes ~ See Disclaimer (Page 24)

Bear Creek

Per Cup (Prepared)

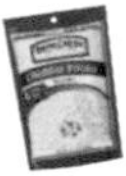

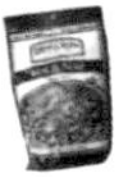

	C	F	Cb
Cheddar Potato	180	7	28
Chicken Noodle	120	1.5	22
Creamy Potato	150	3.5	27
Hot & Sour	80	1	16
Minestrone	110	0	23
Navy Bean	130	0.5	26
Split Pea	110	2	19
Tortilla	90	0.5	22
Vegetable Beef	110	0.5	22

Campbell's

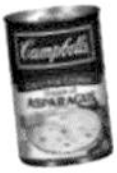

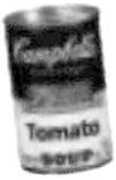

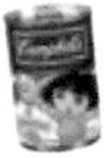

	C	F	Cb
Condensed Soup: *Per ½ Cup*			
Bean w. Bacon	160	3	25
Beef w/ Vegs & Barley; Minestrone, av.	90	1.5	15
Cheddar Cheese	100	5	11
Chicken & Dumplings	70	2.5	10
Chicken Won Ton	60	1	8
Cream of Asparagus	110	7	9
Cream of Broccoli	90	3.5	12
Cream of Chicken & Mushroom	80	6	7
Cream of Mushroom	70	2	10
Cream of Onion	100	6	10
Cream of Potato	90	2	15
Cream of Shrimp	100	6	8
Creamy Chicken Noodle	120	7	11
French Onion	45	1.5	6
Green Pea	180	3	28
Manhattan Clam Chowder	60	0.5	12
New England Clam Chowder	90	2.5	13
Old Fashioned Vegetable	80	1.5	14
Split Pea with Ham & Bacon	180	3.5	27
Tomato	90	0	20
Tomato Bisque	130	3.5	23
Vegetable	100	0.5	20
Healthy Request Condensed: *Per ½ Cup*			
Chicken Rice	70	1.5	13
Vegetable Beef	90	1	15
Kids Condensed Soup: *Per ½ Cup*			
Dora; Jimmy Neutron	80	2	13
Chicken Alphabet; Chicken & Stars	70	2.5	12
Chicken Noodle O's	90	2.5	15
Curly Noodle	80	2	11
Goldfish Pasta	80	2	12
Goldfish Pasta & Meatballs	90	3	11

Campbell's (Cont)

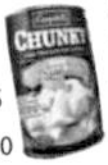

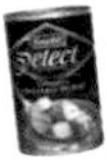

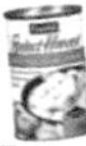

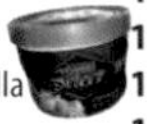

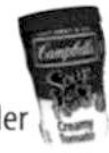

	C	F	Cb
Chunky: *Per 8 fl.oz Cup*			
Baked Potato with Cheddar & Bacon Bits	160	6	23
Chicken Corn Chowder	200	10	20
Classic Chicken Noodle	120	3	14
Fajita Chkn with Rice & Beans	130	1.5	23
Gr. Chicken & Sausage Gumbo	140	3	21
Select Harvest: *Per 8 fl.oz Cup*			
Beef w. Roasted Barley	130	1	21
Carmelized French Onion	80	2	12
Chicken Vegetable Medley	120	1	20
Chicken w. Egg Noodles	100	3	11
Creamy Chicken Alfredo	220	13	15
Creamy Potato with Rstd Garlic	180	10	20
Harvest Tomato with Basil	100	0	22
Italian Sausage w/ Pasta & Pepperoni	160	7	18
Italian-Style Wedding	130	5	13
New England Clam Chowder	170	10	15
Potato Broccoli Cheese	150	9	15
Savory Chicken & Rice	110	0.5	20
Savory Bean with Roasted Ham	170	1.5	30
Slow Roasted Beef & Vegetable	100	0.5	16
Split Pea with Roasted Ham	150	1	29
Tomato Garden; Vegetable Medley	100	0.5	20
Select Harvest Bowls: *Per Cup*			
Chicken with Egg Noodles	120	4	12
Italian-Style Wedding	130	4	16
Mexican-Style Chkn Tortilla	130	2.5	19
Minestrone	100	1	19
Savory Chicken & Rice	110	0.5	20
98% Fat-Free, New Eng. Clam Chowder	110	2.5	17
Microwavable Bowls: *Per Cup*			
Chicken Noodle Soup	70	2	10
Creamy Tomato Soup	160	5	25
Tomato Soup	110	0	24
Soup at Hand: *Per Container*			
Chicken with Mini Noodles	80	2	11
Cream of Broccoli	150	7	17
Creamy Tomato	180	4	32
New England Clam Chowder	160	10	13
Vegetable Beef	70	1	11

Dr McDougall's

	C	F	Cb
Big Cup Soups/Meals: *Per Cup*			
Black Bean & Lime	340	2	60
Hot & Sour Noodle	320	1	34
Minestrone & Pasta	200	1	40
Miso Soup with Noodles	180	1	34
Pad Thai Noodle, average	200	1	42
Ramen Chicken Flavor	200	1	40
Split Pea with Barley	240	1	42
Tamale Soup with Baked Chips	200	2	36
Tortilla Soup with Baked Chips	200	2	34
Light Sodium: *Per Container*			
Chicken Noodle, Vegan	140	0.5	28
Chinese Chicken Noodle	140	1	28
Lentil Couscous	190	1	37
Split Pea	200	1	35
Tomato, Basil Pasta	100	0.5	21
White Bean & Pasta	170	1	34
Ready To Serve: *Per Cup, 8.6 fl.oz*			
Black Bean	120	1	23
Chunky Tomato	90	0	20
Lentil	115	0.5	21
Minestrone	70	0.5	14
Roasted Pepper Tomato	80	0	19
Split Pea	100	0	19
Vegetable	75	0.5	14

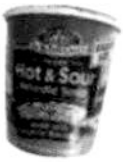

Fantastic Cup Soups

	C	F	Cb
Simmer Soups: *Per Cup, Prepared*			
Blarney Stone Creamy Potato	220	4.5	15
Dutch Split Pea	120	1	21
New England Vege. Chicken Noodle	90	1	14
Vegetarian Soup Cups: *Per Container*			
Baja Black Bean Chipotle	130	0.5	31
Buckaroo Bean Chili	160	2	33
Classic French Onion	90	2.5	15
Creamy Potato Leek	120	2.5	22
Great Lakes Cheddar Broccoli	100	3	15
Green Onion Miso with Tofu	140	1.5	26
Hot & Sour	170	2	33
Mama's Minestrone	160	2.5	30
Sesame Miso	140	2	27
Spicy Thai	150	0.5	32
Split Pea	140	0.5	28
Three Onion Noodle	180	2	36
Vegetarian Chicken Noodle	90	1	17

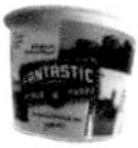

Health Valley

	C	F	Cb
Per Cup, Prepared			
Broths: Chicken: Fat-Free	20	0	0
Low-Fat	35	1.5	0
Vegetable, Fat-Free	20	0	5
Fat-Free Soup:			
Chicken Flavored Noodles with Veggie	110	0	24
Creamy Potato with Broccoli	80	0	17
Lentil with Couscous	130	0	28
Zesty Black Bean with Rice	100	0	22
Low-Sodium: 14 Garden Vegetable	80	0	18
Corn & Vegetable	80	0	20
Lentil & Carrot	110	0	24
Vegetable Barley	80	0	20
No Salt Added: Minestrone	70	0	17
Split Pea	110	0	23
Tomato	80	0	18
Vegetable	90	2	16

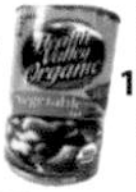

Healthy Choice

	C	F	Cb
Canned: *Per Cup*			
Bean & Ham	180	2	29
Chicken & Dumplings	140	2.5	21
Chicken with Rice Soup	110	1.5	17
Chicken Tortilla Style	160	2	25
Country Vegetable	110	1	19
Fiesta Chicken	120	2	20
Garden Vegetable	120	0.5	24
Hearty Chicken	130	2	20
New England Clam Chowder	110	1	19
Old Fashioned Chicken Noodle	100	1.5	13
Microwavable Containers: *Per 14 oz Container*			
Hearty Vegetable Barley	245	2	53
Tomato & Basil	225	1	49
Traditional Lentil	260	4	47

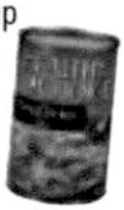

Imagine

	C	F	Cb
Per Cup			
Bistro: Corn Chipotle	100	1	22
Cuban Black Bean	170	3.5	30
Fire Roasted Tomato	120	2.5	24
Canned Organic:			
Chicken Pot Pie	160	4.5	22
Classic Minestrone	120	3.5	20
Country Split Pea	180	2.5	30
Italian White Bean	160	2.5	28
Roasted Garlic Potato	120	3	22
Tortilla	160	4	25

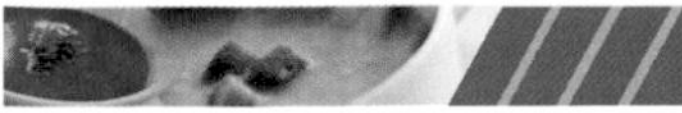

Imagine (Cont)

Per Cup

	C	F	Cb
Garden Natural Soup, Creamy:			
Acorn Squash & Mango	70	1.5	14
Chicken	70	1.5	12
Portobello Mushroom	80	3	10
Potato Leek	110	3	18
Sweet Corn	120	3	20
Sweet Pea	80	1.5	14
Tomato	80	1	15
Tomato Basil	90	1.5	17

Kikkoman

Dry Mixes, Prepared as Directed

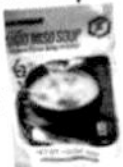

	C	F	Cb
Chinese Style Egg Flower: 1⅓ tsp	40	1	7
Hot & Sour, 1⅓ tsp	30	0	6
Instant Miso:			
Shiro (White): 1 packet	35	1	4
With Tofu, 1 packet	35	1	3

Knorr

	C	F	Cb
Recipe Mix: *Dry Mix*			
Cream of Spinach, 2 Tbsp	60	1.5	11
French Onion, 2 Tbsp	45	1	8
Tomato with Basil, 3 Tbsp, 0.7 oz	70	1	15
Vegetable, 2 Tbsp, 0.3 oz	25	0	6
Bouillon Cubes: *Per ½ Cube, 1 Cup, Prepared*			
Beef; Chicken, average	15	0.5	1

Lipton

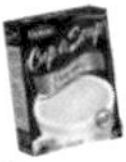

	C	F	Cb
Cup-a-Soup: *Per Envelope*			
Cream of Chicken	70	1.5	14
Chicken Noodle	80	0.5	17
Recipe Secrets: *Per Dry Mix*			
Beefy Onion, 1 Tbsp	25	0.5	5
Onion, 1 Tbsp	20	0	4
Onion Mushroom, 1⅔ Tbsp	25	0	7

Manischewitz

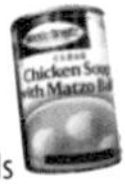

	C	F	Cb
Condensed: *Per ½ Cup*			
Chicken Broth, Clear	15	0	2
Chicken with Kreplach	40	1	6
Chicken with Matzo Balls	80	3.5	9
Quart Jars: *Per 6 fl.oz, Prepared*			
Borscht with Beets	50	0	13
Borscht, Low Calorie	15	0	4
Ready To Serve: Matzo Balls in Broth	220	9	27
Dry Mixes: *Per Cup*			
Matzo Ball & Soup Mix	40	0.5	9
Split Pea Cello	140	0	25
Vegetable Soup	120	0	22

Maruchan

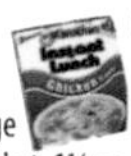

	C	F	Cb
Instant Lunch, Av. all flavors, 1 package	290	12	38
Ramen, all flavors, ½ packet, 1½ oz	190	7	26

Miso Cup

Per Cup, Prepared as Directed

	C	F	Cb
Golden Vegetable; Savoury Seaweed	30	1	3
Savory Seaweed	30	1	3
Traditional with Tofu	35	1	4
Reduced Sodium	25	1	3

Nile Spice ~ *Per Cup*

	C	F	Cb
Black Bean; Lentil	195	1.5	35
Couscous Lentil Curry	200	1	39
Couscous Minestrone	170	1.5	36
Potato Leek	120	3	17
Low-Fat: Split Pea	190	1	33
Chicken Flavored Vegetable	110	2.5	21

Nissin ~ *Per Whole Package*

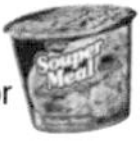

	C	F	Cb
Souper Meal: Per ½ Container			
Chicken	290	13	38
Picante Shrimp	270	11	37
Top Ramen: Beef Flavor	380	14	54
Chicken Flavor	380	14	52

Pacific Foods ~ *Per Cup*

	C	F	Cb
Beef Broth	20	0	1
Chicken Broth	15	0	1
Vegetable Broth	15	0	3
Creamy Organic: French Onion	30	1	5
Butternut Squash	90	2	17
Cashew Carrot Ginger	120	5	19
Curried Red Lentil	140	4.5	19
Tomato	100	2	16
Light Sodium: Roasted Pepper & Tomato	110	2	16
Tomato	100	2	17
Hearty Artisan Soups:			
Chicken Fajita	160	2.5	26
Savory White Beans with Bacon	220	7	27

Pritikin ~ *Per Cup*

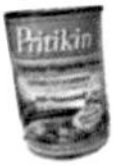

	C	F	Cb
Fat-Free Chicken Broth	5	0	0
Hearty Vegetable	80	0	15
Split Pea	180	0.5	32
Vegetarian Vegetable	80	0	17

Progresso

	C	F	Cb
Microwaveable Bowls: *Per Cup*			
Chicken & Wild Rice	100	1.5	16
Minestrone Soup	90	1.5	17
Vegetable Soup	80	0.5	15
Rich & Hearty: *Per Cup*			
Chicken & Homestyle Noodles	110	2.5	14
Chicken Corn Chowder	200	9	23
Chicken Pot Pie Style	140	4	19
New England Clam Chowder	180	8	22
Savory Beef Barley Vegetable	130	2.5	17
Slow Cooked Vegetable Beef	140	2	20
Steak & Homestyle Noodles	110	2.5	14
Steak & Vegetables	130	2	19
Other varieties, average	125	2	21
Traditional: *Per Cup*			
Beef Barley	120	2.5	17
Chicken & Herb Dumpling	100	2.5	13
Hearty Chicken & Rotini	100	2	13
Homestyle Chicken with Vege & Pasta	100	2	14
Italian-Style Wedding	120	4	11
Roasted Garlic Chicken	100	2	13
Southwestern Style Chkn Chowder	120	2	18
Split Pea with Ham	140	1	24
Vegetable Classic: *Per Cup*			
French Onion	50	1	9
Green Split Pea with Bacon	160	2	28
Garden Vegetable	90	0	20
Hearty Tomato	110	0.5	24
Lentil; Tomato Basil, average	155	2.5	29
Minestrone	100	2	20
Tomato Rotini	130	0.5	28
Vegetable	80	0	15
Light, Low-Fat/Low-Carb:			
Beef Pot Roast	80	1	12
Southwestern-Style Vegetable, 8.5 oz	60	0.5	12
Vegetable & Noodle, 8.75 oz	60	0.5	13

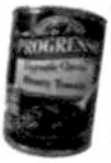

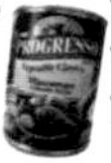

Shelton's

Broth, Chicken, Regular	35	2.5	0

Signature (Safeway)

	C	F	Cb
Signature Soups: *Per Cup*			
Baked Potato	420	33	20
Bistro Mushroom Trio	170	11	14
Broccoli & Cheesy Cheddar	280	21	14
Chunky Chicken Noodle	130	3.5	13
Fiesta Chicken Tortilla	100	3	11
Italian-Style Wedding	160	7	17
Pacific Coast Clam Chowder	330	24	19
Stompin' Steakhouse Chili	260	8	22
Tuscan Tomato & Basil Bisque	310	26	17

Simply Asia

Noodle Soup Bowls: *Per Bowl*			
Miso Tofu	220	1.5	42
Spring Vegetable	210	1	44
Szechwan Hot & Sour	280	5	51
Rice Noodle Soup Bowls: *Per Bowl*			
Sesame Chicken	260	3	55
Shitake Mushroom	270	3	56

Spice Hunter

Mixes ~ Per Bowl			
Beef Barley	180	2	32
Chicken Noodle	140	1.5	25
Chicken Vegetable	160	1	31
Creamy Thai Noodle	200	5	34
Miso Udon	160	1.5	31
Split Pea	250	1.5	43

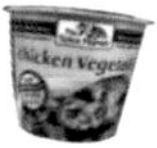

Swanson

Per Cup			
Vegetable Broth	15	0	3
99% Fat Free, Chicken Broth	10	0.5	1
Organic: Beef Broth	15	0.5	1
Chicken Broth	15	0.5	1

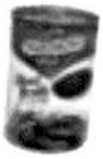

Tabatchnick

Per Pouch			
101 Calories: *Per Pouch*			
Cabbage	90	1	21
Barley Mushroom; Wild Rice, average	80	1	17
Onion	60	1.5	11
Broths: *Per ½ Pouch*			
Chicken with Noodles & Dumplings	150	6	19
New York Style Chicken	70	1	13
Dairy: *Per Pouch*			
Corn Chowder	130	4.5	21
Cream of Broccoli	90	4	12
New England Potato	140	4	24

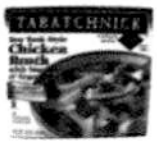

Updated Nutrition Data ~ www.CalorieKing.com
Persons with Diabetes ~ See Disclaimer (Page 24)

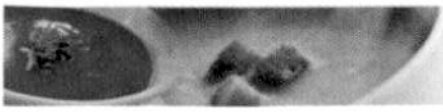

Tabatchnick (Cont)

	C	F	Cb
Gluten Free: *Per Pouch*			
Old Fashioned Potato	**100**	1.5	21
Split Pea	**140**	0	34
Southwest Bean	**220**	5	35
Vegetarian Chili	**180**	3.5	28
Low Sodium: *Per Pouch*			
Barley Mushroom	**80**	1	17
Pea	**140**	0	34
Vegetable	**90**	1.5	17
Meat: *Per Pouch*			
Frenchman's Onion	**60**	1.5	11
Wilderness Wild Rice	**80**	0.5	16
Parve: *Per Pouch*			
Balsamic Tomato & Rice	**110**	3.5	18
Black Bean	**230**	2.5	39
Minestrone	**100**	1.5	18
Vegetable	**90**	1.5	17

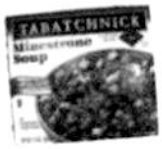

Thai Kitchen

	C	F	Cb
Rice Noodle Soup Bowls: *Per Bowl*			
Hot & Sour	**250**	3	52
Lemongrass & Chili	**250**	2.5	52
Thai Ginger	**260**	3	52

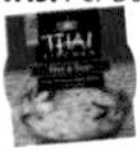

Trader Joe's

	C	F	Cb
Canned: *Per 8 fl.oz Cup Unless Indicated*			
Condensed, Clam Chowder, ½ cup	**80**	2	11
Organic: Black Bean	**130**	1.5	25
Lentil Vegetable, ½ can	**130**	3.5	19
Split Pea	**100**	0	19
Light Sodium, Tomato Bisque	**130**	4	21
Low Sodium: Minestrone, 10¾ can	**200**	4	37
Chkn & Mafalde Pasta, 10¾ can	**110**	3	19
Low Fat, Chicken Noodle	**90**	1	14
Cartons, 32 fl.oz:			
Butternut Squash	**90**	2	16
Carrot Ginger	**80**	1	17
Creamy Corn & Roasted Pepper	**110**	2	23
Garden Patch Veggie	**60**	0	14
Latin Style Black Bean	**70**	1	12
Sweet Potato Bisque	**130**	1	28
Organic: Butternut Squash	**70**	0	17
Creamy Tomato	**90**	3.5	15
Tomato & Roasted Red Pepper	**100**	3.5	15
17.6 fl.oz: Beef Barley with Veggies	**100**	0.5	16
Chicken Noodle with Veggies	**100**	1	16

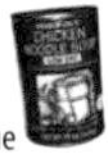

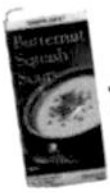

Whole Foods

	C	F	Cb
Per Cup			
Canned: Chicken Noodle	**110**	3	16
Chicken with Wild & Red Rice	**110**	2.5	17
Italian Style Wedding	**150**	6	19
Vegetable	**90**	1	21
Vegetable Beef	**130**	3.5	21
365 Organic: Black Bean	**150**	1	25
Chicken Noodle	**90**	2	11
Cream of Mushroom	**100**	6	11
Lentil	**120**	1	16
Minestrone	**120**	2	21
Tomato	**90**	3.5	11
Vegetable	**70**	1	11

Wolfgang Puck

	C	F	Cb
Per Cup			
Original: Chicken and Egg Noodles	**130**	6	11
Chicken and Dumpling	**220**	13	17
Chicken with Broccoli	**180**	10	14
Chicken with Sweetcorn	**200**	10	20
Chicken Tortilla	**140**	5	17
Creamy Roast Chicken with Rice	**200**	10	16
New England Clam Chowder	**170**	7	18
Old Fashioned Beef Barley	**120**	3.5	17
Organic: Butternut Squash	**200**	11	22
Chicken with Egg Noodle	**110**	5	11
Chicken with White & Wild Rice	**130**	4	18
Corn Chowder	**210**	13	20
Classic Tomato with Basil	**130**	6	18
Creamy Tomato	**250**	16	23
Old Fashioned Potato	**200**	14	17
Thick & Hearty Lentil & Vegetable	**140**	0	28
Tortilla	**160**	3.5	27
Organic Broths: Beef	**20**	0	4
Free Range Chicken	**20**	0.5	4
Vegetable	**10**	0	2

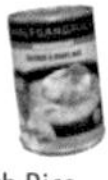

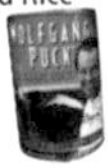

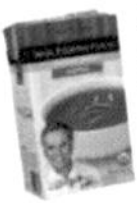

Wylers

	C	F	Cb
Dry Mix: Mrs Grass Onion, 0.25 oz	**20**	0	4
Homestyle Vegetable, 0.4oz	**35**	0	7
Mrs Grass Soup Mix:			
Chicken Noodle, 1 cup	**70**	1.5	10
Beef Vegetable, 1 cup	**90**	0.5	18

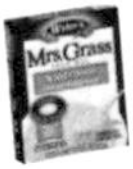

Soybean Products

	C	F	Cb
Cheeses (Soy): *See Page 80*			
Miso Soy Bean Paste			
Cold Mountain: Light Yellow, 1 tsp	10	0	1
Mellow Red, 1 tsp	15	0	3
Red, 1 tsp	10	0	1
Miso Soup (dry mix), av.			
1 Tbsp., dry mix	35	1	5
1 cup, prepared	35	1	5
Natto, ½ cup, 3 oz	160	7	14
Okara (Tofu fiber residue), ½ cup, 2 oz	47	1	8
Tempeh: 1 piece, 3 oz	180	8	12
Fried, 3 oz	250	14	14
Seitan *(White Wave),* Traditional, 3 oz	90	1	3
Soybean Protein *(TVP),* 1 oz	95	0	8
Soy Bean Paste, 1 tsp	10	0	2
Soy Beans: *See Page 167*			
Soy Drinks: *See Page 48*			

Tofu ~ Packaged

	C	F	Cb
Tofu Stir-Fried, average all, 4 oz	120	8	3
Azumaya Tofu: Soft (Silken), 3.2 oz	40	2	1
Firm; Extra Firm, 2.8 oz	70	4	2
Light Extra Firm, 2.8 oz	60	2	3
House Foods			
Premium Tofu: Soft (Silken), 3 oz	50	2.5	2
Medium Firm (Regular), 3 oz	60	3	1
Firm, 3 oz	70	3.5	2
Extra Firm, 3 oz	80	4	1

Tofu ~ Packaged (Cont)

	C	F	Cb
House Foods (Cont)			
Organic Tofu: Firm, 3 oz	60	3.5	0
Extra Firm, 3 oz	70	4	0
House Tofu: Tokusen Kinugoshi, 3 oz	90	4	3
Sukui; Soon (Extra Soft), 3 oz	45	2	2
Yaki Tofu (Broiled), 3 oz	90	5	2
Seasoned Tofu Steak: Grilled, 3 oz	90	5	2
Garlic & Pepper, 3 oz	90	4	1
Mori-Nu Tofu (Silken)			
Soft, 3 oz, 1" slice	45	2.5	2
Firm, 3 oz, 1" slice	50	2.5	2
Extra Firm, 3 oz, 1" slice	45	1.5	2
Organic Firm 3 oz, 1" slice	60	2.5	2
Lite, Firm, 3 oz, 1" slice	30	0.5	1
Nasoya: Soft, ⅕ package, 2.8 oz	60	3	1
Silken, 3.2 oz	45	2	1
Firm, ⅕ package, 3.2 oz	70	3	2
Extra Firm, ⅕ pkg, 2.8 oz	80	4	2
Silken Style Creations: *Per ½ Cup*			
Chocolate; Vanilla, average	120	1.5	24
Strawberry	110	1	22
WestSoy, Firm, 2.8 oz	95	5	3

Spices & Herbs

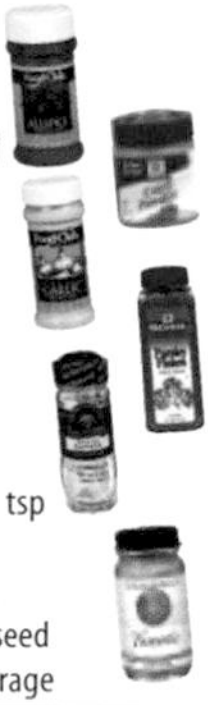

	C	F	Cb
Per Teaspoon: Average all types	5	0	1
All Purpose, 1 tsp	0	0	0
Allspice, ground	5	0	1
Chili Powder	8	0	1
Cinnamon, ground	6	0	2
Curry Powder	6	0	1
Garlic Powder	9	0	2
Nutmeg, ground	12	0	1
Onion Powder	7	0	2
Parsley, dried	4	0	1
Pepper, average	6	0	1
Saffron	2	0	0
Salt-Free Blends, 1 tsp	0	0	0
Tumeric, ground	8	0	1
Seeds: Fenugreek	12	1	2
Mustard, Poppyseed	15	1	1
Other types, average	7	0	1

Seasonings & Flavorings

	C	F	Cb
Accent Flavor Enhancer, 1 tsp	0	0	0
Angostura Bitters, 1 tsp	15	0	4
Bacon Bits, average, 1 Tbsp	35	2	2
Bacon Chips (Durkee), 1 Tbsp	30	1	2
Bac-Os (Betty Crocker), 1½ Tbsp	20	1	1.5
Bragg Liquid Aminos, 1 tsp	0	0	0
Butter Buds, 1 tsp	5	0	2
Garlic Bread Sprinkle, 1 tsp	8	0.5	1
Garlic Salt, 1 tsp	2	0	0
Italian Seasoning, 1 tsp	4	0	1
Lemon Pepper Seasoning, 1 tsp	7	0	1
Meat Tenderizer, average, 1 tsp	7	0	1
Molly McButter, 1 tsp	5	1	1
Mrs Dash Blends, 1 tsp	0	0	0
Salad Crunchies *(McCormick)*, 1 tsp	10	0.5	2
Salt: Regular, Sea Salt, Lite Salt	0	0	0
Seasoning Mixes, av., ¼ package	70	1	9
Taco Seasoning, av., ¼ package	30	0.5	4
Old El Paso: Chili Season. Mix, 1 T.	8	0.5	1.5
Cheesy Taco Seasoning Mix, 1 Tbsp	10	0.5	2
Taco/Burrito Seasoning Mix, 2 tsp	15	0	4
Fajita Seasoning Mix, 1 tsp	5	0	1.5
Vegit Seasoning Mix, ¼ tsp	0	0	0

Supplements

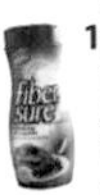

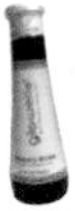

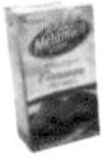

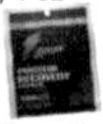

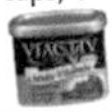

	C	F	Cb
Aloe Vera Juice, undiluted, 2 fl.oz	5	0	1
Brewer's Yeast: Tablets, 2 tabs	4	0	0.5
Flakes, 1 heaping Tbsp, ⅓ oz	30	0.5	4
Powder, 1 heaping Tbsp, ½ oz	50	0.5	6
Calcium Chews: *CVS*, 1 chew	20	0	3
Trader Joe's, Choc., 1 chew	20	1	3
Cod Liver Oil, 1 Tbsp	125	13	0
Fiber Choice, 2 tabs	15	0	4
Fibersure, 1 heaping tsp	25	0	6
Fish Oil Capsules, average, 1	10	1	0
Flax Oil: Capsules, 2	10	1	0
Barlean's, 3 softgels	110	11	0
Garlic Tablets/Capsules, each	3	0	0
Glowelle:			
Beauty Drink, 8 fl.oz	100	0	24
Powder Stick (1)	50	0	12
Lecithin Granules, 1 Tbsp	55	4	0.5
***Metamucil* Powder:**			
Orange (Smooth Texture)			
1 rounded Tbsp	45	0	12
Sugar-Free, 1 rounded tsp	20	0	5
Pink Lemonade, Sugar-Free, 1 rounded tsp	20	0	5
Fiber Wafers (2)	120	5	17
Capsules:			
Heart & Digestive (6)	10	0	3
Strong Bones (5)	10	0	3
Protein, Powders, average, 1 oz	100	0.5	0
Seaweed: Dried, 1 oz	85	0.5	22
Soaked, drained, 1 oz	15	0.5	3
Spirulina, 1 tablet	2	0	0.5
Vitamins/Minerals: Tabs/Caps, 1	2	0	0
Vitamin E Capsules, each	5	0.5	0
***Viactiv* Chews** (1)	20	0.5	4

Cough & Pharmaceutical

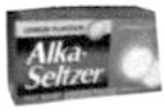

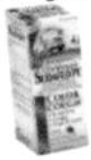

	C	F	Cb
Antacids: Av., 1 tablet	4	0	1
Liquid, 1 Tbsp	6	0	1

(Antacid Sodium Counts *~ See Page 293)*

	C	F	Cb
Cough/Cold Syrups:			
Regular: With sugar, 1 Tbsp	35	0	9
With alcohol, 1 Tbsp	46	0	9
Sugar-Free *(Diabetic Tussin)*, 1 T.	0	0	0

Cough Drops/Lozenges*: See Page 77*

	C	F	Cb
***Sudafed* Syrup,** 1 tsp	14	0	3
***Tylenol* Liquid**: Child, 1 tsp	17	0	4
Extra Strength, 1 tsp	11	0	3

Sugar

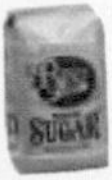

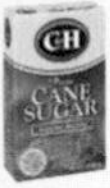

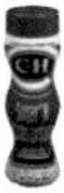

	C	F	Cb
White Sugar, granulated:			
1 level teaspoon	15	0	4
1 heaping teaspoon	25	0	6
Single portion, 1 packet	10	0	3
1 Tablespoon	50	0	12
1 ounce, 1 oz	110	0	28
1 cup, 7 oz	770	0	200
1 pound	1760	0	464
Single Portion Packages:			
1 stick	15	0	4
Square Package	25	0	6
Starbucks, 0.3 oz	30	0	8
1 cube, ½"	25	0	6
Brown Sugar: 1 Tbsp	50	0	13
1 ounce, 1 oz	110	0	28
1 cup, not packed, 5 oz	540	0	140
1 cup, packed, 7¾ oz	845	0	218
Powdered/Confectioners:			
Sifted, 1 cup, 3½ oz	385	0	98
Unsifted, 1 cup, 4¼ oz	460	0	117
Cinnamon Sugar, 1 tsp	15	0	4
Dextrose, 1¼ tsp	15	0	4
Fructose: Dry, 1 tsp	15	0	4
Liquid, 1 oz	80	0	21
Glucose, 1 oz	110	0	27
Glucose Tablets (1)	20	0	5
Palm Sugar, 3 Tbsp	45	0	11
Piloncillo (Brown Sugar), 3oz cone	325	0	81
Turbinado Sugar, 2 Tbsp, 1 oz	110	0	27
Unrefined Cane Sugar, 1 oz	110	0	27

Sugar Substitutes

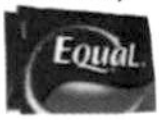

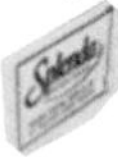

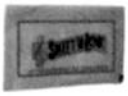

	C	F	Cb
DiabetiSweet, 1 teaspoon *(Carbohydrate as Sugar Alcohol)*	9	0	4
Equal: Tablet (2)	4	0	0.5
Granular, 1 tsp	4	0	0.5
Packet (1)	4	0	0.5
Flavored, 1 stick	4	0	0.5
Natra Taste; Sweet One, 1 packet	4	0	1
NutraSweet, 1 tsp	4	0	0
Splenda:			
Granular: 1 tsp	5	0	0.5
1 cup	95	0	24
Packet, all flavors	5	0	0.5
Sugar Blend,Orig/Brown, ½ cup	385	0	96
Stevia, Single Serving	0	0	0
Sugar Twin: 1 packet	3	0	0.5
Sweet 'N Low, 1 packet	2	0	0.5
Walgreens Wal-Sweet, 1 packet	0	0	0
Weight Watchers, 1 packet	4	0	1
Whey Low, 1 tsp	3	0	3

Syrups, Molasses, Agave

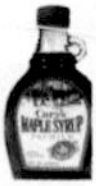

Syrups: ***Average All Brands***
(Corn/Rice/Maple/Pancake/Sundae/Waffle)
Includes Aunt Jemima, Cary's, Karo, Hershey's, Hungry Jack, Log Cabin, Mrs Butterworth's

	C	F	Cb
Regular/Dark/Light Color:			
1 Tbsp, ½ fl.oz	55	0	14
¼ cup (4 Tbsp)	220	0	55
Single Portion: 1½ oz package	170	0	42
Lite: 1Tbsp	25	0	6
¼ cup (4 Tbsp)	100	0	25
Sugar-Free: *Cary's,* 2 Tbsp, 1 oz	18	0	5
Cozy Cottage, 2 Tbsp, 1 oz	10	0	3
Da Vinci, 2 Tbsp, 1 oz	5	0	1
Honey Cream Syrup, ¼ cup, 2 oz	220	0	55
Molasses: Dark/Light: 1 Tbsp, ¾ oz	55	0	14
1 cup, 11½ oz	880	0	224
Blackstrap, 1 Tbsp, ¾ oz	47	0	13
Agave Nectar, average, 1 Tbsp, ¾ oz	60	0	15

Ice Cream Toppings

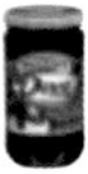

Average All Types & Brands: *Per 2 Tbsp (Hershey's, Smuckers)*

	C	F	Cb
Butterscotch; Caramel	140	1	30
Chocolate: Hot Fudge	140	4	22
Fat Free Chocolate	100	0	23
Pineapple, Strawberry	110	0	28
Smuckers: Lite	90	0	23
Magic Shell	210	15	18
Milky Way	130	4	23

Honey, Jam, Preserves

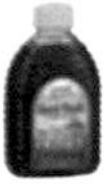

Average All Brands	C	F	Cb
Honey: 1 tsp, ¼ oz	22	0	5.5
1 Tbsp, ¾ oz	65	0	17
1 ounce, 1 oz	85	0	23
1 cup, 12 oz	1030	0	269
Single Portion, ½ oz package	45	0	11
Jams/Jellies/Marmalade/Preserves:			
Regular, 1 tsp, ¼ oz	20	0	5
1 Tbsp, ¾ oz	55	0	14
1 ounce, 1 oz	80	0	20
Single Portion, ½ oz pkg	40	0	11
Apple/Fruit Butters, 1 Tbsp, 0.6 oz	20	0	6
Fruit Spreads: Regular, 1 tsp	15	0	4
Low Sugar, 1 tsp	8	0	2
Low Calorie *(Featherweight),* 1 tsp	8	0	2
Jelly: Regular, average, 1 tsp	18	0	4.5
Imitation, Low Calorie, 1 tsp	4	0	1

Updated Nutrition Data ~ www.CalorieKing.com
Persons with Diabetes ~ See Disclaimer (Page 24)

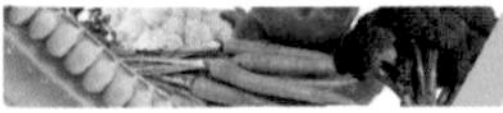

Vegetables

Vegetables	C	F	Cb
Alfalfa Sprouts, ½ cup, ½ oz	5	0	0.5
Artichokes, Globe/French:			
1 medium, 4½ oz	60	0	13
1 large, 5.7 oz	75	0	17
Artichoke Heart, plain, 2 pieces	15	0	3
Asparagus, raw/frozen:			
3 medium spears	10	0	2
Cuts & Tips *(Del Monte)*, ½ cup, 4.3 oz	20	0	3
Bamboo Shoots, cooked, ½ cup, 2 oz	7	0	1
Beans: Green/Snap/String, ½ cup, 2 oz	20	0	4
10 beans (4" long), 2 oz	20	0	4
Dried Beans, *average all types:*			
(Kidney, Brown, Lima, Navy, Pinto, White)			
Raw: 2 Tbsp, 1 oz	95	0.5	18
1 cup, 7 oz	665	3	126
Cooked: 1 oz	35	0	7
½ cup, 3 oz	105	0	21
Bean Sprouts, average, ½ cup, 2 oz	15	0	3.5
Beets (Beetroot):			
Raw, 1 beet (2" diam), 4 oz	35	0	8
Cooked, 1 cup, slices, 3 oz	35	0	8
Canned ~ *See Page 168*			
Beet Greens, cooked, ½ cup, 2½ oz	20	0	4
Bell Pepper: *See Peppers*			
Bitter Melon/Gourd, 1 cup, pces, 1½ oz	15	0	1.5
Blackeye Peas, cooked, ½ cup, 3 oz	100	0.5	18
Bok Choy (Chinese Chard), cooked, 3 oz	10	0	1.5
Breadfruit, ¼ small fruit, 3 oz	100	0	26
Broadbeans (Fava Beans):			
Green (in pod), raw: 4 pods			
(3½ oz with shells; 1.2 oz beans)	30	0	6
1 cup beans (w/o shell), 4½ oz	110	1	22
Mature Seeds: Raw, 1 cup, 5.3 oz	510	2.5	87
Cooked, ½ cup, 3 oz	95	0	17
Broccoflower, ⅕ head, 3½ oz	35	0	7
Broccoli: Raw, chopped, 1 cup, 3 oz	30	0	6
3 Florets, 2½ oz	25	0	5
1 Spear (5" long), 1.1 oz	10	0	2
1 Whole: Medium size, 14 oz	135	1.5	26
Large, 21 oz	205	2	40
1 Head (no stalk), 11 oz	105	1	21
1 Stalk, small (5" long), 5.3 oz	50	0.5	10
Brocco Sprouts, ½ cup, 1 oz	15	0	2
Brussels Sprouts: cooked, ½ cup, 2.8 oz	30	0.5	6
2 Sprouts, 1½ oz	15	0	3
Butterbeans, cooked, ½ cup, 3 oz	90	0	16
Cabbage, all types/colors, average			
Raw: 1 Leaf, large, 1 oz	5	0	2
Shredded, 1 cup, 2½ oz	15	0	4
½ Large Head (7" diam), 22 oz	150	1	35
Cooked, shredded, ½ cup, 2½ oz	15	0.5	3.5

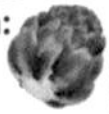

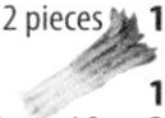

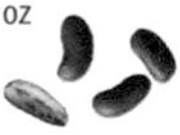

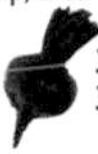

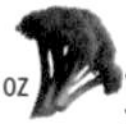

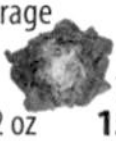

Vegetables (Cont)

Vegetables (Cont)	C	F	Cb
Cactus Leaf (Nopales)			
1 leaf, 4½ oz	20	0	4
1 cup (slices), 3 oz	15	0	3
Carrots, Regular thick variety,			
1 small, 4 oz	45	0	11
1 medium, 6 oz	70	0	16
1 large, 8 oz	95	0	22
Chopped, 1 cup, 4½ oz	50	0	12
Grated, 1 cup, 4 oz	45	0	11
Slices, 1 cup, 4½ oz	50	0	12
Sticks (4"), 4-5, 1½ oz	20	0	4
Long thin variety, 1 medium, 2.2 oz	25	0	6
Baby: Snack size, 3 medium, 1 oz	10	0	2.5
Snack Pack, 3 oz	30	0	7
Cauliflower, Raw: 1 cup (pieces), 3½ oz	25	0	5
½ medium head, 10 oz	70	0	15
Cooked, 3 florets, 2 oz	10	0	2
Celeriac, ½ cup, raw, 2¾ oz	35	0	7
Celery: 1 large stalk, 11", 2.2 oz	10	0	2
1 small stalk, 5", ½ oz	2	0	0.5
4 Strips, thin sticks, ½ oz	5	0	1
Chopped, 1 cup, 3½ oz	15	0	3
Chard (Swiss), ½ cup, cooked, 3 oz	20	0	3.5
Chayote Squash: 1 medium, 7 oz	40	0	9
1 cup (pieces), 4½ oz	25	0	6
Chick Peas			
Dry, 1 cup, 7 oz	730	12	121
Cooked, 1 cup, 6 oz	270	4	45
Chicory Greens, 1 cup, 1 oz	7	0	1.5
Chili Peppers: *See Peppers*			
Chinese Long Bean, sliced, 1 cup, 3.2 oz	45	0	8
Chives, chopped, 1 Tbsp	1	0	0
Choy Sum, 3 oz	15	0	3
Cilantro (Coriander), 1 cup	5	0	0.5
Collards, cooked, ½ cup, 3 oz	25	0	5
Corn, yellow/white:			
Raw: Kernels, ½ cup, 3 oz	80	0.5	19
Ear (5"x 1¾"), 5½ oz	153	1	37
Cooked, Kernels, ½ cup, 3 oz	77	0.5	18
Cob, cooked: Small, 2¼ oz	60	0.5	14
Large ear, 5½ oz	120	1	28
Courgette: *See Zucchini*			
Cowpeas: *See Blackeye Peas*			
Cress, garden, raw, 1 cup, 1¾ oz	15	0	3
Cucumber: 1 whole, 11 oz	45	0.5	11
½ cup slices, 2 oz	10	0	2
Mini/Lebanese (1), 3 oz	15	0	3
Daikon Radish, ½ cup, slices, 2 oz	9	0	2
Dandelion Greens, raw, ½ cup, 1 oz	10	0	2.5
Edamame *(Immature green soybeans):*			
Shelled, ½ cup, 2.6 oz	110	5	8
With shells, 10 pods, 1¼ oz	30	1	3

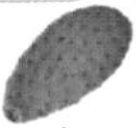

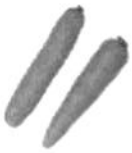

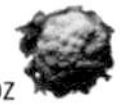

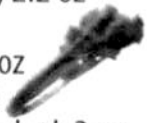

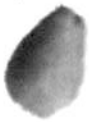

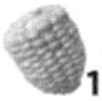

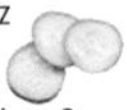

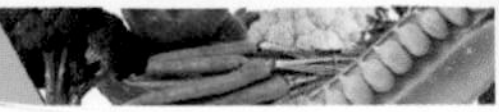

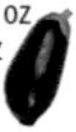

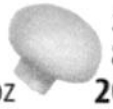
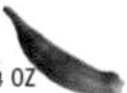
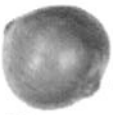

Vegetables (Cont)	C	F	Cb
Eggplant: Raw, ¼ medium, 4 oz	30	0	7
Raw, ½ cup, 1" pieces, 1½ oz	10	0	2
1 slice, fried, 1 oz	75	4	10
Endive, Belgian/French: Raw,			
1 medium head (6"), 2½ oz	12	0	3
Fennel, 1 cup, sliced, 3 oz	25	0	7
Gai Choy Cabbage, cooked, 1 cup, 6 oz	20	0	3
Gai Lan (Chinese Kale), cooked, 1 cup	35	0.5	7
Garlic, 1 clove	4	0	1
Ginger: ¼ cup slices, 1 oz	20	0	5
Crystallized (sugared), 7 pieces, 1½ oz	130	0	35
Horseradish, raw, 1 pod, ½ oz	5	0	1
Jerusalem Artichoke, raw, ½ cup	55	0	13
Jicama, raw, sliced, ½ cup, 2¼ oz	25	0	6
Kale, 1 cup, chopped, 2½ oz	35	0.5	7
Kohlrabi, ½ cup, cooked, 1¾ oz	17	0	5
Leek, cooked, 1 whole, 4½ oz	40	0	9
Lentils, green/brown: Dry, 1 oz	100	0.5	17
Dry, 1 cup, 6¾ oz	680	2	115
Cooked, ½ cup, 3½ oz	115	0.5	20
Lettuce: 1 cup, chopped/shredded, 2 oz	7	0	1
Butterhead, 2 leaves, ½ oz	2	0	0.5
Cos/Romaine, shredded, 1 cup, 1.7 oz	10	0	2
Iceberg: 1 outer leaf, ½ oz	2	0	0.5
1 medium head, 16 oz	75	1	16
Lima Beans, baby, cooked, ½ cup, 3 oz	105	0	20
Lotus Root, 10 slices, cooked, 3 oz	60	0	14
Mung Bean Sprouts, ½ cup, 2 oz	15	0	3
Mushrooms: Raw, 1 medium, 0.6 oz	4	0	0.5
Raw, 1 large, sliced, ¾ oz	5	0	1
Raw, ½ cup pieces, 1¼ oz	8	0	1
Cooked, ½ cup pieces, 2½ oz	20	0.5	4
Fried/Sauteed, 6 oz	220	16	11
Mustard Greens, Raw, ½ cup, 1 oz	7	0	2
Nopales: *See Cactus Leaf*			
Okra: Raw, 8 pods, 4 oz	30	0	7
Cooked, ½ cup, slices, 2¾ oz	20	0	4
Onions, Raw: 1 small, 2½ oz	30	0	7
1 medium, 4 oz	50	0	11
1 large, 5½ oz	65	0	15
1 jumbo, 16 oz	190	0.5	46
Chopped: Raw, ½ cup, 3 oz	35	0	8
1 Tbsp, 0.4 oz	5	0	1
Slices: 1 cup, 4 oz	50	0	12
1 medium slice (⅛"), ½ oz	5	0	1
1 large slice (¼"), 1⅓ oz	15	0	4
Dehydrated flakes, ¼ cup, ½ oz	50	0	12
Rings, breaded & fried, 2 rings	80	5	9
Scallions, ½ cup, 2 oz	15	0	3
Spring, ½ cup, chopped, 2 oz	15	0	3
(*French's* Fried Onions: *See Page 114)*			
Blossom/Blooming: See Fast-Foods (Chili's/Outback)			

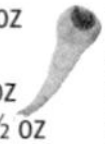
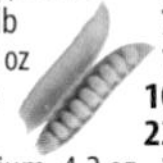
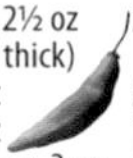
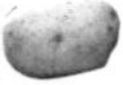
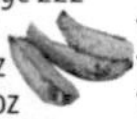

Vegetables (Cont)	C	F	Cb
Parsley, chopped, ½ cup, 1 oz	10	0	2
Parsnip: 1 medium, 4 oz	85	0	20
Cooked, ½ cup slices, 2¾ oz	55	0	13
Peas: Raw, Green, ¼ cup, 1½ oz	30	0	5
Raw, with pods, ½ lb	70	0	13
Snow Peas, 10 pods, 1.2 oz	15	0	3
Split: Dry, hulled, 1 oz	100	0.5	17
Cooked, 1 cup, 7 oz	230	1	42
Peppers: Sweet, 1 medium, 4.2 oz	30	0	7
Bell: 1 medium, 4.2 oz	30	0	7
½ cup, chopped, raw, 2½ oz	20	0	5
2 rings (5" diam. x ¼" thick)	3	0	1
Chili: Green/Red, 1½ oz	20	0	5
Habanero, 1 only, 0.3 oz	10	0	2
Pigeon Peas, cooked, ½ cup, 3 oz	95	1	17
Pimientos, 3 medium, 3½ oz	25	0	5
Poi, ½ cup, 4.2 oz	135	0	33
Potatoes: Raw (with skin)			
1 Baby, 2 oz	45	0	10
1 Small, 6 oz	135	0	30
1 Medium, 8 oz	180	0	40
1 Large, 12 oz	270	0	60
1 Extra large, 16 oz	360	0	80
Baked (no added fat): large, 10 oz (raw wt):			
Plain: With skin, 7 oz (ckd wt)	185	0	42
Without skin, 5½ oz (ckd wt)	145	0	34
With Skin/Toppings:			
+ 2 tsp fat	270	8	58
+ Sour Cream & Chives, 2 Tbsp	320	6	60
+ Plain Yogurt, 2 Tbsp	260	1	60
+ Grated Cheese, 1 oz	370	9	58
Mashed:			
With milk plus fat, ½ cup, 4 oz	120	4.5	18
KFC Style without gravy, 4 oz	100	3	16
Loaded (fat/cream/cheese/bacon):			
Side serving, 6 oz	180	9	22
Large serving, 12 oz	360	18	44
Potato Skins: (Baked with cheese topping),			
½ whole, 4 oz	240	13	22
French Fries: Small serving, 2.6 oz	250	13	30
Medium serving, 4 oz	380	20	47
Frozen, uncooked, 18 fries, 4 oz	165	5.5	28
Oven-heated, 18 fries, 4 oz	165	5.5	28
Take-Out, 1 cup, 5 oz	440	25	60
McDonald's ~ See Page 222			
Fried, 18 pieces, 4 oz	165	5.5	28
Au Gratin, ½ c., 4.3 oz	160	9	14
Pancakes, 2 small, 2 oz	120	6.5	12
Puffs, fried, 4 puffs, 1 oz	55	2.5	8
Scalloped: 1 cup, 8½ oz	220	9	26
Ore-Ida Frozen Potatoes: See Page 168			

Updated Nutrition Data ~ www.CalorieKing.com
Persons with Diabetes ~ See Disclaimer (Page 24)

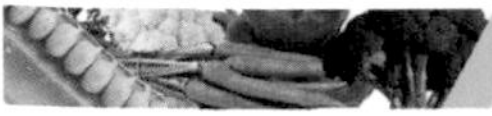

Vegetables (Cont)

Vegetables (Cont)	C	F	Cb
Potato Salad, ½ cup, 4½ oz	180	10	14
Pumpkin:			
Raw, 1" cubes, 1 cup, 4 oz	30	0	7
Cooked:			
Mashed: 1 scoop, 2 oz	10	0	2
½ cup, 4⅓ oz	25	0	6
Baked, without fat, 4 oz	90	7	9
Pumpkin Flowers, 1 cup, 1.2 oz	5	0	1
Purslane: Cooked, ½ cup, 2 oz	10	0	2
Raw, 1" cubes, 1 cup, 1.5 oz	5	0	1.5
Radicchio: 2 leaves, ½ oz	5	0	1
Shredded, 1 cup, 1½ oz	20	0	4
Radishes: 1 small	0	0	0
10 medium/5 large, 1.6 oz	5	0	1
½ cup (slices), 2 oz	10	0	2
Rhubarb, raw, ½ cup, 2 oz	15	0	3
Rutabaga, cooked, ½ cup, (cubes), 3 oz	30	0	7
Salsify, ckd, ½ cup, (slices), 2½ oz	50	0	11
Sauerkraut, ½ cup, 2½ oz	15	0	3
Seaweed: Dried, 1 oz	5	0	2
Soaked, drained, 1 oz	15	0	4
Nori/Laver, dried, 6 sheets, ½ oz	35	0	5
Shallots, 1 Tbsp, (Chopped), ½ oz	5	0	1
Sorrel, raw, ½ cup, 4 oz	20	0	4
Soybeans: Mature, dry, 1 oz	120	5.5	9
Dry, ½ cup, 3.3 oz	390	18	28
Cooked, ½ cup, 3 oz	150	7.5	8
(Soy Products/Tofu/Tempeh: See Page 162)			
Spinach: Cooked, ½ cup, 3 oz	20	0	4
Raw: 3 leaves/1 cup, 1 oz	7	0	1
1 Bunch, 12 oz	80	1.5	12
Creamed, average, ½ cup, 4½ oz	190	15	8
Squash: Summer, raw, ½ cup, 2½ oz	10	0	2
Cooked, ½ cup slices, 3 oz	15	0	3
Winter, cooked,			
Acorn, ½ cup cubes, 3½ oz	35	0	9
½ medium (10 oz raw weight)	115	0	30
Butternut, ½ cup, (cubes), 3½ oz	40	0	10
¼ medium (9 oz raw weight)	115	0	30
Spaghetti, ½ cup, 1¾ oz	15	0	3
Succotash, cooked, ½ cup, 3⅓ oz	110	1	23
Sweetcorn: *See Corn*			
Sweet Potatoes:			
Cooked with skin (w/o fat)			
1 medium, 4 oz	105	0	24
Without skin, mashed, ½ cup, 5½ oz	125	0	29
Swiss Chard, cooked, chopped, 1 c., 6 oz	35	0	7
Taro, cooked, ½ cup, 2⅓ oz	95	0	23

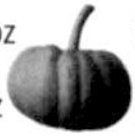
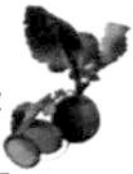
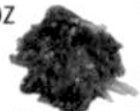
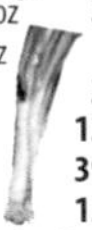
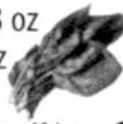
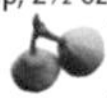
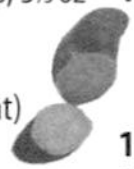

Vegetables (Cont)	C	F	Cb
Tomatoes: 1 small (2¼" diameter), 3 oz	15	0	3
1 medium (2¾" diameter), 5 oz	25	0	5
1 large (3½" diameter), 8 oz	40	0.5	9
1 extra large (3" diam.), 12 oz	60	0.5	14
Chopped, 1 cup, 6½ oz	35	0.5	7
Extra Listings: *Page 103*			
Tomatillo, 1 medium, 1.2 oz	10	0	2
Turnip: cooked, ½ cup, 2¾ oz	15	0	4
Greens, cooked, ½ cup, 2½ oz	15	0	3
Water Chestnuts: 5-6 nuts, 1 oz	56	0.5	13
½ cup, (slices), 2¼ oz, raw	60	0	15
Canned, 1 oz	15	0	3
Watercress, 10 sprigs, 1 oz	3	0	0.5
Yams: Cooked, ½ cup, 2½ oz	80	0	19
Baked, 1 medium (6") 8 oz	265	0.5	63
1 large (9") 12 oz	400	0.5	94
Yardlong Bean, 1 pod, ½ oz	5	0	1
Yucca Root, ½ cup, 3½ oz	165	0.5	39
Zucchini: 1 medium, 7 oz, raw	30	0.5	7
Cooked, ½ cup, (slices), 3 oz	15	0	4

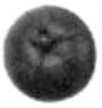
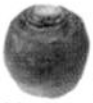
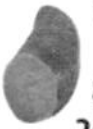

Frozen Vegetables

Frozen Vegetables	C	F	Cb
Birds Eye			
Baby Varieties:			
Peas: ⅔ cup, 3 oz	70	0	12
with Pearl Onions, ⅔ cup	60	0	12
Gold & White Corn, ⅔ cup, 3.2 oz	100	1	20
Brussels Sprouts, (10), 3 oz	45	0	8
White Pearl Onions, ⅔ cup, 3 oz	30	0	6
Whole Green Beans, 1 cup, 3 oz	35	0	5
Steamfresh:			
Mixtures: Brocc & Cauliflower, 1 cup	30	0	4
with Carrots, ¾ cup, 3 oz	30	0	5
Brocc., Crts., Peas, Water Ches., ¾ cup	35	0	6
Premium Selects:			
Sugar Snap Peas, ⅔ cup	40	0	7
Whole Green Beans, 1 cup, 3 oz	35	0	5
Singles: *Per 3.25 oz Bag*			
Baby Brussels Sprouts	50	0	9
Super Sweet Corn	80	1	14
Sweet Peas	70	0	13
Specially Seasoned:			
Asian Medley, 1 cup, 3.3 oz	50	2	6
Garlic Baby Peas & Mushroom, ¾ cup	80	2	12
Lightly Sauced: Broccoli with Cheese	60	2	7
Roasted Red Potato with Chive Butter	140	1.5	29

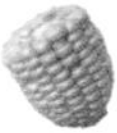

V Vegetables

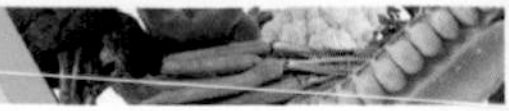

Frozen Vegetables (Cont)

	C	F	Cb
Green Giant			
Just for One,			
Broccoli & Cheese Sauce, 4.25 oz	40	1	7
Vegetables: Asparagus Cuts, ⅔ cup	20	0	3
Corn: Nibblers, ½ ear, 2.2 oz	80	1.5	15
Extra Sweet Niblets, ⅔ cup	70	1	13
Shoepeg, without sauce, ½ cup	80	0.5	17
Honey-Glazed Carrots, 1 cup	90	3	15
Spinach, w/o sauce, ½ cup, 3½ oz	25	0	3
Rice & Vegetables: *Per ½ Package, Prepared*			
Cheesy Rice & Broccoli	150	2.5	28
Rice Medley	125	2	24
Rice Pilaf	105	1.5	20
White & Wild Rice	140	3	25
Valley Fresh: *Per ½ Cup, Prepared*			
Rsted Red Pot., Green Beans w/ Sauce	80	1	16
Ore-Ida (As Purchased):			
Fries: *Per 3 oz*			
Classic: Golden Crinkles	120	3.5	20
Golden; Shoestring, average	135	4	22
Steak	110	3	19
Easy,			
Extra Crispy: Crinkles; Golden	180	8	25
Extra Crispy: Fast Food Fries	160	6	23
Golden Crinkles	170	7	24
Seasoned Crinkles	150	6	22
Premium: Cottage; Country Style	130	4.5	21
Crispers	220	13	23
Golden Twirls	160	6	24
Pixie Crinkles; Texas Crispers, average	145	5	21
Hash Browns: Golden Patties (1)	170	8	15
Potatoes O'Brien, ¾ cup, 3 oz	60	0	14
Southern Style, ⅔ cup, 3 oz	70	0	16
Toaster Patties (2), 3.65 oz	220	12	25
Onion Rings: Gourmet, 2.7 oz	180	8	25
Onion Ringers (6), 3 oz	180	10	21
Steam n' Mash: Cut Russet, ¾ cup	80	0	17
Garlic Seasoned Potatoes, ¾ cup	110	4	17
Three Cheese Potatoes, ¾ cup	80	0.5	16
Tater Tots: 9 pieces, 3 oz	170	8	20
ABC (9), 3 oz	160	8	22
Extra Crispy, 12 pieces, 3 oz	170	9	20
Ultimate Bake: With Butter, 5 oz	170	5	27
With Cheese, 5 oz	190	6	28

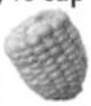

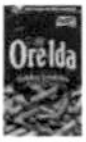

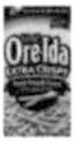

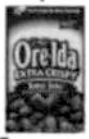

Canned/Bottled

	C	F	Cb
Solids & Liquid			
Artichoke Hearts *(Fanci Foods):*			
Plain, 1 oz (1)	8	0	1
Marinated, ¼ bottle, 1 oz	25	1.5	2
Asparagus: Drained, 3 spears	10	0	1.5
Pieces, ½ cup, 4.3 oz	25	0.5	3
Bamboo Shoots, 1 cup, 4½ oz	25	0	4
Bean Salad, ½ cup, 4⅓ oz	90	0	20
Beans: Green, ½ cup, 2½ oz	15	0	3
Baked Beans, ½ cup, 4½ oz	120	0.5	27
Butter Beans, ½ c., 4½ oz	90	0	16
Italian, ½ cup, 4½ oz	30	0	6
Kidney Beans, ½ cup 3½ oz	105	0.5	19
Lima Beans, ½ cup, 4½ oz	80	0	15
Pinto Beans, ½ cup, 4½ oz	105	1	18
Beets: Sliced, ½ cup, 3 oz	25	0	6
Crinkle/Pickled *(Del Monte)* ½ cup	80	0	20
Carrots: Sliced, ½ cup, 2½ oz	20	0	4
Honey Glazed *(Del Monte)* ½ cup	75	0	18
Corn: Kernels, ½ cup, 4½ oz	80	0.5	18
Creamed style, ½ cup, 4½ oz	90	0.5	23
Garbanzo/Chick Peas, ½ cup, 4.2 oz	145	1.5	27
Green Chilies, diced, 2 Tbsp, 1 oz	6	0	1.5
Hearts of Palm (1), 1.2 oz	7	0	1
Mushrooms: ½ cup, 2½ oz	20	0	4
in Butter Sauce, 2 oz	20	1	2
Onions: Pickled, 1 medium, ½ oz	10	0	2
Cocktail, 1 onion	0	0	0
French's Fried Onions: *See Page 114*			
Peas, ½ cup, 3 oz	60	0.5	10
Peppers: Hot Chili, Jalapeno, (1), 1 oz	5	0	1
Sweet, undrained, 2½ oz	13	0	3
Jalapeno, with liquid, ½ cup chopped	20	0.5	3
Fried, drained, 2 Tbsp, 1 oz	60	5	3
Salsa, average all types, 2 Tbsp	10	0	2
Sauerkraut, drained, 1 cup, 5 oz	25	0	6
Spinach, ½ cup, 3½ oz	25	0.5	3.5
Succotash: Cream Style, ½ cup	100	0.5	23
w/ whole kernels, undrained, ½ cup	80	0.5	18
Sweetcorn: *See Corn*			
Sweet Potato: ½ cup, 3½ oz	90	0	24
Tomatoes, Sundr.: Natural, 5-6 pieces	20	0	5
In Oil, drained, 6 pieces, ½ oz	40	2.5	4
Tomato Products: *See Page 148*			
Vegetables, mixed, ½ cup, 4 oz	45	0	8
Yams: in Light Syrup, ½ cup, 4 oz	105	0	25
Candied, ½ cup, 5 oz	170	0	46
Zucchini in Tomato Sauce., ½ cup, 4 oz	30	0	8

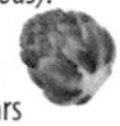

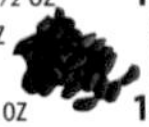

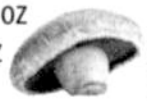

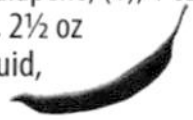

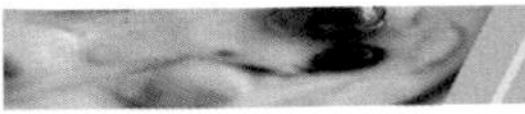

Quick Guide

	C	F	Cb
Yogurt			
Average All Brands: *Per 8 oz Cup*			
Plain Yogurt: Whole	**140**	8	10
Low-Fat	**145**	3.5	16
Fat-Free	**125**	0.5	17
Fruit Flavored: Whole, 8 oz	**225**	8	32
Low-Fat	**230**	3	43
Fat-Free, regular	**215**	0.5	43
Fat-Free, no sugar added	**80**	0	15

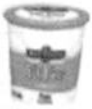

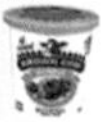

	C	F	Cb
Yogurt Parfait/Deli Cups			
With Fruit Pieces:			
(⅔ Yogurt + ⅓ Fruit)			
Small, 8 oz cup	**140**	3	20
Large, 12 oz cup	**210**	4.5	30
With Fruit + Granola:			
Small, 8 oz cup (+ ¾ oz Granola)	**235**	7	30
Large, 12 oz cup (+ 1½ oz Granola)	**400**	13	58

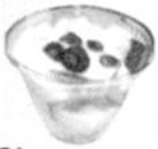

Yogurt ~ Brands

	C	F	Cb
Alta Dena: Low-Fat: Plain, 8 oz	**170**	4.5	20
All Natural, average all flavors	**215**	2	41
Non-Fat: Fruit, average all flavors	**185**	0	38
Plain, 8 oz	**110**	0	16
Vanilla, 8 oz	**160**	0	30
Blue Bunny			
Light, average fruit flavors, 6 oz	**85**	0	14
No Sugar Added, 6 oz	**80**	0	14
Breyers			
Creme Savers, av. all flavors, 6 oz	**165**	1.5	31
Fruit On The Bottom, av. all flav., 6 oz	**160**	1.5	32
Inspirations: Choc Chip/Mint, 4 oz	**140**	3.5	23
Strawberry; Vanilla Bean, 4 oz	**110**	1	22
Light, average all flavors, 6 oz	**80**	0	12
Smooth & Creamy, av. all flav., 6 oz	**170**	1.5	34
YoCrunch: Light, av. all flavors, 6 oz	**120**	1	22
Low-Fat w/ Granola, fruit, average	**190**	2	38
M&M's; Reese's; Crunch, average	**200**	4.5	35
100 Calorie Pack: Strawberry	**100**	0.5	23
Vanilla, Cheesecake	**100**	2	21
Brown Cow			
Cream Top: Plain, 6 oz	**130**	7	9
Fruit Flavors, average, 6 oz	**175**	6	27
Low-Fat: Plain, 8 oz cup	**130**	3	15
Flavors, average, 6 oz	**150**	2	27
Non-Fat: Plain, 8 oz cup	**110**	0	16
Fruit Flavors, av., 6 oz	**135**	0	26
Greek: Plain, 5.3 oz cup	**80**	0	6
Strawberry, 5.3 oz cup	**130**	0	18

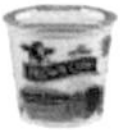

	C	F	Cb
Cabot			
Non-Fat: Plain, 8 oz	**100**	0	19
Fruit flavors, 6 oz	**120**	0	23
Greek Style: Plain, 8 oz	**290**	23	12
Low-Fat (2%), 6 oz	**160**	3	25
Cascade Fresh:			
Low-Fat, all flavors, 6 oz	**140**	2	23
Fat-Free, all flavors, 6 oz	**110**	0	20
Whole Milk: Plain, 8 oz	**170**	8	12
Flavors, average, 8 oz	**200**	7	24
Colombo			
Light, all flavors, 6 oz	**90**	0	16
Classic: Banana Strawb.	**180**	0	39
Vanilla, 6 oz	**130**	0	25
Fat-Free, Plain, 8 oz	**100**	0	15
Dannon:			
Activia Yogurt:			
Plain, 8 oz	**170**	4.5	20
Light, av. all flav., 4 oz	**70**	0	13
Fiber, all flavors., 4 oz cup	**110**	2	19
Drinks, all flavors 5.75 fl.oz	**160**	3	27
All Natural:			
Average all flavors, 6 oz	**150**	2.5	25
Low-Fat, Plain, 6 oz	**100**	2.5	12
Non-Fat, Plain, 6 oz	**80**	0	12
Danimals: Crush Cups, all flavors, 4 oz	**100**	1.5	17
Drinkables, 3.1 fl.oz	**70**	0.5	15
Fruit On The Bottom, av., 6 oz	**150**	1.5	28
Light & Fit: All flavors, 6 oz	**80**	0	16
Quarts, Strawb.; Vanilla, 8 oz serving	**110**	0	21
Smoothies, 7 fl.oz	**70**	0	14
Carb & Sugar Control: 4 oz cup	**50**	1.5	3
Emmi Swiss (Low-Fat): *Per 6 oz cup*			
Berry Pomegranate	**180**	3	30
Coffee	**170**	3	27
Muesli	**110**	2.5	10
Pink Grapefruit; Van. Bean	**110**	2.5	10
Fage			
Classic: Peach; Cherry; Strawb., 5.3 oz	**210**	12	18
Honey, 5.3 oz	**250**	12	28
0%, 8 oz	**120**	0	9
2%: Plain 8 oz	**150**	4.5	9
Fruit, 5.3 oz	**130**	2.5	18
Honey, 5.3 oz	**180**	2.5	29

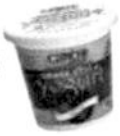

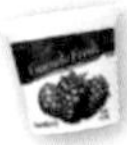

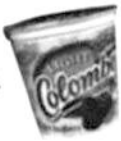

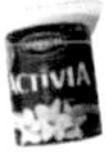

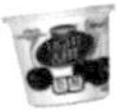

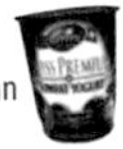

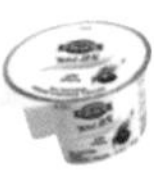

Brands (Cont)	C	F	Cb
Horizon Organic			
Fruit on Bottom, all flavors, 6 oz	140	0	27
Low-Fat: Blended, av. all flav., 6 oz	150	1.5	27
Yogurt Tuberz (1)	60	0.5	11
Jewel: *6 oz Carton (Lowfat)*			
Blended, average all flavors	150	1.5	30
Fruit On The Bottom, average	165	1.5	33
Light, average all flavors	110	0	19
32 oz Tubs: *Per 8 oz*			
Lowfat, average fruit flavors	205	2	39
Plain, Non-Fat	120	0	18
Kemps:			
'Light '80 Calories', 6 oz carton	80	0	16
Yo-J Drink, average, 8.3 fl.oz	150	0	35
Kirkland, Low-Fat:			
Blueberry; Peach; Strawberry, 8 oz	240	2	48
Knudsen: 70 Calories, 6 oz	70	0	11
Free, average, 6 oz	170	0	33
Kroger:			
Blended, Flavors: 6 oz	190	2	35
Carb Master, average all flavors, 6 oz	80	1.5	4
Fruit On The Bottom, av. all fl., 6 oz	170	2	30
Lite, average all flavors, 6 oz	80	0	13
La Yogurt:			
Original, average, 6 oz	150	2.5	27
Light, average, 6 oz	90	0	15
Rich & Creamy, 6 oz	190	2	35
Enriched, average, 6 oz	170	1.5	32
Sabor Latino: Dulche De Leche, 6 oz	190	1.5	36
Fruit Flavors, average, 6 oz	190	1.5	37
LALA, Classic Blended:			
Fruit Flavors, average, 6 oz	150	3	26
Smoothies, average, 9 fl.oz	200	4	34
Lucerne			
Low-Fat:			
Fruit flavors, average, 6 oz	170	2	32
Vanilla, 6 oz	170	2	33
Fat-Free: Plain, 6 oz	80	0	13
Light Fat-Free, fruit, 6 oz	90	0	17

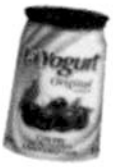

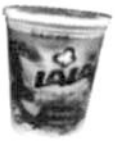

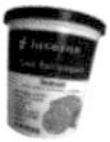

Mountain High	C	F	Cb
Original Style: Plain, 8 oz	180	8	17
Strawb./Vanilla, 8 oz	210	7	28
Low-Fat: Plain, 8 oz	140	2.5	18
Lemon; Raspberry, 8 oz	190	2	33
Strawberry; Vanilla, average, 8 oz	175	2.5	29
Fat-Free: Plain, 8 oz	120	0	18
Strawberry; Vanilla, average, 8 oz	160	0	30
Nancy's			
Whole Milk: Honey, plain, 8 oz	170	8	17
With Fruit on Top, average, 8 oz	230	5	41
Low Fat: Plain/Lemon, average, 8 oz	150	3	16
Average other flavors, 8 oz	175	3	27
Non-Fat: Plain, 8 oz	120	0	17
Vanilla (32 oz carton), 8 oz	220	0	40
Soy Cultured: Plain, 6 oz	150	3	25
Berry flavors, average	140	3.5	24
O Organics (Safeway),			
Low-Fat, average, 6 oz	140	2.5	23
Oikos, Greek Yogurt:			
Plain, 5.3 oz cup	80	0	6
1 cup, 8 oz	130	0	9
Blueberry, 5.3 oz cup	120	0	16
Honey, 5.3 oz cup	120	0	18
Vanilla, 5.3 oz cup	110	0	12
Publix: Fat-Free, Plain, 8 oz	140	0	23
Swiss Style, Low-Fat, 8 oz	240	2.5	41
Ralphs: *Same as Kroger*			
Roberts:			
Low-Fat, average all flavors, 6 oz	165	1.5	32
Fat-Free, all flavors, 6 oz	90	0	14
Silk (Soy): Plain, 8 oz	150	4	22
Vanilla, 6 oz	150	3	25
Average other flavors, 6 oz	155	2	30
Stater Bros: Plain, 6 oz	105	1.5	14
Fruit on the Bottom, Strawb., 6 oz	170	1.5	34
Blended Low-Fat, Strawb., 6 oz	150	1.5	29
Stonyfield Farm (Organic)			
Fat-Free: Plain, 6 oz	80	0	11
Chocolate Underground, 6 oz	180	0	37
Fruit Flavors, average, 6 oz	120	0	24

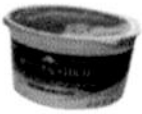

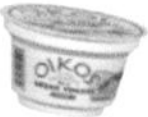

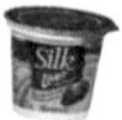

Brands (Cont)

	C	F	Cb
Stonyfield Farm (Cont):			
Lowfat Smooth & Creamy:			
Apple Pie, 6 oz	**130**	**1.5**	21
Plain, 6 oz	**90**	**1.5**	11
Average other fruit flavors, 6 oz	**130**	**1.5**	22
Whole Milk Cream Top: Plain, 8 oz	**170**	**9**	13
French Vanilla, 8 oz	**230**	**8**	31
O'Soy Smooth & Creamy			
Chocolate; Vanilla, 6 oz	**155**	**3**	25
Fruit On The Bottom, av. all flav, 6 oz	**170**	**2.5**	29
YoKids, all flavors, 4 oz cups	**80**	**1**	13
Trader Joe's:			
French Village: Non-Fat, all flav., 6 oz	**130**	**0**	26
32 oz Containers, Plain, 8 oz	**170**	**10**	12
Greek Style: *Per 8 oz Container Unless Indicated*			
Apricot Mango; Honey	**300**	**15**	28
Non-Fat: Plain, 5.3 oz	**90**	**0**	7
Pomegranate, 5.3 oz	**130**	**0**	20
Honey, 5.3 oz cup	**130**	**0**	18
Low-Fat Pre-Stirred, Fruit Flavors, 8 oz	**220**	**3**	40
Weight Watchers, all flavors, 6 oz c.	**100**	**0.5**	17
Wildwood: Soyogurt Plain, 6 oz	**110**	**3.5**	14
Average other flavors, 6 oz	**160**	**3**	28
Whole Foods (365)			
365: Non-Fat, Plain, 6 oz	**90**	**0**	13
Fruit flavors, average 6 oz	**145**	**0**	30
Vanilla, 6 oz	**130**	**0**	23
365 Organic:			
Fruit flavors, average, 6 oz	**150**	**0**	29
Whole Soy: Plain, 6 oz	**150**	**3.5**	27
Berry; Strawb. Banana, 6 oz	**180**	**3.5**	35
Other flavors, average, 6 oz	**160**	**3.5**	30
YoCrunch: *Low-Fat, 6oz Cup*			
Cookies n' Cream	**180**	**3.5**	33
With Granola, all flavors	**190**	**2**	38
Yoplait			
Original, av. all flav., 6 oz	**170**	**1.5**	33
Fiber One, average all flavors, 4 oz	**50**	**0**	13
Go-Gurt!, 2.25 oz tube	**70**	**0.5**	13
Light, Fruit Flavors, 6 oz	**100**	**0**	19

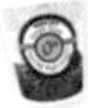
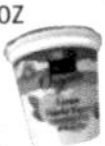
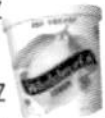
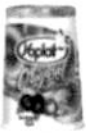

Brands (Cont)

	C	F	Cb
Yoplait (Cont):			
Thick & Creamy, all flavors, 6 oz	**190**	**3.5**	32
Light, 6 oz	**100**	**0**	20
Large 2lb Container, 99% Fat-Free, 1 cup, 8 oz	**200**	**1.5**	39
Yo-Plus, average all flavors, 4 oz	**110**	**1.5**	21
Trix, Fruit Flavors, 4 oz	**115**	**0.5**	18
Whips!: Choc. Flavors, 4 oz	**160**	**4**	26
Fruit Flavors, 4 oz	**140**	**2.5**	25
Yoplait Kids: 4 oz cup	**80**	**1**	13
Squeezers, 2 oz	**60**	**1**	11

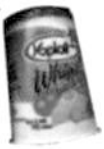

Yogurt Drinks & Probiotics

	C	F	Cb
Cacique:			
Yonique: *Per 6 fl.oz Container*			
Low-Fat: Guava	**140**	**1.5**	27
Mango	**140**	**1.5**	28
Pina Colada	**160**	**3.5**	26
Strawberry Banana	**140**	**1.5**	28
Strawberry, 7 oz	**200**	**1.5**	36
Dannon: Activa, all flavors, 3.1 fl oz	**160**	**3**	27
Danimals, all flavors, 3.1 fl.oz	**70**	**0.5**	15
DanActive, average all flavors, 3.1 fl.oz	**80**	**1.5**	13
Light 'n Fit Smoothies, Non-Fat, all flavors, 7 fl.oz	**70**	**0**	14
Glen Oaks, average all flavors, 8 fl.oz	**190**	**3.5**	35
Good Belly Probiotic, 2.7 fl.oz bottle	**50**	**0**	12
Kemps, Yo-J Drink,			
Orange Cream, 8.3 fl.oz	**150**	**0**	34
Raspberry Orange, 8.3 fl.oz	**150**	**0**	34
Strawberry Banana, 8.3 fl.oz	**150**	**0**	34
Wild Berry, 8.3 fl.oz	**150**	**0**	34
Ralphs:			
Smoothies:			
Peach, 7 fl.oz	**200**	**2.5**	37
Raspberry, 7 fl.oz	**210**	**2.5**	40
Strawberry, 7 fl.oz	**190**	**2.5**	35
Stonyfield Farm			
Smoothies, av., 10 oz	**230**	**3**	40
Wildwood, av., 8 fl.oz	**185**	**2.5**	32
Yoplait Smoothies, All Flavors, 8 fl.oz	**220**	**3**	43

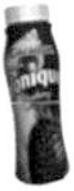
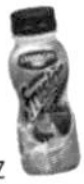
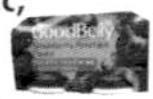

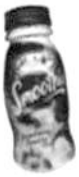

Cafeteria-Style Foods

Average All Preperations	C	F	Cb
Beef Stroganoff, 5 oz	**195**	13	7
Beef Stroganoff with 4 oz noodles	**350**	14	36
Chicken Lasagna, 1 piece	**300**	11	32
Chicken Chop Suey with 4 oz rice	**245**	4	37
Deep Dish Burrito, 7 oz	**265**	13	20
Grnd Beef Casserole, 2 scoops, 6 oz	**245**	13	17
Italian Meat Sauce for Spaghetti, 5 oz	**150**	9	9
with 5 oz Spaghetti	**350**	10	49
Lasagna, 1 piece	**275**	11	25
Meatloaf, 3 oz	**205**	13	4
Ranch Beans, 2 scoops, 6 oz	**350**	11	45
Red Beans & Rice, 7 oz	**280**	9	37
Scalloped Potato/Ham, 2 scoops, 6 oz	**160**	6	20
Stuffed Shells in Sauce (1)	**105**	3	17
Swedish Meatballs (3)	**205**	12	9
Sweet & Sour Pork/Rice, 9 oz	**240**	3	40
Swiss Steak with Mushr. Gravy, 6 oz	**280**	11	4
Tator Tot Casserole, 2 scoops, 6 oz	**260**	15	20
Tenderloin Tips/Mushroom Gravy, 5 oz	**210**	13	3
with 5 oz noodles	**395**	15	38
Tuna Noodle Casserole, 2 scoops, 6 oz	**180**	6	17
Turkey Tetrazzini, 2 scoops, 6 oz	**195**	7	17
Vegetable Lasagna, 1 piece	**250**	13	21

Croissants

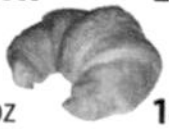

	C	F	Cb
Unfilled: Medium 1½ oz	**180**	10	21
Filled: With Ham (2 oz), garnish	**280**	14	24
With Ham (2 oz), Cheese (2 oz)	**470**	30	20
With Chick (2 oz) Cheese (2 oz)	**470**	30	20
With Turkey/Ham/Cheese (2 oz ea.)	**580**	36	20
Au Bon Pain: Ham & Cheese	**340**	10	46
Spinach & Cheese	**250**	9	32

7-Eleven: *Page 244*

Bagels

	C	F	Cb
Plain: Large, 4 oz (without filling)	**320**	2	65
With 2 oz Cream Cheese	**500**	27	54
With 2 oz Lox (Smoked Salmon)	**400**	4	65

Also see Bagels Section: *Page 58*
Fast-Foods Restaurants: *Page 183*
Au Bon Pain: *Page 185*
Bruegger's: *Page 192*
Einstein Bros Bagels: *Page 206*

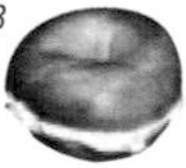

Sandwiches

No Spreads Unless Indicated (Includes 2 Slices Bread ~ 3 oz)	C	F	Cb
BLT (5 strips Bacon, 2 Tbsp Mayo)	**600**	40	46
Breaded Chicken & Garnish	**540**	28	46
Chicken Salad with Mayo., 5 oz	**580**	30	49
Chopped Liver, Egg, Mayonnaise	**630**	25	44
Corned Beef with Mustard, 5 oz	**560**	28	44
Egg Salad with Mayonnaise	**570**	29	49
Egg Salad Club with Bacon & Mayo.	**780**	53	49
Grilled Cheese (3 oz)	**540**	30	44
Ham (4 oz); Cheese (4 oz), & Mayo.	**910**	56	44
Lobster Salad (4 oz) with Mayonnaise	**530**	25	45
Overstuffed Tuna Salad (7 oz)	**870**	39	75
Philadelphia Cheese Steak Sandwich	**550**	23	42
Reuben (6 oz Beef/Pastrami, 2 oz Cheese, 2 Tbsp Dressing)	**920**	60	28
Roast Beef (4 oz) with Mustard	**460**	12	45
Roast Pork (4 oz) with Apple Sauce	**500**	16	55
Shrimp Salad Club with Bacon & Mayo.	**800**	57	48
Sloppy Joe with Sauce (7 oz)	**600**	30	45
Steak Sandwich (5 oz cooked)	**680**	32	41
Triple Cheese Melt (4 oz)	**720**	45	46
Tuna Salad with Mayonnaise, 5 oz	**610**	30	49
Turkey Breast (5 oz) with Mayonnaise	**460**	18	44
Turkey Breast (5 oz) with Mustard	**360**	7	44
Turkey Club with Bacon, Mayonnaise	**830**	38	31
Vegetarian with Avocado & Cheese	**820**	49	72

7-Eleven: *Page 244*
Schlotzsky's: *Page 246*
Subway: *Page 257*

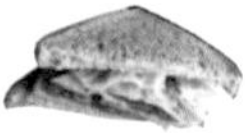

Wraps & Roll-Ups

Average All Types (Meat/Chicken/Fish/Veggie)	C	F	Cb
Small size, approximately 9 oz	**500**	25	48
Regular, approximately 15 oz	**830**	40	80
Large, approximately 22 oz	**1400**	70	134

Fast-Foods Restaurants: *Page 182*
Au Bon Pain: *Page 185*
Sonic Drive-In: *Page 251*
Subway: *Page 257*
WAWA: *Page 266*

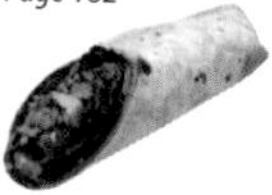

Updated Nutrition Data ~ www.CalorieKing.com
Persons with Diabetes ~ See Disclaimer (Page 24)

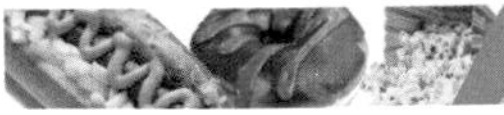

Fair & Carnival Foods

	C	F	Cb
Mexican			
Burrito with Bean/Beef, 17 oz	1100	41	104
Carne Asada, 14.5 oz	820	44	58
Chicken Taco, 3.3 oz	210	12	16
Fish Taco, 5 oz	270	13	31
Nachos with Cheese, 9″ plate	860	59	70
Tamale (1), 3.5 oz	180	8	21
Taquito, 5 oz	370	17	43
Greek			
Baklava, 2″ square	245	13	32
Falafel, 11.6 oz	660	27	85
Greek Salad, 14 oz	520	48	17
Gyro, 7.5″, 12 oz	680	40	55
Spanakopita, 8 oz	200	7.5	23
Italian			
Garlic Bread, ½ loaf, 10 oz	1135	40	147
Pizza Bread, Pepperoni, ½ loaf, 12 oz	1115	32	151
Pizza on a Stick, 1 piece	535	28	55
Personal Pizza, 7″: Cheese (1)	670	24	80
Pepperoni (1)	795	35	80
Ham & Pineapple (1)	800	31	87
Low Carb			
Beef Patty, wrapped in lettuce, 4 oz	480	33	0
Sandwiches: *Per 7½″ Roll*			
Ham, 11 oz	645	39	47
Hot Pastrami, 9 oz	760	17	62
Roast Beef, 11 oz	620	36	46
Philadelphia Cheese Steak, 13 oz	680	36	49
Tuna, 12 oz	830	60	46
Turkey, 11 oz	665	24	65
Veggie, 11 oz	490	23	49
Oriental: Fried Egg Roll, 6 oz	400	19	44
Rice Bowl: Beef, 6″ Bowl	880	13	136
Chicken, 6″ Bowl	870	15	135
Hamburgers			
⅓ Pound Burger, 7.5 oz	670	41	26
Cheeseburger, 6 oz	550	36	25
Hot Dogs/Franks: *With Bun*			
Hot Dog: Regular, (1)	215	14	28
With Chili, 6 oz	450	32	32
With Chili & Cheese, 7.3 oz	500	36	31
⅓ Pound Hot Dog	550	41	31
Foot Long Hot Dog	470	26	41
Corn Dog: Regular, 4 oz	250	14	23
Jumbo, 6 oz	375	21	36
Jumbo Franks with Bun:			
Bratwurst; Sausage; Kielbasa, av.	800	60	28

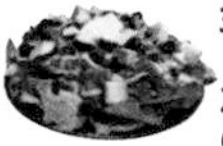

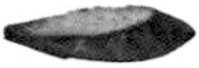

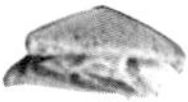

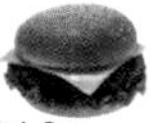

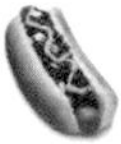

Fair & Carnival Foods (Cont)

	C	F	Cb
Barbeque Items *(Weights with Bone)*:			
Chicken, 15 oz	740	24	34
Corn on the Cob, 8″ (1), 16 oz	200	1	42
Pork Ribs, 18 oz	1360	68	21
Smoked Turkey Legs (with skin), 19 oz	1135	54	0
Beef Stew over Rice, 2 cups	440	14	61
Cheese Curds, Breaded & Fried, *(Culver's)*, 6.7 oz	670	38	54
Potatoes & Fries			
Australian Battered Potato, 12 oz	1290	66	155
Baked Potato, 14 oz	435	0.5	100
Fries: French, 7 oz	560	24	70
Cheese Fries, 10 oz	645	38	62
Chili Fries, 10 oz	700	36	83
Curly Fries, 7 oz	620	30	78
Tasti Chips, 40 chips, 6.5 oz	780	33	117
Sweet Potato, 14 oz	405	0.5	97
Ranch Dip, 3 oz	165	14	9
Finger Foods			
Artichoke: Steamed, 6 pieces	65	0	16
Fried, 9 pieces	250	14	24
Chicken Nuggets (6)	340	17	26
Chicken Strips (4), 4.5 oz	445	21	33
Finger Steaks (2), 4 oz	400	20	26
Mushrooms, Fried, 10-12 pieces	395	26	34
Onion Rings, 3 rings	310	13	40
Onion Flower	1320	72	140
Shrimp, Fried, 10-12 pieces, 5 oz	555	30	36
Sweet Potato Strips, Fried, 4 pieces	750	30	106
Zucchini, Fried, 4 slices	620	40	42
Salads/Sides			
Baked Beans, 4 oz	140	2	38
Chili, 1 cup	280	11	24
Cole Slaw, 5 oz	350	21	37
Pickle, whole (6″)	30	0	8
Potato Salad, 5 oz	290	15	35
Popcorn:			
Plain: Small, 3 oz	450	24	48
Large, 6 oz	900	48	96
Kettle Corn:			
Small, 5 oz	600	15	110
Large, 10 oz	1200	30	220
Cakes, Donuts, Cookies			
Funnel Cake: Plain (1)	760	44	80
Toppings: Cinnamon & Sugar, 2 tsp	30	0	8.5
Apple Cinnamon, 2 oz	85	3	36
Strawberries & Cream, 2 oz	70	0	16
Cinnamon Roll, large (1)	730	24	114
Churro (1), 1½ oz	165	8	21
Donuts, Jumbo Twist, (1), 7.5 oz	905	49	109

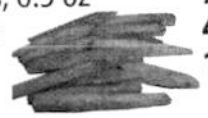

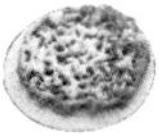

Fair & Carnival Foods (Cont)

Cakes, Donuts, Cookies (Cont)	C	F	Cb
Fried Snicker Bar, 5 oz	**445**	**29**	42
Fried Oreos, 3 cookies	**300**	**10**	33
Fried Twinkie, 1	**420**	**34**	45
Cotton Candy, 5½ oz bag	**625**	**0**	156
Red Rope Licorice, (24"), 2 oz	**200**	**0**	46
Cream Puff, 4.3 oz	**500**	**43**	22
Puff-on-a-Stick (4), 8.6 oz	**995**	**86**	44
Strawberry Crepe, 4.3 oz	**280**	**14**	36
Choc. Dipped Strawberry, 1 piece	**125**	**7**	15
Fudge, 1.5 oz	**200**	**11**	25
Twinkie Dog (Sundae)	**500**	**14**	89
Key Lime Pie Bar, 6 oz	**635**	**40**	59
Cheesecake on a Stick, 6 oz	**655**	**47**	56
Cobbler, 5 oz	**350**	**10**	62
Soft Pretzel, 4.5 oz	**340**	**2**	70
Candied Apple, 7 oz	**330**	**0.5**	80
Ice Cream & Frozen Treats			
Dippin' Dots Ice Cream: Small, 4 oz	**150**	**7**	17
Medium, 8 oz	**305**	**14**	35
Large, 16 oz	**600**	**28**	70
Snow Cone (includes 3 oz syrup)	**270**	**0**	68
Frozen Yogurt in sugar cone, 14 oz	**475**	**2**	94
Ice Cream: Small, sugar cone, 10 oz	**775**	**42**	83
Large, sugar cone, 14 oz	**935**	**54**	96
Sherbet, 8 oz	**270**	**4**	59
Frozen Banana, chocolate coated, 5 oz	**240**	**4**	53
Drinks			
Lemonade, 18 fl.oz	**210**	**0**	52
Orange Julius, 20 fl.oz	**490**	**10**	96
Strawberry Julius, 20 fl.oz	**430**	**0**	98
Icee, 16 fl.oz	**235**	**0**	59
Malt, 16 fl.oz	**690**	**33**	85
Slushies, 16 fl.oz	**260**	**0**	65
Soft Frozen Lemonade, 12 fl.oz	**300**	**0**	78
Smoothies: Berry Flavors, 16 fl.oz	**350**	**1**	80

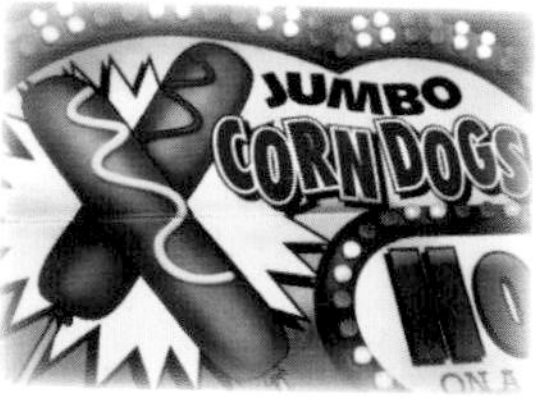

Stadium Foods

	C	F	Cb
Sandwiches			
Bacon Burger, 8.3 oz	**470**	**25**	34
Cheeseburger, 8.3 oz	**450**	**23**	33
Chicken Sandwich: With Cheese, 8.3 oz	**510**	**29**	40
Without Cheese, 7.7 oz	**460**	**25**	40
With Bacon, 8.3 oz	**530**	**31**	41
Hamburger, 7.8 oz	**400**	**19**	33
Polish Sausage Sandwich, 7 oz	**565**	**33**	46
French Fries, 6.4 oz	**470**	**34**	39
Fruit Cup, 6 oz	**80**	**0**	20
Hot Dogs			
Chili Dog, 7.7 oz	**520**	**29**	45
Hot Dog, 6.4 oz	**465**	**21**	50
Jumbo Dog, 6 oz	**440**	**25**	38
Kraut Dog with Sauerkraut , 7.8 oz	**490**	**27**	41
Nachos, 40 chips with 4 oz cheese	**1100**	**59**	132
Individual Pan Pizza (6"): *Per 10 oz Pizza*			
BBQ Chicken	**630**	**24**	71
Cheese	**630**	**27**	71
Pepperoni	**660**	**30**	70
Snacks			
Brownie, 2.5" x 4.5"	**360**	**18**	44
Cheese Sauce, 1.25 oz	**100**	**8**	4
Cheetos, 2.75 oz package	**440**	**28**	42
Chocolate Chip Cookie, 2.3 oz	**280**	**12**	40
Churros, 8", 3 oz	**325**	**15**	42
Doritos, Nacho, 2.75 oz package	**390**	**20**	48
King Size Candy:			
Butterfinger, 3.75 oz	**485**	**18**	75
Nestle Crunch, 2.75 oz	**390**	**21**	85
Lays Chips, 2.75 oz package	**440**	**28**	42
Peanuts in shell, 8 oz	**930**	**80**	24
Popcorn: Small (9 cup size)	**575**	**35**	56
Large (15 cup size)	**950**	**58**	93
Red Vines, 5.5 oz box	**560**	**0**	136
Soft Pretzel: Regular, 5.5 oz	**490**	**3.5**	101
Giant, 8 oz	**710**	**5**	147
Beverages: Orange Juice, 12 fl.oz	**180**	**0**	2
Beer: Heineken, 16 fl.oz	**200**	**0**	16
Light Miller, 16 fl.oz	**165**	**0**	10
Miller Draft, 16 fl.oz	**205**	**0**	18
Jack Daniels Punch, 12 fl.oz	**235**	**0**	34
Wine, White, 9 fl.oz	**190**	**0**	6
Soda (with ½ ice), average: 20 fl.oz	**160**	**0**	40
32 fl.oz	**260**	**0**	65
Snow Cone, 18 oz (incl. 3 oz syrup)	**270**	**0**	68
Starbuck's Frappuccino, 12 fl.oz	**195**	**2.5**	39

Updated Nutrition Data ~ www.CalorieKing.com
Persons with Diabetes ~ See Disclaimer (Page 24)

Chinese & Asian Dishes

Appetizers	C	F	Cb
Crab Cake, 2¼ oz	125	10	1
Dumplings: Pork, steamed, 1	80	4.5	5
Pork, fried, 1 dumpling	90	6	5
Vegetable, steamed, 1	35	1	5
Egg Rolls, mini, 3 rolls	100	3	11
Spring Roll: Small, 1½ oz	85	4	9
Medium, 3 oz	170	8	17
Large, 5 oz	290	15	29
Wonton, 1 only	75	4	5
Soup: Egg Flower, bowl 12 oz	90	2	16
Hot & Sour Soup, bowl 12 oz	110	3.5	14
Rice: Plain, 1 cup (½ Pint), 6½ oz	320	2	66
2 cups (1 Pint), 13 oz	640	4	132
Fried: 1 cup, 5 oz	365	11	55
Large dish, 16 oz	950	28	67
Noodles: Chinese Egg, cooked, 1 cup	200	4	37
Entrees & Mains: *Per Serving*			
Almond Chicken, 6 oz	270	10	21
BBQ Pork, 5.5oz	440	23	15
Beef in Black Bean Sauce, 8.5 oz	390	17	17
Broccoli Beef, 6 oz	370	21	13
Chicken & Broccoli, 5.5 oz	160	8	10
Chicken Skewers, 3 oz	210	9	18
Chop Suey: Chicken, 5 oz	140	9	2
Pork, 5 oz	170	12	3
Chow Mein, Beef/Chicken, 8 oz	390	12	59
Crab Puff/Rangoon, 1 dumpling	190	11	13
Crispy Fried Chicken, 8 oz	485	33	12
Egg Drop Soup: With Noodles, 1 cup	110	3	16
Without Noodles, 1 cup	60	3	4
Egg Foo Yung with Sauce, 1 cup	270	15	16
Kung Pao Chicken, 5.5 oz	240	15	12
Lemon Chicken, 5 oz	525	21	57
Lo Mein (stir-fried) 8 oz	705	42	49
Moo Shu Chicken (2)	360	19	25
Omelet, Chicken/Shrimp, 16 oz	990	82	10
Orange Chicken, 5.5 oz	500	27	42
Steamed Whole Fish, ½ Sockeye Salmon	646	36	23
Sweet & Sour: Fish, 20 oz	1160	58	106
Pork, 5.5 oz	400	23	35
Vegetable Combination, with oil, 6 oz	367	5	66
Vegetables, Steamed, without oil, 6 oz	137	1	29
Sauces: Mandarin Sauce 1.5 oz	70	0	17
Potsticker Sauce 1.5 oz	35	0	8
Bubble Tea, average, 12 fl oz	280	0.5	68
Fortune Cookie: Each	32	0.5	7

Cajun & Creole

	C	F	Cb
Alligator, 4 oz cooked	160	2	0
Baked Herb Chicken, 1 serving	850	53	2
Bouillabaisse	400	15	10
Cajun Fried Turkey, 1 serving	630	25	0
Cocktail Sauce, 2 Tbsp	30	0	6
Couche-couche, ½ cup	80	0	17
Crawfish Bisque, 1 serving	500	10	10
Crawfish, cooked, 2 oz	45	0.5	0
Creole Jambalaya, 1 serving	550	30	15
Frog Legs, steamed (2)	45	0	0
Guinea Fowl, flesh, 4 oz, cooked	160	4	0
Hogshead Cheese, ¼ cup	80	5.5	0
Jambalaya, Shrimp & Crabmeat	520	14	12
Red Beans & Rice, 1 serving	400	17	52
Roasted Quail, with Bacon on Toast	550	25	15
Remoulade Sauce, 2 Tbsp, 1 oz	110	11	2
Shrimp Creole, 1 serving	450	20	10
Stuffed Smothered Steak, with 1 cup Rice	890	50	50
Turtle, cooked, 3 oz	120	3	0

Cuban

	C	F	Cb
Bl. Beans w/ Rice (Moros con Cristianos)	510	22	76
Black-Eyed Pea Fritters (Bollitos de Carita)	80	5	6
Casserole Corn Tamale	445	20	55
Chicken w/ Yellow Rice (Arroz con Pollo)	925	49	87
Cuban Bread (Pan Cubano)	80	1.5	15
Donuts in Syrup (Bunuelos)	170	5	10
with Melado	100	5	10
Grilled Plantains	145	0	40
Gypsy's Arm Cake (Brazo Gitano)	260	18	42
Roast Pork S'wich (Pan con Lechon)	640	30	62
Seasoned Beef with Olives & Raisins (Picadillo)	435	36	10
Shredded Beef (Ropa Vieja)	550	35	10
Taro Root Mash (Pure de Malanga)	315	3	69
Yuca with Citrus Garlic Dressing (Yuca con Mojo)	190	9	25

French Foods

	C	F	Cb
Blanquette d'Agneau (Lamb Stew)	800	30	17
Brioche, 1 cake	280	14	34
Bouillabaisse (Fish Stew)	400	15	10
Coq au Vin (Chicken in Wine)	800	30	16
Coquilles St. Jacques	320	13	36
Crème Brulée, 1 serving	460	40	21

French Foods (Cont)

	C	F	Cb
Baguette, 3 slices, 2.2 oz	150	1	35
Creme Caramel (Caramel Custard)	260	10	38
Crepe Suzette, 1x6" crepe with sauce	220	10	13
Duck a l'Orange	780	35	47
Escargot (Snails), garlic butter (6)	200	10	4
Frog Legs, fried, 4 med. pairs	400	20	10
Lamb Noisettes, fried, 2 chops	500	40	1
Potage Creme Crecy (Carrot Soup)	360	18	14
Salade Nicoise (Tuna/Olives/Vegs)	450	13	14
Veal Cordon Bleu (Veal/Ham)	650	25	18
Vichyssoise (Potato /Leek Soup), 1 c.	200	9	15

Baguette & French Stick: *Page 56*
Croissants: *Pages 136, 172, 205*

German

	C	F	Cb
Bavarian Bread Dumpling, 3 small	330	10	28
Beef Goulash with Veggies	520	20	46
Black Forest Cake, 1 slice	380	16	30
Bratwurst, grilled, 1 medium, 6 oz	450	37	2
Chicken: Fried, Viennese-style	530	20	28
Livers with Apple/Onion, 6 oz	460	28	10
Herring, Pickled: Rollmops, 4 oz	260	16	3
With Sour Cream, 4 oz	310	20	3
Hot Sausage Curry	300	7	6
Kugelhupf Cake, 1 large slice, 4 oz	400	23	40
Sauerbraten Pork (Pot Roast)	650	35	15
Torte: Linzer (Almond/Raspb. Jam)	430	18	58
Sacher (Chocolate/Apricot Jam)	260	12	23
Weiner Schnitzel, 1 medium	750	35	38

Greek

	C	F	Cb
Baklava Pastry: Small	240	13	32
Large, 3¾ oz	400	21	45
Calamari, deep fried, 1 cup	300	13	17
Chicken Kebob Plate	345	13	8
Dolmades (Stuffed Grape Leaves) 2 rolls, 6 oz	200	5	13
Galactobureko, 1 only (Filo, Custard, Pastry in Syrup)	360	15	48
Greek Chicken Salad	400	18	9
Gyros: 6" Pita, 8 oz	475	32	35
7½" Pita, 12 oz	680	40	55
Hummus & Pita, 4 oz	260	12	30
Kataifi, (Filo, Nut, Pastry in Syrup)	350	11	56
Moussaka: Small serving, 8 oz	350	22	22
Large serving, 16 oz	700	44	44
Soup: Avgolemono (Egg Lem. Soup with Chicken & Rice), 1 cup	85	6	5
Souvlaki (Lamb), each, 2 oz	120	6	1

Greek (Cont)

	C	F	Cb
Stuffed Tomatoes, 2 only	250	12	17
Taramosalata, 1 Tbsp, ½ oz	40	3	2
Tyropita (Filo/Egg/Cheese Pastry)	350	26	31
Tzatziki (Cucumber/Yog. Dip), 1 oz	40	2	2

Daphne's Greek Cafe: *See Fast-Foods Section*

Hawaiian

	C	F	Cb
Ahi Tuna, grilled w/o fat, (6 oz fillet)	220	2	0
Chicken Long Rice, 1 cup, 7 oz	240	14	12
Gyoza, 1 only	55	2	6
Haupia (Coconut Pudd.), 1 pce (4"x 2½")	120	6	17
Hawaiian Sweet Bread, ½" sl., 2 oz	180	4.5	29
Kalua Chicken, 4 oz	280	16	0
Pork, 4 oz	350	24	0
Kim Chee (pickled cabbage), ½ c., 4 oz	20	0	5
Kulolo (Taro Pudding), 1 slice	125	5	19
Lau Lau: Chicken (1) 7 oz	280	21	3
Pork (1) 7 oz	320	26	5
Loco Moco (rice/burger/egg/gravy)	650	27	63
Lomi Salmon, ¼ cup, 4 oz	20	1	2
Malasadas (Donut), 2 oz	240	13	26
Manapua (Char Siu Pork Bun), 2.3 oz	180	8	25
Poi (mashed cooked taro), 1 c., 8½ oz	270	0.5	65
Poke, average all types, 3 oz	90	1	0
Portuguese Sausage, 2 oz	180	15	2
Potato Salad, ½ cup, 5 oz	170	10	17
Shave Ice *(Matsumoto)*, all flavors:			
With Icecream, 1 large	300	4	64
With Beans, 1 large	290	0	72
Spam Musubi: with Regular Spam (4 oz rice+1.3 oz Spam/7-Eleven Hawaii)	265	11	34
Homemade: w/ Lite Spam (50% less fat)	220	5	34
Taro Pancake Mix, ⅓ cup (makes 2)	140	2	26
Plate Lunches:			
Chicken Katsu (9 oz) with 2 scps Rice	1110	48	108
+ Macaroni Salad, ¾ cup	1360	68	123
or Tossed Salad + Fr. Dress. (2 T.)	1240	61	111
Hamburger (5 oz) w/ 2 scoops Rice	710	24	81
Gravy + Macaroni Salad	1135	49	112
MahiMahi (7 oz) with 2 scps Rice	650	12	90
+ Macaroni Salad + Tartar Sce	1150	58	109
or Macaroni Salad, w/o Tartar ce	935	34	108
or Tossed Salad + Fr. Dress. (3 T.)	815	27	96
or Tossed Salad, without dressing	670	12	93
Teri Beef (5 oz) with 2 scps Rice	790	23	94
+ Macaroni Salad, ¾ cup	1095	47	113
or Tossed Salad, without dressing	800	23	95

Updated Nutrition Data ~ www.CalorieKing.com
Persons with Diabetes ~ See Disclaimer (Page 24)

Indian & Pakistani

Per Serving
(Meat dishes allow 4 oz meat/serving)

	C	F	Cb
Aloo Samosa, each	**155**	12	12
Alu Gosht Kari (Meat/Potato Curry)	**600**	40	23
Chicken Korma	**500**	35	6
Chicken Pilaf (Murgh Biriyani)	**700**	53	50
Chicken Tikka	**260**	16	2
Chicken Vindaloo	**400**	20	8
Chapati/Roti, 7" diameter, 1 piece	**60**	0.5	11
Dahl (Lentil Puree): 1 cup, without oil	**230**	1	37
1 Tbsp Tadka (oil topping)	**120**	13	0
Dhakla (Lentil Dish), 1" square, 1 oz	**105**	5	13
Dhansak, ½ cup	**105**	3.5	11
Gosht Kari (Meat Curry/Tomato/Pot.)	**460**	25	17
Lamb Pilaf	**520**	35	40
Lassi (Sweet or Mango), 1 cup, 8 oz	**160**	4	24
Masala Gosht (Beef/Tomato/Gravy)	**400**	25	18
Mulligatawney Soup, average	**300**	15	8
Murgh Tikka, 1 cup	**300**	4	7
Naan Bread, ¼ (8" x 2"), 1 oz	**75**	2	11
Pappadum, 1 large/2 small	**50**	3	5
Pesrattu (Lentil Crepe), 9", 2.6 oz	**130**	5	15
Pork Vindaloo Curry without Rice	**620**	47	3
Rajmah (Kidney Bean Curry), 1 cup	**225**	5	35
Rogan Josh (Lamb/Yogurt Sauce), without Rice/Potatoes	**500**	30	3
Shahi Korma (Braised Lamb)	**430**	28	3
Tandoori Chicken: Breast	**260**	13	5
Leg/Thigh portion	**300**	17	6

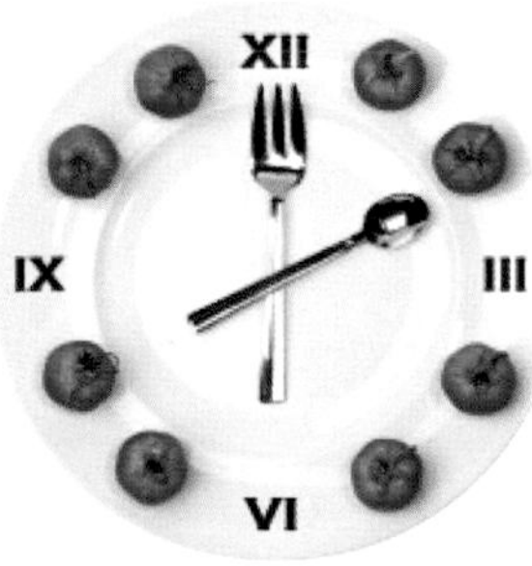

Italian Dishes

	C	F	Cb
Baked Ziti: Small	**370**	27	32
Regular	**575**	42	49
Breadstick (1), 2 oz	**120**	2.5	25
Broccoli Fettucine Alfredo, regular	**815**	23	125
Bruschetta, 2 slices	**380**	17	53
Calzones, average, all types	**840**	34	101
Cannelloni, 1 tube, 6 oz	**280**	15	18
Cheese Breadstick (1), 2.4 oz	**180**	8	20
Cheese Ravioli with Sauce	**495**	17	65
Chicken Alfredo	**775**	29	82
Chicken Parmigiana, 11 oz	**520**	22	16
Chicken Scallopine, dinner	**1110**	71	68
Eggplant Parmigiana	**900**	39	78
Fettucine Alfredo: Small	**525**	15	80
Lunch	**775**	22	119
Dinner	**1130**	81	68
Linquine & Seafood, dinner	**1130**	71	79
Manicotti Formaggio	**800**	38	57
Meat Lasagne: Small, 10 oz	**440**	23	39
Large, 16 oz	**700**	36	60
Meat Ravioli	**725**	22	102
Minestrone Soup, 1 bowl	**110**	2	18
Penne Rustica: Lunch	**1300**	71	76
Dinner	**1540**	80	101
Ravioli, over-stuffed, average	**990**	67	57
Spaghetti & Meatballs:			
With Tomato Sauce: Kids	**500**	20	58
Medium/Lunch	**1080**	63	89
Large/Dinner	**1430**	81	119
With Meat Sauce: Kids	**550**	25	56
Medium/Lunch	**1300**	79	84
Large/Dinner	**1700**	103	110
Veal Marsala, dinner	**1320**	66	132
Veal Parmigiana, dinner	**1270**	65	116
Vegetable Primavera	**610**	8	116
Macaroni & Cheese ~ *Page 135*			
Panini S'wich (Restaurant):			
Chicken, 16 oz	**900**	38	81
Meats, average, 18 oz	**940**	39	81
Vegetarian, 15 oz	**750**	31	83
Pizza: Ready-To-Eat ~ *Page 137*			
Gourmet Deep Dish (*Gino's East*) ~ *Page 209*			
Desserts: Lemon Ice	**180**	0	45
Gelato: Vanilla (Milk Base), ½ cup	**200**	15	18
Choc. Hazelnut (Milk), ½ cup	**370**	29	26
Water Base, ½ cup	**100**	0	25
Tiramisu, 1 piece, 5 oz	**400**	29	30

For more listings see Fast-Foods Section

Japanese

Japanese	C	F	Cb
Sushi Rice: cooked, 1 Tbsp	**25**	**0**	5
1 cup, 5¼ oz	**380**	**3**	82
Sushi (Maki) Rolls: *Per Piece*			
Average all types (California Rolls; Cream Cheese with Crab; Eel; Salmon; Shrimp; Tuna; Yellowtail; Vegetable)			
Small (1⅛" diameter x 1⅛" high), 0.8 oz	**25**	**0.5**	3.5
Medium (1¾" diam. x 1¾" high), 1.6 oz	**50**	**1**	7
Large (2¼" diameter x ⅞" high), 2 oz	**60**	**1.5**	9
Sushi Packs: *Per Pack*			
Average all types: 6 large pieces	**370**	**5**	55
9 medium pieces	**360**	**6**	60
12 small pieces	**265**	**3**	45
Futomaki (thick roll), 6 pieces	**380**	**5**	72
Hand Roll (Cone) 4 oz	**120**	**2**	18
Inari (rice filled soybean pocket), 4 pces	**420**	**9**	73
Sushi-Nigiri (fish on rice):			
average all types, 1 piece	**70**	**0.5**	12
Sushi Plate: Assorted, 6 pieces	**420**	**3**	36
Combination (Sushi & Sushi Rolls)			
2 Sushi + 6 small & 3 medium rolls	**400**	**7**	72
Sashimi (Sliced Raw Seafood/Beef)			
Ika (Squid), 4 oz	**105**	**2**	0
Hamachi (Yellowtail), 4 oz	**165**	**6**	0
Maguro (Yellowfin Tuna), 4 oz	**120**	**1**	0
Niku (Beef), 5 oz	**200**	**10**	0
Saba (Mackerel), 4 oz	**160**	**7**	0
Suzuki (Sea Bass), 4 oz	**110**	**0.5**	0
Tako (Octopus), 4 oz	**95**	**1**	0
Dipping Sauces: Average, 2 Tbsp	**30**	**0**	7
Ginger Vinegar Dressing, 2 Tbsp	**20**	**0**	5
Edamame (young green soybeans):			
Steamed (in pods), 4 oz	**60**	**3**	5
Boiled beans (no pods), 4 oz	**160**	**7**	12
Katsu-don Pork with Rice	**1100**	**39**	141
Miso Soup with Tofu pieces, 1 cup	**85**	**3**	11
Seaweed Salad, 1.5 oz	**20**	**2**	0
Sukiyaki (Beef/Tofu/Veg.), 8 oz	**400**	**24**	32
Tempura (Batter-fried Shrimp & Veggies)			
3 large shrimp & veggies	**320**	**18**	25
1 shrimp only	**60**	**4**	3
Teppan Yaki (Steak, Seafood & Veggies)			
10 oz serving	**470**	**30**	15
Teriyaki: Beef, 4 oz serving	**350**	**25**	4
Chicken, 4 oz serving	**260**	**9**	7
Salmon, medium, 6 oz serving	**270**	**8**	3
Sake Wine (16% alcohol), 3 fl.oz	**115**	**0**	7
Yakatori, 1 skewer, 2½ oz	**140**	**5**	1

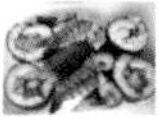

Kosher/Deli Foods

Kosher/Deli Foods	C	F	Cb
Bagel/Bialy, 1 small, 2 oz	**160**	**2**	32
Beiglach (Cheese Knish)	**350**	**17**	35
Blintzes: Average, 1 only	**120**	**1**	25
With Sour Cream & Preserves	**370**	**10**	30
Borscht: (Without Sour Cream), 1 cup	**85**	**3**	14
Diet/Reduced Calorie, 1 cup	**30**	**1**	7
Cabbage Roll (meat/rice), 5 oz	**170**	**6**	21
Chicken Broth: 1 cup	**80**	**8**	0
With vegetables	**100**	**8**	5
With noodles	**150**	**9**	16
Lowfat, plain, 1 cup	**25**	**1**	0
Cholent, 1 medium serving, 1 cup	**350**	**16**	48
Chopped Liver: 1 serving, 3 oz	**110**	**6**	5
With Egg Salad, ¼ cup	**100**	**7**	3
Farfel, dry, ½ cup	**90**	**0.5**	21
Hallah (Yeast Bread), 1 slice, 1 oz	**85**	**2**	14
Gefilte Fish Balls: Regular, medium, 2 oz	**55**	**2**	4
With Jelled Broth	**80**	**2**	6
Cocktail size, 1 oz	**30**	**1**	2
Sweet, medium, 2 oz	**65**	**2**	4
With Jelled Broth	**95**	**2**	9
Herring: Smoked, 2 oz	**120**	**8**	0
In Sour Cream, 2 oz	**150**	**10**	0
Kasha, cooked, ½ cup	**100**	**0.5**	20
Kipfel (Vanilla/Almdond Cookie), 1 piece	**60**	**2**	7
Knaidlach ~ See Matzo Balls			
Knish: Kasha/Potato, 1 only	**130**	**4**	22
Cheese, 1 only	**350**	**17**	35
Kreplach, beef, 1 piece	**40**	**1**	6
Kugel, potato/noodle, 1 serving	**300**	**20**	25
Latkes (Potato Pancake), 2 oz	**200**	**11**	22
3 Latkes with Sour Cran Apple Sauce	**750**	**25**	95
Lochshen: Plain, 1 cup	**130**	**2**	26
Pudding, 1 cup	**380**	**13**	48
Lox (Smoked Salmon), 2 oz	**65**	**2**	0
Mandelbrot (Almond Bread), 1 slice, ¼" thick	**45**	**2**	5
Matzo *(See Page 90)*, 1 oz board	**110**	**0.5**	21
Matzo Balls: 2 small, or 1 large, 2"	**90**	**3**	12
Extra large ball, 3"	**180**	**6**	24
Matzo Ball Soup:			
Cup with 2 small or 1 large ball	**150**	**5**	27
Bowl with Chicken & Noodles	**325**	**13**	34
Jerry's Deli, large bowl	**560**	**17**	56
New York Cheesecake, 4 oz	**350**	**24**	26
Pierogi, potato/cheese, 1 piece	**90**	**4**	11
Reuben S'wich with ½ lb Corned Beef	**920**	**60**	28
Schmaltz (Rend'd Chicken Fat), 1 Tbsp	**90**	**10**	0

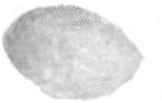

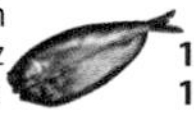

Updated Nutrition Data ~ www.CalorieKing.com
Persons with Diabetes ~ See Disclaimer (Page 24)

Korean Food

	C	F	Cb
Bibimbab (Veggies & Beef on Rice), 1 cup	**565**	**15**	89
Bulgogi (Barbeque Beef), 3.5 oz	**325**	**12**	15
Galbi (Short Ribs), 16 oz	**975**	**61**	16
Gujeolpan (Pancake with Meat & Vegetables), 1 cup with 1 pancake	**340**	**11**	39
Japchae (Noodle with Veggies & Meat), 1¼ cup	**365**	**19**	34
Sides:			
Kimchee (Cabbage Relish), ½ cup	**30**	**0**	6
Namool (Assorted Veggies) 1 cup	**125**	**6.5**	9
Soups: *Per Serving*			
Muguk (Radish & Chive Soup), 6 oz	**105**	**7**	6
Samgyetang (Ginseng Chicken Soup), Without Chicken Skin, 1 cup	**520**	**11**	60
With Chicken Skin, 1 cup	**725**	**35**	60
Yuk Gae Jang (Spicy Beef Soup), 1¼ cup	**180**	**13**	5

Lebanese/Middle East

	C	F	Cb
Baba Ghannouj, 2 Tbsp, 1 oz (Eggplant/Sesame Dip)	**70**	**6**	2
Baklava, 1 pastry, 1¾ oz (Pastry, Nuts, Syrup)	**245**	**18**	18
Cabbage Rolls, 1 roll, 3 oz (Cabbage Leaf, Meat, Rice)	**100**	**3**	12
Cous Cous, 1 serving (Semolina, Milk, Fruit, Nuts)	**400**	**21**	43
Felafel (Chick Pea Fritter): Fried, 1 medium, 1 oz	**60**	**4**	4
Hummus, ¼ cup, 2.2 oz	**105**	**3**	5
Fried Kibbi, 1 piece, 3 oz (Wheat, Meat, Pinenuts)	**180**	**8**	15
Kafta, 1 skewer, 1½ oz (Ground Lamb Sausage on Skewer)	**85**	**5**	2
Kibbeh Naye, 1 cup, 9 oz (Raw Lamb, Bulgur & Spices)	**450**	**18**	28
Lebanese Omelet, 1 serving, 4 oz (Egg, Spinach, Pinenuts, Onion)	**200**	**12**	13
Pilaf, 1 cup (Rice, Onion, Raisins, Apr., Spice)	**400**	**11**	60
Shawourma, 1 serving, 4 oz (Spit-Roast Beef)	**280**	**15**	2
Shish Kabob, 1 stick, 2½ oz	**130**	**7**	2
Spinach Pie, 1 piece, 3½ oz	**290**	**21**	20
Sweet Almond Sanbusak, 1 piece (Pastry, Almonds, Spices)	**200**	**15**	11
Tabouli, 1 serving, 4 oz	**125**	**7**	13
Tahini Sauce, average, 1 Tbsp	**90**	**8**	2

Mexican

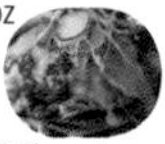

	C	F	Cb
Black Bean Soup, 1 bowl	**200**	**3**	34
Burritos *(Taco Bell):* Bean	**370**	**10**	55
Supreme® Beef	**440**	**18**	50
Chili, plain, ¼ cup	**90**	**6**	8
Chili con Carne: With Beans, 1 cup	**310**	**17**	15
Without Beans, 1 cup	**370**	**28**	10
Chimichangas, Beef, 5 oz	**400**	**19**	43
Chorizo Sausage, 2 oz	**265**	**23**	0
Churros, 1½ oz	**150**	**8**	18
Corn Chips, ½ cup, 1 oz	**160**	**10**	17
Costillas Ribs, 6 oz	**675**	**52**	0
Enchilada, average	**330**	**10**	49
Fajitas, Chicken	**200**	**7**	20
Guacamole, average, 2 Tbsp, 1 oz	**45**	**4**	2
Horchata: *Don Jose,* 1 cup, 8 fl. oz	**140**	**4**	25
Cacique, 1 pint bottle, 16 fl. oz	**320**	**7**	62
Margarita (with 1½ oz Tequila)	**160**	**0**	6
Masa (Pre-mixed for Tamales), 1 oz	**80**	**5**	9
Menudo, ½ cup	**55**	**1.5**	10
Nachos: *Del Taco,* Regular	**395**	**24**	40
Macho Nachos	**1145**	**63**	113
Taco Bell: BellGrande®	**760**	**43**	80
Supreme®	**470**	**26**	42
Nachos: With cheese, peppers, 1 portion (6-8 nachos), 7 oz	**600**	**33**	60
With cheese, beans, ground beef, peppers, 1 portion (6-8 nachos), 9 oz	**570**	**31**	56
Nopal Cactus Salad, 1 serving	**130**	**9**	11
Papas Fritas (Fried Potatoes) (1), 6 oz	**325**	**18**	40
Piloncillo (Brown Sugar): 1 Tbsp, 0.46 oz	**50**	**0**	13
Cone, small, 3", 3 oz	**325**	**0**	81
Quesadilla, Cheese *(Taco Bell)*	**490**	**28**	39
Queso Fresco, ¼ cup	**80**	**4.5**	8
Refried Beans, ¾ cup, 6 oz	**160**	**3**	26
Rice Pudding (Arroz Con Leche), 4 oz	**140**	**3**	24
Sopes (Gorditas), 2 oz	**120**	**0**	27
Taco *(Taco Bell)*: Regular, Crispy	**170**	**10**	13
Ranchero Chicken	**270**	**15**	21
Taco Supreme®	**220**	**14**	14
Double Decker® Taco	**340**	**14**	39
Taco Salad with Salsa	**840**	**52**	85
Taco Sauce, average, ¼ cup	**15**	**0**	3
Taco Shell, regular	**50**	**2**	8
Tamales, Beef/Chicken, average 4.5 oz	**250**	**11**	27
Taquitos, Beef & Cheese, 4.5 oz	**330**	**15**	36
Tostada *(Taco Bell)*	**250**	**10**	29
Tortilla, Corn, 6" diameter	**70**	**1**	14
Tortilla Chips, 1 oz	**150**	**8**	18

Extra Listings of Mexican Dishes:

- **Fast-Foods Section** *(Taco Bell, Del Taco)*
- **Canned Bean/Chili Products:** *See Pages 113-118*

Mexican (Cont)

	C	F	Cb
Breads: Bolillos, 1 roll, 3½ oz	**240**	**4**	42
Telera, 2 oz	**150**	**1.5**	19
Mexican Cornbread, 4" square	**210**	**11**	19
Cakes, Cookies, Pastries			
Banderilla (Pastry Puff), 1 shell	**140**	**10**	8
Bigotes, 7"	**570**	**22**	44
Calvos, 2½ oz	**320**	**18**	38
Capirotada (Bread Pudding), 10 oz	**810**	**38**	107
Cinnamon Cookies, 2	**125**	**8**	13
Cocadas, 1 oz	**120**	**6**	15
Cortadillo, 1 cookie, 1.9 oz	**300**	**11**	48
Concha (All Colors):			
Small (3" diameter), 2½ oz	**250**	**8**	38
Medium (4" diameter), 3½ oz	**350**	**11**	53
Large (5" diameter), 5½ oz	**550**	**18**	84
Cream Puff with Custard, 4¼ oz	**255**	**14**	25
Cuerno, 2 oz	**200**	**4.5**	34
Cuerno Fine, 2¾ oz	**330**	**17**	40
Donut, large, 4", 3½ oz	**440**	**21**	58
Elotes, 3½ oz	**450**	**24**	51
Empanadas (Average all types):			
Small, 2 oz	**230**	**10**	28
Regular, 3 oz	**300**	**14**	42
Fiesta Cookie, 2¼ oz	**280**	**8**	47
Galletas Mixtas (1), 1 oz	**100**	**2.5**	16
Guayaba, 3¼ oz	**360**	**14**	53
Jelly Rolls, 3¼ oz	**240**	**4**	46
Mantecadites (Almond Shortbread), 4½ oz	**670**	**42**	64
Mini Pound Cake, 3 oz	**260**	**12**	33
Mini Cupcakes, 1¾ oz	**180**	**8**	25
Muffins/Nino Enbuelto, large, 6 oz	**465**	**11**	48
Nuez, 3¼ oz	**380**	**17**	52
Ojo De Buey, 4 oz	**360**	**15**	55
Oreja (Elephant Ear), 3 oz	**310**	**15**	38
Pan Dulce (Mexican Sweet Bread), 1 bun	**330**	**10**	45
Panquecitos, 2½ oz	**260**	**11**	36
Piedras, 4 oz	**470**	**15**	76
Polvorones, 3 oz	**370**	**18**	48
Puerquitos, 5 oz	**600**	**24**	88
Rebanadas, 3½ oz	**390**	**18**	51
Roles De Canela (Cinn. Roll), 4½ oz	**490**	**15**	81
Roscas, 2¾ oz	**360**	**18**	44
Semitas, 3 oz	**300**	**10**	46
Sopapillas (flaky pastry puffs), 1 piece	**100**	**7**	10
with Honey & Cream	**200**	**14**	18
Strawberry Crema Roll (⅙), 2½ oz	**240**	**5**	45

Extra Food Listings ~ See CalorieKing.com

Polish

	C	F	Cb
Cabbage Rolls with Sour Cream, 2 sm.	**220**	**10**	30
Chicken Casserole w/ Mushrooms, 1 cup	**520**	**27**	5
Kielbasa (Sausages, Onions, fried), 2 large	**350**	**28**	2
Meatballs in Sour Cream, 3 x 1½" balls	**300**	**16**	11
Pierogi, Fruit/Vegetables, 3" ball	**80**	**2**	15
Pork Goulash (Pork/Vegetable Stew)	**550**	**21**	38
Pot Roast with Vegetables	**630**	**21**	28

Soul Foods

	C	F	Cb
Breakfast Sausage, fried, 2 patties	**250**	**17**	0
Brunswick Stew, 1 cup, 8.5 oz	**320**	**14**	19
Cornbread, homemade, 3 oz	**200**	**7.5**	28
Fatback, raw, ¼ oz	**60**	**6.5**	0
Ham Hock	**90**	**6.5**	2
Hog Maw	**45**	**2.5**	0
Hominy, cooked, ¾ cup	**110**	**0.5**	25
Hush Puppies, 5 pieces	**260**	**12**	35
Kale, cooked, ½ cup	**20**	**0.5**	4
Oxtail	**70**	**3.5**	0
Pig's Ear, ¼ ear	**50**	**3**	0
Pig's Foot, ½ foot	**70**	**4.5**	0
Pig's Tail, ⅓ tail	**115**	**10**	0
Poke Salad, cooked, ½ cup	**16**	**0.5**	3
Pork Brains	**40**	**2.5**	0
Pork Chitterlings, simmered, 3 oz	**260**	**25**	0
Pork Cracklings, ½ oz	**80**	**6**	0
Pork Neck Bones	**65**	**4**	0
Pork Skin, 1 cup	**70**	**4.5**	0
Pork Tongue, ⅓ tongue	**75**	**5.5**	0
Possum	**65**	**3**	0
Sousemeat	**60**	**4.5**	0
Succotash, ½ cup	**80**	**1**	17
Sweet Potato Pie, ⅛ of 9" pie	**250**	**12**	34
Tripe, 2 oz	**55**	**2**	0
Vienna Sausage, 2 small	**90**	**8**	1
1 small	**45**	**4**	0.5

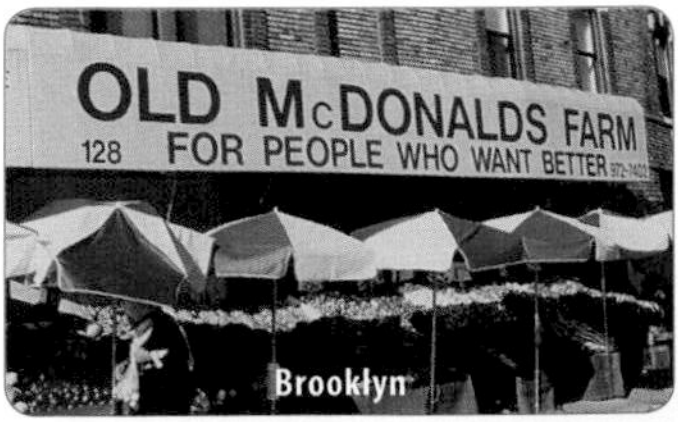

Spanish

	C	F	Cb
Arroz Abanda (Fish with Rice)	**340**	8	31
Arroz Con Pollo (Rice/Chicken Salad)	**500**	23	50
Clams Marinara, 8 clams	**330**	16	22
Cochifrito (Lamb with Lemon/Garlic)	**650**	25	5
Cochinillo Asado, 2 slices (Rst Suckling Pig)	**300**	15	3
Cocido Madrileno (Madrid-Style Boiled Dinner)	**450**	27	18
Flan de Leche (Caramel Custard)	**325**	9	52
Fritadera de Ternera (Sauteed Veal)	**450**	27	2
Gazpacho, 1 bowl	**60**	0	15
Paella a la Valenciana (Chicken & Shellfish Rice)	**900**	42	70
Pollo a la Espanola (Chicken)	**475**	30	4
Ternera al Jerez (Veal with Sherry)	**660**	29	6
Zarzuela (Fish & Shellfish Medley)	**530**	27	40

Thai Foods

	C	F	Cb
Appetizers: Satay Pork, 1 oz	**100**	4	2
Spring Roll, 1¼ oz	**110**	6	13
Soups: Tom Yam (Hot & Sour):			
Spicy Shrimp/Seafood, 1 cup	**100**	4	6
1 bowl	**160**	7	10
Vegetarian, 1 cup	**50**	0	11
Curries: Chicken with Ginger, 1 cup	**390**	34	4
Thick Red Curry withBeef, 1 cup	**600**	50	7
Thai Chicken Curry, 1 cup	**340**	23	4
Massaman Curry, 1 cup	**680**	57	8
Green Curry with Pork, 1 cup	**480**	44	5
Pad Thai, Large serving, 18 oz	**990**	38	125
Fish: Steamed with Spicy Thai Sce	**450**	8	46
Crispy Fried, 5 oz	**290**	15	9
Spicy Chicken (with veggies), stir-fry	**450**	22	14
Spicy Garlic Tofu with veggies, stir-fry	**340**	18	18
Sticky Thai Rice: Plain 1 cup, 6 oz	**170**	0.5	36
With Coconut & Sesame Seeds, 1 cup	**880**	28	120
Stir-fried Rice Noodles, 1 cup, 5½ oz	**270**	9	40
Stir-fried Vegetables, 1 cup	**100**	3	18
Salads: Green Papaya Salad	**160**	0	40
Spicy Prawn, 9 shrimp	**170**	3	15
Thai Chicken, 1 serving	**330**	9	17
Thai Beef Salad, 1 serving	**260**	9	15
Thai Noodle, 1 serving	**410**	13	45
Satay Chicken & Peanut Sauce:			
1 satay stick	**390**	24	20
Sauces: Peanut Satay, ½ cup, 4 oz	**160**	10	13

Vietnamese

	C	F	Cb
Banh Cuon (Steam Rice with Pork), 1 roll	**105**	7	8
Bo Nuong (Beef Satay), 2 sticks	**265**	9	4
Bo Xao Dau Phong (Ginger Beef with Onion, Fish Sauce)	**750**	30	10
Ca Chien Gung (Whole Snapper/Ginger)	**600**	16	6
Canh Chay (Vegetable/Tofu Soup)	**80**	3	13
Cari (Curry) Chicken, 1 cup	**475**	29	16
Cari (Curry) Chicken with Rice Noodle, cup curry & cup cooked noodles	**660**	29	60
Cari (Curry) Chicken, with Steamed Rice, cup curry & cup rice	**650**	29	55
Cuu Xao Lan (Curried Lamb, Veggies in Coconut)	**900**	40	80
Ga Chien (Crisp Chick + Plum Sauce)	**900**	40	105
Ga Nuong (Chicken Satay + Sauce)	**240**	10	4
Ga Xao Rau (Marinated Chicken Braised with Vegetables)	**800**	26	100
Gio Lua (Lean Pork Pie), ⅙ of pie	**245**	12	0
Goi Cuon (Cold Spring Rolls), each	**60**	1	7
Rau Cai Xao Chay (Stir Fried Veges)	**400**	15	65
Thit Bo Vien (Beef Balls), 6 balls	**225**	14	2
Thit Heo Goi Baup Cai, each (Spicy Cabbage Rolls with Pork)	**200**	7	11
Soup: *Per Bowl (1½ Cup)*			
Bun Bo Hue (Hot & Spicy Soup			
Without Pork Feet	**340**	9	35
With Pork Feet	**830**	45	35
Chicken & Rice Noodle Soup	**400**	3	55
Pho Bo (Beef Noodle Soup)	**410**	7	59
Pho Ga (Chicken Noodle Soup)	**460**	6	58
Pho Tai (Rare Beef & Noodle Soup)	**440**	7	73
Salad: *Per ½ Cup*			
Goi Du Du (Green Papaya Salad)	**155**	3	29
Sauce: Nuoc Cham (Hot Sauce)	**5**	0	1

Gourmet & Miscellaneous

	C	F	Cb
Ants Eggs/Larvae, 1 Tbsp	**20**	0	0
Ants, chocolate coated, 3 Tbsp	**140**	7	2
Bee Maggots, canned, 3 Tbsp	**65**	2	0
Caviar, black/red, 1 Tbsp	**40**	3	0
Caterpillars, canned, 2 oz	**60**	2	0
Frog Legs, fried, 1 pair (large)	**125**	7	0
Haggis, boiled, 4 oz	**350**	24	22
Locusts, roasted, 1 oz	**35**	1	0
Silkworms, raw, 1 oz	**60**	2	0
Snails in garlic butter, 6 large	**200**	10	4
Snake, roasted, 4 oz	**160**	6	0

FOR MORE RESTAURANTS
See www.CalorieKing.com

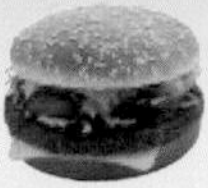

For Complete Menu Listings
& Extended Nutritional Data
~ See CalorieKing.com

A&W® (May '10)

Burgers:	C	F	Cb
Hamburger	380	19	33
Cheeseburger	420	21	37
Double Cheeseburger	680	38	44
Bacon Cheeseburger	530	30	39
Bacon Double Cheeseburger	760	45	45
Papa Burger	690	39	44
Papa Single Burger	470	25	38
Sandwiches: Crispy Chicken	550	25	52
Grilled Chicken	400	15	31
Chicken Strips: 3 pieces	500	29	32
Hot Dogs: Plain	310	19	23
Coney Chili Dog	340	20	26
Coney Chili Cheese Dog	380	23	28
Corn Dog Nuggets: 5 pieces	180	8	20
8 pieces	280	13	32
Fries/Sides:			
French Fries: Small/Kids, 2.5 oz	200	8	28
Regular, 4 oz	310	12	45
Large, 5.5 oz	430	17	61
Cheese Fries: 6 oz	390	18	50
Chili Cheese Fries, 7 oz	410	17	52
Cheese Curds, Breaded/Fried, 5 oz	570	40	27
Onion Rings: Reg., Breaded, 4 oz	350	16	45
Large, 5.5 oz	480	27	62
Dipping Sauces: BBQ, 1 oz	40	0	10
Honey Mustard, 1 oz	100	6	12
Ranch, 1 oz	160	17	2
Desserts: *Per Small Serving*			
Polar Swirl: M&M/Oreo, average	700	25	107
Reese's	740	31	97
Sundaes: Choc.;Caramel; Fudge, av.	340	9	55
Strawberry	300	8	47
Soft Serve, Vanilla cone, 5.5 oz	260	7	41
Milkshakes: Strawb., small, 16 fl.oz	670	29	90
Choc.; Vanilla, av., Small, 16 fl.oz	710	30	100
Medium, 20 fl.oz	890	38	123
Floats:			
A&W Root Beer: 20 oz	350	5	77
Large, 32 fl.oz	640	10	136
Diet, 20 oz	170	5	30
Freeze, A&W Root Beer, 16 oz	430	9	79
Sodas:			
Sodas/Pepsi, average, Sml,11.5 fl.oz	140	0	39
Medium, 14 fl.oz	180	0	49
Large, 22 fl.oz	280	0	77
A&W Root Beer: Medium, 14 fl.oz	290	0	76
Diet, 20 fl.oz	0	0	0
Tea: Lipton Raspberry, Med., 14 fl.oz	140	0	37

Updated Nutrition Data ~ www.CalorieKing.com
Persons with Diabetes ~ See Disclaimer (Page 24)

Applebee's® (May '10)

Shareable Appetizers: *As Served*	C	F	Cb
Buffalo Chicken Wings: Classic	710	49	7
Honey BBQ	790	35	59
Hot	720	49	8
Boneless: Classic	1170	69	66
Honey BBQ	1240	55	117
Hot	1170	70	67
Chili Cheese Nachos	1680	107	133
Crunchy Onion Rings	1230	59	161
Dynamite Shrimp	730	54	40
Mozzarella Sticks (9)	940	46	84
Quesadillas: Cheese Grande	1300	87	85
Chicken Grande	1460	90	90
Chicken: *Includes Standard Sides*			
Chicken Fried Chicken	1250	60	114
Chicken Tenders: Basket	1000	59	81
Platter	1300	77	104
Fiesta Lime Chicken	1230	67	97
Margherita Chicken	750	27	67
Combos: *Without Sides or Toppings*			
Steak: with Fried Shrimp	630	31	35
with Grilled Shrimp	390	19	2
with Honey BBQ Chicken	530	13	25
with Riblets	950	47	38
Pasta Bowls: *As Served*			
Chicken Broccoli Alfredo	1200	58	104
Crispy Orange Chicken	1900	73	231
Shrimp Fettuccine Alfredo	1220	62	105
Three-Cheese Chicken Penne	1310	61	120
Realburgers: *Without Fries*			
Bacon Cheddar Cheeseburger	940	60	48
Cheeseburger	850	52	47
Cowboy Burger	1120	67	74
Fire Pit Bacon Burger	1070	73	50
Hamburger	770	46	47
Quesadilla Burger	1420	104	45
Steakhouse Burger with A1 Sauce	1190	82	63
Ribs & Fajitas: *Includes Standard Sides*			
Applebees Riblets: Basket	1110	57	89
Platter	1700	88	130
Sizzling Fajitas: Chicken	1470	57	163
Combo	1520	61	163
Steak	1560	66	164

Applebees® cont... (May '10)

Under 500 Calories: Includes Sides	C	F	Cb
Asiago Peppercorn Steak	390	14	26
Asian Crunch Salad with Dressing	490	9	57
Grilled Dijon Chicken & Portobello	450	16	32
Grilled Shrimp & Island Rice	380	4.5	59
Spicy Shrimp Diavolo	500	10	79
***Sandwiches:** Without Sides*			
Bacon, Cheese Chicken Grill	720	33	47
California Turkey Club	1050	63	62
Seafood: As Served			
Double Crunch Shrimp	1280	70	129
Garlic Herb Salmon	750	37	59
Hand-Battered Fish & Chips	1560	105	106
***Sliders:** Without Fries*			
BBQ Pulled Pork	1020	48	89
Cheeseburger	1240	80	81
French Dip	830	49	74
***Sigature Steaks:** Without Sides*			
Bourbon Street w/ Mshrms & Onions	600	38	9
Shrimp 'N Parmesan Sirloin	540	28	5
***Steak & Toppers:** Without Sides*			
House Sirloin, 9 oz	310	13	0
New York Strip, 12 oz	590	39	1
Ribeye, 12 oz	590	39	0
***Salads:** Regular, Without Dressing Unless Indicated*			
Apple Walnut Chicken	440	19	17
Grilled Shrimp 'N Spinach	720	53	25
Oriental Grilled Chicken w/ Dressing	1240	77	87
Santa Fe Chicken	900	54	51
Sides: Chili bowl	540	32	24
Loaded Baked Potato	450	35	28
Loaded Mashed Potato	430	29	30
Salads: Caesar, small	90	3.5	10
House, small	230	15	12
***Soup:** Per Bowl*			
French Onion	280	16	19
Tomato Basil Soup	250	14	27
***Desserts:** As Served*			
Maple Butter Blondie	990	52	116
Shooters: Chocolate Moose	450	31	44
Hot Fudge Sundae	340	18	45
Triple Chocolate Meltdown	810	46	91

Arby's® (May '10)

Sandwiches:	C	F	Cb
Beef 'n Cheddar Sandwiches:			
Regular	430	19	42
Medium	530	25	42
Large	650	33	44
Roast Beef Sandwiches:			
Regular, 3 oz Beef	350	13	37
Medium, 5 oz Beef	450	19	37
Roastburgers: All American	390	16	40
Bacon Cheddar	430	18	39
Bacon Bleu	450	21	39
Chicken:			
Chicken Bacon & Swiss: Crispy	590	27	54
Roast	470	19	43
Chicken Fillet: Crispy	520	24	51
Roast	400	16	40
Melts:			
Arby's Melt	320	11	38
Ham & Swiss Melt	300	8	37
Market Fresh Sandwiches:			
Corned Beef Reuben	690	32	65
Pecan Grilled Chicken Salad	870	44	88
Roast Ham & Swiss	750	30	85
Roast Turkey Ranch & Bacon	850	37	84
Ultimate BLT	880	46	84
Popcorn Chicken:			
Regular, 4.75 oz	360	16	27
Large, 6.5 oz	490	22	38
Toasted Subs:			
Classic Italian	590	30	57
French Dip & Swiss	500	17	59
Philly Beef	570	27	55
Turkey Bacon Club	570	24	56
***Regular Combos:** Includes Medium Curly Fries & 22 fl.oz Pepsi Without Ice*			
Beef 'n Cheddar Sandwich	1245	48	183
Chicken Bacon & Swiss Crispy	1405	56	195
Corned Beef Reuben Sandwich	1505	61	206
Pecan Grilled Chicken Salad S'wich	1645	73	223
Popcorn Chicken	1150	45	160
Roast Turkey & Swiss Sandwich	1525	57	219
***Market Fresh Chopped Salads:** Without Dressing*			
Italian	390	31	10
Turkey Club	250	14	9
Sides & Sidekickers:			
Curly Fries: Small, 4.5 oz	410	22	48
Medium, 6 oz	540	29	64
Large, 7 oz	640	34	76
Jalapeno Bites, regular, 5 bites	300	17	32
Loaded Potato Bites, regular,5 bites	340	20	29
Mozzarella Sticks, regular, 4 sticks	430	23	36
Onion Petals, regular, 3.5 oz	330	18	38
Potato Cakes, small, 2 cakes	260	14	16

Updated Nutrition Data ~ www.CalorieKing.com
Persons with Diabetes ~ See Disclaimer (Page 24)

Arby's® cont... (May '10)

	C	F	Cb
Kids Menu:			
Curly Fries, 2.7 oz	240	13	29
Popcorn Chicken, 3.5 oz	260	12	20
Jr Roast Beef Sandwich, w/o Mayo	300	9	37
Breakfast: *Per Serving*			
Blueberry Muffin, 3 oz	280	14	33
Biscuits: Plain	250	11	32
Bacon, Egg & Cheese	450	26	34
Ham, Egg & Cheese	420	22	34
Sausage, Egg & Cheese	590	42	35
Croissants: Bacon, Egg & Cheese	390	24	24
Ham & Cheese	270	14	22
Ham, Egg & Cheese	360	20	24
Sausage, Egg & Cheese	530	40	24
Sourdoughs: Bacon, Egg & Cheese	540	27	46
Egg & Cheese	440	19	45
Ham, Egg & Cheese	480	20	46
Sausage Egg & Cheese	530	40	24
Wraps: Bacon, Egg & Cheese	620	33	45
Sausage, Egg & Cheese	740	47	45
Sauces: Cheddar Cheese, side, 1½ oz	45	3	3
Marinara, 1½ oz	35	1.5	5
Tangy Southwest, 1½ oz	230	24	3
Dipping Sauces: Tangy BBQ, 1 oz	45	0	11
Buffalo, 1 oz	10	0.5	2
Honey Dijon Mustard, 1 oz	130	12	5
Desserts:			
Turnovers: Apple with Icing	340	15	48
Cherry Turnover with Icing	340	15	47
Shakes: *17 fl.oz*			
Chocolate; Jamocha, average	620	17	108
Vanilla	540	17	85
Drinks:			
Iced FruiTea: Mandarin Peach, 11 fl.oz	90	0	23
Passion Fruit, 11 fl.oz	100	0	25
Mountain Dew, 22 fl.oz	300	0	84
Pepsi, 22 fl.oz	275	0	77

Arthur Treachers® (May '10)

	C	F	Cb
Meals: *With Triple Chips*			
Boats: Chicken, 9.8 oz	520	33	53
Fish, 10.2 oz	560	29	57
Shrimp, 9.8 oz	610	29	72
Sides: *Per Ala Carte Serving*			
Baked Potato, 8 oz	210	0	48
Batter Dip't Chicken, 2.6 oz	260	7	35
Batter Dip't Fish, 3.7 oz	190	6	26
Chips: 1 Regular, 6.5 oz	370	20	46
1 Triple, 15 oz	850	45	105
Cole Slaw, 3.5 oz	140	9	15
Hushpuppies, 6 pieces, 7 oz	830	30	127
Onion Rings, 1 regular, 4.6 oz	260	1.5	56

Atlanta Bread Co® (May '10)

	C	F	Cb
Sandwiches:			
Chicken Salad on Sourdough	440	19	42
Honey Maple Ham on Honey Wheat	410	5	64
Kid's Peanut Butter & Jelly on French	550	15	89
Kid's Grilled Cheese on French	390	15	46
Tuna Salad on French	630	33	57
Turkey on Nine Grain	370	6	50
Veggie on Nine Grain	500	25	52
Signature Sandwiches: *On Focaccia Unless Indicated*			
ABC Special on French Baguette	750	38	57
Bella Chicken	610	38	34
California Avocado	930	50	98
Chicken Waldorf	450	29	26
NY Hot Pastrami on Rye	660	29	59
Turkey Bacon Rustica	960	56	62
Paninis: Chicken Pesto	710	26	80
Chicken Cordon Bleu	670	19	80
Cubano	650	19	80
Italian Vegetarian	570	16	84
Turkey Club	710	24	81
Salads: *Without Dressing*			
Caesar	150	9	7
Balsamic Bleu Salad	330	18	35
Chopstix Chicken Salad	240	10	22
Greek Salad	240	16	15
House Salad	90	2	13
Salsa Fresca Salmon Salad	560	29	40
Soups: *Per 1¼ Cup*			
Broccoli Cheese	250	17	14
Chicken & Sausage Gumbo	190	6	24
Chili, Beef/Frontier, average	290	10	30
Tomato Fennel & Dill	290	23	18
Wisconsin Cheese	290	15	24

For Extra Menu Items ~ see CalorieKing.com

Au Bon Pain® (May '10)

	C	F	Cb
Bagels: *Per Bagel*			
Asiago Cheese	370	8	57
Cinnamon Crisp	410	7	77
Everything	320	4	60
Jalapeno Double Cheddar	340	10	53
Honey 9 Grain	350	4	69
Cream Cheese Spreads: *Per 2 oz*			
Lite Cream Cheese	120	9	5
Honey Pecan, 2.5 oz	200	16	10
Vegetable	170	16	3

Continued Next Page...

Au Bon Pain® cont... (May '10)

Breakfast Sandwiches:	C	F	Cb
Egg on a Bagel	430	12	58
With Bacon	490	16	58
With Bacon & Cheese	570	23	59
With Cheese	510	18	59
Smkd. Salm. & Wasabi/Onion Dill Bagel	430	11	64
Café Sandwiches			
Arizona Chicken	710	29	62
Baja Turkey	700	27	71
Caprese	680	32	65
Chicken Pesto	660	24	66
Mozzarella Chicken	680	24	67
Pastrami	590	23	52
Spicy Tuna	470	16	60
Hot Sandwiches and Melts			
Baked Turkey	720	26	79
Eggplant & Mozzarella	670	30	73
Steakhouse on Ciabatta	640	23	73
Wraps: Chicken Caesar Asiago	610	28	61
Mediterranean Wrap	610	29	73
Southwest Tuna	760	41	66
Thai Peanut Chicken	530	15	79
Harvest Rice Bowls:			
Angus Steak Teriyaki	660	18	101
with Brown Rice	620	19	86
Mayan Chicken	550	11	87
with Brown Rice	510	13	72
Breads: *Per Piece*			
Artisan Honey Baguette, 4.7 oz	340	5	66
Bread Bowl , 9.2 oz	620	3	123
Farm House Rolls, 4.5 oz	360	7	63
Focaccia, 4.6 oz	360	7	62
Rosemary Garlic Bread Stick, 2 oz	190	5	31
Soups: *Per Medium 12 oz Bowl*			
Baked Stuffed Potato	350	20	29
Carrot Ginger	140	5	22
Chicken Gumbo	180	8	21
Corn & Green Chili Bisque	260	15	27
Cream of Chicken & Wild Rice	240	14	22
Italian Wedding	170	7	19
Southern Black-Eyed Pea	170	2	29
Tomato Florentine	130	3	18
Vegetarian Chili	220	2	39
Wild Mushroom Bisque	190	9	22
Kid's Menu, Macaroni & Cheese	330	10	24
Salads: *Without Dressing*			
Apple & Goat Cheese, 10 oz	290	13	39
Caesar Asiago Salad, 6 oz	220	12	18
Chef's Salad, 8.9 oz	250	15	7

Au Bon Pain® cont... (May '10)

Salads (Cont): *Without Dressing*	C	F	Cb
Garden, 6.5 oz	70	2	12
Grilled Chicken Caesar Asiago, 8.5 oz	300	13	18
Mandarin Sesame Chicken, 9.7 oz	310	17	29
Mediterranean Chicken, 10.3 oz	290	16	12
Thai Peanut Chicken, 11 oz	240	8	19
Tuna Garden, 10.5 oz	240	12	15
Turkey Cobb, 11 oz	330	19	14
Dressing: Caesar, 2 oz	270	28	4
Hazelnut Vinaigrette, 2 oz	270	25	11
Sesame Ginger, 2 oz	230	20	12
Bakery: *Per Item*			
Brownie, Blondie, 4 oz	460	33	59
Cookies: English Toffee, 1.6 oz	250	14	27
Shortbread, 2.3 oz	340	20	37
Croissants: *Per Croissant, Filled*			
Almond	600	38	55
Apple	280	11	44
Apple Almond	460	23	59
Chocolate	440	22	58
Raspberry Cheese	370	17	46
Sweet Cheese	400	19	49
Desserts: Creme de Fleur	500	25	56
Lemon Pound Cake, 5 oz	520	25	67
Mint Chocolate Pound Cake, 5 oz	530	29	64
Strudel: Apple; Cherry, average	450	25	50
Muffins: Blueberry	490	17	74
Carrot/Cranberry Walnut	550	26	69
Low-Fat Triple Berry	300	3	65
Raisin Bran	480	11	85
Beverages: Caffe Latte, 16 fl.oz	260	14	21
Hot Chocolate, 16 fl.oz	460	15	74
Peach Iced Tea, 22 fl.oz	240	0	61
Coffee Blast, 16 fl.oz	440	21	71
Strawberry Smoothie, 16 fl.oz	310	1	66

For Complete Nutritional Data ~ see CalorieKing.com

Auntie Anne's® (May '10)

Pretzels: *With Butter*	C	F	Cb
Almond	390	6	74
Cinnamon Sugar	470	12	84
Garlic	350	5	65
Jalapeno	330	5	63
Original	340	5	65
Original Stix, 6 sticks	340	5	65
Sesame	400	10	67
Sour Cream & Onion	360	5	68

Updated Nutrition Data ~ www.CalorieKing.com
Persons with Diabetes ~ See Disclaimer (Page 24)

Auntie Anne's® cont... (May '10)

Pretzels: Without Butter	C	F	Cb
Almond Pretzel	350	2	74
Cinnamon Sugar	380	1	84
Garlic Pretzel	310	1	65
Jalapeno	300	1	63
Original	310	1	65
Original Stix, 6 sticks	310	1	65
Sesame	360	6	67
Dipping Sauces			
Caramel Dip, 1.5 oz	130	3	23
Cheese Sce; Hot Salsa Cheese, av., 1.1 oz	90	7	3
Cream Cheese, 1¼ oz	80	6	1
Heated Marinara Sauce, 2 oz	45	0	7
Sweet Dip, 1.4 oz	130	0	32
Sweet Mustard, 1¼ oz	60	2	10
***Beverages:** Per Serving*			
Auntie Anne's Lemonade, 21 fl.oz	260	0	66
Dutch Ice (20 fl.oz): Blue Raspberry	240	0	62
Kiwi-Banana	220	0	53
Lemonade	300	0	76
Mocha	390	12	73
Pina Colada	300	0	73
Strawberry	230	0	58
Wild Cherry	280	0	69
Dutch Smoothie: *Per 20 fl.oz*			
Blue Raspberry	440	15	72
Kiwi-Banana	420	15	66
Lemonade	470	15	81
Mocha	540	22	79
Pina Colada	470	15	79
Strawberry	430	15	69

Back Yard Burgers® (May '10)

Burgers:	C	F	Cb
American Cheeseburger ⅓ lb	730	44	47
Back Yard Burger ⅓ lb	680	39	47
Black Jack	780	49	48
Bleu Cheeseburger: ⅓ lb	780	47	47
⅔ lb	1270	86	47
Cheddar Cheeseburger: ⅓ lb	790	48	47
⅔ lb	1290	88	47
Jr Burger	530	27	47
Mushroom Swiss	790	49	45
Pepper Jack, ⅓ lb	740	45	47
Swiss Cheeseburger: ⅓ lb	790	48	47
⅔ lb	1290	88	47
Chicken Sandwiches:			
Blackened Chicken	540	24	53
Crispy Chicken	590	26	65
Grilled Chicken	350	4.5	47
Hawaiian Chicken	450	11	59

Back Yard Burgers® (May '10)

Specialities:	C	F	Cb
Big Dog	500	33	32
Bak-Pak: Chicken Tender Meal	1110	71	91
Dog	320	18	29
Chicken Tender Meal	1260	79	102
Chili Cheese Big Dog	630	44	34
Garden Veggie Burger	400	8	57
***Sides:** Per Serving*			
Chili	150	9	8
Seasoned Fries: regular, 6 oz	640	45	58
large, 9 oz	960	68	87
***Salads:** Without Dressing*			
Blackened Chicken	330	15	25
Fried Chicken	410	19	41
Garden Fresh	100	2	20
Grilled Chicken	220	4	23
Side Salad	30	0	6
***Dressings:** Per Serving*			
Bleu Cheese	220	24	1
Honey Mustard	240	23	7
Ranch	150	15	2
***Desserts:** Per Serving*			
Cobblers: Apple	360	14	59
Blackberry	290	8	51
Cherry	350	12	59
Peach	330	11	56
***Shakes:** Per 12 fl.oz*			
Chocolate; Strawberry	630	29	83
Vanilla	620	28	71

For Complete Nutritional Data ~ see CalorieKing.com

Baja Fresh® (May '10)

Burritos: As Served	C	F	Cb
Baja Burrito: With Chicken	790	38	65
With Steak	850	46	67
Bare Burrito: With Charbroiled Chkn	640	7	97
Veggie and Cheese	580	10	101
Bean & Cheese Burrito: With Chicken	970	35	96
With Steak	1030	43	97
Vegetarian	840	33	96
Burrito Mexicano: With Chicken	790	13	117
With Steak	860	21	118
Burrito Ultimo: With Chicken	880	36	84
With Steak	950	44	85
Grilled Vegetarian	800	33	94
***Fajitas:** As Served, Without Tortilla Chips*			
Chicken with Corn Tortillas	860	24	105
Chicken with Flour Tortillas	1140	33	147

Continued Next Page . . .

Baja Fresh® cont... (May '10)

	C	F	Cb
Nachos: *: As Served*			
With Charbroiled Chicken	**2020**	110	164
With Charbroiled Steak	**2120**	118	163
With Cheese	**1890**	108	163
Quesadillas: *As Served*			
With Charbroiled Chkn	**1330**	80	84
With Charbroiled Steak	**1430**	87	84
With Cheese	**1200**	78	84
Vegetarian	**1260**	78	96
Tacos: *As Served*			
Baja Fish Taco, Fried	**250**	13	27
Grilled Mahi Mahi Taco	**230**	9	26
Original Baja Style Taco: W/ Chicken	**210**	5	28
With Charbroiled Shrimp	**200**	5	28
Salads: *As Served, Without Dressing*			
Baja Ensalada:			
With Charbroiled Chicken	**310**	7	18
With Charbroiled Shrimp	**230**	6	18
With Charbroiled Steak	**450**	18	18
Tostadas: Charbroiled Fish	**1130**	55	99
Charbroiled Shrimp	**1120**	55	99
Charbroiled Steak	**1230**	63	98
Savory Pork Carnitas	**1180**	62	100

For Complete Nutritional Data ~ see CalorieKing.com

Baskin Robbins® (May '10)

	C	F	Cb
Ice Creams: *Per 4 oz Scoop*			
Classic Flavors: Cherries Jubilee	**240**	12	30
Chocolate	**260**	14	33
Jamoca Almond Fudge	**270**	15	31
Mint Chocolate Chip	**270**	16	28
Old Fashioned Butter Pecan	**280**	18	24
Oreo Cookies 'n Cream	**280**	15	32
Pralines 'n Cream	**280**	14	35
Rainbow Sherbet	**160**	2	34
Reese's P'nut Butter Cup	**300**	18	31
Vanilla	**260**	16	26
Very Berry Strawberry	**220**	11	28
World Class Chocolate	**280**	16	31
Premium Churned: *Per 2.5 oz Scoop*			
Light: Aloha Brownie	**150**	5	26
Cappuccino	**140**	5	20
Raspberry Chip	**140**	4	24
Frozen Yogurt, Fat-Free Van., 4 oz	**150**	0	32
Fruit Blast Bars, all flavors, average	**50**	0	14
Sorbets: *Per 4 oz Scoop*			
Lemon; Strawberry	**130**	0	34
Mango	**120**	0	32

Baskin Robbins cont... (May '10)

	C	F	Cb
Sundaes:			
Classic Sundaes: Banana Royale	**620**	28	87
Brownie	**920**	47	119
Banana Split	**1010**	34	173
Premium Sundaes:			
Chocolate Chip Cookie Dough	**990**	43	138
Reese's Peanut Butter Cup	**1220**	80	109
Soft Serve Sundaes: *Per 10 oz Regular*			
Caramel	**580**	21	89
Strawberry	**450**	18	59
Sundae Cups: Oreo	**330**	15	45
Reese's Peanut Butter Cup	**390**	24	36
Pralines 'n Cream	**330**	16	44
Soft Serve:			
'31 Below' Blends: *Per 16 oz Cup*			
Chocolate Oreo	**1290**	55	187
Fudge Brownie	**1390**	58	199
Heath	**1160**	54	151
Jamoca Oreo	**860**	33	128
Oreo	**1000**	41	143
Reese's Peanut Butter Cup	**1220**	67	134
Strawberry Banana	**710**	23	112
Cups: Vanilla: Kid's, 3 oz cup	**140**	6	19
Regular, 6 oz cup	**280**	11	37
Large, 9 oz cup	**430**	17	58
Fruit Cream:			
Strawberry: Medium, 16 fl.oz	**630**	19	102
Large, 24 fl.oz	**860**	25	144
Mango, Medium, 16 fl.oz	**635**	18	110
Large, 24 fl.oz	**870**	23	153
Beverages			
Freezes with Orange Sherbet:			
Small	**370**	4	82
Medium	**510**	5	112
Cappuccino Blast: *Per Medium, 24 fl.oz*			
Original	**480**	19	72
Mocha	**610**	19	104
Fruit Blast: *Per Medium, 24 fl.oz*			
Peach Passion Fruit	**370**	0.5	94
Strawberry Citrus	**330**	0	83
Wild Mango	**470**	1.5	116
Fruit Blast Smoothie: *Per Medium, 24 fl.oz*			
Mango	**620**	2	148
Peach Passion Banana	**540**	1	131
Milk Shakes: *Per Medium, 24 fl.oz*			
Choc Chip Cookie Dough	**1030**	42	137
Vanilla	**980**	45	125
Chocolate with Vanilla Ice Cream	**990**	44	131
Strawberry w/ Strawb. Ice Cream	**770**	31	105
Cones: Cake	**25**	0	5
Sugar	**45**	0.5	9
Waffle	**160**	4	28

For Complete Nutritional Data ~ see CalorieKing.com

Updated Nutrition Data ~ www.CalorieKing.com
Persons with Diabetes ~ See Disclaimer (Page 24)

Big Apple Bagels® (Feb '10)

Bagels:	C	F	Cb
All types, average, 5 oz	340	2	68
½ bagel, 2.5 oz	170	1	34
Choice Bagels: *Per Bagel*			
Blueberry Cobbler	390	8	70
Cheddar Nacho	350	6	60
Cinnamon Apple Pie	385	8	68
Cinnamon Bun	400	8	70
Cinnamon Danish	395	8	72
French Toast	370	4	74
Quiche Lorraine	355	8	54
Strawberry White Chocolate	365	4	72
Swiss Melt	370	8	58
White Chocolate Swirl	395	8	70
Cream Cheese: *Per 2 Tbsp , 1 oz*			
Plain	90	9	2
Plain, Lite	60	4.5	3
Other varieties, average	90	8	2
Whipped: Classic Plain	70	7	1
Brown Sugar Cinnamon	70	5	5
Reduced-Fat Spring Veggie	60	5	2
My Favorite Muffin: *Per Jumbo, 5.8 oz*			
Regular: Blueberry	505	24	66
Chocolate Chip	635	33	81
Cinnamon Swirl Cheesecake	640	33	84
Pumpkin Spice	545	24	78
Fat Free: Blueberry	325	0	78
Chocolate Marble	375	0	87
Cinnamon Bun	505	0	126
Sandwiches:			
Big Apple Club	795	37	75
Classic Reuben, Overstuffed	960	43	57
Grilled Chicken Bruschetta Pizzaah	345	21	24
Morning Classic	485	11	73
Roast Beef Parmesan Grinder	585	15	76

For Complete Nutritional Data ~ see CalorieKing.com

Biggby Coffee (Feb '10)

Hot Drinks: *Per 16 fl.oz, Without Sugar Unless Indicated*	C	F	Cb
Caffe Latte: With 2% Milk	175	7	16
With Non-Fat Milk	115	0	16
With Soy	160	5	19
Cappuccino: With 2% Milk	105	4	10
With Non-Fat Milk	70	0	9.5
With Soy	95	3	11
Chai Latte: With 2% Milk	345	8	53
With Non-Fat Milk	285	0	53
Cocoa Carmella: *With Sugar*			
With 2% Milk	310	9	49
With Whipped Cream	390	15	53
Mocha Mocha: *With Sugar*			
With 2% Milk	275	7.5	46
With Whipped Cream	355	14	50

Biggby Coffee cont... (Feb '10)

Cold Drinks: *16 fl.oz, Without Sugar*	C	F	Cb
Big Chill: Chai with 2% milk	430	6	86
Mocha with Whipped Cream	410	14	65
Original	330	6	69
Creme Freeze: Banana	375	5	84
Berry Fruizen-T w/ Whipped Crm	465	10	90

Extra Menu Listings ~ See CalorieKing.com

Blimpie® (Apr '10)

Cold Deli Subs: *Per 6" Sub on White, Includes Dressing*	C	F	Cb
Blimpie Best, with Provolone	450	17	49
BLT, without Cheese	430	22	43
Club, with Swiss	410	13	49
Cuban, with Swiss	410	11	43
Ham & Swiss Cheese	420	14	49
Roast Beef & Provolone	430	14	46
Tuna without Cheese	470	21	43
Turkey & Provolone	410	13	49
Wraps: Chicken Caesar	560	24	56
Southwestern	530	22	61
Hot Deli Subs: *Per 6" Sub on White*			
Meatball, with Provolone	580	31	50
Pastrami, with Swiss	430	16	42
VegiMax, with Provolone	520	20	56
Salads: *Regular, Without Dressing*			
Buffalo Chicken	220	9	10
Garden Salad	30	0	6
Macaroni Salad, Side	330	22	28
Tuna Salad	270	19	6
Dressings & Sauces: *Per 1.5 oz*			
Creamy Caesar	210	21	2
Creamy Italian	180	18	4
Soups: *Per 8.6 oz Serving*			
Chicken Noodle	130	4	18
Cream of Broccoli with Cheese	250	19	13
Harvest Vegetable	100	1	19
Minestrone	90	3	14
New England Clam Chowder	170	3	28
Desserts:			
Brownie	230	10	28
Cookies: Oatmeal Raisin	180	7	27
Sugar	320	16	42

For Complete Nutritional Data ~ see CalorieKing.com

Bob Evans® (May '10)

Breakfast	C	F	Cb
Bowls: Border Scramble, 18.5 oz	1030	57	75
Sausage, 19.5 oz	1025	63	78
Spinach, Bacon & Tomato, 18.4 oz	1040	62	81
Country Biscuit	650	45	39
Pot Roast Hash	680	45	30
Hotcakes: Buttermilk (1), w/o topping	335	10	56
Cinnamon (1), without topping	380	12	62
Omelets: Three Cheese	530	40	5
Border Scramble	635	46	14
Egg Lites	420	24	13
Farmer's Market	630	45	14
Western	530	36	8
Crepes: Plain (1)	255	14	27
Blueberry (1)	305	14	40
***Dinners:** As Served*			
Beef: Meatloaf with Gravy	435	22	22
Pot Roast Beef Stew, 20 oz	715	34	67
Pot Roast Stroganoff, 24 oz	815	43	65
Chicken: Chicken & Brocc. Alfredo	870	46	62
Chicken-N-Noodles: Deep-Dish	700	29	66
Slow-Roasted, 13.2 oz	225	4	30
Chicken Parmesan, w/ Sce, 28 oz	1175	58	96
Fried Chicken Strips (1), 1½ oz	135	8	10
Garlic Butter Grilled Chkn Breast	180	6	1
Fish: Fried Haddock, 6½ oz	365	18	27
Garlic Butter Salmon, 8 oz	255	9	1
Potato-Crusted Flounder, 5 oz	175	7	9
Salmon, 7 oz	245	8	0
Wildfire Salmon, 8½ oz	310	9	15
Pork, Cranb. Apple Pork Loin, 11½ oz	390	22	30
Turkey, Slow-Roasted, 4 oz	135	5	3
Seniors: *Without Sides Unless Indicated*			
Chicken Parmesan with Meat Sauce	845	44	57
Country Fried Steak with Gravy	550	37	37
Meatloaf with Gravy	435	22	22
Open-Faced Roast Beef with Gravy	475	24	22
Farm Fresh Wraps:			
Chicken Caesar, 11.4 oz	605	29	55
Chicken Salad, 10.1 oz	605	29	66
Turkey Club, 10.2 oz	695	34	58
Fit from the Farm:			
Breakfast: Egg Lites with Tomato	60	0	2
Blueberry-Banana French Toast	325	6	36
Fresh Fruit Plate:			
With Low Fat Cottage Cheese	345	4	69
With Low Fat Strawb. Yogurt	355	2	84
Veggie Omelet	270	2	43

Bob Evans® cont... (May '10)

Fit From The Farm (Cont)	C	F	Cb
Dinners: *Includes Menu-Listed Sides, Condiments*			
Chicken, Spinach & Tomato Pasta	525	16	67
Grilled Chicken Breast, 23 oz	480	9	58
Potato Crusted Flounder, 20½ oz	415	8	67
Salads: *With Reduced-Fat Raspberry Dressing*			
Apple-Cranberry Spinach, regular	390	15	49
Savor Size, 8.3 oz	380	15	47
Sandwiches & Burgers			
Burgers: Bacon Cheeseburger	720	38	35
Cheeseburger	650	31	35
Hamburger	540	22	34
Sandwiches: Fried Chicken Club	635	31	47
Bob-B-Q Pulled Pork	595	24	65
Grilled Chicken Club	510	23	34
Grilled Chicken, plain	370	10	33
Pot Roast	575	28	50
Turkey Bacon Melt	590	28	49
***Salads:** Large, Without Dressing Unless Indicated*			
Cobb, 14½ oz	515	31	10
Country Caesar w/ Drssg,16.7 oz	745	53	20
Country Spinach, 10.7 oz	430	25	12
Heritage Chef ,12½ oz	400	25	11
Wildfire Grilled Chicken, 13½ oz	390	13	37
Side Dishes:			
Baked Potato, 10 oz	195	0	50
Bread & Celery Dressing, 6 oz	295	16	31
Coleslaw, 3½ oz	210	14	19
Grilled Mushrooms, 7 oz	85	5	10
Home Fries, 5 oz	165	6	24
Loaded Baked Potato, 11½ oz	395	16	53
Mashed Potatoes, 5½ oz	190	7	16
Gravy/Sauces			
Gravy: Beef, 2 oz	25	1	3
Chicken/Pork Roasted, 2 oz	60	4.5	3
Sauces: Tartar, 0.7 oz	115	2	1
Wildfire BBQ, 1 oz	60	0	15
Kid's Menu:			
Mac & Cheese, 6½ oz	320	8	41
Mini Cheeseburger (1)	285	15	22
Plenty-O-Pancakes, 5½ oz	335	12	52
Smiley Face Potatoes, 3 oz	270	16	29
Sundae, Fudge Blast, 4 oz	215	9	31
Dessert:			
Pie: Apple Pie, N.S.A., 6.8 oz slice	500	30	56
Coconut Cream Pie, 7 oz slice	515	29	59

Updated Nutrition Data ~ www.CalorieKing.com
Persons with Diabetes ~ See Disclaimer (Page 24)

Bojangles® (May '10)

Cajun & Southern Style Chicken	C	F	Cb
Breast, average	280	17	12
Leg, average	120	16	11
Thigh, average	310	23	11
Wing, average	160	25	11
Sandwiches			
Cajun Filet: Without Mayonnaise	335	11	41
With Mayonnaise	435	22	41
Grilled Filet: Without Mayonnaise	235	5	25
With Mayonnaise	335	16	25
Snacks: Buffalo Bites	180	5	5
Chicken Supremes, 4 pieces	335	16	26
Biscuit Sandwiches: Plain	245	12	29
Bacon	290	17	26
Bacon, Egg & Cheese	550	42	27
Cajun Filet	455	21	46
Country Ham	270	15	26
Egg	400	30	26
Sausage	350	23	26
Smoked Sausage	380	26	27
Steak	650	49	37
Fixins': Botato Rounds	235	11	31
Cajun Pintos	110	0	18
Dirty Rice	165	6	24
Green Beans	25	0	5
Macaroni & Cheese	200	14	12
Marinated Cole Slaw	135	3	26
Potatoes, without Gravy	80	1	16
Seasoned Fries	345	19	39
Sweet Biscuits: Bo Berry	220	10	29
Cinnamon	320	18	37

For Complete Nutritional Data ~ see CalorieKing.com

Boston Market® (May '10)

Sandwiches & Burgers:	C	F	Cb
Boston Chicken Carver	750	29	64
Boston Turkey Carver	700	26	65
Classic Chicken Salad	800	41	65
Half Boston: Chicken Carver	375	15	32
Turkey Carver	350	13	32
Meatloaf Open-Faced	670	38	48
Roasted Turkey Open-Faced	330	6	43

Boston Market® cont... (May '10)

Individual Meals: Without Sides	C	F	Cb
Beef Brisket, 4 oz	230	13	0
Half Rotisserie Chicken, 12 oz	610	29	1
Pastry Top Chicken Pot Pie, 15 oz	810	48	60
Family Meals: *Without Sides*			
Meatloaf, 7.7 oz	480	36	21
Roasted Turkey, 5 oz	180	3	0
Salads: *Entree Size*			
Caesar Salad: W/o dressing, 6 oz	140	8	7
With 2 oz Caesar Dressing	430	38	9
With 1.5 oz Lite Ranch Dressing	210	12	15
Market Chopped Salad:			
Without Dressing	190	9	22
With 2 oz Dressing	480	40	24
Add Extra for:			
5 oz Rotisserie Chicken	180	3	0
3 oz Roasted Turkey	110	2	0
Sides			
Cinnamon-Apples, 5 oz	210	3	47
Creamed Spinach, 6.7 oz	280	23	12
Fresh Steamed Vegetables, 4.8 oz	60	2	8
Fresh Vegetable Stuffing, 4.8 oz	190	8	25
Garlic Dill New Potatoes, 5.5 oz	140	3	24
Gravy: Beef, 3 oz	35	1.5	4
Poultry, 4 oz	50	2	7
Green Beans, 3.2 oz	60	3.5	7
Macaroni & Cheese, 7.8 oz	300	11	35
Mashed Potatoes, 7.8 oz	270	11	36
Potato Salad, 7 oz	390	29	26
Seasonal Fresh Fruit Salad, 5 oz	60	0	15
Sweet Corn, 6.2 oz	170	4	37
Sweet Potato Casserole, 7 oz	460	16	77
Soups			
Chicken Noodle, 14 oz	250	8	23
Chicken Tortilla: With Toppings	410	26	30
Without Toppings	160	8	13
Desserts			
Apple Pie, 5.7 oz	580	30	74
Chocolate Cake, 5.1 oz	580	34	67
Choc. Chip Fudge Brownie, 3 oz	320	13	49

For Complete Nutritional Data ~ see CalorieKing.com

Boston Pizza® (May '10)

Starters: Per Order	C	F	Cb
Cactus Cut Potatoes with Dip, 10 oz	830	70	38
Boston's Pizza Bread, w/o Sauce,	500	12	84
Oven Roasted Wings, 9.3 oz	430	30	6
Burgers & Sandwiches:			
Burgers: Prime Rib Original	940	68	47
With Bacon	1000	73	47
Sandwiches: BBQ Pulled Pork	780	15	131
Beef Dip	860	27	108
Boston Brute	810	21	116
Boston Cheesesteak	1140	49	113
Buffalo Chicken	910	33	118
Ciabatta Chicken	750	42	58
Pizzas (Medium): *Per Slice*			
BBQ chicken	190	6	25
Bacon Double Cheeseburger	250	10	25
Cajun Shrimp	290	16	23
Deluxe	220	7	25
Hawaiian	210	5	28
Meateor	260	11	25
Pepperoni	200	7	24
Szechuan	200	5	27
Tropical Chicken	250	11	26
Tuscan	250	10	29
Pastas: *Full Order, Without Garlic Bread*			
Boston's Lasagna, 17.2 oz	670	19	90
Chicken & Mushroom Fettuccini	1460	79	139
Spicy Italian Penne	1530	88	137
Salads: *Includes Dressing*			
Caesar, starter size	210	19	7
Greek, starter size	270	27	7
Desserts:			
Apple Crisp, 14.4 oz	740	19	138
Chocolate Brownie Addiction, 8.6 oz	570	18	99

For Complete Nutritional Data ~ see CalorieKing.com

Braum's® (May '10)

Frozen Yogurt: Per ½ Cup	C	F	Cb
Chocolate Peanut Butter Cup	180	10	19
Average Fruit Flavors	130	5	19
***Ice Cream:** Per ½ Cup*			
Carb Watch: Chocolate Chip	180	10	17
Other flavors, average	155	11	17
Light: Average all varieties	130	4	19
Premium: Peanut Butter Cup	190	12	18
Other flavors, average	150	6	18

For Complete Nutritional Data ~ see CalorieKing.com

Bruegger's Bagels® (May '10)

Bagels	C	F	Cb
Average all flavors, 4.3 oz	320	3	65
***Breakfast S'wiches:** With Plain Bagel*			
Egg & Cheese	470	14	63
with Bacon	480	21	63
with Sausage	560	23	63
Smoked Salmon	460	10	66
Spinach & Cheddar Omelet	500	16	64
Western	760	56	66
***Deli Sandwiches:** Plain Bagel Unless Indicated*			
BLT on Hearty White Bread	720	42	62
Chicken Breast	550	6	81
Garden Veggie	360	2	72
Ham On Honey Wheat Bread	540	16	64
Roast Beef on Hearty White Bread	560	18	59
Turkey	440	8	64
Signature & Classic Sandwiches:			
Herby Turkey/Sesame Bagel	530	14	73
Leonardo da Veggie/Plain White Bread	560	15	76
Roma Roast Beef/Hearty White Bread	770	44	62
Tarragon Chkn Salad/Hrty White Bread	750	37	75
Thai Peanut Chicken/Plain Bagel	580	11	91
Turkey Chipotle Club/Hon. Wheat Bread	800	51	57
***Salads:** With Dressing*			
Caesar	270	17	22
Chicken Caesar	380	20	23
Mandarin Chicken Medley	450	21	37
Sesame Chicken	490	29	30
Cookies: Chocolate Chip	390	17	52
Double Chocolate	390	19	51
Everything	380	18	49
Dessert Bars: Seven Layer	650	43	58
Chocolate Chunk Brownie	310	18	38
Toffee Almond	400	19	53

For Complete Menu & Data ~ see CalorieKing.com

Burgerville® (May '10)

Burgers:	C	F	Cb
Cheeseburger	380	20	30
Classic Hamburger	530	30	42
Double Beef Cheeseburger	450	27	30
Half Pound Colossal	750	45	43
Hamburger	320	17	30
Tillamook Cheeseburger	640	39	42
Sandwiches: Crispy Chicken	460	19	54
Deluxe Crispy Chicken	600	30	54
Grilled Chicken, Low-Fat	330	5	45
Nine Grain Turkey Club	540	32	36
French Fries: Regular, 5 oz	360	15	52

For Complete Menu & Data ~ see CalorieKing.com

Updated Nutrition Data ~ www.CalorieKing.com
Persons with Diabetes ~ See Disclaimer (Page 24)

Burger King® (May '10)

Breakfast:	C	F	Cb
Cheesy Bacon BK Wrapper	380	24	28
Ham Omelet Sandwich	270	12	29
French Toast Sticks: 5 Pieces	380	18	49
Cini-minis with Icing (4)	490	18	74
Biscuits			
Bacon, Egg & Cheese	420	25	34
Ham, Egg & Cheese	400	22	33
Sausage, Egg & Cheese	550	37	34
Burritos: *Includes Salsa*			
Bacon, Egg & Cheese	300	16	24
Potato, Egg & Cheese	320	17	29
Croissan'wich: Bacon Egg & Chse	340	19	26
Egg & Cheese	300	16	26
Ham Egg & Cheese	330	16	27
Double Croissan'wich			
with Bacon, Egg & Cheese	420	25	27
with Ham, Bacon, Egg & Cheese	420	24	28
with Ham, Sausage, Egg & Chse	550	35	28
with Sausage, Egg & Cheese	680	49	29
Hash Browns: Small, 2.5 oz	400	26	39
Medium	540	35	52
Sourdough Sandwich:			
Ham, Egg & Cheese	420	19	40
Sausage, Egg & Cheese	560	34	41
Chicken			
BK Chicken Fries, *without Buffalo Sauce:*			
6 pieces	250	15	16
9 pieces	380	22	24
Kid's:			
Crown Shaped Chicken Tenders:			
4 pces	180	11	13
8 pieces	360	21	25
Macaroni & Cheese	160	5	22
Sandwiches & Burgers:			
Burgers:			
BK Stackers: Double	570	37	29
Triple	750	51	30
Quad	930	65	31
Cheeseburger	310	15	28
Double Cheeseburger	460	27	28
Hamburger	260	11	27
XT: A1 Steakhouse	970	61	55
Steakhouse	770	46	53
BK Veggie Burger with Cheese	450	20	44
Chicken & Fish Sandwiches: *With Mayo or Sauce*			
BK Big Fish	640	31	67
Original Chicken	630	39	46
Spicy Chick'N Crisp	460	30	34
TenderCrisp Chicken	800	46	68
TenderGrill Chicken	520	19	49

Burger King® cont... (May '10)

Sandwiches & Burgers (Cont)	C	F	Cb
Whopper Sandwiches: *With Mayo*			
Original	670	40	51
Double Whopper	920	58	51
Triple Whopper	1160	76	51
Whopper JR.	340	20	28
Salads: Without Dressing or Croutons			
Garden: with TenderCrisp Chicken	410	23	27
with TenderGrill Chicken	230	8	9
Sides:			
BK Fresh Apple Fries w/ Dipping Sce	70	0.5	16
French Fries: Small, 4.3 oz	340	17	44
Medium, 5.8 oz	440	22	56
Large, 7 oz	540	27	69
Onion Rings: Small (15)	310	17	36
Medium (20)	400	21	47
Large (24)	490	26	57
Sauces & Condiments: Per 1 oz Container			
Dipping Sauces: Buffalo	80	8	2
Honey Mustard	90	6	8
Ranch	140	15	1
Sweet & Sour	45	0	11
Zesty Onion	150	15	3
Dressings: Ken's Creamy Caesar, 2 oz	210	21	4
Ken's Fat Free Ranch, 2 oz	60	0	15
Desserts/Pies:			
Dutch Apple Pie	320	14	46
Funnel Cake Sticks with Icing (9)	300	11	49
Hershey's Sundae Pie	300	18	31
Beverages:			
Mocha Iced Coffee, 16 fl.oz	340	7	63
Frozen Coca-Cola: Small, 16 fl.oz	110	0	31
Medium, 22 fl.oz	140	0	40
Shakes:			
Chocolate: Small, 16 fl.oz	440	11	78
Medium, 22 fl.oz	650	16	119
Large, 32 fl.oz	960	23	176
Strawberry: Small, 16 fl.oz	430	11	77
Medium, 22 fl.oz	630	15	116
Large, 32 fl.oz	930	21	172
Vanilla: Small, 16 fl.oz	370	12	60
Medium, 22 fl.oz	520	16	84
Large, 32 fl.oz	760	24	124
Oreo Sundae Shakes: *Per Medium, 22 fl.oz*			
Chocolate	920	28	159
Vanilla	790	28	124

For Complete Nutritional Data ~ see CalorieKing.com

California Pizza Kitchen

~ See CalorieKing.com

Captain D's Seafood® (May '10)

Dinners/Platters: Includes Cole Slaw, French Fries & Hush Puppies	C	F	Cb
Bite Size Shrimp Dinner	1140	61	120
Catfish Feast	995	57	88
Clam Platter, ½ lb	1450	87	133
Country Style Fish Dinner	1070	59	97
Deluxe Seafood Platter	1610	94	114
Fried Flounder	1530	93	115
Oyster Dinner	1000	58	100
Ultimate Premium Shrimp Platter	1290	65	69
Salads:			
Fried Chicken Salad	205	10	18
Side Salad	20	0	3
Wild Alaskan Salmon Salad	175	1	8
Sides			
Baked Potato, plain	240	0	54
Broccoli, 3.5 oz	40	1	5
Macaroni & Cheese, 4 oz	160	7	17
Desssert, Cheesecake w/ Strawb.	430	26	45

Caribou Coffee® (May '10)

Without Whipped Cream Unless Indicated

Classic Hot Beverages: *Per Medium*	C	F	Cb
Coffee, with Steamed 2% Milk	90	3.5	9
Coffee Of The Day, with 2% Milk	20	0.5	1
Espresso, 1 medium, 3 shots, 6 fl.oz	0	0	0
Breve	510	45	17
Cappuccino, with 2% Milk	70	3	6
Macchiato, with 2% Milk, 6 fl.oz	20	1	1
Cold Beverages: *Per Medium*			
Iced Americano	5	0	0
Iced Coffee, Cold Pressed	5	0	0
Iced Latte, with 2% Milk	150	6	14
Iced Mocha , Milk Choc., 2% Milk	350	11	51
Coolers: *Per Medium With Whipped Cream*			
Caramel	500	16	88
Coffee	420	17	67
Espresso	370	16	57
Smoothies: *Per Medium*			
Passion Fruit Green Tea	290	0	70
Pom-a-Mango	350	0.5	85
Strawberry Banana, 22 fl.oz	350	0	84
Snowdrift: *Per Medium With Milk Chocolate*			
Cookies & Cream, with 2% Milk	630	18	103
Mint, with 2% Milk	510	13	84
Wild: *Per Medium With Whipped Cream*			
Hot Apple Blast	400	11	76
Mint Cond. Milk Choc., 2% Milk	580	40	67

For Complete Menu & Data ~ see CalorieKing.com

Carl's Jr.® (May '10)

Charbroiled Burgers:	C	F	Cb
Big Hamburger	460	17	54
Chili Cheeseburger	780	41	58
Famous Star with Cheese	660	39	53
Kids Hamburger	230	10	24
Super Star with Cheese	920	58	54
The Big Carl	920	59	51
The Six Dollar Burger: Original	890	54	58
Bacon Cheese	950	62	49
Chili Cheese	1000	56	59
Guacamole Bacon	1040	70	53
Low-Carb	570	43	7
Teriyaki	840	43	69
Western Bacon	1020	53	81
Chicken Sandwiches:			
Charbroiled: BBQ Chicken	380	7	49
Chicken Club	560	27	44
Santa Fe Chicken	630	35	44
Bacon Swiss Crispy Chicken	750	40	62
Spicy Chicken Sandwich	420	27	33
Chicken Strips, 5 pieces	610	43	32
Chicken Stars, 6 pieces	320	24	14
Fish: Fish & Chips	730	39	72
Carl's Catch Fish Sandwich	710	37	74
Breakfast: Bacon & Egg Burrito	550	32	37
Breakfast Burger	780	41	64
French Toast Dips, 5 pcs, w/o syrup	460	21	60
Hash Brown Nuggets, 4 oz.	350	23	32
Loaded Breakfast Burrito	780	49	51
Sourdough Breakfast Sandwich	470	25	37
Steak & Egg Burrito	650	36	43
Sunrise Croissant Sandwich	590	44	27
Fries: Chili Cheese, 12.1 oz	980	56	88
CrissCut Fries, 4.9 oz	450	29	42
Natural Cut: Small, 4.2 oz	320	15	42
Medium, 6 oz	460	22	60
Large, 6.5 oz	500	24	65
Onion Rings, 4½ oz	530	28	61
Salads: *Without Dressing or Croutons*			
Cranb. Apple Walnut Gr. Chicken	300	11	25
Original Grilled Chicken	200	6	13
Dressings: *Per 2 oz Pkg*			
Blue Cheese	320	34	1
House	220	22	3
Low-Fat Balsamic	35	1.5	5
Shakes: Van.;Choc.;Strawb. av.	710	33	86
Oreo	730	38	81
Malts, average all flavors	780	35	99

Updated Nutrition Data ~ www.CalorieKing.com
Persons with Diabetes ~ See Disclaimer (Page 24)

Carvel® (May '10)

Ice Creams: Per Small, 7.5 oz	C	F	Cb
Cups: Chocolate	410	21	48
Vanilla	450	26	47
No Sugar Added, Vanilla	260	7	51
Dashers: *Per Small 12 oz*			
Mint Chocolate Chip	770	42	95
Peanut Butter Cup	1060	60	95
Strawberry Shortcake	580	29	74
Novelties: Brown Bonnet	390	23	43
Deluxe Flying Saucer with Sprinkles	350	16	49
Flying Saucer, Chocolate	230	10	33
Classic Sundaes: *Small*			
Caramel	700	36	84
Hot Fudge	540	30	60
Strawberry	610	34	67
Beverages			
Blended Drinks: *Per Small, 16 fl.oz*			
Arctic Blender: Cookie Dough	920	40	126
Fried Ice Cream	670	31	85
Peanut Butter	870	33	88
Carvelanche: Butterfinger	730	38	92
M&M; Reece's, average	755	39	87
Smoothies, average all flav.,16 fl.oz	315	0	78
Thick Shake, Strawberry	600	31	70
Thick ShakeFloats: Chocolate	790	34	109
Strawberry	750	39	85
Vanilla	810	39	102

Checkers®

Same Menu & Data as Rally's ~ See Page 239

Cheesecake Factory® (Dec '09)

(Author Estimates)

10" Cheesecake: Per Slice	C	F	Cb
Adam's P'nut B'cup Fudge Ripple	930	59	93
Banana Cream	860	63	70
Brownie Sundae	970	63	96
Choc Chip Cookie Dough	1910	72	102
Dulce de Leche Caramel	1010	74	83
Kahlua Cocoa Coffee	840	55	80
Key Lime Cheesecake	710	49	64
Original Cheesecake	630	45	53
Vanilla Bean Cheesecake	870	64	69
White Choc. Raspberry Truffle	900	62	80
Appertizer: Avocado Eggrolls, 1 roll	435	27	48
Dinners: *Complete Meal*			
Cajun Jambalaya Pasta	1960	43	290
Chicken Madeira	1430	76	82
Famous Factory Meatloaf	1955	96	162
Fresh Fish Tacos	1130	23	160
Herb Crusted Filet of Salmon	1040	60	68
Lemon-Herb Roasted Chicken	1790	108	94
Salad: BBQ Ranch Chkn, no bread	1415	113	65

Charley's Grilled Subs® (May '10)

	C	F	Cb
Subs: *Regular 7¾" Includes Standard Toppings, Without Sauce or Dressings Unless Indicated*			
BBQ Cheddar, with Sauce	580	20	69
Bacon 3 Cheese Steak	635	32	54
Buffalo Chicken, with Sauce	530	16	60
Chicken Bacon Club	570	25	53
Chicken Cordon Blue	570	18	54
Chicken Teriyaki with Sauce	520	16	58
Italian Deli	585	25	53
Mushroom Swiss Steak	520	19	57
Philly Cheesesteak	520	19	55
Philly Chicken	515	15	67
Philly Ham & Swiss	515	15	59
Philly Steak Deluxe	525	19	58
Philly Veggie	450	15	62
Sicilian Steak	640	31	53
Turkey Cheddar Melt	470	12	53
Ultimate Club	560	23	54
Salads: *Cheese/Dressings not included*			
Chicken, Teriyaki; Buffalo, average	210	7	13
Fresh Garden Salad	60	2	9
Grilled Steak Salad	210	10	10
Dressings, Italian/Ranch, av., 1 oz	150	16	1
Mayo, 1 Tbsp., ½ oz	100	11	0
Original Lemonade, 16 fl.oz	165	0	40

Extra Menu Items & Data ~ www.CalorieKing.com

Chevys Fresh Mex® (May '10)

	C	F	Cb
Sizzling Fajitas: *As Served*			
Original Famous Chicken	930	32	95
Sizzling Steak	1030	46	94
Mesquite Grilled Tacos: *As Served*			
Chicken	1050	35	125
Fish	1060	39	125
Steak	1110	44	124
Fresh Mex Specialties: *As Served*			
Chili Verde	1030	44	113
Crispy Chicken Flautas	1510	76	156
Red Chile Pork Taquitos	1350	69	136
Signature Enchiladas: *As Served*			
Chicken Mole	950	51	84
Chipotle Chicken	1070	64	87
Shrimp & Crab	1360	97	87
Grande Salads: *With Dressing Unless Indicated*			
Grilled Chicken Caesar	860	69	32
Grilled Fajita	1585	128	70
Santa Fe Chopped, w/o Dressing	670	39	30
Tostada without Dressing	1680	115	105
Soup, Tortilla, 1 bowl	390	17	35
Tamalito (Sweetcorn), 2	190	7	29
Tortilla (El Machino), 2	140	4	22

Chick-fil-A® (May '10)

Chick-fil-A Sandwiches: *W/o Sauce*	C	F	Cb
Chargrilled Chicken	300	3.5	38
Chargrilled Chicken Club	410	12	39
Chicken Salad	500	20	52
Cool Wraps: *Without Dressing*			
Chargrilled Chicken	410	12	50
Chicken Caesar	460	15	47
Spicy Chicken	410	12	48
Breakfast: Chicken Biscuit	450	20	48
Bacon, Egg & Cheese Biscuit	520	29	44
Sausage Biscuit	590	41	42
Burritos: Chicken	450	20	43
Sausage	510	29	40
Chick-n-Minis, 1 box, 3 pieces	260	10	30
Chicken, Egg & Cheese Bagel	530	23	50
Cinnamon Cluster	400	15	61
Hash Browns, 2.7 oz	280	19	25
Salads: *Without Dressing & Condiments*			
Chargrilled Chicken & Fruit	230	6	23
Chargrilled Chicken Garden	180	6	11
Chick-n-Strips	470	23	27
Southwest Chargrilled Chicken	240	9	18
Salad Dressings, Sauces & Condiments:			
Garlic & Butter Croutons, ½ oz	60	2	9
Tortilla Strips,½ oz	80	4	8
Dressings: Blue Cheese, 1 oz	150	16	1
Buttermilk Ranch; Caesar, 1 oz	160	17	1
Light Italian, 1.1 oz	15	0.5	2
Thousand Island, 1.1 oz	150	14	5
Sauces: BBQ; Honey Mustard, 1 oz	45	0	11
Buffalo, ¾ oz	10	0	1
Buttermilk Ranch, ¾ oz	110	12	1
Chick-fil-A, 1 oz	140	13	6
Honey Roasted BBQ, 0.4 oz	60	5	2
Sides: Carrot & Raisin Salad, 6 oz	260	12	39
Chicken Salad Cup, 6 oz	350	24	6
Cole Slaw, 10.5 oz	580	50	31
Side Salad w/o Croutons or Dress., 4 oz	70	4.5	5
Waffle Potato Fries: Small, 3 oz	290	16	34
Medium, 4 oz	380	21	45
Large, 4.5 oz	430	23	50
Desserts:			
Cheesecake, 3.2 oz	310	23	22
Fudge Nut Brownie, 2.8 oz	370	19	45
Lemon Pie, 1 slice, 4.23 oz	360	13	58
Icedream Cone w/o Toppings	170	4	31
Milkshake, Chocolate, 18.25 oz	750	28	113

Chili's® (May '10)

Appetizers: *As Served*	C	F	Cb
Bottomless Tostada Chips with Salsa	480	39	26
Crispy Onion Str. & Jalap. Stack/Ranch	1020	86	49
Loaded Nachos: Beef (12)	1690	122	60
Chicken (12)	1570	97	64
Skillet Queso with Tostada Chips	920	73	46
Southwestern Eggrolls with Dressing	910	57	72
Triple Dipper: Big Mouth Bites w/ Dress.	740	48	46
Buffalo Boneless Wings, with Dress.	750	60	27
Chicken Crispers without Dress.	600	39	29
Hot Spin. & Artichoke Dip with Chips	570	45	20
Burgers: *As Served, On white Bun with Fries*			
Big Mouth Bites with Dressing	1810	110	140
Classic Bacon Burger	1520	88	115
Jalapeno Smokehouse with Dressing	2130	139	127
Everything Is Better On The Grill			
Cajun Pasta: *As Served*			
With Grilled Chicken	1350	70	104
With Shrimp	1310	75	105
Chicken: *As Served*			
Margarita Grilled Chicken	530	8	67
Monterey Chicken	870	47	53
Fajitas: *Without Tortillas & Condiments*			
Beef	470	25	26
Buffalo Chicken	1040	76	43
Classic Chicken	360	12	23
Trio	530	26	28
+ Condiments only (1)	230	19	7
+ Flour Tortillas only (3)	380	10	62
Quesadillas: *As Served*			
Bacon Chicken Ranch	1550	94	93
Jalapeno Steak	1520	102	99
Steaks: *Without Sides*			
Classic Sirloin, 8 oz	450	26	19
Flame-Grilled Ribeye, 12 oz	900	68	18
Hand Battered: *As Served*			
Chicken Crispers w/ Honey Mustard	1750	109	136
Country-Fried Steak	1440	83	123
In-House Smoked Ribs: *Full Rack Without Sides*			
Original	1110	81	33
Memphis Dry Rub	1180	87	34
Shiner Bock BBQ	1230	81	58
Salads: *Large, Includes Dressing Unless Indicated*			
Asian: With Grilled Chicken	930	50	71
With Salmon	1120	69	71
With Steak	1050	63	74
Sweet Endings:			
Cheesecake, 1 slice	710	42	68
Chocolate Chip Paradise Pie, 1 slice	1290	68	163
Molten Chocolate Cake, 1 slice	1070	51	143

For Complete Menu & Data ~ see CalorieKing.com

Chipotle® (May '10)

Breads	C	F	Cb
Crispy Taco Shells (3)	180	6	27
Flour Tortillas (Burrito), (1)	290	9	44
Flour Tortillas (Taco), (3)	270	8	39
Meal Components			
Barbacoa, 4 oz	170	7	2
Black Beans, 4 oz	120	1	23
Carnitas, 4 oz	190	8	1
Cheese, 1 oz	100	9	0
Chicken, 4 oz	190	6.5	1
Cilantro-Lime Rice, 3 oz	130	3	23
Lettuce, 1 oz	5	0	0
Pinto Beans, 4 oz	120	1	22
Steak, 4 oz	190	7	2
Condiments			
Salsa: Corn, 4 oz	80	1.5	15
Green Tomatillo, 2 oz	15	0	3
Red Tomatillo, 2 oz	40	1	8
Tomato, 3½ oz	20	0	4
Sour Cream, 2 oz	120	10	2
Vinaigrette, 2 fl.oz	260	25	12
Extras: Chips, serving, 4 oz	570	27	73
Guacamole, 3½ oz	150	13	8

Chuck E. Cheese® (May '10)

Appetizers: *Includes Condiments*	C	F	Cb
Buffalo Wings (12)	900	60	48
Italian Bread Stick (1)	175	9	18
Mozzarella Stick (1)	95	6	6
Pizzas: *Per Medium Slice*			
BBQ Chicken	185	6	24
Cheese	155	5	21
Super Combo	185	8	22
Veggie Combo	160	6	22
Oven Baked Sandwiches:			
Ham & Cheese	685	27	79
Italian Sub	790	39	78
Roasted Chicken Ciabatta	715	28	80
French Fries:			
With Ketchup & Ranch: 4 oz	420	20	55
8 oz	840	40	110
Hot Dog, with Mustard & Relish	310	19	35
Desserts: Apple Dessert Pizza, 1 slice	190	5	33
Chocolate Cake (8"), 1 slice	290	13	41
Cinnamon Stick, w/ Toppings, 1 stick	70	2	11

Church's Chicken® (May '10)

Chicken: *Per Serving*	C	F	Cb
Original: Breast, 1 piece	200	11	3
Leg, 1 piece	110	6	3
Thigh, 1 piece	330	23	8
Wing, 1 piece	300	19	7
Spicy: Breast, 1 piece	320	20	12
Leg, 1 piece	180	11	8
Thigh, 1 piece	480	35	20
Wing, 1 piece	430	27	17
Tender Strips: 1 piece	120	6	6
Spicy, 1 piece	135	7	7
Sides: *Per Regular Serving*			
Cajun Rice, 6 oz	130	7	16
Cole Slaw, 6 oz	150	10	15
Corn on the Cob (1)	140	3	24
French Fries, 3½ oz	290	14	38
Honey Butter Biscuits (1), 1.7 oz	190	10	22
Jalapeno Cheese Bombers, 4 pces	240	10	29
Macaroni & Cheese, 6 oz	220	10	24
Mashed Potatoes & Gravy, 6 oz	70	2	12
Okra, 3.4 oz	350	22	36
Whole Jalapeno Peppers (2)	10	0	2
Sauces: *Per Packet*			
BBQ; Sweet & Sour	25	0	6
Creamy Jalapeno	80	9	1
Honey Mustard	90	9	3
Purple Pepper	45	0	12
Ranch	105	10	1

Cici's Pizza® (May '10)

Buffet: *Per 1/10 of 12" Pizza*	C	F	Cb
Alfredo	120	3.5	18
Bacon Cheddar	110	4.5	19
Bar-B-Que	150	2.5	25
Beef	150	4	20
Cheese	150	4	19
Ham & Pineapple	150	3.5	21
Pepperoni & Jalapeno	150	4.5	20
Sausage	140	5	20
Spinach Alfredo	120	3.5	19
Zesty Ham & Cheddar	120	4	19
To-Go: *Per 1/10 of 15" Pizza*			
Alfredo	170	6	23
Bar-B-Que	240	6	36
Beef	190	8	24
Pepperoni & Jalapeno	210	7	24
Sausage	220	8	25
Spinach Alfredo	170	6	23
Zesty Ham & Cheddar	160	7	23
Zesty Pepperoni	170	9	23
Zesty Veggie	140	6	24

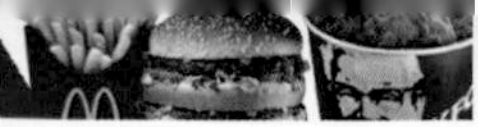

Cinnabon® (May '10)

	C	F	Cb
Caramel Pecanbon (1)	1100	47	156
Cinnabon Bites (6)	520	16	78
Cinnabon Stix (5)	410	23	46
CinnaPretzel (1)	750	6	156
Classic Cinnabon (1)	815	32	117
Cup Cakes: 24-Carrot; Cinnacake (1) av.	470	25	55
Average all others (1)	515	25	70
Sweet Roll Icing: Frosting Cup, 1.4 oz	180	11	25

Claim Jumper® (May '10)

	C	F	Cb
Appetizers: *As Served*			
Cheese Potatocakes (3)	1055	65	96
Southwest Eggrolls	1160	48	108
Burgers & Sandwiches: Motherlode	1540	81	75
Widow Maker	1595	105	94
Meals: *Per Whole Dish, Unless Indicated*			
Favorites: Giant Stuffed Baker	1235	59	106
Meatloaf & Mashed Potatoes	1700	106	139
Whiskey Apple Glazed Pork Loin	2185	136	140
Pasta: Black Tie Chicken, large	3775	233	269
Spaghetti & Meatballs, large	1790	83	190
Spicy Jambalaya w/ Rice, large	1995	128	129
Rotisserie: *Includes Roasted Vegetables Only*			
BBQ Baby Back Pork Ribs	1215	48	138
Roasted Tri-Tip & Gravy	720	42	23
Seafood: Oaxacan Style Sea Bass	780	26	88
Tilapia Veracruz	910	34	92
Entree Salads: *Per Large Size, Includes Dressing*			
Chicken Citrus, Charbroiled	2550	147	224
Salmon Caesar, Broiled	1520	113	56
Soups: *Per Bowl, Without Cheese Toast*			
Baked Potato Cheddar	540	40	33
New England Clam Chowder	440	33	25
Desserts: Choc. Motherlode Cake	2725	140	339
Lemon Bar Brulee	1075	48	144

For Complete Menu & Data ~ see CalorieKing.com

Coldstone Creamery® (May '10)

	C	F	Cb
Ice Creams			
Amaretto: Like it	330	20	33
Love it	530	31	53
Gotta have it	790	47	80
Sorbet: *Average all flavors*			
Like it	155	0	38
Love it	250	0	62
Gotta have it	370	0	93

Cosi® (May '10)

	C	F	Cb
Flatbread Pizza, *Individual:*			
Margherita	705	31	96
Pepperoni	805	40	95
Traditional Cheese	685	29	95

Cosi® cont... (May '10)

	C	F	Cb
Melts: *With Rustic Bread*			
Chicken TBM	695	31	49
Pesto Chicken	670	31	52
Steakhouse Gonzola	750	47	49
Tuna Melt	875	40	51
TBM Melt	635	32	49
Sandwiches: *With Rustic Bread*			
Buffalo Bleu	565	25	47
Fire Roasted Veggie	325	8	44
Italiano	745	42	49
TBM	530	30	46
Soup: *Per 10 oz Bowl Unless Indicated, w/o Flatbread*			
Pollo e Pasta	160	4	14
Tomato Basil Aurora	225	15	18
Salads: *Includes Dressing*			
Cosi Cobb, 12½ oz	710	55	16
Greek Salad, 14 oz	515	47	19
Grilled Chicken Caesar, 11 oz	620	44	20
Signature Salad, 11¼ oz	610	45	44
Steakhouse, 14 oz	615	49	14

Costco Food Court (May '10)

	C	F	Cb
Pizza: *Per Slice*			
Combo, 11oz	680	29	72
Cheese, 10 oz	700	28	70
Pepperoni , 9 oz	620	24	68
Dogs, average, 8 oz	560	32	46
Salad, Chicken Caesar, 20.5 oz	670	40	35
Meals: Cheese Burger Fry Combo	860	45	72
Chicken Bake 11.5 oz	770	25	78
Ital. Sausage Sandwich, 12.6 oz	700	42	46
Beverages: Hot Latte, 9.6 fl oz	190	5	24
Hot Mocha, 11.3 fl oz	310	9	45
Mocha Freeze, 16.3 fl .oz	320	7	49
Latte Freeze, 15.3 oz	240	7	32
J&JChurro, 5.2 oz	470	22	61
Smoothies: Fruit Smoothie, 16 fl.oz	290	0	72
Desserts: Ice cream Bar, 8 oz	870	65	60
Berry Sundae, 12.3 oz	410	0	87
Yogurt, 12 oz	390	0	82

Cousins Subs® (May '10)

	C	F	Cb
7½" Subs			
BLT with Mayo	590	38	47
Cheese Steak	505	19	49
Chicken Cheddar Deluxe w/ Mayo	670	39	51
Club with Mayo	645	35	51
Double Cheese Steak	745	36	49
Italian Special with Dressing	815	51	50
Meatball & Provolone with Sauce	725	38	54
Philly Cheese Steak with Sauce	530	19	55
Roast Beef with Mayo	605	30	50
Seafood with Crab & Mayo	640	38	60

Updated Nutrition Data ~ www.CalorieKing.com
Persons with Diabetes ~ See Disclaimer (Page 24)

Cousins Subs® cont... (May '10)

7½" Subs (cont)	C	F	Cb
Three Cheese with Mayo	685	44	50
Tuna with Mayo Blend	645	38	49
Turkey Breast with Mayo	530	28	50
Better Bunch, 5" Mini Subs: *Without Mayo & Cheese*			
Club	190	2	26
Garden Veggie; Hot Veggie, average	140	1	27
Ham; Turkey Breast	175	2	26
French Fries: Small, 2.8 oz	250	13	30
Medium, 4 oz	365	19	43
Large, 5.3 oz	485	25	57
Salads: *Without Dressing*			
Chef Salad	325	14	25
Italian	405	24	24
Tuna Salad	625	46	23

For Complete Nutritional Data ~ see CalorieKing.com

Culver's® (May '10)

Butter Burgers:	C	F	Cb
Original: Single; Kids	345	12	35
Double	480	20	36
Triple	615	28	37
Cheddar with Bacon, Single	540	30	31
Cheese: Single; Kids	400	17	36
Double	580	29	37
Culver's Bacon Deluxe: Single	575	35	34
Double	750	47	34
Culver's Deluxe: Single	495	28	35
Double	670	40	34
Mushroom & Swiss, Single	430	20	32
Sourdough Melt, Single	415	20	33
Corn Dog, Kids	260	14	26
Chicken Tenders, 4 pieces	440	20	32
Hot Dog	460	27	46
Kids	435	27	38
Sides			
Crinkle Cut Fries: Kids	275	12	38
Regular	385	17	53
Large	495	22	68
Chili Cheddar Fries, 8.82 oz	605	30	71
Dairyland Cheese Curds, 6.7 oz	670	38	54
Mashed Potatoes with Gravy	140	2	26
Sandwiches: Angus Philly Steak	470	21	35
Beef Pot Roast	365	12	33
Crispy Chicken Filet	580	35	50
Flame Roasted Chicken	310	9	36
Grilled Reuben Melt	590	31	41
North Atlantic Cod Filet	665	41	47
Pork Tenderloin (Breaded)	595	26	62
Shaved Prime Rib	505	28	35
Turkey Sourdough BLT	560	32	36

Culver's® cont... (May '10)

Dinner Plates: *Per Serving*	C	F	Cb
Beef Pot Roast	745	36	73
Butterfly Crispy Shrimp, 6 pieces	1320	68	152
Chopped Steak	850	50	63
Fried Chicken, 2 pieces	1790	100	141
4 Pieces	2220	122	159
North Atlantic Cod, Fried, 2 pces	1865	122	136
Salads: *Without Dressing*			
Chicken Cashew w/ Flame Rstd Chkn	445	24	20
Classic Caesar w/ Flame Roasted Chkn	340	16	14
Garden Fresco	230	10	20
Side Caesar	55	2	5
Side Salad	55	2	6
Desserts:			
Frozen Custard: Chocolate, 1 scoop	295	14	35
Vanilla, 1 scoop	310	18	30
Concrete Mixers: *Medium*			
Chocolate	995	49	122
Turtle	1155	71	114
Classic Sundaes: *Per 2 Scoops Unless Indicated*			
Bananas Foster	785	41	93
Turtle	980	60	97
Beverages: Choc. Malt, medium	970	45	122
Chocolate Shake, medium	910	44	114
Root Beer Float, medium	550	18	90

For Complete Nutritional Data ~ see CalorieKing.com

D'Angelo's® (May '10)

Sandwiches:	C	F	Cb
Cheeseburger: Pokket	460	23	35
Sub	530	25	49
Wrap	600	31	52
Chicken Stir Fry: Pokket	400	10	39
Sub	470	12	53
Wrap	550	19	57
Classic Vegetable: Pokket	360	13	43
Wrap	520	22	61
Roast Beef: Sub	320	5	46
Wrap	410	12	50
Turkey Breast: Pokket	260	1	31
Sub	330	3	45
Grilled Quesadillas: Number 9	380	19	31
Chicken Stir Fry	360	15	31
Veggie	290	13	33
Salads: *Entree Size With Dressing Unless Indicated*			
Caesar	620	54	28
Chicken Caesar	670	53	21
Chicken Cobb , without Dressing	330	18	14
Greek	320	22	20
Tossed, without Dressing	60	0	13
Turkey, without Dressing	170	1	10

Extra Menu Items ~ www.CalorieKing.com

Dairy Queen® (May '10)

Burgers & Sandwiches:	C	F	Cb
GrillBurgers:			
Bacon Cheddar, ¼ lb	650	35	41
½ lb Burger	720	40	42
½ lb Flame Thrower	1060	75	41
Original: Bacon Dbl Cheeseburger	730	41	35
Cheeseburger	400	18	34
Hamburger	350	14	33
Double	540	26	33
Sandwiches: Crispy Chicken	560	28	48
Grilled Chicken	370	16	32
Baskets:			
Chkn Strips: 4 piece w/ Gravy	1360	63	103
6 piece, with Country Gravy	1640	74	121
Iron Grilled Chicken Quesadilla	1070	50	117
Hot Dogs: All Beef	250	14	21
With Chili & Cheese	430	22	39
Salads: *Without Dressing*			
Crispy Chicken	460	19	31
Grilled Chicken	280	11	14
Sides			
DQ French Fries, Regular, 4 oz	310	13	43
DQ Onion Rings, Regular, 4 oz	360	16	47
Desserts: *Per Medium*			
Blizzard Treats: Banana Cream Pie	780	30	115
Butterfinger	740	26	114
Cappuccino Heath	870	38	122
Chocolate Chip	880	50	96
Cookie Dough	1010	40	148
Oreo Cookies	680	25	100
Reese's Peanut Butter Cups	760	31	101
Strawberry CheeseQuake	690	28	92
DQ Blizzard Cakes (10"): *Per 1/10 Cake*			
Oreo	720	31	97
Reese's Peanut Butter Cup	730	34	93
Strawberry CheeseQuake	630	27	84
DQ Dipped Cones: *Per 7¾ oz Cone*			
Butterscotch	490	23	59
Chocolate	470	22	60
DQ Sundaes: *Per Medium, 8.2 oz*			
Caramel	430	11	75
Hot Fudge	440	14	66
Strawberry	350	10	56
Malts: *Per Medium*			
Caramel	960	24	163
Chocolate	900	22	154
Strawberry	770	20	128
Moo Latte: *Per 16 fl.oz*			
Cappuccino	500	18	71
French Vanilla	560	18	88
Mocha	590	23	82

For Complete Nutritional Data ~ see CalorieKing.com

Daphne's® Greek Cafe (May '10)

Starters:	C	F	Cb
Hummus & Pita	330	17	37
Fire Feta & Pita	335	19	31
Pita Sandwiches: *Without Fries, Rice or Salad*			
Crispy Shrimp	430	23	39
Fresh Carved Gyros	665	46	42
Grilled Chicken	480	18	33
Spicy Grilled Chicken	600	29	36
Plates: *Without Sides, Pita Bread or Tzatziki*			
Grilled Chicken Ka-bobs	325	7	6
Grilled Steak Ka-bobs	220	11	9
Greek Salads: *Without Dressing*			
Classic	195	6	14
Crispy Shrimp	360	16	20
Falafel	670	40	52
Grilled Chicken	365	11	14
Dressings: Original	105	12	2
Lite Greek	60	6	2
Sides: Falafel, (3 pieces)	280	19	23
French Fries	270	12	37
Grilled Chicken Ka-bob	160	4	3
Pita Bread	230	8	28
Salad & Rice with Orig. Dressing	385	12	50
Spanakopita	220	18	11
Tzatziki	45	4	3

Davanni's® (May '10)

Half Hoagies: Includes 6" White Bun, Cheese, Salad, Butter, Dressing, Mayo & Sauce	C	F	Cb
Assorted	390	29	21
BLT	595	48	22
Chicken & Bacon with Honey Mustard	440	22	30
Chicken Parmigiana	365	17	22
Club	385	25	22
Italian Sausage	525	37	28
Pastrami	445	25	22
Pizza	315	18	22
Southwestern Chicken	480	27	25
Three Cheese	385	28	21
Tuna Melt	550	42	24
Turkey	355	22	22
Turkey Bacon Chipotle	465	30	22
Veggie	350	23	25
Calzones: Sausage Green Peppers	790	42	69
Pepperoni Sausage	825	49	66
Pizzas			
5 Meat: Thin Crust, 1 slice	240	12	18
Traditional Crust, 1 slice	300	12	30
Solo, Thin Crust	1010	63	45
The Works: Thin Crust, 1 slice	250	13	18
Traditional Crust, 1 slice	310	14	30
Veggie: Thin Crust, 1 slice	210	9	18
Traditional Crust, 1 slice	265	9	30

Updated Nutrition Data ~ www.CalorieKing.com
Persons with Diabetes ~ See Disclaimer (Page 24)

Del Taco® (May '10)

	C	F	Cb
Breakfast			
Breakfast Burrito	**280**	13	26
Bacon & Egg Quesadilla	**430**	20	37
Egg & Cheese Burrito	**400**	18	35
Steak & Egg Burrito	**520**	25	35
Hash Brown Sticks (5)	**210**	15	18
Burgers: Cheeseburger	**430**	22	40
Double Del Cheeseburger	**560**	35	35
Triple Del Cheeseburger	**950**	66	40
Burritos:			
Del Beef	**470**	20	37
Del Classic Chicken	**510**	33	37
Deluxe Combo	**570**	25	64
Deluxe Del Beef	**510**	23	39
Half Pound Red/Green, averag	**440**	10	67
Macho Beef	**1010**	44	82
Macho Chicken	**920**	30	111
Macho Combo	**990**	34	112
Shredded Beef Combo	**500**	20	55
Spicy Chicken; Veggie Works, av.	**615**	16	96
Nachos: 4 oz	**330**	22	28
Del, 7.27 oz	**440**	23	45
Quesadillas:			
Cheddar; Spicy Jack	**480**	25	37
Chicken Cheddar; Spicy Jack Chkn	**570**	30	40
Tacos: Big Fat Chicken	**330**	14	34
Big Fat Steak	**390**	18	33
Chicken Del Carbon	**150**	5	19
Chicken, Soft	**220**	12	16
Classic	**200**	12	10
Crispy Fish	**300**	17	29
Macho	**300**	17	16
Steak Taco Del Carbon	**210**	8	18
Salad:			
Deluxe Taco Salad	**850**	46	70
Sides:			
Chips & Salsa, 3 oz	**140**	8	15
Fries: Small, 5 oz	**270**	16	31
Macho, 10 oz	**550**	31	63
Chili Cheese, 10.5 oz	**570**	33	46
Deluxe Chili Cheese, 12 oz	**610**	36	48
Nachos, Macho, 17 oz	**1000**	56	94
Shakes: Chocolate, 13.4 fl.oz	**630**	13	117
Strawberry, 13.4 fl.oz	**600**	13	108
Vanilla, 13.4 fl.oz	**560**	13	100

Denny's® (May '10)

	C	F	Cb
Breakfast: *Without Sides*			
Favorites: T-Bone Steak & Eggs, 16 oz	**780**	36	4
Country Fried Steak & Eggs, 11 oz	**660**	42	29
Moons Over My Hammy, 13 oz	**780**	42	50
Southwest Steak Burrito	**910**	52	76
Omelettes: Ham & Cheddar, 10 oz	**590**	44	4
Ultimate, 12 oz	**670**	54	8
Veggie-Cheese, 13 oz	**500**	37	10
Scrambles: Heartland, 20 oz	**1150**	66	97
Meat Lovers, 19 oz	**1130**	66	80
Slams: All American, 10 oz	**820**	69	5
French Toast, 15 oz	**940**	53	68
Grand Slamwich, w/o Hash Browns	**1320**	90	71
Lumberjack, 15 oz	**850**	46	60
Sides: Biscuit & Sausage Gravy, 8 oz	**580**	34	57
English Muffin, with Margarine, (1)	**180**	3	25
Hash Browns, 5 oz	**210**	12	26
Oatmeal, with 8 oz milk, 16 oz	**270**	7	37
Sweets:			
Fabulous French Toast Platter (3)	**1010**	52	93
Pancakes: *Without Margarine, Syrup or Toppings*			
Buttermilk (3)	**510**	6	102
Chocolate Chip (3)	**720**	18	129
Toppings: Maple-flav Syrup, 1.5 oz	**145**	0	36
Sugar-free, 1.5 oz	**25**	0	9
Cherry Topping, 3 oz	**85**	0	21
Whipped Margarine, 1 Tbsp	**50**	0	6
Appetizers:			
Mozzarella Cheese Sticks, 8 oz	**750**	40	195
Smothered Cheese Fries, 10 oz	**840**	50	74
Burgers & Sandwiches: *Without Sides*			
Better Burgers:			
Bacon Cheddar, 15 oz	**940**	52	49
Classic Cheeseburger, 15 oz	**870**	46	51
Without Cheese, 14 oz	**790**	40	50
Double Cheeseburger, 23 oz	**1480**	88	52
Mushroom Swiss, 18 oz	**910**	49	55
Slamburger, 15 oz	**990**	54	59
Sandwiches: BLT, w/ Mayo, 7 oz	**520**	35	35
Club, with Mayo, 11 oz	**640**	33	55
Grilled Chicken, w/ dressing, 15 oz	**880**	51	64
Super Bird, without dressing, 12 oz	**700**	37	53
Melts: *Without Dressing*			
Chicken Ranch, 12 oz	**800**	30	80
Spicy Buffalo Chicken, 15 oz	**870**	41	82
Dinner Meals: *W/o sides, sauce or bread unless indicated*			
Amerian Classics: Chicken Strips, 8 oz	**560**	24	41
Country Fried Steak w/ Gravy, 13 oz	**1000**	65	54
Homestyle Meatloaf w/ Gravy, 7 oz	**600**	46	14
Sizzlin' Skillets: Grilled Chicken	**770**	34	72
Prime Rib, 19 oz	**900**	42	77

Continued Next Page...

Denny's® cont... (May '10)

Dinner Meals (Cont) *Without Sides, Sauce Or Bread Unless Indicated*	C	F	Cb
Steak & Seafood:			
Fit Fare Grilled Tilapia, 17 oz	600	11	66
Grilled Shrimp Skewers, 10 oz	370	10	39
Lemon Pepper Tilapia, 13 oz	640	27	41
T-Bone Steak: 12 oz	740	56	0
With Breaded Shrimp, 13 oz	920	64	20
With Shrimp Skewer, 12 oz	830	60	0
Tilapia Ranchero, 19 oz	470	17	57
***Salads:** Without Dressing or Bread*			
Chicken Strip Deluxe, 18 oz	590	29	44
Cranberry Pecan Chicken, 9 oz	250	8	11
Grilled Chicken Deluxe, 17 oz	290	10	15
Prime Rib & Bleu, 10 oz	270	16	6
***Dressings:** Per 1 oz*			
Bleu Cheese	130	13	1
Caesar	100	10	0
French	75	5	8
Honey Mustard	160	15	5
Ranch	130	14	1
Sides (Dinner)			
Coleslaw, 5 oz	260	22	15
Country-Fried Potatoes, 5 oz	390	28	30
Dinner Rolls, 2 pcs	260	9	38
Garlic Bread, 2 pcs	170	9	21
Ranchero Mashed Potatoes, 4 oz	140	6	50
***Soups:** Without Bread*			
Chicken Noodle, 12 oz	165	4	19
Clam Chowder, 12 oz	265	17	24
Vegetable Beef, 12 oz	125	1	18
Desserts			
Cheesecake, 7 oz	640	41	58
French Silk Pie, 7 oz	770	57	59
Hot Fudge Brownie a la Mode, 9 oz	830	37	122
Oreo Blender Blaster, 14 oz	890	44	113
Oreo Sundae, 9 oz	760	37	103
Beverages			
Flav. Cappuccino; Hot Choc., 8 fl.oz	100	2	28
Milkshakes, Van/Choc, 12 fl.oz	560	26	76
Raspberry Nestea, 16 fl.oz	80	0	21

For Complete Nutritional Data ~ see CalorieKing.com

Dippin' Dots® (Feb '10)

Flavored Ices	C	F	Cb
All flavors, ½ cup, 3 oz	90	0	23
Frozen Yogurt:			
Strawberry Cheesecake, ½ cup	100	0	21
***Ice Cream:** Per ½ Cup*			
Banana Split	170	10	16
Chocolate Chip Cookie dough	215	11	26
Peanut Butter Chip	165	10	15
Strawberry	170	10	16
Fat-Free, Fudge, No Sugar Added	90	0	18
Red.-Fat, Vanilla, No Sugar Added	125	6	13

Donato's® Pizza (May '10)

***Thin Crust Pizza:** ¼ Large Pizza*	C	F	Cb
Chicken Vegy Medley	495	20	51
Classic Trio	675	37	52
Founder's Favorite	700	38	52
Hawaiian	590	27	56
***Thicker Crust Pizza:** ¼ Large Pizza*			
Founder's Favorite	860	42	78
Mariachi Beef	795	36	81
Mariachi Chicken	805	35	81
Pepperoni	800	39	76
Serious Cheese	800	38	77
The Works	845	41	81
Vegy	715	29	83
No Dough Pizza - Individual			
Chicken Vegy Medley	495	29	20
Classic Trio	530	37	18
Founder's Favorite	560	38	18
Hawaiian	435	26	22
Mariachi Beef	530	34	23
Mariachi Chicken	495	30	21
Pepperoni	500	35	17
Pepperoni Zinger	585	42	17
Serious Cheese	455	31	17
Serious Meat	655	46	19
The Works	545	37	21
***Stromboli:** 3 Meat*	690	31	67
Cheese	695	31	66
Deluxe	615	25	68
Pepperoni	715	34	67
Vegy	605	24	69
Desserts:			
Apple Timpano, 2 slices	405	9	72
Cinnamon Timpano, 2 slices	525	22	73

For Complete Nutritional Data ~ see CalorieKing.com

Updated Nutrition Data ~ www.CalorieKing.com
Persons with Diabetes ~ See Disclaimer (Page 24)

Domino's® Pizza (Feb '10)

	C	F	Cb
***12" Hand-Tossed**: Per Slice, ⅛ Pizza*			
Beef	205	9	23
Cheese Only	180	6	23
Green Peppers, Onion & Mushroom	180	6	23
Ham	190	6	23
Ham & Pineapple	195	6	24
Pepperoni	205	8	23
Pepperoni & Sausage	235	11	24
Sausage	210	9	24
***14" Thin Crust:** Per Slice, ⅛ Pizza*			
Beef	230	14	18
Cheese Only	190	11	18
Green Pepper Onion & Mushroom	190	11	18
Ham	200	11	18
Ham & Pineapple	210	11	20
Pepperoni	220	14	18
Pepperoni & Sausage	265	17	19
Sausage	235	14	19
***12" Deep Dish:** Per Slice, ⅛ Pizza*			
Beef	245	12	26
Cheese Only	220	10	26
Green Pepper Onion & Mushroom	220	10	26
Ham	230	10	26
Ham & Pineapple	235	10	27
Pepperoni	245	12	26
Pepperoni & Sausage	275	14	27
Sausage	250	12	27
***12" Feast Hand-Tossed:** Per Slice, ⅛ Pizza*			
America's Favorite Feast	120	14	10
Bacon Cheeseburger Feast	260	12	25
Barbecue Feast	240	10	30
Deluxe Feast	220	9	26
ExtravaganZZa Feast	280	13	27
Hawaiian Feast	210	7.5	27
MeatZZa Feast	270	13	26
Philly Cheese Steak Feast	220	9	23
Ultimate Pepperoni	250	13	24
Vegi Feast	210	7.5	26
***14" Feast Thin Crust:** Per Slice, ⅛ Pizza*			
America's Favorite Feast	180	10	19
Bacon Cheeseburger Feast	310	20	21
Barbecue Feast	280	16	27
Deluxe Feast	250	15	21
ExtravaganZZa Feast	320	20	22
Hawaiian Feast	230	13	23
MeatZZa Feast	310	20	21
Philly Cheese Steak Feast	240	14	18
Ultimate Pepperoni	290	19	19
Vegi Feast	220	13	22

Domino's® Pizza cont... (Feb '10)

	C	F	Cb
***12" Feast Deep Dish:** Per Slice, ⅛ Pizza*			
America's Favorite Feast	160	5	24
Bacon Cheeseburger Feast	300	15	28
Barbecue Feast	280	13	30
Hawaiian Feast	250	11	29
Philly Cheese Steak Feast	260	12	25
Ultimate Pepperoni	290	15	27
Oven Baked Sandwiches			
Chicken Bacon Ranch	880	46	70
Chicken Parm	760	31	72
Italian	880	45	71
Philly Cheese Steak	690	27	72
***BreadBowl Pasta:** Per ½ Bowl*			
Chicken Alfredo, 10.85 oz	700	25	93
Chicken Carbonara, 11.65 oz	740	28	94
Italian Sausage Marinara, 11.9 oz	735	27	98
Pasta Primavera, 11 oz	670	24	94
***Salads:** Per 2 Servings*			
Garden Fresh, 8.45 oz	140	7	10
Grilled Chicken Caesar, 9.5 oz	180	7	10
***Salad Dressings & Condiments:** Per 1.5 oz Package*			
Blue Cheese	240	25	2
Buttermilk Ranch	230	24	2
Creamy Caesar	210	21	2
Golden Italian	210	22	2
Light Italian	20	1	3
Bread Side Items			
Breadsticks: 1 stick, without sauce	105	6	11
8 sticks, without sauce	850	48	88
Cheesy Bread:			
1 stick, without sauce	110	6	11
8 sticks, without sauce	880	48	88
Bread Dipping Sauces: *Per Container*			
Garlic	250	28	0
Marinara	25	0	5
Cinna Stix:			
1 stick, without icing	120	6	14
8 sticks, without icing	960	48	112
Sweet Icing, Dipper Cup	250	2.5	57
Chicken Side Items			
Buffalo Chicken Kickers			
without Dipping Sauce (2)	100	4.5	7
Buffalo Wings:			
Barbecue, 2 wings, without sauce	230	14	6
Hot, 2 wings, without sauce	200	14	2
Chicken Dipping Sauces: *Per 1.5 oz Container*			
Blue Cheese	240	25	2
Hot	50	4.5	3
Ranch	200	21	2

Don Pablos® (May '10)

Appetizers: Per Whole Plate, Includes Queso & Garnish, without Guacamole	C	F	Cb
Beef Taquitos (6)	625	45	27
Chicken Flautas (6)	565	36	39
Dips: *Per 6 oz Cup, Without Chips*			
Queso Blanco	540	45	6
Prairie Fire Bean	355	21	27
Nachos: *Per Whole Plate, w/ Garnish w/o Guacamole*			
Acapulco Beef (9 chips)	1385	87	69
Cheese (9 chips)	1145	84	39
Quesadillas: *With Garnish, without Guacamole*			
Mesquite Grilled: Chicken, 4 slices	825	50	62
Steak, 8 slices	1630	100	104
Burritos: *Entree, Per Burrito, Beans Not Included*			
Chicken	1180	58	105
Spicy Ground Beef & Bean	1285	68	97
Carnitas: *Entree, Beans Not Included*			
Pork	985	34	120
Cold Set, Side	160	11	18
Chimichangas: *Entree, Beans Not Included*			
Chicken	1100	61	91
Spicy Ground Beef De Oro	1475	80	112
Classic Fajitas: *Entree, w/ On., Peppers & Lime, w/o Fajita*			
Combo - Steak & Chicken	625	31	47
Grilled Chrimp	425	38	22
Mesquite - Grilled: Chicken	570	27	58
Steak	680	36	36
Add Fixin's: Flour Tortillas (3)	1120	33	180
Corn Tortillas (4)	235	4	48
Guacamole, 1 scoop	70	6	4
Tacos: Crispy Beef (3)	870	41	65
Crispy Chicken (3)	725	31	66
Lunch:			
Combos: *Entree, w/o Beverage, Soup or Side Salad*			
Don Pablo's	790	36	70
Dos Beef Tacos (Soft)	1085	48	192
Fajitas: *Entree, w/ On., Peppers & Lime, w/o Fajita*			
Chicken	280	13	29
Steak	335	17	18
Quesadilla & Salad Combo: *Entree, w/o Dressing*			
Cheese	1045	69	64
Chicken	1045	56	75
Salads:			
Chicken Caesar, with Dressing	1285	76	114
Steak Caesar, with Dressing	1360	82	99
Sides: French Fries, w/o Ketchup, 7 oz	345	10	60
Mexican Rice, 3 oz	120	2	23
Monterey, Jack & Cheddar Chse, 1 oz	110	9	1
Refritos, 5 oz	215	7	27
Sour Cream, 1 scoop	80	8	2

Dunkin Donuts® (May '10)

	C	F	Cb
Donuts: Apple N' Spice	240	11	32
Bavarian Kreme	250	12	31
Boston Kreme	280	12	38
Chocolate Frosted	230	10	32
Chocolate Kreme Filled	310	16	37
French Cruller	250	20	18
Jelly Filled	260	11	36
Old Fashioned Cake	280	18	27
Powdered Cake	300	18	30
Strawberry Frosted	230	10	33
Sugar Raised	190	9	22
Vanilla Kreme Filled	320	17	37
Fancies: Apple Fritter	400	15	63
Bow Tie Donut	310	15	39
Chocolate Iced Bismark	350	14	53
Coffee Roll: Original	370	18	49
Chocolate Frosted	380	19	50
Eclair	350	14	53
Fritter: Apple	400	15	63
Glazed	400	15	63
Munchkins: Plain Cake (4)	200	12	20
Glazed, average all varieties (4)	240	12	32
Jelly Filled (5)	300	13	40
Powdered Cake (4)	240	14	24
Sugar Raised (5)	200	13	25
Sticks: Plain Cake	300	20	26
Cinnamon Cake	310	20	30
Glazed: Cake	340	20	38
Chocolate Cake	390	25	40
Jelly	400	20	54
Powdered Cake	320	20	31
Bagels: Plain; Salt	320	2.5	63
Cinnamon Raisin	330	3.5	65
Everything; Poppy Seed, average	350	5	65
Multigrain	390	8	65
Onion; Wheat, average	315	3	62
Sesame	360	6	63
Danish: Apple Cheese	330	16	41
Cheese	330	17	39
Strawberry Cheese	320	16	40
Muffins: Chocolate Chip	630	23	98
Blueberry	510	16	87
Reduced Fat	450	10	86
Coffee Cake	660	26	98
Corn	510	17	84
Honey Bran Raisin	500	14	86

Continued Next Page ...

Dunkin Donuts® cont... (May '10)

Breakfast	C	F	Cb
Oven Toasted Breakfast Sandwiches:			
Bagels: Egg & Cheese	**470**	14	66
Bacon Egg & Cheese	**510**	17	66
Ham Egg & Cheese	**510**	16	67
Sausage Egg & Cheese	**640**	29	67
Biscuits: Bacon Egg & Cheese	**470**	29	36
Sausage Egg & Cheese	**610**	40	36
Croissant: Bacon Egg & Cheese	**510**	31	39
Ham Egg & Cheese	**510**	30	39
Sausage Egg & Cheese	**640**	43	39
English Muffin:			
Bacon Egg & Cheese	**360**	16	34
Ham Egg & Cheese	**360**	15	35
Sausage Egg & Cheese	**490**	28	35
Sandwiches			
Dunkin' Deli Sandwiches			
Cravings: Chicken Bruschetta	**580**	26	49
Chipotle Chicken	**600**	25	50
Pastrami Supreme	**750**	39	51
Pressed Cuban	**680**	33	50
Deli Classics: Tuna (Albacore)	**660**	19	56
Turkey & Cheese	**450**	13	52
Favorites: Steak & Cheese	**470**	16	50
Toasted Italian	**560**	25	52
Turkey & Bacon Club	**440**	13	51
Salads: *With Dressing*			
Dunkin' Deli: Caesar	**320**	29	11
Chicken Caesar	**440**	33	11
Garden	**180**	6	21
Soups: Broccoli Cheddar, 1 cup	**190**	11	14
Chicken Noodle	**130**	3	19
Beverages			
Cappuccino, without sugar, 10 fl.oz	**80**	4	7
Coolatta:			
Coffee: with Skim Milk, 16 fl.oz	**210**	0	51
With Cream, 16 fl.oz	**400**	23	49
With Milk, 16 fl.oz	**240**	4	50
Strawberry Fruit, 16 fl.oz	**300**	0	72
Tropical Orange, 16 fl.oz	**220**	0	52
Hot Chocolate: Small, 10 fl.oz	**210**	7	39
White, 1 medium, 14 fl.oz	**340**	13	56
Iced Coffee: 16 fl.oz	**10**	0	2
Flavored Coffee: Caramel, 10 fl.oz	**10**	0	2
Toasted Almond, 10 fl.oz	**10**	0	1

Eat 'N Park® (May '10)

Breakfast	C	F	Cb
Fruit Cup	**60**	0.5	15
Hash Browns	**200**	8	28
Home Fries	**210**	12	24
Oatmeal with Milk	**200**	4	33
Omelette: Cheese	**390**	30	2.5
Chicken Fiesta	**565**	37	10
Ham & Cheese	**535**	35	4
Veggie	**415**	30	8
Western	**345**	21	7
Pancakes, Buttermilk: Plain (1)	**75**	1	15
Blueberry (1)	**85**	1	16
Waffles: Belgian (1)	**280**	12	35
Strawberry (1)	**375**	18	48
Appetizers:			
Buffalo Chicken Tenders	**635**	42	27
Fried Cheese Sticks	**535**	36	26
Grilled Chicken Quesadillas	**905**	55	51
Onion Rings	**245**	16	23
Burgers:			
Black Angus: American Grill	**610**	37	31
BBQ Bacon Cheddar	**865**	53	53
Mushroom & Onion	**710**	41	45
Superburger	**1085**	73	28
Classic: Black Angus	**420**	21	22
Bacon Cheeseburger	**530**	31	22
Cheeseburger	**465**	25	22
Garden Burger	**220**	4	33
Original, Superburger	**565**	38	27
Sandwiches:			
BLT	**490**	15	66
Buffalo Chicken	**740**	41	59
Chargrilled Chicken	**320**	6	32
Chicken Portabella Hoagie	**845**	56	47
Hot Turkey	**500**	9	71
Reuben on Rye	**730**	50	31
Santa Fe Turkey & Bacon	**880**	60	45
Shredded Pot Roast	**530**	31	28
Turkey Club	**835**	50	52
Whale of a Cod Fish	**880**	41	76
Dinners: Baked Lemon Sole, 1 filet	**195**	10	6
Chargrilled Chicken, 2 pieces	**350**	9	0
Chicken Fillets (5)	**530**	26	28
Chkn Parmigiana: With Marinara Sce	**960**	37	100
With Meat Sauce	**985**	40	95
Chicken Stir-Fry	**390**	8	47
Cod Floridian, 2 filets	**240**	3	8
Ground Sirloin with Fried Onion Ring	**425**	26	5
Spaghetti Marinara	**695**	9	129
Spaghetti with Meat Sauce	**830**	16	145
T Bone Steak	**575**	39	1

Continued next page...

Eat 'N Park® cont... (May '10)

Salads: Without Dressing	C	F	Cb
Buffalo Chicken Salad	610	35	42
Chicken Fajita	410	12	35
Garden Salad	95	3	15
Grilled Chicken	445	20	30
Grilled Chicken & Strawberry	215	6	13
Grilled Chicken Portobella	310	10	23
***Dressings:** Per 2 fl.oz*			
Bleu Cheese	245	25	3
French Fat Free	75	0	18
Italian Fat Free	20	0	5
House Ranch	215	21	4
Thousand Island	190	19	4
Desserts:			
Grilled Stickies a la Mode	725	39	81
Ice Cream, 2 scoops	230	12	27
Pies: *Per Slice*			
Apple	525	27	67
Cherry	520	28	63
Peachberry	390	19	51
Strawberry	295	12	45

Edo Japan® (May '10)

***Meals:** Per Bento Box w/o Teriyaki*	C	F	Cb
Beef Yakisoba, 20.28 oz	830	30	102
Chicken Yakisoba, 20.53 oz	800	25	102
Seafood Grill, 23 oz	860	16	129
Sizzling Shrimp, 22.05 oz	800	16	122
Sukiyaki Beef, 20.14 oz	900	28	120
Specialties: *Without Teriyaki Sauce*			
Curry Chicken Bowl, 13.23 oz	500	21	27
Ginger Pork, 14.6 oz	650	23	82
Hawaiian Chicken, 15.52 oz	590	12	85
Seafood Grill, 17.71 oz	570	4	89
Sukiyaki Beef, 14.85 oz	610	16	80
Teriyaki Chicken, 15.1 oz	580	12	80

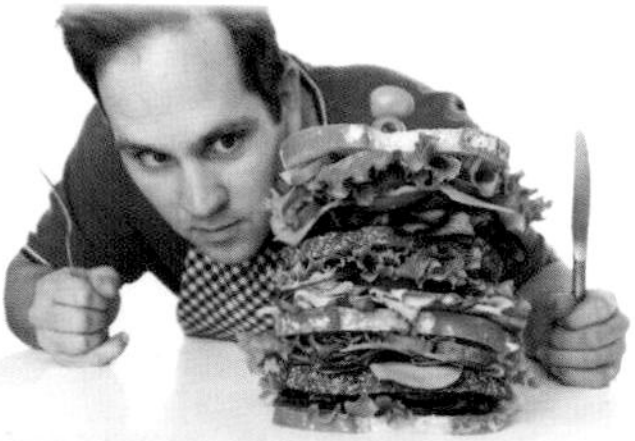

Einstein Bros®/Noahs® (May '10)

Bagels:	C	F	Cb
Asiago Cheese	310	5	56
Blueberry	300	1	65
Chocolate Chip	280	2.5	56
Cinnamon Sugar Chicago Style	310	2.5	66
Egg	300	5	54
Everything	270	2	56
Garlic Dip'd	270	2.5	56
Honey Whole Wheat; Plain	260	1	57
Onion Dip'd	270	2.5	56
Poppy Dip'd	280	3	56
Potato	270	4	52
Power Bagel, Fruit & Nut	310	5	61
Sesame Dip'd	280	3	56
Sundried Tomato	260	1.5	54
Gourmet Bagels: Dutch Apple	350	7	66
Green Chile	350	8	58
Spinach Florentine	340	8	57
Six-Cheese	330	6	56
Breakfast Sandwiches			
Egg Way: Original	530	20	62
With Bacon	580	24	59
With Black Forest Ham	570	21	62
Spinach Mushroom & Omelette	540	20	65
Bacon & Spinach Panini	860	51	66
Sausage Ranchero Panini	680	29	64
Vegetable Panini	730	36	68
Wraps: California Chicken	630	28	63
Chipotle Turkey	730	37	70
***Bagel Dogs:** With Cheddar Cheese*			
Original	550	26	56
Original Asiago	560	27	56
Pizza Bagels: Cheese	420	12	63
Pepperoni	470	16	63
***Cream Cheese:** Per 2 Tablespoons, Whipped*			
Reduced Fat: Blueberry	70	5	6
Garlic Herb/Garden Veggie	60	5	3
Honey Almond; Strawberry, av.	70	5	6
Plain; Sun Dried Tomato & Basil	60	5	2
Onion and Chive	70	6	3
Smoked Salmon	60	6	2
***Salads:** With Dressing*			
Bros Bistro	820	68	38
Bros Bistro with Chicken	940	71	39
Chipotle	590	38	53
Chicken Chipotle	710	41	54
Caesar Salad with Chicken	820	66	20
***Coffee, Specialty:** Per Regular, 12 fl.oz*			
Americano Regular 8 fl.oz	1	0	0
Café Latte	140	5	13
Non-Fat	100	1	14
Cappuccino, Whole Milk	150	8	13
Espresso, Regular 2 fl.oz	1	0	0
Mocha, Whole Milk	270	9	38

Updated Nutrition Data ~ www.CalorieKing.com
Persons with Diabetes ~ See Disclaimer (Page 24)

El Pollo Loco® (May '10)

Burritos:	C	F	Cb
BRC	440	12	68
Classic Chicken	550	17	69
Ultimate Grilled	710	23	86
Flame-Grilled Chicken: *Skin On*			
Breast	220	9	0
Leg	90	4	0
Thigh	220	15	0
Wing	90	5	0
Bowls: Chicken Caesar	490	22	44
The Original Pollo	690	10	106
Ultimate Pollo	1050	34	110
Loco Value Menu:			
Chicken Taquito with Avocado Salsa	230	12	20
Chips & Guacamole	250	14	26
Cheese Quesadilla	420	23	35
Loco Salad with Cilantro Dressing	170	14	7
Taco al Carbon	150	5	17
Mexican Favorites:			
Grilled Chicken Nachos	810	40	70
Grilled Chicken Tortilla without Sauce	390	16	37
Soup:			
Chicken Tortilla w/ Tortilla Strips, reg.	210	9	18
Large	450	20	37
Tacos: Crunchy Chicken	190	8	16
Soft Chicken	260	12	18
Salads: Chicken Tostada w/o Dressing	840	42	74
Garden Salad, small, w/o Dressing	70	3.5	8
Dressings: *Per Packet*			
Creamy Cilantro, 3 oz	440	46	3
Light Creamy Cilantro, 2 oz	70	5	6
Light Italian, 2 oz	20	1	2
Ranch, 2 oz	230	24	2
Thousand Island, 2 oz	220	21	6
Condiments			
Guacamole, 1.3 oz	70	6	3
Salsa: Avocado, 1.5 oz	40	3.5	2
House, 1.5 oz	10	0	2
Pico de Gallo, 1.5 oz	15	1	2
Sides			
Corn Cobbette, 5 oz	90	0.5	19
French Fries, 6 oz	330	17	42
Fresh Vegetables w/ Marg., 4.1 oz	60	3	8
Macaroni & Cheese, 5.5 oz	280	17	28
Mashed Potatoes with Gravy, 6 oz	120	1.5	25
Pinto Beans, 6 oz	200	4	29
Refried Beans with Cheese, 6.3 oz	270	7	36
Spanish Rice, 4½ oz	220	2	45
Desserts: Caramel Flan, 5.1 oz	260	12	34
Churros (2)	300	18	32

For Complete Nutritional Data ~ see CalorieKing.com

Fatburger® (May '10)

Burgers: *Without Extras*	C	F	Cb
Baby Fat	400	21	37
Fatburger	590	31	46
Kingburger	850	41	69
Turkeyburger	480	21	50
Veggieburger	510	20	60
Sandwiches: *Without Extras*			
Crispy Chicken	560	27	53
Grilled Chicken	430	14	42
Fish	560	31	55
Sides and Fries			
Fries: Fat Fries; Skinny Fries, av.	*385*	*17*	*53*
with Chili, average	485	23	57
with Chili & Cheese, average	595	32	58
Sides: American Cheese, 1 slice	70	5	1
Cheddar Cheese, 1 slice	110	9	1
Chili Cup	200	11	10
with Cheese & Onions	320	20	12
Mayonnaise	90	10	1
Onion Rings	540	29	64
Relish	20	0	5
Shakes: Chocolate	910	45	115
Peanut Butter	950	53	114
Strawberry; Vanilla, average	885	44	112

***For* Complete Nutritional Data ~ see CalorieKing.com**

Fazoli's® Italian Food (May '10)

Pasta Bowl: *Per Serving*	C	F	Cb
Fettuccine with Alfredo, 19.9 oz	900	27	126
Fettuccine with Marinara, 20.5 oz	660	3	129
Ravioli with Marinara Sce, 12.3 oz	490	15	69
Ravioli with Meat Sauce, 13.1 oz	570	21	70
Spaghetti w/ Marinara Sce, 20.5 oz	660	3	129
Sampler Platter: *Per Serving*			
Classic Sampler Platter, 22.8 oz	880	30	110
Ultimate Sampler Platter, 29.9 oz	1130	34	153
Oven-Baked Pasta: *Per Serving*			
Chicken Broccoli Penne	920	42	77
Chicken Parmigano, 21.6 oz	1000	39	108
Baked Spaghetti, 15.5 oz	640	22	80
With Meatballs, 18.5 oz	890	39	86
Penne with Creamy Basil Chkn, 18.7 oz	970	51	73
Rigatoni Romano, 17.3 oz	880	44	76
Tortellini Robusto, 17.6 oz	1020	50	80
Twice-Baked Lasagna, 18.4 oz	700	39	47
Pizzas: *Per Slice*			
Cheese, 4 oz	270	11	32
Pepperoni, 4.3 oz	310	14	32

Continued next page...

Fazoli's® cont... (May '10)

Submarinos	C	F	Cb
Club Italiano, 13 oz	780	36	68
Fazoli's Original, 12.8 oz	880	50	68
Ham 'n' Swiss Supremo, 12.1 oz	690	31	68
Italian Four Chse & Tomato, 11.6 oz	710	37	59
Rstd Red Pepper Chicken, 11.8 oz	780	36	59
Smoked Turkey Basil, 12.8 oz	750	37	68
***Salads:** Without Dressing*			
Caesar Side Salad, 4.2 oz	40	2	4
Chicken & Pasta Caesar, 13.3 oz	470	15	38
Cranberry & Walnut Chicken	390	14	27
Crispy Chicken BLT	480	26	31
Grilled Chicken Artichoke	240	4.5	11
Italian Side Salad, 4.2 oz	80	4.5	4
Pasta Side Salad, 6 oz	300	12	38
***Salad Dressing:** Per 1.5 oz*			
Caesar	230	25	1
Italian	160	14	7
Fat Free	25	0	6
Honey French	220	18	14
Ranch	220	24	2
Lite Ranch	120	12	2

For Complete Nutritional Data ~ see CalorieKing.com

Firehouse Subs® (May '10)

***Subs:** Per Medium, Without Mayo or Cheese*

	C	F	Cb
Chicken Salad	760	46	63
Engine Company	390	6	52
Engineer	380	5	55
Ham	410	7	58
Hero	430	7	54
Hook & Ladder	410	7	68
Italian	560	25	55
NY Steamer	410	12	48
Roast Beef	410	6	48
Tuna Salad	610	28	62
Turkey	370	4	54
Veggie	300	5	56
***Chili and Salads:** Includes Meat, Cheese and Egg, w/o Dressing*			
Chili	370	28	17
Chief's Salad: With Chicken Salad	740	58	16
With Tuna Salad	610	40	16
With Ham	360	18	16
With Turkey	300	15	12
Desserts: Brownie (1)	420	18	63
Chocolate Chip Cookie	290	14	37

Five Guys (May '10)

Burgers	C	F	Cb
Bacon Burger	780	50	39
Bacon Cheeseburger	920	62	40
Cheeseburger	840	55	40
Hamburger	700	43	39
Little: Bacon Burger	560	33	39
Bacon Cheeseburger	630	39	40
Cheeseburger	550	32	40
Hamburger	480	26	39
Dogs			
Bacon Dog	625	42	40
Bacon Cheese Dog	695	48	41
Cheese Dog	615	41	41
Hot Dog	545	36	40
Fries: Regular 8.6 oz	620	30	78
½ Regular Order	310	15	39

Freshens® (May '10)

***Frozen Yogurt:** Per Serving*	C	F	Cb
Soft Serve Yogurt, 1 oz	35	0	7
***Smoothies:** 100% Juice (21 fl.oz)*			
Blended Fruit: Caribbean Craze	290	0	73
Citrus Mango	490	7	108
Jamaican Jammer	350	0	77
Maui Mango	290	0	74
Orange Sunrise	360	3	82
Peach Sunset	270	0	67
Strawberry: Kiwi	320	0	81
Shooter	250	0	64
Squeeze	310	0	68
Tropical Pineapple	310	4	97
High Protein: Peanut Butter	540	12	84
Chocolate Oreo	610	7	11
Low Calorie: No Sugar Added			
Average all flavors	80	0	50
(Note: Carbs include 35g Erythritol Sweetener)			
Nature's Energy: Acai Energy	320	3	71
Mangosteen	320	0	89
Tart Berry	320	0	82
Yerba Mate	320	0	68
Fro-Yo Blasts:			
Cap'n Crunch & P'nut Butter	510	12	82
Cookie Dough	570	7	112
Oreo Overload	430	3.5	83
Indulgent Shakes: Chocolate	530	4	103
Oreo Cream	610	7	115
Strawberry	490	4	94

Updated Nutrition Data ~ www.CalorieKing.com
Persons with Diabetes ~ See Disclaimer (Page 24)

Gino's East® ® (May '10)

	C	F	Cb
Deep Dish Pizza: *Medium 11" Per ⅙ Slice of Pizza*			
Cheese	410	11	58
Crumbled Sausage	420	21	38
Pepperoni	450	15	57
Spinach	410	11	59
Deep Dish Pizza: *Small 6" ~ Per Whole Pizza*			
Cheese	720	16	116
Crumbled Sausage	800	22	116
Pepperoni	780	20	116

Godfather's™ Pizza May '10)

	C	F	Cb
Golden Pizza: *Per Slice*			
Cheese: Medium, ⅛ pizza	220	8	25
Large,1/10 pizza	250	9	28
Combo: Medium, 1/8 pizza	290	13	27
Large, slice, 1/10 pizza	330	15	30
Original Pizza			
Cheese: Mini, ¼ pizza	150	4	20
Medium, ⅛ pizza	260	7	34
Jumbo, 1/12 pizza	350	10	44
Combo: Mini, ¼ pizza	200	8	21
Medium, ⅛ pizza	350	14	36
Jumbo, 1/12 pizza	480	20	47
Thin Pizza			
Cheese: Medium, ⅛ pizza	170	8	15
Large, 1/10 pizza	210	10	17
Combo: Medium, ⅛ pizza	240	13	17
Large, 1/10 pizza	280	16	20
Sides			
Breadstick (1)	110	2	20
Cheesestick,1 piece, ⅙	130	3.5	18
Potato Wedges, 4 oz	175	8	24

Gold Star Chili® (May '10)

	C	F	Cb
Meals			
Bowls: Low Carb Coney, 10.5 oz	570	47	7
Veggie Chili, 9 oz	160	2	29
Coney, 5.15 oz	285	14	30
Cheese Coney, 5.64 oz	345	18	31
Chili: 8 oz	215	12	8
Tex Mex, 8 oz	210	9	17
Chili Cheese Nachos, 8.47 oz	410	25	30
Regular: 2-Way	420	11	58
Bean	490	12	71
Onion	435	11	62
Onion Bean	505	12	75

Gold Star Chili (Cont)® (May '10)

	C	F	Cb
Meals (Cont)			
Bowls (Cont): Regular 3-Way	650	30	59
Regular 4-Way	665	30	63
Regular 5-Way	735	30	76
Super 5-Way	1140	51	109
Sandwiches: Chili	210	5	32
Chili Cheese	290	12	30
Salads: *Without Dressing*			
Cafe: 7.9 oz	160	10	15
With Crispy Chicken	310	15	24
With Grilled Chicken, 10.4 oz	250	12	15
Caesar Salad, 5.95 oz	130	6	12
With Crispy Chicken, 8.4 oz	280	11	22
With Grilled chicken, 8.4 oz	210	8	12
South of the Border Chili, 16.7 oz	640	39	55
Sides: Fries, 5 oz	365	19	44
Chili Cheese, 9.5 oz	595	36	46
Garlic Bread: Without Cheese, 2 oz	215	13	19
With Cheese, 2½ oz	270	18	19

Golden Corral® (May '10)

	C	F	Cb
Breakfast:			
Bacon & Cheese Quiche, 1 sl., 4 oz	280	19	15
Corned Beef Hash, 1 cup	420	30	22
French Toast, 1 slice	240	8	23
Hash Browns, 1 cup	205	14	16
Sausage Links (3)	160	14	1
Sausage Patties (1)	245	21	0.5
Scrambled Eggs, 3.5 oz	160	11	2
Split Smoked Sausage (1)	250	23	2
Meals:			
Hot Bar: *Without Sides*			
Awesome Pot Roast, 3 oz	100	4.5	5
Baked Fish with Shrimp & Sauce	160	10	2
Baked Florentine Fish, 3 oz	180	12	2
BBQ: Chicken Leg Quarter, 7.8 oz	490	22	21
Pork, 3 oz	170	8	5
Bone-In Breaded Catfish, 3 oz	210	14	7
Bourbon Street Chicken, 3 oz	170	9	4
Breaded Scallops (10), 2.57 oz	140	6	13
Coconut Shrimp (5), 2 oz	200	12	16
Crab Cakes (1), 1.95 oz	180	15	8
Grilled Lemon Pepper Fish (1), 3 oz	180	11	5
Meatloaf, w/ Topping,1 slice, 4.05 oz	220	11	12
Sirloin Steak, 4.5 oz	230	9	1
Cold Bar: Per ½ Cup			
Cajun Potato Salad	230	17	15
Coleslaw	110	9	6
Salads: Seafood	140	10	9
Spinach Applewood Bacon , 1 cup	150	11	7
Tuna	200	14	5

(The) Great American Bagel Co® (May '10)

	C	F	Cb
Bagels: 4-Grain Honey	390	4	80
Apple Cinnamon Sugar	390	4	78
Asiago Cheese	520	16	72
Banana Nut	410	9	69
Blueberry	370	3.5	75
Cheddar Bacon	600	23	71
Chocolate Chip	420	8	78
Cinnamon Delight	640	18	108
Jalapeno Cheddar	370	7	63
Onion	380	4	74
Plain; Pumpernickel; Salt	360	4	71
Stuffed Pepperoni	570	17	78
Stuffed Spinach	640	20	86
Sun-Dried Tomato Basil	390	4	74
Tomazzo	520	13	77
Veggie	310	3.5	61
Sandwiches: BLT	550	17	72
Chicken Parmigiana	740	22	81
Ham	460	9	71
Roast Beef	465	8.5	71
Cream Cheese Filling: *Per 1 oz*			
Apple Cinnamon; Blueberry	60	4.5	4
Caramel Apple; Choc. Chip, average	70	4	7.5
Garlic Herb; Plain, average	60	5	1
Salsa; Scallion; Spinach, average	50	4.5	1
Strawberry	55	5	1

Green Burrito (May '10)

	C	F	Cb
Burritos: Bean & Cheese	780	36	94
Grilled Chicken	880	46	81
The Green Burrito with Steak	850	32	109
Specialties:			
Super Nachos: Chicken	920	48	93
Ground Beef	1060	61	95
Taco Salad: Chicken	780	44	66
Ground Beef	920	56	69
Steak	810	46	69
Tacos: Fish	320	15	36
Hard Shell: Chicken; Steak, average	195	9	15
Ground Beef	240	14	15
Soft Shell: Chicken	200	7	17
Ground Beef	250	13	18
Sides: Chips, 2 oz	300	17	35
Chips & Cheese, 5 oz	700	42	62
Guacamole, 1.4 oz	60	5	3
Pinto Beans & Cheese, 8.5 oz	320	16	43
Rice, 6 oz	290	9	50
Sour Cream, 1.4 oz	50	3.5	3

(The) Great Steak & Potato Company® (May '10)

	C	F	Cb
Breakfast Sandwiches			
Bacon, Egg & Cheese	600	36	39
Egg and Cheese	500	29	39
Ham and Cheese	430	22	41
Ham, Egg and Cheese	570	32	42
Sausage, Egg and Cheese	700	47	39
Steak, Egg & Cheese	600	34	40
Breakfast Sides:			
Potatoes: Deluxe Home	390	23	44
Fresh Cut Home	380	23	42
Sandwiches: *7"*			
Chicken Philly	620	22	62
Great Steak Cheesesteak	740	37	62
Ham Delight	710	33	71
Ham Explosion	710	34	70
Philly Cheesesteak	650	26	62
Super Steak Cheesesteak	750	37	64
Veggie Delight	610	31	66
Sides			
Baked Potato, Plain, 6 oz	160	0	36
Chicken Nuggets, Kids, 2.8 oz	165	9	10
Great Fry: Kids, 6.17 oz	270	13	36
Regular, 10.3 oz	440	20	60
Large, 12.42 oz	540	25	72
Potato Skins, 6.46 oz	390	26	24
Meat: *Per 4 oz Serving, without Sides*			
Chicken	140	3	0
Corned Beef, 3 oz	135	8	0
Gyro	210	12	5
Ham	120	4	6
Steak	160	7	0
Turkey	90	1	2
Salads: *Without Dressing*			
Chef Salad	260	11	15
Garden	60	1	13
Grilled Steak	400	23	18
Sauces: Buffalo 1 oz	10	0	2
Teriyaki , 1 oz	25	0	3
Tzatziki, 1 oz	50	4	2
Breads/Pita			
Bread, 12" White, 7 oz	420	4	82
Bread, 7" Wheat, 4 oz	310	4	56
Pita, 2.8 oz	220	5	38

Updated Nutrition Data ~ www.CalorieKing.com
Persons with Diabetes ~ See Disclaimer (Page 24)

Haagen-Dazs® (May '10)

Ice Cream: Per ½ Cup	C	F	Cb
Amaretto Almond Crunch	270	17	24
Baileys Irish Cream	260	17	21
Bananas Foster	240	13	27
Banana Split	280	16	31
Butter Pecan	310	23	21
Caramel Cone	320	19	32
Cherry Vanilla	240	15	23
Chocolate	270	18	22
Chocolate Chip Cookie Dough	310	20	29
Chocolate Chocolate Chip	300	20	26
Coffee	270	18	21
Cookies & Cream	270	17	23
Creme Brulee	280	19	23
Dark Chocolate	160	17	21
Dark Chocolate Mint	250	17	19
Dulce de Leche	290	17	28
Mango	250	14	28
Midnight Cookies & Cream	290	17	30
Pineapple Coconut	230	13	25
Pistachio	290	20	22
Frozen Yogurt: *Per ½ Cup*			
Coffee	200	4.5	31
Dulce de Leche	190	2.5	35
Peach	170	2	31
Vanilla Raspberry Swirl	170	2.5	32
Wildberry	180	2	34
Sorbet: *Per ½ Cup*			
Cranberry Blueberry	100	0	25
Raspberry; Strawberry	120	0	31
Zesty Lemon	110	0	28

Ice Cream Bars ~ See Page 111

Hardee's® (May '10)

Breakfast	C	F	Cb
Biscuits: Bacon, Egg & Cheese	530	36	36
Biscuit 'N' Gravy	530	34	47
Chicken Fillet	600	34	50
Cinnamon 'N Raisin	300	15	40
Country Ham	440	26	36
Country Steak	630	43	45
Loaded Omelet	610	42	36
Made from Scratch	370	23	35
Monster	770	55	37
Sausage	530	38	36
Sausage and Egg	610	44	36
Smoked Ssge with Egg & Cheese	750	56	38

Hardee's® cont... (May '10)

Breakfast Bowls:	C	F	Cb
Loaded Biscuit 'N' Gravy	740	52	49
Low Carb	620	50	6
Breakfast Burrito, Loaded	760	49	39
Breakfast Croissants:			
Sunrise: With Bacon	450	29	28
with Ham	400	23	27
with Sausage	550	38	29
Breakfast Sandwiches:			
Frisco	400	18	27
Texas Toast: Bacon, 4.73 oz	380	21	31
Ham, 6.35 oz	390	18	31
Sausage, 5.5 oz	480	30	32
Breakfast Sides:			
Grits, 5 oz	110	5	16
Hash Rounds: Small, 3 oz	250	16	25
Medium, 4.23 oz	390	26	36
Large, 5.75 oz	530	35	49
Burgers:			
Big Shef, 7.5 oz	660	46	36
Cheeseburger: Regular, 4.62 oz	350	16	36
Double, 7.35 oz	530	32	34
Hamburger, Small, 4.44 oz	310	15	32
Thickburger: Original, ⅓ lb	770	48	53
Bacon Cheese, ⅓ lb	850	57	49
Little Thick Cheeseburger, 5.9 oz	450	23	38
Low-Carb ⅓ lb	420	32	5
Monster, ⅔ lb	1320	95	46
Mushroom 'N' Swiss ⅓ lb	650	36	47
Six Dollar Burger, ½ lb	930	59	57
Chicken Strips: *Without Sauce*			
3 Strips, 3.8 oz	370	26	19
5 Strips, 8.5 oz	610	43	32
Sandwiches:			
Big Hot Ham 'N' Cheese	460	20	40
Chicken: Charbroiled BBQ Chicken	400	6	62
Big Chicken Fillet	710	38	62
Charbroiled Chicken Club	630	32	54
Fish, Supreme	630	38	51
Kids Meals: *Incl. Kid's Fries & Small Drink*			
Cheeseburger	560	29	59
Crispy Chicken Strips (2), w/o sauce	450	27	40
Hamburger	520	25	59

Continued next page...

Hardee's® cont... (May '10)

Sides	C	F	Cb
Beer Battered Onion Rings, 4.5 oz	410	24	45
Fries:			
Crispy Curls: Small 3 oz	340	17	43
Medium 4.7 oz	410	20	52
Large 5.4 oz	480	23	60
Natural Cut: Small, 4.3 oz	320	14	45
Medium, 5.7 oz	430	19	60
Large, 6.2 oz	470	21	65
Dessert, Apple Turnover	290	15	36
Drinks: Hot Chocolate	150	3	18
Malts: *Per 16 fl.oz*			
Chocolate	780	35	97
Strawberry	775	35	98
Vanilla	710	35	97
Shakes: *Per 16 fl.oz*			
Chocolate	700	34	85
Strawberry	700	33	86
Vanilla	710	33	87

Harvey's® (May '10)

Sandwiches & Burgers	C	F	Cb
Angus Burger	560	26	47
Angus Burger, with Cheese	640	32	49
Angus Patty, 1 patty	320	23	4
Cheeseburger	460	23	39
Hamburger	380	16	37
Grilled Chicken Sandwich	290	5	28
VeggieBurger	290	10	33
Hot Dog, *(1)*	300	13	32
Breakfast:			
Bacon, 3 Strips	40	3.5	0
Extra Egg (1)	90	6	0
Homefries	300	19	29
Sandwich: Breakfast Club	400	19	36
Breakfast Club Deluxe	530	28	39
Toast, White, 2 slices	180	2	35
Sides:			
Chicken Strips, 3 pieces	320	15	27
French Fries: Regular, 4.2 oz	320	13	49
Large, 5.3 oz	410	16	61
Value, 3.1 oz	240	10	37
Onion Rings: Regular, 2.8 oz	270	15	33
Large, 5.1 oz	550	29	65

Harvey's® cont... (May '10)

Garnishes:	C	F	Cb
Barbecue Sauce, 1 oz	50	0	12
Canadian Cheddar Cheese, 1 slice	80	6	1
Ketchup, 0.3 oz	10	0	2
Light Mayonnaise, ½ oz	45	5	1
Relish, 0.71 oz	20	0	5
Dipping Sauce: Barbecue. 1.52 oz	90	0	21
Honey Mustard, 1.52 oz	160	12	13
Plum, 1.52 oz	80	0	21
Sweet n' Sour, 1.52 oz	80	0.5	17

Heavenly Ham® (May '10)

Meats: *Per 3 oz Serving*	C	F	Cb
Bone-In Hams: Glazed	190	11	4
Fat Removed	160	3	4
Boneless Hams: Glazed	120	4	4
Fat Removed	90	1	4
Classic Sandwiches: Roast Beef	635	36	50
Swiss Philly	700	46	49
Salads: *Without Dressing*			
Chicken	260	17	14
Taste of Italy	310	20	14
Bread: Croissant	230	12	27
French Batard	210	0.5	46
Multigrain Batard	250	3.5	46
Sliced Wheat Bread	300	5	54
Sauces: BBQ, 1.75 oz	260	26	4
Bistro, 0.75 oz	120	13	1
Dill, 1.5 oz	170	19	1
Mayonnaise, 1 oz	200	24	0
Ranch, 1.5 oz	220	23	2
Spicy Brown Mustard, 1 oz	30	0	0
Sweet Café Spread, 1 oz	100	10	4
That Mustard, 1 oz	150	0	30

Hot Dog on a Stick® (May '10)

Menu Items	C	F	Cb
American Cheese on a Stick	270	14	26
Beef Hot Dog on a Bun	460	29	37
Turkey Hot Dog on a Stick	240	11	28
Veggie Dog on a Stick	250	5	35
Pepperjack Cheese on a Stick	260	13	25
French Fries, 4.48 oz	390	15	60
Lemonade (16 fl.oz): Original	150	0	38
Sugar Free Lemonade	15	0	3
Cherry	210	0	53

Updated Nutrition Data ~ www.CalorieKing.com
Persons with Diabetes ~ See Disclaimer (Page 24)

Hungry Howie's Pizza® (May '10)

Counts may vary in Florida.

Pizzas: Per Slice	C	F	Cb
Cheese: Small, ⅙ pizza	**160**	**3.5**	20
Medium, ⅛ pizza	**190**	**5.5**	23
Large, 1/10 pizza	**210**	**5**	25
X-Large, ⅛ pizza	**395**	**9**	42
Oven Baked Subs: *Per ½ Sub*			
Deluxe Italian	**505**	**18**	61
Ham & Cheese	**475**	**15**	61
Steak & Cheese	**490**	**15**	64
Turkey Club	**555**	**15**	63
Vegetarian	**530**	**21**	64
Sides: Chicken Tenders, 2 pieces	**140**	**4.5**	11
Howie Wings, 5 wings	**180**	**13**	0
Salads: *Per Small Size, Without Dressing*			
Antipasto	**230**	**15**	6
Chef	**230**	**13**	8
Garden	**40**	**0.5**	7
Greek	**250**	**15**	16
Dressings: Creamy Italian, 1 oz	**120**	**12**	2
Greek, 1 oz	**110**	**11**	2
Ranch, 1 oz	**180**	**19**	1
Thousand Island, 1 oz	**140**	**14**	4

In-N-Out Burger® (May '10)

Burgers: Hamburger with Onion	**390**	**19**	39
w/ Mustard/Ketchup, w/o Spread	**310**	**10**	41
Protein Style w/ Lettuce Wrap, no Bun	**240**	**17**	11
Cheeseburger with Onion	**480**	**27**	39
w/ Mustard/Ketchup, w/o Spread	**400**	**18**	41
Protein Style w/ Lettuce Wrap, no Bun	**330**	**25**	11
Double Double® with Onion	**670**	**41**	39
w/ Mustard/Ketchup, no Spread	**590**	**32**	41
Protein Style w/ Lettuce Wrap, no Bun	**520**	**39**	11
French Fries, 4.4 oz	**400**	**18**	54
Drinks: Milk, 10 fl.oz	**180**	**6**	18
Coca-Cola®,16 fl.oz	**200**	**0**	54
Lemonade, 16 fl.oz	**180**	**0**	40
Root Beer,16 fl.oz	**220**	**0**	60
Shakes: Chocolate, 15 fl.oz	**690**	**36**	83
Strawberry, 15 fl.oz	**690**	**33**	91

IHOP® (Jan '10)

Counts may vary between locations	C	F	Cb
Pancakes: *With Toppings Unless Specified*			
Buttermilk Without Butter Or Syrup:			
Full Stack (5)	**750**	**n/a**	100
Short Stack (3)	**450**	**n/a**	60
Chocolate Chip (4)	**610**	**n/a**	100
Double Blueberry (4)	**690**	**n/a**	120
Strawberry Banana (4)	**690**	**n/a**	130
Syrup: Regular, 1 Tbsp	**50**	**0**	12
Sugar-Free, 1 Tbs	**10**	**0**	2
Whipped Butter/Margarine, 1 Tbsp	**80**	**9**	0
French Toast & Waffles: *W/ Toppings Unless Indicated*			
Belgian Banana Pecan Waffle	**700**	**n/a**	77
French Toast, 6 pcs, w/o butter/syrup	**680**	**n/a**	90
Viva La French Toast Combo	**750**	**n/a**	60
International Crepes: *With Toppings*			
Chicken Florentine (2)	**880**	**n/a**	80
Garden Stuffed (2)	**800**	**n/a**	90
Nutella (3)	**990**	**n/a**	170
Swedish (4)	**1080**	**n/a**	90
Omelettes: *Full Platter, Without Butter/Syrup*			
Big Steak	**920**	**n/a**	160
Colorado	**1890**	**n/a**	130
Garden	**1350**	**n/a**	140
Hearty Ham & Cheese	**1630**	**n/a**	130
Spinach & Mushroom	**1620**	**n/a**	130
Classic Combos			
Biscuits w/ Gravy & Sausage	**1410**	**n/a**	98
Eggs Benedict	**980**	**n/a**	100
Smokehouse Combo	**1290**	**n/a**	90
Top Sirloin Steak & Eggs	**1210**	**n/a**	80
Two x Two x Two, average	**670**	**n/a**	55
Signature Favorites: *Without Butter/Syrup*			
Big Country Fried Steak & Eggs	**1620**	**n/a**	160
Breakfast Sampler	**1250**	**n/a**	90
Ham Steak & Eggs	**1130**	**n/a**	90
Rooty Tooty with toppings, average	**950**	**n/a**	80
Split Decision	**1120**	**n/a**	90
T-Bone Steak & Eggs	**1160**	**n/a**	70
IHOP For Me			
Balsamic-Glazed Chicken	**510**	**20**	36
Blueberry Harvest Combo	**570**	**20**	76
Simply Chicken Sandwich	**440**	**6**	42
Spinach/Mushroom/Tomato Omelette	**350**	**14**	24
Tilapia Hollandaise	**370**	**13**	15
Turkey Bacon Omelette	**470**	**25**	17
Two-Egg Breakfast	**380**	**11**	40
Veggie Omelette	**360**	**14**	34
Whole Wheat French Toast Combo	**470**	**14**	51

Jack in the Box® (May '10)

Sandwiches & Burgers	C	F	Cb
Bacon Ultimate Cheeseburger	940	66	45
Hamburger: Original	290	12	32
With Cheese	330	15	32
Deluxe	360	19	33
With Cheese	440	26	34
Jumbo Jack: Original	540	32	45
With Cheese	620	39	45
Junior Bacon Cheeseburger	420	24	32
Sirloin Cheeseburger w/ Bacon	960	64	52
Sourdough Jack	680	46	40
Ultimate Cheeseburger	870	61	44
Chicken & Fish			
Chicken Breast Strips, crispy, (4) w/o sce	560	24	53
Chicken Sandwich	440	23	42
With Bacon	480	26	42
Fish & Chips, small, w/o sce, 8.47 oz	670	35	68
Jack's Spicy Chicken Sandwich	570	25	60
With Cheese	650	31	62
Sourdough Grilled Chicken Club	550	29	38
Breakfast			
Biscuit: Bacon, Egg & Cheese	420	24	36
Sausage, Egg & Cheese	570	39	37
Breakfast Jack: Regular	280	11	30
With Bacon	300	13	30
Croissant: Sausage	570	40	32
Supreme	440	26	32
Sandwiches: Extreme Sausage	660	47	32
Sourdough	410	21	34
Ultimate	510	24	41
Hash Brown Sticks (5)	280	19	26
Meaty Burrito, without salsa	600	37	38
Snacks & Sides:			
Bacon Cheddar Potato Wedges, 9.17 oz	710	45	58
Beef Taco, regular, (1)	180	10	17
Egg Rolls, without sauce, (3)	440	22	46
Mozzrella Cheese Sticks (3)	280	16	22
Mozzrella Cheese Sticks (6)	560	33	43
Pita Snack: Crispy Chicken (1)	410	19	43
Grilled Chicken, without salsa, (1)	330	14	31
Stuffed Jalapenos, (3)	220	12	21
Stuffed Jalapenos, (7)	510	29	49
Onion Rings, (8), 4.2 oz	450	28	45
Seasoned Curly Fries, med., 4.6 oz	430	25	46

Jack in the Box® cont... (May '10)

Bowls:	C	F	Cb
Teriyaki: Chicken, 17.6 oz	690	6	133
Steak, 17.6 oz	750	11	133
Salads: *No Dressing or Condiments*			
Chicken Club with Grilled Chicken	350	18	13
Grilled Chicken	240	8	15
Side Salad	20	0	4
Southwest Chicken w/ Gr. Chkn Strips	340	14	29
Sauces & Dressings			
Dipping Sauce: Barbecue, 1 oz	40	0	10
Buttermilk House, 1 oz	130	13	3
Frank's Red Hot Buffalo, 1 oz	10	0	2
Sweet & Sour, 1 oz	45	0	11
Tartar, 1½ oz	210	22	2
Sauce: Mayo-Onion, ½ oz	90	10	1
Soy, 0.3 oz	5	0	1
Taco, 0.3 oz	0	0	0
Cheese: American, 1 slice	40	3.5	0
Real Swiss, 1 slice	70	6	0
Condiments			
Ketchup, 0.57 oz	20	0	4
Mustard, 0.2 oz	5	0	0
Sour Cream, 1 oz	60	5	2
Desserts			
NY Style Cheesecake, 3.25 oz	310	17	32
Chocolate Overload Cake, 3.3 oz	300	7	57
Ice Cream Shakes: *Per 16 fl.oz With Whipped Topping*			
Chocolate Ice Cream	800	38	101
Oreo Cookie Ice Cream	810	43	92
Strawberry Ice Cream	780	38	95
Vanilla Ice Cream	700	38	76

For Complete Nutritional Data ~ see CalorieKing.com

Jack's® (May '10)

Sandwiches: Big Bacon Burger	610	41	31
Big Jack Burger	530	33	35
Cheeseburger	380	21	31
Chicken Fillet Sandwich	500	25	43
Double Big Jack Cheese Burger	850	59	35
Double Cheeseburger	540	34	31
Grilled Chicken Sandwich	380	16	32
Hamburger	340	18	31
Chicken, Chicken Fingers, 3 pieces	420	23	28
Fries, regular	310	13	42
Breakfast, Egg & Cheese Biscuit	360	21	31

Additional Listings ~ see CalorieKing.com

Updated Nutrition Data ~ www.CalorieKing.com
Persons with Diabetes ~ See Disclaimer (Page 24)

Jamba Juice® (May '10)

Breakfast	C	F	Cb
Ideal Meals: Berry Topper, 16 fl oz	480	9	91
Chunky Strawberry, 16 fl oz	570	17	92
Mango Peach Topper, 16 fl oz	500	9	95
Hot Oatmeal: *With Fruit & Sugar*			
Apple Cinnamon	290	4	60
Blueberry & Blackberry	290	3.5	58
Grab N Go Food:			
California Flat Bread: *With Dressing*			
Four Cheesy, 5.7 oz	420	16	46
MediterraneYum, 6 oz	320	8	49
Smokehouse Chicken, 6 oz	390	10	53
Baked Goods			
Cheddar Tomato Twist, 3.2 oz	240	4.5	38
Orange Chocolate Chip Scone, 3.2 oz	380	15	57
Tart Cherry Scone, 3.2 oz	360	12	58
All Fruit: *Original, 22 fl oz*			
Mega Mango	320	1	80
Peach Perfection	300	0.5	75
Pomegranate Paradise	340	0.5	85
Strawberry Whirl	300	0.5	75
Blended With A Purpose: *Per 16 fl.oz*			
Acai Super-Antioxidant	260	4	53
Coldbuster	240	1.5	56
Protein Berry Workout: With Whey	280	0	52
With Soy Protein	270	1	51
Strawberry Energizer	280	1	67
Classics: *Per 16 fl.oz*			
Aloha Pineapple	290	1	67
Caribbean Passion	250	1	57
Mango-a-go-go	280	1	65
Strawberry Surf Rider	300	1	72
Creamy Treats: *Per 16 fl oz*			
Chocolate Moo'd	430	4	86
Orange Dream Machine	350	1.5	75
Peanut Butter Moo'd	470	10	82
Fresh Squeezed Juices: *Per 16 fl oz*			
Carrot	130	0.5	30
Orange	220	1	52
Jamba Light: *Per 16 fl oz*			
Berry Fulfilling	150	0.5	32
Mango Mantra	150	0.5	31
Strawberry Nirvana	150	0	31
Shots: *Single*			
Matcha Energy Shot-Soymilk, 4 fl.oz	70	0	14
Wheatgrass, 1 fl oz	5	0	1

Jersey Mike's Subs® (May '10)

Cold Subs: *Per Regular, on Wheat, Without Vinegar, Oil or Mayo*	C	F	Cb
#1 BLT	530	24	55
#2 Jersey Shore Favorite	520	16	59
#3 American Classic	520	16	57
#5 Super Sub	540	17	59
#6 Roast Beef & Provolone	680	23	56
#7 Turkey Breast & Provolone	500	14	56
#8 Club Sub with Mayonnaise	850	50	58
#9 Club Supreme w/ Mayonnaise	900	50	58
#10 Albacore Tuna	870	57	58
#13 Original Italian	640	25	60
#14 Veggie	680	31	57
Hot Subs/Cheese Steaks: *Per Regular on Wheat Roll*			
#15 Meatball & Cheese	850	50	64
#17 Chicken Philly	590	23	57
Steak Philly	580	22	56
#43 Chipotle Chicken	870	54	60
Chipotle Steak	860	53	58
#18 Chicken Parmesan	610	20	69
#19 BBQ Beef	670	14	75
#20 Pastrami & Swiss	540	16	52
#56 Big Kahuna Steak	630	26	57
#56 Big Kahuna Chicken	640	27	58
Cold Wraps: *With Flour Tortilla, w/o Vin./Oil or Mayo*			
#1 BLT	590	29	60
#2 Jersey Shore Favorite	580	22	64
#3 American Classic	580	22	63
#5 Super Sub	600	22	65
Salads: *Without Dressing*			
Chef, 16 oz	240	10	12
Grilled Chicken Caesar, 12.5 oz	510	35	11
Tossed, 12 oz	50	0.5	11
Tuna, 18 oz	690	60	15
Dressings: *Per 2 Tbsp, 1 oz*			
Caesar	150	15	2
Chipotle Mayo	180	20	0
Golden Italian	110	11	3
Ranch	120	12	2
Russian	160	16	4
Condiments: Oil, regular, 1 oz	270	30	0
Mustard, ½ oz	0	0	0
Desserts: Cookie, Choc Chip, 1.5 oz	200	11	24
Brownie, Chocolate, 4 oz	440	20	60
Drinks: Mountain Dew, 22 oz	310	0	84
Mug Root Beer, 22 oz	290	0	79
Tropicana Twister Orange, 22 oz	360	0	96

Jimmy John's® (May '10)

Subs (8")	C	F	Cb
Figures Based on French Bread w/ Standard Toppings & Mayo, Unless Indicated			
#1 Pepe	615	31	50
#2 Big John	535	24	49
#3 Totally Tuna without dressing	650	31	54
#4 Turkey Tom	515	22	50
#5 Vito with Italian Vinaigrette	600	28	52
#6 Vegetarian	580	30	53
JJBLT	635	35	49
Giant Club Sandwiches: *Figures Based on French Bread w/ Standard Toppings & Mayo, Unless Indicated*			
#7 Gourmet Smoked Ham	775	32	69
#8 Billy	800	34	68
#9 Italian Night with Mayo & Vinaig.	950	51	70
#10 Hunter's	805	35	67
#11 Country	770	31	69
#12 Beach Club	730	31	71
#13 Gourmet Veggie Club	775	38	71
#14 Bootlegger	685	25	67
#15 Club Tuna without dressing	845	39	72
#16 Club Lulu	755	33	67
#17 Ultimate Porker	765	39	67
Plain Slims: *Figures Based on French Bread without Toppings, Dressing or Mayo*			
Slim 1 Ham & Cheese	510	10	66
Slim 2 Roast Beef	425	3	64
Slim 3 Tuna Salad	720	31	68
Slim 4 Turkey Breast	400	0.5	65
Slim 5 Salami Capicola & Cheese	600	20	66
Slim 6 Double Provolone	545	16	65
The J.J. Gargantuan	990	54	54
Low Carb Options: *With Standard Toppings & Mayo, without Bread*			
Hunter's Club Unwich	470	35	4
The JJ Gargantuan Unwich	740	54	7
Low-Fat Options: *W/o Standard Toppings, Dressing or Mayo*			
#4 Turkey Tom	305	0.5	48
Slim 4 Turkey Breast	400	0.5	65
Sides			
Jimmy Chips: BBQ, 1 oz	160	9	17
Jalapeno, 1 oz	150	7	18
Regular, 1 oz	160	8	18
Sea Salt & Vinegar, 1 oz	140	8	16
Skinny, 1 oz	130	5	19
Pickle: Spear	5	0	1
Whole	20	0	4
Cookies, average	420	17	64

Johnny Rockets® (May '10)

Original Hamburgers	C	F	Cb
Hamburger #12	900	59	55
Original Burger	820	53	52
Chili Cheese	850	50	53
Patty Melt	690	37	49
Rocket: Single	710	44	45
Double	1020	63	52
Route 66	920	60	55
Smoke House: Single	950	55	68
Double	1360	80	99
St Louis	990	56	53
Streamliner	410	8	57
Sandwiches: Chicken Club	930	51	58
Grilled Breast of Chicken	560	25	47
Grilled Cheese	540	29	48
Philly Cheese Steak	715	46	48
Tuna Melt	900	62	40
Tuna Salad	800	50	41
Other Favourites			
Chicken Tenders without Sauce	610	33	39
Chili Dog	810	55	48
Hot Dog	370	20	34
Extras: Bacon, 2 slices, 0.6 oz	90	7	1
Chili, 3 oz	155	12	5
Grilled Mushrooms, 1 oz	35	3	1
Grilled Peppers & Onions, 1 oz	20	1	3
Starters			
Chili Bowl, 13 oz	870	73	24
American Fries, 8 oz	550	22	78
Cheese Fries, 10 oz	780	44	72
Chili Fries, 15 oz	1010	62	85
Onion Rings, 8 oz	790	36	80
Rocket Wings, 9 oz	640	36	26
Desserts: Apple Pie, 10 oz	800	33	119
A la Mode, scoop, 4 oz	250	16	25
Super Sundae, 13 oz	1110	74	120
Beverages: *20 fl.oz*			
Root Beer	170	0	49
Coke	170	0	28
Sprite	170	0	45
Lemonade	170	0	49
Shakes: *Original, 16 fl.oz*			
Chocolate	890	44	102
Strawberry	750	44	77
Vanilla	840	44	100

Updated Nutrition Data ~ www.CalorieKing.com
Persons with Diabetes ~ See Disclaimer (Page 24)

KFC® (May '10)

	C	F	Cb
Original Recipe:			
Breast: 1 piece, 5.78 oz	**320**	15	4
without skin or breading, 4.1 oz	**150**	2.5	0
Drumstick, 1 piece, 1.85oz	**120**	7	3
Thigh, 1 piece, 3.3 oz	**220**	15	5
Whole Wing, 1 piece, 2 oz	**140**	8	4
Spicy Crispy: Breast, 1 piece, 6.2 oz	**420**	25	12
Drumstick, 1 piece, 2 oz	**160**	10	5
Thigh, 1 piece, 3.9 oz	**360**	27	13
Whole Wing, 1 piece, 1.75 oz	**170**	12	6
Grilled :			
Breast, 4.35 oz	**190**	6	0
Drumstick, 1.48 oz	**70**	3.5	0
Thigh, 2.5 oz	**150**	9	0
Whole Wing, 1.3 oz	**80**	4.5	0
Strips & Filets:			
Crispy, 2 Strips, 3.56 oz	**250**	15	8
3 Strips, 5.36 oz	**380**	22	12
Original Filets, 3.4 oz	**170**	7	4
Popcorn Chicken: Kids, 3 oz	**290**	19	16
Individual, 4 oz	**400**	26	22
Large, 5.6 oz	**550**	35	30
Sandwiches: *With Sauce*			
Crispy Twister, with Crispy Strips	**590**	31	49
Double Crunch, with Crispy Strip	**520**	28	35
Double Down: Original	**540**	32	11
Grilled	**460**	23	3
Filet Sandwich: Original	**480**	24	37
Grilled	**390**	15	27
KFC Snackers:			
Crispy Strip: Regular	**300**	14	28
Buffalo	**260**	9	30
Ultimate Cheese	**280**	11	29
Tender Roast Sandwich	**410**	15	29
Toasted Wraps: *With Sauce*			
With Crispy Strip	**360**	20	27
With Grilled Filet	**300**	14	24
With Tender Roast Filet	**310**	15	24
Wings: *Per Wing Without Dipping Sauce*			
Boneless: Fiery Buffalo; Honey BBQ, av.	**80**	3.5	6
Bone In: Fiery Buffalo; Honey BBQ, av.	**80**	5	4
Hot Wings: Regular	**70**	5	3
Fiery Buffalo	**80**	5	5
Honey BBQ	**90**	5	7

KFC® cont... (May '10)

	C	F	Cb
Dipping Sauces			
Fiery Buffalo, 1 oz	**25**	0	6
Creamy Ranch, 1 oz	**140**	15	1
Honey BBQ, 1 oz	**40**	0	9
Honey Mustard, 1 oz	**120**	10	6
Sweet & Sour, 1 oz	**45**	0	12
KFC Famous Bowls & Pot Pie			
Bowls: Snack Size, 8 oz	**320**	15	34
Mashed Potato with Gravy, 18½ oz	**700**	32	77
Chicken Pot Pie, 13 oz	**690**	40	57
Sides: *Per Single Portion*			
BBQ Baked Beans, 4.6 oz	**200**	1.5	39
Biscuit, 2 oz	**180**	8	23
Cole Slaw, 4.6 oz	**180**	10	19
Corn on the Cob (3"), 2.5 oz	**70**	0.5	16
Cornbread Muffin, 2 oz	**210**	9	28
Macaroni & Cheese, 4.8 oz	**180**	9	20
Mashed Potatoes with Gravy, 5.1 oz	**120**	4	19
Potato Wedges, 3.6 oz	**260**	13	33
Salads: *Without Dressing or Croutons*			
Crispy Chicken BLT	**340**	19	14
Crispy Chicken Caesar	**320**	19	12
House Side Salad	**15**	0	2
Grilled Chicken BLT	**220**	7	6
Grilled Chicken Caesar	**200**	6	4
Dressings:			
Original Ranch Fat Free, 1½ oz	**35**	0	8
Creamy Parmesan Caesar, 2 oz	**260**	26	4
Light Italian, 1 oz	**10**	0.5	2
Croutons, Parm. Garlic, Pouch (1)	**70**	3	8
Desserts:			
Lil' Buckets Parfait Cups:			
Chocolate Cream, 4 oz	**280**	14	37
Lemon Creme, 4.5 oz	**390**	14	60

Kilwin's® ~ see CalorieKing.com

Koo•Koo•Roo® ~ see CalorieKing.com

Kohr Bros® ~ see CalorieKing.com

Kolache® ~ see CalorieKing.com

Krispy Kreme® (Feb '10)

Doughnuts	C	F	Cb
Apple Fritter	380	20	47
Caramel Kreme Crunch	380	19	49
Chocolate Glazed Cruller	290	15	37
Chocolate Iced Cake	280	14	36
Chocolate Iced Custard Filled	300	17	35
Chocolate Iced Glazed	250	12	33
Chocolate Iced Kreme Filled	350	20	39
Chocolate Iced with Sprinkles	270	12	38
Cinnamon Apple Filled	290	16	32
Cinnamon Bun	260	16	28
Cinnamon Twist	240	15	23
Dulce de Leche	300	18	31
Glazed: Chocolate Cake	300	15	42
Cinnamon	210	12	24
Cruller	240	14	26
Kreme Filled	340	20	39
Lemon Filled	290	16	35
Maple Iced	240	12	32
Original	200	12	22
Raspberry Filled	300	16	36
Sour Cream	300	13	43
Powdered: Cake	290	14	37
Strawberry Filled	290	16	33
Sugar Doughnut	200	12	21
Traditional Cake Doughnut	230	13	25
Doughnut Holes: Orig. Glazed (4)	200	11	25
Glazed Cake, Regular/Choc. (4)	210	10	29
Chiller Beverages: No Cream Topping			
Fruity Chillers:			
Average all flavors, 12 fl.oz	175	0	43
20 fl.oz	295	0	71
Kremey Chillers: *Includes Whipped Cream Topping*			
Orange & Kreme: 12 fl.oz	630	28	92
20 fl.oz	970	40	150
Lemon Sherbert: 12 fl.oz	630	28	95
20 fl.oz	980	40	155
Choc./Mocha: Average, 12 fl.oz	670	29	104
average 20 fl.oz	1050	41	171
Lotta Latte: 12 fl.oz	670	28	49
20 fl.oz	1050	40	79

For Complete Nutritional Data ~ see CalorieKing.com

Krystal® (Feb '10)

Burgers:	C	F	Cb
B.A. Burger	470	27	39
B.A. Double Bacon Cheese	800	53	41
Krystal: Burger	130	6	20
Double Burger	290	13	33
Bacon Cheese	200	11	20
Cheese Burger	160	8	20
Double Cheese	350	17	34
Chik Burger	300	16	27
Pups: Chili Cheese Pup	230	14	16
Corn Pup	240	14	22
Plain Pup	150	8	15
Sampler Combo: Krystal, Chik, Pup, Med Fries + Coca Cola, 16 fl.oz	1010	43	140
French Fries			
Medium, 4.2 oz	470	20	53
Chili Cheese Fries, 8.18 oz	570	29	62
Sides			
Large Chili, 12 oz	300	11	33
Chik'n Bites, Small, 3.1 oz	200	7	20
Salad, Crispy Chicken, 11 oz	370	21	20
Breakfast Items			
Krystal Sunriser Sandwich	200	11	16
Biscuits: Bacon, Egg & Cheese	440	24	34
Chik	400	18	43
Gravy	350	18	41
Plain	260	17	32
Sausage	420	28	32
Scramblers: Original with Bacon	330	16	27
with Sausage	420	26	27
4-Carb Scramblers: With Bacon	450	31	2
with Sausage	620	52	3
Kryspers	150	7	19
Desserts: Apple Turnover, fried	220	8	34
Lemon Icebox Pie	320	9	56
Drinks: Per 16 fl.oz with ¼ ice			
Coca-Cola Classic	120	0	32
Diet Coke	0	0	0
Sprite	110	0	31

For Complete Nutritional Data ~ see CalorieKing.com

For Menu Updates, Check Author's Website www.CalorieKing.com

La Rosa's Pizzeria® (Feb '10)

	C	F	Cb
Focaccia Style: *Per 1/10 of Medium Pizza*			
Florentine	240	13	24
Roma,	300	18	23
Hand Tossed: *Per Slice, 1/8 of Medium Pizza*			
Cheese	230	8	29
Double Pepperoni	300	14	29
Big 4 Meat	325	15	29
Big 4 Pick 4	280	11	30
Big 4 Veggie	240	7	30
Pan Crust: *Per Slice· 1/8 of Medium Pizza*			
Cheese	300	16	30
Double Pepperoni	370	22	30
Big 4 Meat	325	15	29
Big 4 Pick 4	275	11	30
Big 4 Veggie	235	7	30
Traditional Crust: *Per Slice, 1/8 of Medium Pizza*			
Cheese	200	10	19
Double Pepperoni	280	16	20
Big 4 Meat	285	16	20
Big 4 Pick 4	260	13	21
Big 4 Veggie	200	8	21
Calzones: *Per Calzone, No Dipping Sauce*			
3 Meat & 3 Cheese	1080	55	102
3 Veggie & 3 Cheese	860	34	105
Cheese & Pepperoni	960	45	101
Cheese	840	34	101
Philly Cheesesteak	870	39	90
Sausage Pelucci	1040	52	92
Pasta Dinner: *Without Sides*			
Cheese Ravioli	660	26	80
Lasagna with Meat Sauce	735	38	61
Spaghetti: With Meatballs	870	28	119
with Alfredo Sauce	975	50	104
with Meat Sauce	700	18	104
with Traditional Sauce	640	12	113
Ziti Chicken Alfredo	980	42	102
Ziti Sausage Pelucci	765	20	115
Appetizers			
Boneless Wings: BBQ (1), 1.6 oz	75	3	8
Hot (1), 1.6 oz	80	5	6
Chicken Tenders, 8.57 oz	540	31	30
Four Taste Sampler, 23.6 oz	1570	99	82
French Fry Basket with Provolone	860	56	73
Mozzarella Cheese Sticks, 6.4 oz	635	43	36
Onion Twists, Regular w/out Sauce	460	27	48

For Complete Nutritional Data ~ see CalorieKing.com

La Salsa Fresh Mexican Grill® (Feb '10)

	C	F	Cb
Appetizers: Salsa & Chips, 14.5 oz	700	32	87
with Guacamole, 14.5 oz	970	55	103
Nachos:			
Black Beans: With Carnitas	1570	83	141
with Chicken	1600	83	148
with Steak	1580	84	142
Pinto Beans: With Carnitas	1560	83	139
with Chicken	1590	83	146
with Steak	1565	84	139
Burritos: Black Beans w/ Cheese	1100	48	132
with Carnitas	1205	51	132
with Chicken	1240	52	139
Pinto Beans with Cheese	1070	48	115
with Chicken	1200	52	122
with Steak	1175	54	115
Baja Fish Burrito	875	53	58
California Steak & Black Beans	815	35	89
Overstuffed Grilled Burrito:			
with Chicken	1260	59	110
with Carnitas	1200	59	108
with Steak	1290	66	109
Grande, Black Beans:			
with Carnitas	810	34	91
with Chicken	810	33	93
with Steak	820	35	91
Tacos: Baja Fish	395	22	29
Baja Shrimp	320	19	30
Guadalajara Carnitas	320	15	30
Quesadillas: *With Chips unless indicated*			
Classic: Carnitas	1160	68	82
Chicken	1155	67	83
Steak	1165	69	82
Grande, Pinto Beans:			
with Carnitas	1335	71	114
with Chicken	1330	71	116
with Steak	1330	72	115
Favorites: *Without Chips*			
Stuffed Fajita Quesadilla:			
with Carnitas	855	51	53
with Chicken	865	52	56
with Steak	885	55	53
with Shrimp	800	49	54
Fire Roasted Bowl			
Black Beans: with Chicken	730	32	74
with Steak	735	34	73
without meat	630	29	71
Pinto Beans: With Chicken	730	32	73
with Steak	720	34	70
without meat	620	29	69

Little Caesars® (Jun '10)

14" Pizza: Per Slice, 1/8 Pizza	C	F	Cb
Original Crust: 3 Meat Treat	350	18	30
Hula Hawaiian: With Ham	270	9	33
With Canadian Bacon	280	9	34
Ultimate Supreme	310	14	31
Vegetarian	270	10	32
Deep Dish:			
Just Cheese	320	13	38
Pepperoni	360	16	38
Hot-N-Ready: Just Cheese	240	9	30
Pepperoni	280	11	30
Baby Pan! Pan!: *Per Pan*			
Cheese & Pepperoni	360	18	33
Caesar Wings: Barbecue, 1 wing	70	4	3
Mild/Hot, 1 wing	60	4.5	1
Oven, Roasted, 1 wing	50	3.5	0
Caesar Dips: *Per 1.5 oz Container*			
Buffalo	140	14	4
Buffalo Ranch	230	24	3
Buttery Garlic	380	42	0
Cheezy	210	21	3
Chipotle	220	24	2
Ranch	250	26	3
Bread: *Per Piece*			
Crazy Bread, 1 stick	100	3	15
Italian Cheese Bread	130	7	13
Pepperoni Cheese Bread	150	8	13
Sauce, Crazy, 4 oz	45	0	10

Lone Star Steakhouse® (Jun '10)

Appetizers: *Per Serving*	C	F	Cb
Chicken Tenders, 12 oz	1095	66	91
Lone Star Wings, 11 oz	955	62	15
Texas Rose, 15.5 oz	1260	83	108
Meals: *Served Without Sides, Toppings & Sauce*			
Mesquite Grilled Steaks:			
Cajun Ribeye, 16 oz	1250	101	0
Chopped Steak, 10 oz	900	71	0
Delmonico, 11 oz	860	69	0
Five Star Filet, 9 oz	740	60	0
NY Strip, 14 oz	1035	80	0
San Antonio Sirloin, 12 oz	770	55	0
T-Bone, 20 oz	1540	124	0
Texas Ribeye, 14 oz	1090	88	0

Lone Star® cont... (Jun '10)

	C	F	Cb
Meals (Cont): *Served Without Sides, Toppings & Sauce*			
Mesquite-Grilled Specialties:			
Baby Back Ribs, 12 oz	970	80	0
Grilled Chicken, 6 oz	185	2.5	0
Grilled Pork Chops, 16 oz	1430	100	0
Shrimp Dinner, 3.5 oz	105	2	1
Sweeet Bourbon Salmon, 6 oz	240	11	0
Slow Roasted, Prime Rib, 16 oz	1250	10	0
Salads: *Per Serving, Without Dressing*			
El Paso Salad	385	23	21
Grilled Chicken Caesar	455	10	31
Lettuce Wedge	505	48	12
Dressings: *Per Serving*			
Bleu Cheese	250	26	4
Honey Mustard	265	27	8
Ranch	210	22	2
Texas Ranch	215	22	3
Thousand Island	200	18	9
Wish Bone	310	32	4
Sides: *Per Serving*			
Baked Potato	665	18	114
Sauteed Mushrooms	115	8	6
Sauteed Onions	95	7	8
Steamed Mixed Vegetables	70	1	14
Texas Rice	80	2	12
Desserts: *Per Serving*			
Big Brownie Blast	1390	69	178
Homemade Cobbler, average all	240	8	43
Homemade Ice Cream	255	19	19

Long John Silver's® (Jun '10)

	C	F	Cb
Sandwiches: *Includes Toppings And Condiments*			
Chicken, 6.63 oz	440	30	47
Fish, 6.2 oz	470	23	49
Ultimate Fish, 7 oz	530	27	50
Seafood			
Battered Fish, 1 piece, 3.2 oz	260	16	17
Battered Shrimp, 3 pieces, 1.5 oz	130	9	8
Breaded Clam Strips, 3 oz	320	19	29
Buttered Lobster Bites, snack box, 3.2 oz	230	9	24
Grilled Pacific Salmon, 2 filets, 4.5 oz	150	5	2
Grilled Tilapia, 1 filet, 4.1 oz	110	2.5	1

Continued next page...

Updated Nutrition Data ~ www.CalorieKing.com
Persons with Diabetes ~ See Disclaimer (Page 24)

Long John Silver's® (Feb '10)

	C	F	Cb
***Sandwiches & Burgers:** Includes toppings and condiments*			
Chicken, 4.8 oz	360	15	40
Fish, 6.2 oz	470	23	49
Ultimate Fish, 7 oz	530	27	50
Seafood			
Battered Fish, 1 piece, 3.2 oz	260	16	17
Battered Shrimp, 3 pieces, 1.5 oz	130	9	8
Breaded Clam Strips, 3 oz	320	19	29
Buttered Lobster Bites, snack box, 3.2 oz	230	9	24
Grilled Pacific Salmon, 2 filets, 4.5 oz	150	5	2
Grilled Tilapia, 1 filet, 4.1 oz	110	2.5	1
Lobster Stuffed Crab Cake, 2.2 oz	170	9	16
Popcorn Shrimp, 1 snack box, 2.9 oz	270	16	23
Shrimp Scampi, 8 pieces	200	13	3
Chicken			
Chicken Plank, 1 piece, 1.8 oz	140	8	9
Bowls:			
Salmon: without Sauce, 13.5 oz	380	8	47
with Sauce, 15 oz	460	8	65
Shrimp: without Sauce, 12.2 oz	310	4.5	47
with Sauce, 13.7 oz	390	5	65
***Freshside Grille:** With Premium Rice & Vegetables*			
Grilled Pacific Salmon, 2 filets	380	8	47
Grilled Tilapia, 1 filet	340	5.5	46
Sauces & Condiments:			
Dipping Sauces: *Per 1 fl.oz*			
Cocktail	25	0	6
Tartar	105	9	4
Ginger Teriyaki Sauce, 1 packet	80	0	18
Louisiana Hot Sauce, 1 tspn	0	0	0
Ketchup, 1 packet	10	0	2
Malt Vinegar, ½ oz	0	0	0
Sides			
Breadstick, 2 oz	170	3.5	29
Broccoli Chse Soup, 1 bowl, 7.4 oz	220	18	8
Cole Slaw, 4 oz	200	15	15
Corn Cobbette w. Butter Oil, 3.4 oz	150	10	14
Crumblies, 1 oz	170	12	14
Fries: Platter Portion, 3 oz	230	10	34
Combo Portion, 4 oz	310	14	45
Hushpuppies, 1 pup, 0.8 oz	60	2.5	9
Rice, 5 oz	180	1	37

For Complete Nutritional Data ~ see CalorieKing.com

Macaroni Grill (Feb '10)

	C	F	Cb
***Appetizers:** Inc. Sauce & Garnish*			
Calamari Fritti	650	43	42
Crab-Stuffed Mushrooms	310	24	4
Romano's Sampler, 3 Choices	800	52	50
Tomato Bruschetta	560	17	77
Meals:			
Amore De Le Grill: *As Served, Includes Sides*			
Grilled Pork Chops	1380	77	96
Grilled Salmon	750	35	55
Honey Balsamic Chicken: Lunch	540	13	54
Dinner	640	15	54
Classico Italian:			
Lunch: Chicken Marsala	620	34	46
Chicken Scaloppine	740	45	46
Eggplant Parmigiana	800	47	65
Parmesan-Crusted Sole	1190	71	101
Spaghetti Bolognese	570	19	72
Dinner: Chicken Marsala	650	33	49
Chicken Scaloppine	910	59	59
Parmesan-Crusted Sole	1710	105	131
Mediterranean Grill: *As Served, Includes Sides*			
Calabrese Strip	1130	65	47
Grilled Chicken Spiedini	360	10	17
Grilled Pork Chops	1380	77	96
Jumbo Shrimp Spiedini	230	5	15
Handcrafted Pasta: *As Served*			
Capellini Pomodoro	390	14	55
Carmela's Chicken Rigatoni	1080	58	100
Lobster Ravioli	520	30	32
Pasta Milano	750	24	93
Penne Rustica	980	38	94
Pollo Caprese	550	20	45
Shrimp Portofino, lunch	560	34	37
Seafood Linguine	650	22	75
Pizzas: *Per Whole Pizza*			
Neapolitan: Italian Sausage	970	39	95
Margherita	720	20	95
Quattro Formaggio	950	34	111
***Salads:** As Served, Includes Dressing*			
Caesar	260	20	14
Chicken Caesar	650	42	29
Parmesan-Crusted Chicken	960	63	49
Scallops & Spinach	360	18	16
***Salad Dressings & Condiments:** Per 1 fl.oz*			
Caesar	150	16	2
Mediterranean Vinaigrette	130	14	3
Parmesan Peppercorn Ranch	120	12	2
***Desserts:** Per Serving*			
Italian Sorbetto with Biscotti	220	2	48
Tiramisu	1120	80	88

For Complete Nutritional Data ~ see CalorieKing.com

McDonald's® (May '10)

Burgers/Sandwiches	C	F	Cb
Hamburger	250	9	31
Cheeseburger	300	12	33
Double Cheeseburger	440	23	34
Big Mac	540	29	45
Big N'Tasty	460	24	37
Big N'Tasty with Cheese	510	28	38
Quarter Pounder	410	19	37
with Cheese	510	26	40
Double with Cheese	740	42	40
Angus: Bacon & Cheese	790	39	63
Deluxe	750	39	61
Mushroom & Swiss	770	40	59
Filet-O-Fish	380	18	38
McChicken	360	16	40
McRib	500	26	44
Southern Style Crispy Chicken Sndwch	400	17	39
Premium Chicken Classic Sandwiches:			
Crispy Chicken	530	20	59
Crispy Chicken Club	630	28	60
Crispy Chicken Ranch BLT	580	23	62
Grilled Chicken	420	10	51
Grilled Chicken Club	530	17	52
Grilled Chicken Ranch BLT	470	12	54
Snack Wraps:			
Chipotle BBQ: With Crispy Chicken	330	15	35
With Grilled Chicken	260	9	28
Honey Mustard: With Crispy Chicken	330	16	34
With Grilled Chicken	260	9	27
Ranch: With Crispy Chicken	340	17	33
With Grilled Chicken	270	10	26
French Fries:			
Small, 2.5 oz	230	11	29
Medium, 4.1 oz	380	19	48
Large, 5.4 oz	500	25	63
Ketchup, 1 package	15	0	3
Chicken McNuggets®			
Chicken McNuggets: 4 pieces	190	12	11
6 pieces	280	17	16
10 pieces	460	29	27
Chicken Selects® Breast Strips			
Strips: 3 pieces	400	24	23
5 pieces	660	40	39
Sauces: Barbecue, 1 oz	50	0	12
Creamy Ranch, 1.3 oz	170	18	2
Spicy Buffalo, 1.3 oz	60	6	1
Sweet 'N Sour, 1 oz	50	0	12
Tangy Honey Mustard, 1.3 oz	60	2	10

McDonald's® cont... (May '10)

Breakfast Menu	C	F	Cb
Biscuit: Regular	260	12	33
Large	320	16	39
Bacon Egg & Cheese: Regular	420	23	37
Large	480	27	43
Sausage with Egg: Regular	510	33	36
Large	570	37	42
Southern Style Chicken, Regular	410	20	41
Big Breakfast, Regular Biscuit	740	48	51
English Muffin	160	3	27
Grape/Strawberry Jam	35	0	9
Hash Brown (1), 2 oz	150	9	15
Hotcakes: Plain (3)	350	9	60
With Margarine (2 pats), no Syrup	430	18	60
With Margarine (2 pats) & Syrup (1)	610	18	105
McGriddles: Bacon, Egg & Cheese	420	18	48
Sausage	420	22	44
Sausage, Egg & Cheese	560	32	48
McMuffin: Egg	300	12	30
Sausage	370	22	29
Sausage with Egg	450	27	30
McSkillet: Burrito with Sausage	610	36	44
Burrito with Steak	570	30	44
Sausage Burrito, 3.9 oz	300	16	26
Sausage Patty, 1.4 oz	170	15	1
Scrambled Eggs (2), 3.3 oz	170	11	1
Happy Meals			
with 4 Chicken McNuggets:			
+ Small Fries + Apple Juice	510	23	63
+ Small Fries + 1% Low Fat Milk	520	25	52
+ Apple Dipper/ Dip + 1% Choc Milk	390	15	46
with Hamburger:			
+ Small Fries + Apple Juice	580	20	84
+ Small Fries + Sprite (12 oz)	590	20	88
+ Apple Dippers/Dip + Low-Fat Milk	460	12	66
with Cheeseburger:			
+ Small Fries & Apple Juice	630	24	85
+ Small Fries + 1% Low-Fat Milk	640	26	74
+ Apple Dippers/Dip & 1% Choc Milk	520	13	80
Mighty Kids Meals			
with 6 Chicken McNuggets:			
+ Small Fries + Apple Juice	610	28	68
+ Apple Dippers/Dip + 1% Choc Milk	550	21	65
with Double Cheeseburger:			
+ Small Fries + Apple Juice	770	34	86
+ Apple Dippers/Dip + Low-Fat Milk	640	26	69

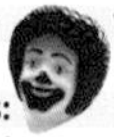

Updated Nutrition Data ~ www.CalorieKing.com
Persons with Diabetes ~ See Disclaimer (Page 24)

McDonald's® cont... (Apr '10)

Premium Salads: Without Dressing	C	F	Cb
Bacon Ranch Salad: W/o Chicken	140	7	10
With Crispy Chicken	370	20	20
With Grilled Chicken	260	9	12
Caesar Salad: Without Chicken	90	4	9
With Crispy Chicken	330	17	20
With Grilled Chicken	220	6	12
Southwest Salad: WithCrispy Chicken	430	20	38
With Grilled Chicken	320	9	30
Fruit & Walnut, Snack Size, 1 pkg	210	8	31
Side Salad, 3.1 oz	20	0	4
Butter Garlic Croutons, ½ oz	60	1.5	10
Salad Dressings: Per Package			
Newman's Own: Ranch, 2 fl.oz	170	15	9
Creamy Caesar, 2 fl.oz	190	18	4
Creamy Southwest, 1.5 fl.oz	100	6	11
Low-Fat: Balsamic Vinaigrette	40	3	4
Family Recipe Italian, 1.5 fl.oz	60	2.5	8
Desserts/Cookies			
Apple Dippers: 1 package, 2.4 oz	35	0	8
With Low-Fat Caramel Dip	105	0.5	23
Baked Hot Apple Pie, 2.7oz	250	13	32
Cinnamon Melts, 4 oz	460	19	66
Cookies: Chocolate Chip Cookie, (1)	160	8	21
McDonaldland® Cookies, 2 oz	260	8	43
Oatmeal Raisin (1), 1.1 oz	150	6	22
Sugar Cookie (1), 1.1 oz	160	7	21
Fruit 'n Yogurt Parfait: Reg., 5.3 oz	160	2	31
Without Granola, 5 oz	130	2	25
Ice Cream: Kiddie Cone, 1 oz	45	1	8
Vanilla Reduced-Fat Cone, 3.2 oz	150	3.5	24
McFlurry™: M&M® Candies, 12 fl.oz	620	20	96
Oreo® Cookies, 12 fl.oz cup	550	17	88
Sundaes: Hot Caramel Sundae, 6.4 oz	340	8	60
Hot Fudge Sundae, 6.3 oz	330	10	54
Strawberry Sundae, 6.3 oz	280	6	49
Peanuts (for Sundaes), 0.3 oz	45	3.5	2
Triple Thick Shakes: *Average all Flavors:*			
12 fl.oz cup	425	10	74
16 fl.oz cup	565	14	98
21 fl.oz cup	750	18	130
32 fl.oz cup	1125	27	197
Fruit Juice			
Apple Juice, 6.8 fl.oz box	100	0	23
Orange Juice: Small, 12 fl.oz	140	0	33
Medium, 16 fl.oz	180	0	42
Large, 21 fl.oz	250	0	57

McDonald's® cont... (Apr '10)

Sodas	C	F	Cb
Coca-Cola or Sprite: *Without Ice*			
Child, 12 fl.oz cup	110	0	29
Small, 16 fl.oz cup	150	0	40
Medium, 21 fl.oz cup	210	0	58
Large, 32 fl.oz cup	310	0	86
Diet Coke	0	0	0
Hi-C Orange Lavaburst: *Without Ice*			
Child, 12 fl.oz cup	120	0	32
Small, 16 fl.oz cup	160	0	44
Medium, 21 fl.oz cup	240	0	64
Large, 32 fl.oz cup	350	0	94
Powerade Mountain Blast: *Without Ice*			
Child, 12 fl.oz	70	0	20
Small, 16 fl.oz	100	0	27
Medium, 21 fl.oz	150	0	39
Large, 32 fl.oz	220	0	58
Milk: 1% Low-Fat, 8 fl.oz	100	2.5	12
1% Chocolate, 8 fl.oz carton	170	3	26
Iced Tea, no added sugar	0	0	0
Coffee Drinks, Black, 16 fl.oz	0	0	0
Coffee Cream 1 package, 0.4 fl.oz	20	2	0
Sugar Packet (1), 0.14 oz	15	0	4
Iced Coffee:			
Regular or flavors (average):			
Small, 8 fl.oz	130	5	21
Medium, 11.5 fl.oz	190	8	29
Large, 17 fl.oz	270	11	45
with Sugar-Free Vanilla Syrup:			
Small, 8 fl.oz	60	5	8
Medium, 11.5 fl.oz	90	8	11
Large, 17 fl.oz	120	11	16
McCafe Coffees			
Cappuccino			
Whole Milk: Small,12 fl oz	120	7	9
Medium, 16 fl oz	140	8	11
Large, 20 fl oz	180	10	13
Nonfat Milk: Small, 12 fl oz	60	0	9
Medium, 16 fl oz	80	0	12
Latte			
Whole Milk: Small, 12 fl oz	150	8	11
Medium, 16 fl oz	180	10	13
Nonfat Milk: Small, 12 fl oz	90	0	13
Medium, 16 fl oz	110	0	15
Mocha			
Whole Milk: Small, 12 fl oz	280	11	40
Medium, 16 fl oz	330	12	48
Nonfat Milk: Small, 12 fl oz	240	5	41
Medium, 16 fl oz	280	6	50

Extra Listings ~ www.CalorieKing.com

Manhattan Bagel® (Feb '10)

Bagel (East Coast): Per Bagel	C	F	Cb
Blueberry, 3.8 oz	270	1	60
Chocolate Chip, 3.8 oz	290	2.5	58
Cinnamon Raisin, 4.1 oz	330	1	70
Egg; Jalapeno Cheddar, 4.1 oz	320	2	67
Pumpernickel, 3.6 oz	250	1.5	55
Salt; Spinach, average, 4.2 oz	320	1	68
Sundried Tomato, 4.1 oz	310	1	66
Cream Cheese: Plain, 1.75 oz	180	16	4
Reduced-Fat, 1.75 oz	150	12	5

For Complete Nutritional Data ~ see CalorieKing.com

Marie Callender's ® (Feb '10)

Tasters: *Per Complete Dish as Served*	C	F	Cb
Crispy Chicken Tenders	1000	68	57
Crispy Green Beans	810	52	74
Loaded Potato Skins	710	43	51
Burgers and Sandwiches: *Without Sides*			
Original Burger	870	59	39
Albacore Tuna Melt	1060	73	55
Roasted Turkey Croissant Club	1450	98	95
Smoked Ham Stack	880	61	49
Main Meals: *Per Complete Meal as Served*			
Americana Classics:			
Braised & Slow Roasted Pot Roast	660	37	37
Roasted Turkey Dinner	820	42	74
From The Grill: Grilled Lemon Chkn	730	44	41
Grilled Atlantic Salmon, Cajun Style	840	60	29
St. Louis BBQ Ribs	1260	82	58
Pasta Perfecto:			
Chkn & Brocc. Fett. w/ Grlc. Bread	1480	87	119
Double Shrimp Pasta	1490	95	97
Pies, Chicken Pot Pie, w/out Sides	1370	102	72
Home-Style Soups & Chili:			
Chili, without Cornbread, 1 cup	280	8	34
Hearty Vegetable, 1 bowl	90	0	8
Fr. Onion, w/ Garlic Bread, 1 crock	710	43	52
Crisp Salads: *Includes Dressing*			
Chicken Ginger-Sesame	1070	47	130
Gorgonzola, Pecan & Field Greens	790	43	88
Traditional Caesar	490	35	28
Sides: Cornbread, 1 piece, 2 oz	170	6	*26*
French Fries, 4 oz	*380*	*20*	*45*
Honey Butter, 1 oz	*180*	*16*	*8*
Desserts: *Per Slice Unless Indicated*			
Pies: Apple	570	31	70
Banana Cream with Meringue	510	24	66
Chocolate Cream with Meringue	570	26	77
Pumpkin, with Whipped Cream	530	23	70
Razzleberry	660	39	71

Breakfast & Other Menu Items ~ see CalorieKing.com

Max & Erma's® (Feb '10)

Appetizers:	C	F	Cb
Black Bean Roll-Ups w/out dressing	575	10	95
Entrees: As Served			
Caribbean Chicken (lunch)	535	20	59
Salads: *No Breadstick*			
Hula Bowl with dressing	585	10	78
Baby Greens Salad, with dressing	120	11	6
Sides:			
Fruit Salad, 4.5 oz	55	0	17
Garlic Breadstick (1)	150	6	20
Fruit Smoothie	125	0.5	29

Mazzio's® (Feb '10)

Appetizers: *Per Serving*	C	F	Cb
Cheese Dippers, w/o sauce, ⅓ order	405	18	47
BBQ Chicken Wings, ⅕ order	190	12	7
Nachos: Beef w/ Jalapenos, ½ order	485	34	20
Cheddar with Jalapenos, ½ order	425	30	19
Calzones: *Per 1/10 Whole*			
Ham Bacon & Cheddar, w/o Sauce	245	7.5	32
Pepperoni	260	10	33
Pastas: *Without Garlic Toast*			
Fettuccine Alfredo	1060	56	107
Spaghetti with Marinara Sauce	640	8	120
Lasagna: with Alfredo Sauce	1265	94	55
with Meat Sauce	950	52	64
Sandwiches: *Without Chips or Pickle*			
Wheatberry:			
Chicken, Bacon & Swiss	1020	70	48
Ham & Cheddar	745	47	47
Mazzio's Sub	770	49	45
Hoagie: Chicken, Bacon & Swiss	1360	72	120
Ham & Cheddar	1090	50	119
Mazzio's Sub	1110	52	117
Turkey & Swiss	1060	40	118
Pizzas: *Per ⅛ Medium Pizza*			
Cheese: Original Crust	235	9	30
Thin Crust	180	9	18
Chicken Club: Original Crust	260	9	31
Thin Crust	205	9	19
Mazzio's Works: Original Crust	305	14	31
Thin Crust	255	15	20
Meatbuster: Original Crust	285	13	30
Thin Crust	235	13	19
Pepperoni: Original Crust	255	11	30
Thin Crust	200	11	18
Sausage: Original Crust	275	12	30
Thin Crust	225	12	19
Sides: Breadsticks, w/o sce, ¼ order	150	3	26
Garlic Toast, w/o sce, 1 pce, 1.4 oz	160	10	15

For Complete Nutritional Data ~ see CalorieKing.com

Updated Nutrition Data ~ www.CalorieKing.com
Persons with Diabetes ~ See Disclaimer (Page 24)

Mimi's Cafe® (Jun '10)

Breakfast	C	F	Cb
Hot Off The Griddle: *Without Sides*			
Belgian Waffle	395	17	50
French Toast	305	13	40
Gourmet: *Without Sides*			
Brie Cheese Lorraine Crepes	550	41	21
Eggs Florentine Benedict	690	50	36
Sandwiches and Burritos: *Without Sides*			
Chipotle Burrito	965	44	84
Ciabatta Breakfast Sandwich	945	53	77
Three Egg Omelettes: *Without Sides*			
Capresse	475	38	8
Mardi Gras	620	45	5
Lunch:			
Burgers: *Without Sides*			
French Quarter	1480	105	68
Turkey Pesto Ciabatta	1250	73	83
Dinner:			
Just Enough Dinner: *As Served, Without Soup or Salad*			
Artichoke Asiago Chicken Spaghettini	1265	76	81
BBQ Pork Chop	850	40	86
Santa Fe Shrimp & Chicken Fettuccine	925	55	70

Miami Subs® (Jun '10)

Burgers	C	F	Cb
Deluxe Burger	785	59	31
Deluxe Cheeseburger	860	65	32
Deluxe Bacon Cheeseburger	920	70	32
Platters: Chicken Breast	745	41	57
Gyros	1420	93	81
10 Wings with Fries & Blue Cheese	1020	67	50
Salads: Caesar with Dressing	460	34	26
Chicken Caesar with Dressing	610	39	28
Chicken Club	490	25	23
Garden	310	18	21
Greek	285	15	24
Cheesesteaks (6"): Original	410	11	45
Classic	420	11	48
Chicken Philly Classic	550	27	47
Works	530	23	51
Pitas: Gyros	660	39	47
Chicken	390	13	34
Subs(6"): Ham & Cheese	450	18	49
Italian Deli	515	25	49
Meatball	490	22	49
Tuna	470	18	44
Turkey	485	19	51
Sides: Mozzarella Sticks	755	57	34
Onion Rings	870	68	56
Spicy Fries: Regular	530	39	39
Large	1040	72	85

Mr. Goodcents® (Jun '10)

	C	F	Cb
Cold Sub: *Per ½ Sub on Wheat Bread*			
Centsable	480	20	58
Italian Sub	640	37	55
Mr. Goodcents Original	510	25	56
Oven Roasted Chicken Breast	350	6	55
Penny Club	350	6	57
Pepperoni & Cheese	740	46	55
Roast Beef	350	6	55
Tuna Salad	490	21	63
Veggie Sub	290	4	58
Hot Sub: *Per ½ Sub on Wheat Bread w/ Cheese*			
Chicken Bacon Ranch w/ Cheddar	630	29	57
Meatball with Mozzarella	670	33	65
Philly Jack 'n Cheese	490	16	60
Pasta:			
Alfredo Sauce on Mostaccioli	1290	80	106
Chicken Alfredo on Mostaccioli	1370	70	112
Chicken Parmesan on Mostaccioli	660	10	100
Red Sauce on Mostaccioli	520	4	100

Mr. Hero® (Jun '10)

7" Hot Subs & Burgers	C	F	Cb
Burgers: Cheeseburger	775	55	47
Romanburger	860	62	48
Meatball Sub	725	47	47
Steak Subs: Tuscan	625	31	42
Hot Buttered Cheesesteak	670	42	45
Zesty Bacon & Swiss	615	32	42
7" Deli Subs: Original Italian	640	39	47
Tuna & Cheese	725	54	44
Turkey	470	20	46
Ultimate Italian	675	40	46
4½" Taste Buddies: *Per Sandwich*			
Bacon Cheeseburger	430	30	33
Grilled Italiano	440	32	32
Tuna 'n Cheese	485	38	31
Zesty Chicken	495	25	48
Pasta, Spag./Rigatoni with Meatballs in Marinara Sauce & Breadstick	1115	36	153
Salads: *Without Dressing Unless Indicated*			
Grilled Chicken	165	2.5	13
Tuna Delight with Mayonnaise	495	48	10
Sides:			
Breadsticks, w/ Marinara Sauce (2)	445	17	64
Cheese Sauce, 1.5 oz	55	4	4
Jalapeno Poppers. 4.5 oz	430	28	37
Mozzarella Sticks, w/ Marinara Sce	565	43	12
Onion Petals, w/ Tangy Sce, 5.7 oz	695	46	64
Fries, Potato Waffer, 5.7 oz	430	30	38
Desserts: Oreo Cookie Cheesecake	260	17	24
Strawberry Swirl Cheesecake	280	19	22

Mrs Fields Cookies® (Feb '10)

Brownies: Per 2.6 oz Brownie	C	F	Cb
Butterscotch Blondie	350	14	52
Double Fudge	360	20	45
Pecan Fudge	360	20	46
Special Walnut Fudge & Blondie	330	16	43
Toffee Fudge	360	19	47
Walnut Fudge	360	20	45
Cake:			
Chocolate Chip, 3 oz piece	350	17	45
Cookies:			
Bite Size Nibblers: Cinn. Sugar (3)	170	8	22
Debra's Special (3)	170	7	23
Peanut Butter (3)	180	10	20
Semi-Sweet Chocolate (3)	170	8	24
Triple Chocolate (3)	170	9	23
White Chunk Macadamia (3)	180	9	23
Butter (1)	200	8	29
Cut Out (1)	400	19	56
Debra's Special (1)	200	9	28
Peanut Butter (1)	210	12	24
Semi-Sweet Chocolate (1)	210	10	29
with Walnuts(1)	220	11	29
Triple Chocolate (1)	210	11	28
White Chunk Macadamia (1)	230	12	27
Muffins: Blueberry (1), ¾ oz	70	3	10
Chocolate Chip (1), ¾ oz	80	4	11
Mandarin Orange (1), ¾ oz	80	3	9
Raspberry (1), ¾ oz	70	3	10

For Complete Nutritional Data ~ see CalorieKing.com

Nathan's Famous® (Feb '10)

Burgers:	C	F	Cb
Burger with Cheese,10.2 oz	705	43	45
Double Burger with Cheese, 15.6 oz	1180	84	45
Bacon Cheeseburger, 10.8 oz	785	50	45
Super Cheeseburger, 13.65 oz	985	72	47
Corn Dog with Stick, 3.2 oz	380	21	39
Nathan's Famous Hot Dogs:			
All Beef (1), 3.5 oz	295	18	24
All Beef Cheese (1), 4.5 oz	340	21	27
All Beef Chili (1, 5.5 oz	400	23	33
Chicken:			
Chicken Tenders (3), 6.2 oz	525	39	24
Chicken Tender Platter, 17.5 oz	1245	90	80
Chkn Wings with Bleu Chse, 12.9 oz	1240	100	23
Grilled Chicken Breast Platter, 15 oz	840	56	58

Nathan's Famous® (Feb '10)

Sides:	C	F	Cb
Fries: French: Medium, 6.5 oz	440	29	36
Large, 9 oz	610	41	50
Super, 14 oz	940	63	78
Cheese: Medium, 8 oz	490	34	41
Large, 9 oz	680	46	56
Super, 17 oz	1070	73	89
Mozzarella Sticks (3), w/ Sauce, 5.5 oz	385	28	20
Onion Rings, regular, 5.6 oz	545	45	36
Wraps:			
Grilled Chicken Caesar	700	34	60
Grilled Chicken Santa Fe	750	39	62

For Complete Nutritional Data ~ see CalorieKing.com

Ninety Nine (Feb '10)

Appetizers: Serves 4	C	F	Cb
Boneless Wings & Skins Sampler (4)	1660	111	70
Calypso Coconut Shrimp (4)	600	32	60
Outrageous Potato Skins (4)	1140	86	43
Steak & Chse Spring Rolls (4), w/ Sce	900	55	62
Sandwiches: *Without Sides*			
Chicken Parmigiana	880	36	92
Triple-Decker Turkey Club	950	37	107
Steakburger: Bacon & Cheese	940	57	46
Mushroom & Cheese	950	58	49
Steakburger	810	47	45
with Cheese	890	53	46
Sweet & Smokey	1060	61	67
Meals: *Without Sides*			
Cape Cod Seafood Trio	650	40	20
Captain's Combo Platter	1410	96	73
Fish & Chips	1160	76	60
Grilled Chicken Fajitas	1350	54	101
Smothered Sirloin Tips	820	40	9
Salads:			
Boneless Buffalo Wing	1030	57	74
Pecan Crusted Chicken	880	44	80
Wild Bleu Chicken & Spinach	1190	79	52
Sides:			
Double Bleu Iceberg Wedge	450	41	9
Garl. Red-Skin Mashed Pot., 2 scoops	260	12	34
Honey Butter Biscuit w/ Honey Butter	230	12	27
Perfect: Rice Pilaf, 2 scoops	260	6	46
French Fries, Kids, 8 oz, raw wt.	510	34	48
Desserts: *Per Serving*			
Apple Fortune	860	38	122
Little Midnight Fudge Hero	430	23	53
Strawberry Mimosa Cake	680	33	85

Updated Nutrition Data ~ www.CalorieKing.com
Persons with Diabetes ~ See Disclaimer (Page 24)

Noodles & Company® (Jun '10)

Meals: Per Regular Order	C	F	Cb
American: Buttered Noodles	620	16	84
Mushroom Stroganoff	780	31	100
Wisconsin Mac & Cheese	900	31	119
Asian Noodles: Bangkok Curry	490	13	85
Indonesian Peanut Saute	950	23	165
Japanese Pan	690	9	133
Pad Thai	700	20	117
Mediterranean: Pasta Fresca	780	22	111
Penne Rosa	810	26	119
Pesto Cavatappi	910	30	124
Whole Grain Tuscan Linguine	770	26	108
Proteins: Braised Beef	190	10	0
Organic Tofu	180	11	4
Parmesan Crusted Chicken Breast	190	8	17
Sauteed Beef	210	12	1
Seasoned Chicken Breast	130	2.5	0
Salads: Cucumber Tomato	80	0	18
Tossed Green	60	6	3
Sides: Potstickers, 3 Pieces	200	4.5	31
Ciabatta Roll (1)	160	1.5	31
Soups: Chicken Noodle, Regular	300	4	44
Tomato Basil Bisque, Regular	420	23	45

Nothing But Noodles® (Jun '10)

Noodle Bowls	C	F	Cb
American: Beef Stroganoff	510	31	33
Buttery Noodles	650	44	46
Santa Fe Pasta	705	54	40
Southwest Chipotle	715	58	41
Spicy Cajun Pasta	660	50	44
Asian: Pad Thai Noodles	600	10	118
Sesame Lo Mein	410	11	64
Spicy Japanese Noodles	420	8	74
Thai Peanut	570	20	89
Italian: Basil Pesto	575	42	36
Cappelini Primavera	500	28	56
Fettuccini Alfredo	725	56	36
Margherita Pasta	475	31	36
Marinara Pasta	485	11	77
Three-Cheese Macaroni	445	21	45
Rice Dishes: General Tso's Chicken	760	44	69
Kung Pao Chicken	935	51	89
Thai Peanut Stir Fry	595	27	59

Extra Menu Items ~ See CalorieKing.com

O'Charley's® (Jun '10)

Appetizers: As Served	C	F	Cb
Barbacoa Quesadillas	1170	73	64
Chicken Tenders, w/ Chipotle BBQ Sce	1040	37	119
Over-Loaded Potato Skins	1260	98	43
Southwestern Twisted Chips	1280	89	111
Spicy Jack Cheese Wedges (7)	880	60	55
Three-Cheese Shrimp Dip	870	49	86
Top Shelf Combo	1880	130	105
Brunch: *With Sides & Rustic Bread*			
Omelettes: Ham & Cheese	1210	76	76
Prime Time Prime Rib, 10 oz	1420	91	78
Spinach & Mushroom	1110	67	80
Meals: *Without Sides Unless Indicated*			
Chicken: Boneless Buffalo Tenders (5)	880	66	27
Teriyaki Sesame, with Rice Pilaf	1030	25	151
Pasta: Chicken Parmesan	1500	77	138
Outrgs. Chckn & Spinach Lasagna	1210	73	72
Prime Rib	1530	101	90
Seafood:			
Catfish Platter with Tartar Sauce	1430	121	46
Gr. Salmon with Rice Pilaf, 6 oz	560	27	32
Gr. Shrimp with Rice Pilaf & Sce	290	7	32
Steak & Ribs: *Per Serving, Without Sides*			
Baby Back Ribs: ½ Rack	740	48	38
1 full rack	1480	96	76
Filet Mignon, 9 oz	450	28	0
Grilled Top Sirloin, 7 oz	430	28	1
Louisiana Sirloin with Cajun Butter	680	40	3
Sides: *Per Serving*			
Potato: Baked, plain	240	5	50
Loaded	480	29	54
Smashed	370	12	47
French Fries, adult/a la carte	390	24	40
Salads: *Without Dressing Unless Indicated*			
Apple Crunch Salad	920	56	79
Black & Bleu Caesar with Dressing	1050	79	22
California Chicken	700	37	48
Tortilla Chicken	610	27	41
Soup: *Per Cup*			
Chicken Harvest	160	8	12
Chicken Tortilla	150	9	12
Creamy Wild Mushroom	150	14	7
Desserts: Cinnamon Sugar Donuts	1130	54	139
Ooey Gooey Caramel Pie, 1 slice	730	28	106
Ultimate Choc. Choc. Cake, 1 sl.	1080	59	151

Extra Menu Items ~ See CalorieKing.com

Old Country Buffet (Jun '10)

~ See CalorieKing.com

Olive Garden® (Jun '10)

Appetizers	C	F	Cb
Bruschetta	610	13	100
Muscles di Napoli	180	8	13
Sicilian Scampi	500	22	43
Stuffed Mushrooms	410	28	19
Entrees:			
Lunch: Eggplant Parmigiana	620	26	70
Fettuccine Alfredo	800	48	69
Five Cheese Ziti al Forno	770	32	89
Lasagna Classico	580	32	35
Dinner: Chicken Parmigiana	1090	49	79
Fettucini Alfredo	1220	75	99
Manicotti Formaggio	940	46	81
Garden Fare Selections (Lower Fat)			
Lunch: Capellini Pomodora, 13 oz	480	11	78
Linguine alla Marinara, 10.6 oz	310	4	55
Shrimp Primavera, 19 oz	510	9	79
Venetian Apricot Chicken	280	3	32
Dinner: Capellini Pomodora, 21 oz	840	17	141
Linguine alla Marinara, 17 oz	430	6	76
Shrimp Primavera, 26 oz	730	12	110
Venetian Apricot Chicken	380	4	32
Desserts: Black Tie Mousse Cake	760	48	73
Chocolate Gelato	620	25	89
Tiramisu	510	32	48

(The) Old Spaghetti Factory® (Jun '10)

Appetizers: *Per Serving*	C	F	Cb
Shrimp, Spinach & Artichoke Dip	150	10	10
Sicilian Garlic Cheese Bread	330	19	28
Toasted: Beef Ravioli, 4 oz	200	4.5	30
Cheese Ravioli, 4 oz	210	6	30
Entrees, Lunch/Dinner:			
Classics:			
Spaghetti: With Clam Sauce, 15 oz	660	14	104
With Marina Sauce, 15 oz	560	5	108
With Meat Sauce, 15 oz	610	9	105
With Sicilian Meatballs, 21 oz	960	31	114
Factory Favorites:			
Chicken Parmigiana, 19 oz	830	32	80
Spinach & Cheese Ravioli, 11 oz	480	16	63
Spinach Tortellini w/ Alfredo Sauce	930	56	86
Signature Selection: Chicken Penne	910	32	105
Crab Ravioli, 11 oz	810	46	73
Lasagna Vegetariano 20¾ oz	830	48	68
Meatloaf, Italian Style, 18½ oz	1180	68	83

On the Border® (Jun '10)

Appetizers: *As Served*	C	F	Cb
Border Sampler	2010	135	105
Fajita Quesadillas: Chicken	1240	85	59
Steak	1230	90	59
Burritos & Chimichangas: *Includes Rice, Without Beans & Sauce*			
Burrito, Classic Shredded Beef	1010	39	105
Chimichangas: Chicken	1300	76	107
Ground Beef	1400	88	107
Dinner: *Includes Rice, Without Beans*			
Enchiladas: Gr. Pepper Jack Chkn	1110	50	104
Ranchiladas	1490	83	106
Suiza	1010	44	111
Fresh Grill: *Served As Listed*			
Carne Asada	930	35	103
Chicken Salsa Fresca	520	9	60
Jalapeno-BBQ Salmon	590	21	45
Queso Chicken	1130	50	115
Tomatillo Chicken	850	24	108
Salads: *Without Dressing*			
House, Side	200	12	20
Sizzling Fajita Chicken	710	46	25
Sides: *Per Serving*			
Mexican Rice	290	5	54
Pico de Gallo	10	1	1
Sour Cream	60	5	2
Sauce: *Per Serving*			
Chipotle Honey	230	4	48
Habanero Fire	120	9	9
Tequila Lime Chile	170	14	6
Dressings: *Per Serving*			
Ranch Dressing	230	23	2
Smoked Jalapeno Vinaigrette	230	23	8

For Complete Nutritional Data ~ see CalorieKing.com

Orange Julius® (Jun '10)

	C	F	Cb
Orange Julius: Small, 16 fl.oz	130	0.5	33
Medium, 20 fl.oz	160	0.5	41
Large, 32 fl.oz	260	1	65
Other Julius Originals: *Per 16 fl.oz*			
Bananarilla	320	7	65
Pina Colada	260	7	52
Raspberry	200	1	59
Strawberry Banana	300	7	60
Premium Fruit Smoothies: *Per 20 fl.oz*			
Blackberry Storm	680	15	128
Orange Swirl	540	12	103
Raspberry Creme	650	15	118
Tropi-Colada	530	10	99
Fat Free: Mango Passion	370	0	86
Strawberry Xtreme	390	0	89
Nutrition Boosts: Fiber Plus, 0.2 oz	5	0	4
Heart Health, 0.15 oz	15	0	3
Joint Care, 0.2 oz	20	0	5
Protein (Soy), 0.67 oz	90	3	8

Updated Nutrition Data ~ www.CalorieKing.com
Persons with Diabetes ~ See Disclaimer (Page 24)

Outback Steakhouse® (Jun '10)

	C	F	Cb
***Aussie-Tizers:** Per Whole Dish, with Sauce/Dressing*			
Alice Springs Chkn Quesadilla, Sm	**1115**	**70**	69
Regular	**2140**	**133**	128
Aussie Cheese Fries: Small	**1210**	**87**	77
Regular	**2135**	**151**	139
Bloomin' Onion	**1565**	**84**	185
Gold Coast Coconut Shrimp	**565**	**22**	68
Kookaburra Wings, Hot	**2145**	**185**	28
Seared Ahi Tunah: Small	**355**	**23**	12
Regular	**480**	**29**	17
Burgers & Sandwiches			
Bacon Cheese Burger	**1130**	**80**	44
with Fries	**1485**	**99**	88
Grilled Chicken & Swiss Sandwich	**695**	**33**	50
with Fries	**1050**	**52**	93
Roasted Filet Sandwich	**765**	**20**	88
with Fries	**1115**	**39**	131
The Bloomin Burger	**1175**	**72**	76
with Fries	**1525**	**91**	119
The Outbacker Burger	**760**	**45**	43
with Fries	**1115**	**64**	86
***Steaks:** Meat Only ~ Add Extra for Sides*			
New York Strip, 14 oz	**715**	**37**	0.5
Outback Special: 6 oz Sirloin	**330**	**19**	0.5
9 oz Sirloin	**445**	**23**	0.5
12 oz Sirloin	**560**	**27**	0.5
Prime Rib, 8 oz	**535**	**45**	2
16 oz	**1060**	**90**	2
Ribeye, 14 oz	**1195**	**99**	0.5
Teriyaki Marinated Sirloin, 9 oz	**420**	**12**	17
The Melbourne, P/house, 20 oz	**1010**	**58**	1
Victoria's Filet: 6 oz	**520**	**42**	0.5
***Outback Favorites:** Per Total Meal as Per Menu*			
Alice Springs Chicken	**1650**	**113**	73
Baby Back Ribs, full rack	**2365**	**179**	67
Grilled Chicken on the Barbie	**585**	**26**	32
New Zealand Rack of Lamb	**1815**	**149**	48
No Rules Parmesan Pasta	**910**	**53**	89
with Chicken	**1355**	**77**	91
with Chicken & Scallops	**1365**	**77**	94
with Chicken & Shrimp	**1365**	**78**	92
with Scallops	**1320**	**76**	97
with Shrimp	**1275**	**77**	92
Sweet Glazed Rstd Pork Tenderloin	**850**	**43**	73

Outback Steakhouse® (Jun '10)

	C	F	Cb
***Fish & Seafood:** Without Sides Unless Indicated*			
Atlantic Salmon	**360**	**21**	1.5
Lobster Tails	**230**	**2**	6
Shrimp en Fuego Fettuccini	**1185**	**55**	95
Tilapia with Lump Crab Meat	**505**	**29**	8
***Perfect Combinations:** Without Sides Unless Indicated*			
Filet & Shrimp Scampi	**615**	**38**	18
Outback Special:			
Grilled Shrimp, with 6 oz Sirloin	**550**	**35**	7
With 9 oz Sirloin	**610**	**33**	9
With 12 oz Sirloin	**725**	**36**	9
Ribs & Alice Spring Chicken	**1270**	**98**	7
with Aussie Fries	**1625**	**18**	50
***Salads:** As Served*			
Chicken Caesar	**1045**	**74**	27
Blue Cheese Pecan, side	**525**	**36**	35
Queensland Salad: w/o Dressing	**840**	**59**	23
with Ranch Dressing	**1050**	**79**	30
Classic Roasted Filet Wedge	**565**	**30**	27
***Soups:** Per Bowl*			
Baked Potato	**775**	**48**	73
Cream of Broccoli	**410**	**30**	24
Onion	**435**	**32**	28
Add On Mates:			
Grilled Scallops with Butter	**320**	**23**	9
Lobster Tail with Butter	**325**	**24**	5
Lobster & Mushroom Topping	**395**	**36**	8
Sauteed Mushrooms	**135**	**3**	18
Sides: Aussie Fries	**355**	**19**	43
Baked Potato: Plain	**330**	**4.5**	65
with Bacon	**380**	**9**	65
with Butter	**520**	**26**	65
with Cheese	**355**	**7**	65
Loaded	**530**	**25**	66
with Sour Cream & Chives	**390**	**10**	66
Fresh Seasonal Veggies with Butter	**145**	**11**	11
Garlic Mashed Potatoes	**370**	**25**	32
Potato Boats	**165**	**2**	32
Sweet Potato	**595**	**21**	99
without butter	**420**	**4**	92
***Desserts:** Per Single Serving*			
Classic Cheesecake without Sauce	**185**	**9**	26
Chocolate Thunder from Down Under	**480**	**38**	34
Nutter Butter Peanut Butter Pie	**880**	**56**	89

Extra Menu Items ~ See CalorieKing.com

Panda Express® (Feb '10)

Appetizers	C	F	Cb
Chicken Egg Roll, (1), 3 oz	200	12	16
Chicken Potsticker (3)	220	11	23
Veggie Spring Roll (2)	160	7	22
Meals			
BBQ Pork, 4.6 oz	360	19	13
Beef & Broccoli, 5.4 oz	150	6	12
Beijing Beef, 5.6 oz	850	50	67
Black Pepper Chicken, 6.1oz	250	14	12
Eggplant & Tofu, 6.1 oz	310	24	19
Kung Pao Chicken, 6.1 oz	300	19	13
Mongolian Beef, 6.9 oz	230	11	17
Orange Chicken, 5.4 oz	400	20	42
Sweet & Sour Pork, 5.6 oz	400	23	36
***Rice & Noodles**: Per Serving*			
Chow Mein, 8.3 oz	400	12	61
Fried Rice, 10 oz	570	18	85
Steamed Rice, 8.7 oz	420	0	93

Panera Bread® (Feb '10)

Bagels: Blueberry	330	1.5	67
Dutch Apple & Raisin	360	3	77
Plain	290	1.5	59
Spreads: Plain Cream Cheese, 2 oz	180	18	2
Reduced-Fat, average, 2 oz	130	12	2
***Sandwiches:** Per Full Sandwich*			
Cafe:			
Sierra Trky on Focc. w/ Asiago Chse	970	54	80
Smoked Ham & Swiss on Rye	700	28	65
Smoked Turkey Brst on Country	560	17	68
Tuna Salad on Honey Wheat	750	47	64
Signature: Asiago Rst Beef w/ Cheese	690	27	64
Bacon Turkey Bravo, on Tom. Basil	840	32	87
Italian Combo, on Ciabatta	1040	45	94
***Salads:** With Dressing*			
Asian Sesame Chicken, 11.25 oz	410	20	30
Caesar, 9.75 oz	390	27	25
Classic Cafe, 9.75 oz	170	11	18
Greek, 13.5 oz	380	34	14
***Soups:** Per 8oz*			
Broccoli Cheddar	190	10	16
Cream of Chicken & Wild Rice	210	11	21
French Onion, w/o Cheese/Croutons	80	3.5	10
Low-Fat: Chicken Noodle	80	3	7
Garden Vegetable with Pesto	110	2	19
Muffins: Choc. Chip Muffie, 2.75 oz	280	12	40
Pumpkin Muffie, 2.75 oz	270	10	42
Wild Blueberry, 4.5 oz	390	15	58

Papa Gino's® (Feb '10)

***Appetizers:** Small, Per ½ Serving*	C	F	Cb
BBQ Chicken Tenders, 4 oz	260	9	28
Buffalo Chkn Tenders 4 oz	225	10	18
Cheese Breadsticks, 6.75 oz	485	20	58
Cinnamon Sticks, 3.6 oz	310	10	50
French Fries, 6 oz	270	12	40
Mozzarella Sticks, 5.5 oz	475	30	35
***Pastas:** Entree Size*			
Papa Platter, Penne; Spaghetti, 19.4 oz	990	32	135
Ravioli, 13.5 oz	590	24	71
Spaghetti & Meatballs, 19.6 oz	890	29	123
Spagh. Chkn Parmigiana, 23.5 oz	1070	39	129
***Pizzas:** Per Slice*			
Large Thin Crust: BBQ Chicken	270	7	38
Buffalo Chicken	240	7	31
Cheese	220	6	31
Chicken and Roasted Garlic	290	10	34
Chicken Pepper	270	9	32
Meat Combo	330	15	32
Papa Roni	320	15	32
Pepperoni	270	11	31
Super Veggie	240	7	35
The Works	300	12	33
***Pizza Slices:** Per Slice*			
Thin Crust: Cheese, 5.6 oz	310	9	42
Pepperoni, 6 oz	380	16	42
***Subs:** Per Small Sub*			
BLT	720	35	71
Italian	910	48	69
Meatball	740	32	76
Meatball Parmesan	840	41	76
Steak	630	25	65
Steak & Cheese	720	32	68
Super Steak	760	32	76
Tuna	740	39	67
Turkey Club	630	23	70
***Salads:** Without Dressing or Bread Stick*			
Buffalo Chicken Tender	330	15	29
Caesar	190	10	19
with Chicken	320	11	14
Chicken Bacon Cheddar	530	33	22
Chicken Tender	320	14	29
Garden	180	8	25
Side: Caesar	70	4	6
Garden	70	3	10
Dressings: Bleu Cheese, 1.1 oz	150	15	2
Caesar, 3 oz	400	44	2
Ranch, 3 oz	280	30	4
Honey Dijon Fat-Free, 1.5 oz	60	0	13

Updated Nutrition Data ~ www.CalorieKing.com
Persons with Diabetes ~ See Disclaimer (Page 24)

Papa John's® (Jun '10)

Original Crust (14"): Per 1/8 Pizza	C	F	Cb
BBQ Chicken & Bacon, 5.3 oz	350	12	44
Spicy Italian, 5.2 oz	380	18	38
Spinach Alfredo, 4.1 oz	290	11	36
The Meats, 3.7 oz	370	17	38
The Works, 5.5 oz	330	14	39
***Thin Crust (14"):** Per 1/8 Pizza*			
BBQ Chicken & Bacon, 4 oz	290	13	29
Spicy Italian, 3.9 oz	320	20	22
Spinach Alfredo, 2.8 oz	230	13	20
The Meats, 3.7 oz	310	19	22
The Works, 4.2 oz	270	15	23
Wings: Without Sauce			
BBQ, 2 wings, 2.6 oz	190	12	6
Buffalo, 2 wings, 2.6 oz	170	13	3
***Dipping Sauces:** Per 1 oz Container*			
Barbeque	45	0	11
Blue Cheese	160	16	1
Buffalo	15	0.5	2
Ranch	100	10	1
***Sides:** Without Dipping Sauce*			
Breadsticks (2)	290	4.5	54
Cheesesticks (4), 4.8 oz	370	16	41
ChickenStrips (2), 2.6 oz	130	4.5	10
Cinnamon Sweetsticks (4), 6.8 oz	580	16	98

Papa Murphy's® (Jun '10)

***Original Crust:** Per 1/12 Family Size Pizza*	C	F	Cb
BBQ Chicken	340	13	37
Cheese	270	11	30
Cowboy	350	18	32
Gourmet: Chicken Garlic	320	14	30
Classic Italian	350	18	31
Vegetarian	300	14	31
Hawaiian	290	11	33
Murphy's Combo	360	18	33
Pepperoni	320	15	31
Rancher	330	16	31
Specialty of the House, average	320	15	32
Veggie Combo	300	13	33
***Stuffed Pizza:** Per 1/16 Family Size Pizza*			
5 Meat	370	16	39
Big Murphy	370	16	40
Chicago Style	370	16	40
Chicken and Bacon	370	15	39

Papa Murphy's® cont... (Jun '10)

	C	F	Cb
***Thin Crust deLITEs:** Per 1/10 Large Pizza*			
Cheese	140	7	13
Hawaiian	160	7	15
Pepperoni	170	9	13
Veggie	160	9	13
***Salads:** Without Dressing or Croutons*			
Club	280	16	12
Garden	200	12	16
Italian	280	20	14

Pei Wei Asian Diner (Jun '10)

***First Tastes:** Per Whole Dish, Without Sauce*			
Crab Wontons	340	20	26
Crispy Potstickers	300	16	24
Edamame	320	14	18
Minced Chicken with Lettuce Wraps	620	22	72
Vegetable Spring Rolls	210	7	35
***Noodles & Rice Bowls:** Per Whole Meal, 2 Servings*			
Dan Dan Noodle, Chicken	780	20	106
Fried Rice: Beef	1040	32	136
Chicken	1000	24	132
Lo Mein Noodles: Chicken	1120	40	134
Beef	1080	40	136
Pad Thai Noodles: Beef	1580	52	218
Chicken	1440	40	210
Teriyaki Bowl: *Includes White Rice*			
Beef	1100	26	162
Chicken	1120	26	160
Shrimp	1060	24	160
Japanese Chili Ramen: Beef	980	32	128
Chicken	1000	32	126
Vegetable Tofu	1080	40	138
***Signature Dishes:** Per Whole Meal, 2 Servings, Without Rice*			
Honey Seared: Chicken	840	24	102
Shrimp	860	30	102
Sweet & Sour: Chicken	720	20	96
Shrimp	740	26	94
***Soup:** Per Serving*			
Hot & Sour: Per Cup	190	8	12
Per Bowl	250	10	16
Thai Wanton: Per Cup	150	8	6
Per Bowl	140	8	7
***Salads:** Per Whole Meal, Serves 2, Without Dressing*			
Asian Chopped Chicken	340	8	24
Spicy Chicken	1010	38	120
***Dressings:** Per 2 oz Serving*			
Lime Vinaigrette	220	20	8
Sesame Ginger	220	21	6
Sauces: Lettuce Wrap	50	3	3
Sweet Chile	140	0	17

Pepe's Mexican® (Feb '10)

Burritos:	C	F	Cb
Beef & Bean	510	24	52
Beef & Bean Suizo	640	34	55
Chicken & Bean	480	21	51
Chicken & Bean Suizo	610	31	54
Pork & Bean	470	19	51
Pork & Bean Suizo	600	29	54
Flauta: Beef, plain	160	9	10
Beef with Cheese & Sauce	190	12	11
Chicken, plain	190	10	16
Chicken with cheese & sauce	230	13	17
Tacos: Beef Crisp	210	11	16
Beef Soft Corn	250	10	28
Beef Soft Flour	250	11	24
Chicken Crisp	190	9	15
Chicken Soft Corn	230	8	27
Chicken Soft Flour	230	9	23
Pork Crisp	170	6	16
Pork Soft Corn	220	6	27
Pork Soft Flour	220	7	24
Tostada			
Beef & Bean	380	23	26
Beef & Bean Suiza	440	29	26
Chicken & Bean	360	21	21
Chicken & Bean Suiza	410	26	25
Pork & Bean	350	20	26
Pork & Bean Suiza	410	25	26
Taco Salads			
Beef: with 4 oz salsa	550	26	52
without Taco Shell	330	19	20
Chicken: with 4 oz salsa	520	23	51
without Taco Shell	300	16	19
Pork: with 4 oz salsa	500	20	52
without Taco Shell	290	13	19

Peter Piper Pizza (Feb '10)

Appetizers	C	F	Cb
Breadsticks (2), 2.45 oz	250	10	36
Chicken Strip (2), 4.85 oz	300	9	26
Wing (2), 1.7 oz	110	8	0
Pizza: *Per Slice*			
Original Crust: *Per ⅛ of 14" Pizza*			
Cheese	300	9	37
Ham & Pineapple	280	7	38
Pepperoni	300	10	36
Pepperoni & Sausage	310	11	37
Sausage	310	10	38

Peter Piper Pizza cont... (Feb '10)

Pizza: *Per Slice*	C	F	Cb
Hand-Tossed Crust: *Per ⅛ of 14" Pizza*			
Cheese	290	9	38
Ham & Pineapple	280	7	39
Pepperoni	290	10	37
Pepperoni & Sausage	310	11	38
Sausage	310	19	39
Pan Crust: *Per ⅛ of 14" Pizza*			
Cheese	290	9	38
Ham & Pineapple	310	7	46
Pepperoni	330	10	44
Pepperoni & Sausage	340	11	45
Sausage	340	11	46
Thin Crust: *Per ⅛ of 14" Pizza*			
Cheese	150	5	14
Ham & Pineapple	130	4	15
Pepperoni	150	6	13
Pepperoni & Sausage	150	7	14
Sausage	150	7	14
Signture Pizzas			
Original Crust: *Per ⅛ of 14" Pizza*			
5 Meat Supreme	350	13	38
California Veggie	200	6	23
Chicago Classic	300	10	38
New York 3 Cheese w. Pepperoni	380	16	38
Smokehouse	370	15	38
The Werx	320	11	38
Hand-Tossed: *Per ⅛ of 14" Pizza*			
5 Meat Supreme	350	13	38
California Veggie	270	7	39
Chicago Classic	300	10	39
New York 3 Cheese w. Pepperoni	380	16	39
Smokehouse	370	15	38
The Werx	310	11	39
Pan: *Per ⅛ of 14" Pizza*			
5 Meat Supreme	380	14	36
Califoria Veggie	300	7	47
Chicago Classic	340	10	46
New York 3 Cheese w. Pepperoni	410	16	46
Smokehouse	400	15	46
The Werx	350	11	46
Thin Crust: *Per ⅛ of 14" Pizza*			
5 Meat Supreme	180	8	14
California Veggie	130	4.5	15
Chicago Classic	150	6	15
New York 3 Cheese w. Pepperoni	200	10	14
Smokehouse	200	9	15
The Werx	160	7	14
Salads: *Without Dressing or Croutons*			
Chicken Caesar, 8 oz	200	8	10
Family, 4 oz	20	0	4
Italian Chef, 13 oz	290	16	14
Side, 5 oz	20	0	4

Updated Nutrition Data ~ www.CalorieKing.com
Persons with Diabetes ~ See Disclaimer (Page 24)

P.F. Chang's® (Feb '10)

Starters: Small Plate, Per Serving	C	F	Cb
Crab Wontons w/o Plum Sauce (2)	165	10	13
Egg Roll (1)	175	8	22
Lettuce Wraps: Chicken (1)	155	7	15
Vegetarian (1)	140	7	10
Peking Dumplings: Pan-Fried (1)	90	5	6
Steamed (1)	75	4	6
Shrimp Dumplings: Pan-Fried (1)	65	2	8
Steamed (1)	60	1	7
Spare Ribs: Northern Style (1)	345	19	11
Changs BBQ, (1)	345	24	7
Spring Rolls (2)	155	8	17
***Meals:** Per Whole Dish without Rice*			
Beef: A La Sichuan, 18 oz	910	36	75
Mongolian, 18 oz	1010	45	60
Orange Peel, 15 oz	850	39	63
Chicken: w/ Black Bean Sce, 27 oz	900	48	42
Chang's Spicy, 18 oz	970	39	69
Kung Pao Chicken, 15 oz	1150	69	42
Orange Peel Chicken, 15 oz	1000	45	60
Philip's Better Lemon, 21 oz	1030	42	90
Sesame Chicken, 24 oz	1030	42	75
Sweet & Sour Chicken, 15 oz	1110	57	114
VIP Duck, 12 oz	1300	58	110
Seafood: Cantonese Scallops, 14 oz	490	28	34
Cantonese Shrimp, 14 oz	430	20	20
Chang's Lemon Scallops, 18 oz	730	30	84
Kung Pao Scallops, 15 oz	920	60	51
Kung Pao Shrimp, 15 oz	840	51	36
Lemon Pepper Shrimp, 18 oz	470	20	38
Shrimp w/ Candied Walnuts, 21 oz	1130	72	75
Vegetarian Plates:			
Buddha's Feast, steamed, 12 oz	110	0	22
Coconut Curry Vegetables, 26 oz	1020	72	52
Ma Po Tofu, 27 oz	1080	72	51
***Lunch Bowls:** Served on White Rice, without Soup*			
Moo Goo Gai Pan, 28 oz	780	22	94
Sesame Chicken, 28 oz	1070	30	152
Shrimp with Lobster Sauce, 24 oz	680	20	90
***Sides:** Small, Per Whole Dish*			
Garlic Snap Peas, 4.5 oz	95	3	11
Green Tea Soba Noodles, 6 oz	425	18	56
Shanghai Cucumbers, 6 oz	60	3	5
Sichuan Asparagus, 6 oz	125	7.5	11
Spinach Stir-Fried with Garlic, 7.5 oz	80	4.5	8
Soups: Hot & Sour, 1 cup, 7 oz	80	3	9
1 bowl, 34 oz	390	15	44
Egg Drop : 1 cup, 7 oz	60	3	8
1 bowl, 34 oz	290	15	39
Desserts: Banana Spring Rolls (4)	940	40	136
Great Wall of Chocolate Cake (4)	1530	72	244
Mini Tiramisu (1)	100	11	10

Piccadilly Cafeteria® (Feb '10)

***Meals:** Without Sides*	C	F	Cb
Beef: Angus Chopped Steak	435	31	0
10 oz	885	65	5
Liver with Onion Sauce	365	20	22
Meatballs & Spaghetti	815	40	80
Chicken: & Dumplings, 8 oz	285	10	7
Breast, Blackened	295	14	3
Florentine, 8 oz	465	9	44
Lemon Pepper, half	1545	105	22
Parmigiana, 1 order	1240	36	135
Sesame Glaze, 9 oz	720	34	57
Tetrazzini, 1 order	375	21	18
Pork:			
Chop: Blackened with Fett. Alfredo	660	30	35
Smothered, 8 oz	730	34	46
Southwest with Mexican Rice	955	31	113
Sausage with Red Beans & Rice	805	42	76
Seafood: Blackened Shrimp Pasta	825	40	73
Cajun Baked Tilapia	335	20	5
Crawfish Etoufee	555	14	84
Tilapia with Shrimp Cream Sauce	280	6	10
Mediterranean Tilapia	240	8	8
New Orleans Sauteed Shrimp	835	40	78
***Salads:** Without Dressing*			
Ambrosia, 6.5 oz	285	14	43
Italian Rotini, 3.5oz	285	19	26
Piccadilly Fruit Salad, 5.75 oz	70	0	18
Potato, 4 oz	170	7	24
Tossed Spinach	95	5	7
Savory Sides:			
Baked Macaroni & Cheese, 5.25 oz	310	17	26
Breaded Okra, 3.25 oz	240	13	26
Broccoli & Rice, 5 oz	385	17	42
Candied Sweet Potatoes, 4.5 oz	305	0	77
Carrot Souffle, 5 oz	390	17	58
Cauliflower with Cheese Sauce	175	10	5
Mashed Potatoes, 5 oz	115	4	19
Turnip Greens, 1 order	60	2	11
***Soups:** Per Cup*			
Seafood Gumbo	225	6	32
Shrimp & Corn	200	10	19
Tomato-Macaroni	110	1	22
Bread:			
Corn Sticks (1)	155	9	16
Garlic Bread, 1 slice	205	10	25
Desserts:			
Buttermilk Chess Pie, 1 slice	635	30	87
Coconut Cream Pie, 1 slice	550	33	59
Peach Cobbler, 8 oz	545	22	82
Red Velvet Cake, 1 slice	835	54	83

Pita Pit (Feb '10)

Breakfast Pitas: Includes White Pita, Specific Ingredients, Eggs, Hashbrowns, Peppers and Onions	C	F	Cb
Awakin' with Bacon	610	27	57
Chicken Classic	555	18	59
Ham n' Eggs	515	17	58
Meat the Day	570	24	59
Morning Glory	505	19	61
Sausage Sunrise	530	21	59
***Meat Pitas:** Includes White Pita and Specific Ingredients*			
Black Forest Ham	320	4.5	43
B.L.T.	440	19	44
Chicken Breast	300	4	43
Chicken Caesar	385	10	44
Chicken Crave	360	6	44
Chicken Souvlaki	355	10	42
Dagwood	385	6.5	44
Gyro	560	29	49
Philly Steak	320	5.5	44
Roast Beef	360	7.5	45
Tuna	330	2.5	41
Turkey	290	1.5	41
***Veggie Pitas:** : Includes White Pita and Specific Ingredients*			
Babaganoush	270	5.5	47
Cheddar	420	19	41
Falafel	455	4	65
Feta	320	8.5	43
Garden	200	0.5	41
Hummus	300	7.5	49
Pita: White (1)	200	0.5	41
Toppings: Avocado	45	4	2
Babaganoush	35	2.5	3
Hummus	50	3.5	4
Pineapple	10	0	2
Lettuce, Tomato, On. & Cucumber	20	0	4
Sauces: BBQ	50	0	14
Caesar	140	15	0
Hot Sauce	0	0	0
Mayo	70	7	2
Ranch	80	8	2
Sour Cream	60	6	2
Teriyaki	35	0	8
Tzatziki	45	4	2
Cheeses: American Swiss	50	4.5	1
Cheddar	220	18	0
Feta	120	8	2
Parmesan	50	3.5	0
Smoothies: Berry Go Round	300	0.5	69
Banana Very Berry	270	0	63
Mango Tango	280	0	65

Pizza Hut® (May '10)

Thin 'n Crispy (12"): Per Slice ⅛ Pizza	C	F	Cb
Cheese Only, 2.3 oz	190	8	22
Ham & Pineapple, 2.5 oz	180	6	23
Meat Lover's, 3 oz	280	16	22
Supreme, 3 oz	240	12	23
Veggie Lover's, 3 oz	180	6	23
***Fit' n Delicious (12"):** Per Slice, ⅛ Pizza*			
Chkn, Mushroom & Jalapeno, 3.3 oz	170	4.5	23
Chicken, Onion & Green Pepper, 3.3 oz	180	4.5	23
Green Pepper, Onion & Tomato, 3.1 oz	150	4	24
Ham, Onion & Mushroom, 3 oz	160	4.5	23
Ham, Pineapple & Tomato, 3 oz	160	4.5	24
Tomato, Mushroom & Jalapeno, 3 oz	150	4	23
Hand-Tossed Style (12"): *Per Slice, ⅛ Pizza*			
Cheese Only, 3 oz	220	8	26
Dan's Original, 3.6 oz	260	12	26
Hawaiian Luau, 3.5 oz	240	10	27
Ham & Pineapple, 3.2 oz	200	7	27
Italian Sausage & Onion, 3.5 oz	240	11	27
Meat Lover's, 3.7 oz	310	16	26
Pepperoni, 3 oz	230	10	25
Pepperoni & Mushroom, 3.2 oz	210	8	26
Spicy Sicilian, 3.5 oz	250	11	26
Supreme, 3.7 oz	260	12	26
Triple Meat Italiano, 3.4 oz	260	12	25
Veggie Lover's, 3.7 oz	200	7	27
***P'Zone:** Per ½ P'Zone*			
Classic, 8.2 oz	630	23	77
Meaty, 8.57 oz	710	31	76
Pepperoni, 7.7 oz	630	24	76
***Pan (12"):** Per Slice, ⅛ Pizza*			
Cheese Only, 3.2 oz	240	11	27
Dan's Original, 3.9 oz	280	14	27
Ham & Pineapple, 3.4 oz	230	9	28
Hawaiian Luau, 3.6 oz	260	12	28
Italian Sausage & Onion, 3.7 oz	270	13	28
Meat Lover's, 4 oz	330	18	27
Pepperoni & Mushroom, 3.4 oz	240	10	27
Spicy Sicilian, 3.7 oz	270	13	27
Supreme, 4 oz	290	14	27
Triple Meat Italiano, 3.6 oz	290	15	27
Veggie Lover's, 3.75 oz	230	9	28

Continued next page...

Updated Nutrition Data ~ www.CalorieKing.com
Persons with Diabetes ~ See Disclaimer (Page 24)

Pizza Hut® cont... (May '10)

Personal Pan (6"): Per Pizza	C	F	Cb
Cheese Only, 7.3 oz	590	24	69
Ham & Pineapple, 7.6 oz	550	20	71
Meat Lover's, 9.3 oz	830	46	68
Supreme, 9 oz	720	36	69
Veggie Lover's, 8.2 oz	550	20	70
Pizza Mia (12"): *Per Slice, ⅛ Pizza*			
Cheese; Pepperoni, average, 2.55 oz	200	7.5	24
Stuffed Crust (14"): *Per Slice, ⅛ pizza*			
Cheese Only, 4.6 oz	350	14	39
Ham & Pineapple, 5 oz	340	13	41
Meat Lover's, 5.8 oz	480	26	39
Supreme, 5.7 oz	420	21	40
Veggie Lover's, 5.5 oz	330	13	40
Appetizers			
Breadsticks (1), 1.5 oz	150	7	19
Cheese Breadsticks (1), 2 oz	180	7	20
Wings: *Per 2 Pieces without Dipping Sauce*			
Baked: Hot, 1.5 oz	100	6	1
Mild, 1.5 oz	110	7	1
Bone Out: Buffalo, 2.6 oz	190	9	18
Honey BBQ, 3 oz	220	8	27
Crispy Bone In: Buffalo, 2.6 oz	230	15	16
Honey BBQ, 3 oz	260	14	24
Traditional: All American, 1.4 oz	80	5	0
Garlic Parmesan, 2 oz	180	16	1
Pastas, Tuscani: *Per ½ Pan*			
Bacon Mac N Cheese, 12.4 oz	520	22	54
Chicken Alfredo, 11.4 oz	630	33	56
Lasagna, 11.3 oz	600	33	43
Meaty Marinara, 11 oz	520	24	50
Sauces			
Dipping: Blue Cheese, 1.5 oz	230	24	2
Marinara, 3 oz	60	0	12
Ranch, 1.5 oz	220	23	2
Desserts			
Cinnamon Sticks, 2 pieces, 1.9 oz	170	6	26
Hershey's Chocolate Dunkers, 2 pcs,	200	9	26
with choc. sauce, 1.5 oz	320	12	50
Dipping Cup, White Icing, 2 oz	170	0	44

Pizza Ranch® (Feb '10)

Pizzas, 12 ": Per Slice (⅛ Pizza)	C	F	Cb
Original: Beef	170	6	21
BBQ Chicken	170	5	23
Bacon Cheeseburger	190	7	21
California Chicken	210	10	22
Canadian Bacon	170	6	21
Cheese	180	7	21
Chicken Broccoli	180	7	21
Garlic Cheese	190	9	21
Italian Sausage	180	8	21
Pepperoni	180	8	21
Prairie	170	6	22
Roundup	190	8	22
Stampede	210	9	22
Sweet Swine	170	6	22
Texan	200	8	26
Skillet: Beef	180	6	23
BBQ Chicken	180	5	24
Bacon Cheeseburger	200	7	23
Bronco	220	10	24
California Chicken	220	10	24
Cheese	190	7	23
Chicken Broccoli	190	7	23
Garlic Cheese	200	9	22
Italian Sausage	190	8	23
Pepperoni	190	8	23
Prairie	180	6	24
Roundup	200	8	24
Stampede	210	9	24
Sweet Swine	180	6	24
Texan	210	8	28
Thin: Beef	130	6	12
BBQ Chicken	130	5	14
Bacon Cheeseburger	140	7	12
California Chicken; Bronco, av	165	9	13
Canadian Bacon, av	120	5	12
Cheese; Chicken Broccoli, av	135	7	12
Garlic Cheese	140	9	11
Italian Sausage; Pepperoni, av	140	7	12
Prairie; Sweet Swine, av	130	6	13
Roundup	150	8	13
Stampede	160	8	13
Texan	160	7	17
Broasted Chicken: Breast, 1 pce	440	23	4
Leg, 1 piece	190	12	2
Thigh, 1 piece	370	26	4
Wing, 1 piece	190	13	2
Sides: Potato Wedges (1)	60	0	13

For Complete Nutritional Data ~ see CalorieKing.com

Planet Smoothie® (Feb '10)

Cool Blended Smoothies Per 22 fl.oz Unless Indicated	C	F	Cb
Captain Kid, 12 fl oz	180	0	46
PB & J	700	32	98
Shag-a-delic	300	0	77
The Last Mango	340	1	85
Twig & Berries	280	0	74
Vinnie del Rocco	370	0	92
Energy Smoothies: *Per 22 fl.oz*			
Berry Bada-Bing	350	0.5	92
Chocolate Elvis	430	17	68
Frozen Goat	220	0.5	55
Grape Ape	210	0	54
Road Runner	300	0	75
Spazz	270	0	69
Workout Smoothies: *Per 22 fl.oz Unless Indicated*			
Big Bang, protein blast	370	0	80
Chocolate Chimp, protein blast	220	1.5	38
Merlin's Mix, Pineapple, 32 fl oz	330	2	29
Strawberry, 32 fl oz	390	2	47

Pollo Tropical® (Feb '10)

¼ Chicken:	C	F	Cb
Dark Meat: with skin	270	17	0
without skin	180	9	0
White Meat: with skin	350	17	0
without skin	230	7	0
Tropichop:			
Chicken, White Rice/Black Beans:			
Regular	530	10	90
Large	1090	27	142
Chicken, Yellow Rice/Vegetables:			
Regular	330	5	51
Large	840	22	93
Pork, White Rice/Black Beans: Reg.	680	22	92
Large	1260	49	145
Pork, Yellow Rice/Vegetables: Reg.	490	18	54
Large	1000	44	97
Vegetarian:Regular	580	12	110
Large	950	21	178
Fajita: *With Sides, Toppings, Tortillas*			
Chicken; Steak, average	1145	38	153
Salad, Caribbean Cobb	950	41	57
Tropical Favorites:			
Cheesy Yuca Bites, 6 pieces	290	14	32
Fried Yuca, 5 pieces	500	24	69
Sweet Plantains, 5 pieces	310	8	63
Wraps: Chicken Caesar	790	39	65
Cuban	680	29	61
Pork	740	25	73

Popeye's® (Feb '10)

Chicken: *Mild & Spicy with Skin*	C	F	Cb
Breast, average	355	21	8
Leg, average	105	6	3
Thigh, average	290	22	7
Wing, average	145	10	5
Big Deals: Delta Mini (1), 3.6 oz	300	13	30
Chicken Biscuit, 3.6 oz	350	20	30
Loaded Chicken Wrap, 6 oz	400	17	44
Sides: Biscuit, 2.1 oz	240	13	26
Cajun Rice, regular, 4.1 oz	170	6	22
Coleslaw, regular, 5 oz	260	23	14
Corn on the Cob (1), 7.8 oz	190	2	37
French Fries, 3 oz	310	17	35
Mashed Potatoes: no Gravy, reg.	100	3	17
w. Gravy, regular, 5 oz	120	4	18
Red Beans & Rice, regular, 6 oz	320	19	31
Desserts: Cinn. Apple Turnover, 3 oz	250	12	34

Port of Subs® (Feb '10)

Figures Based on West Coast Outlets	C	F	Cb
Light Submarine: *Per 5" Sub (Five Grams of Fat or Less)*			
#2 Ham Turkey	330	5	46
#5 Smoked Ham & Turkey	320	5	46
#6 Vegetarian, no Cheese	240	2	44
#7 Roast Beef	315	4	43
#8 Turkey	315	4	47
#9 Peppered Pastrami	295	4	44
#10 Roasted Chicken Breast	305	3	44
#14 Smoked Ham	300	4	44
#18 Roast Beef & Turkey	315	4	45
Cold Submarine S'wiches: *Per 5" Sub w/o Mayo/Mustard*			
#1 Ham, Salami, Capicolla			
& Pepperoni w. Provolone	530	26	45
#2 Ham & Turkey w. Provolone	435	15	46
#3 Salami & Turkey w. Provolone	465	20	46
#4 Ham & Salami w. Provolone	470	21	45
#5 Smkd Ham & Turkey w. Cheddar	430	15	47
#6 Vegetarian w. Avocado & Olives	600	33	49
#7 Roast Beef w. Provolone	420	14	43
#8 Turkey w. Provolone	420	14	47
#9 Peppered Pastrami w. Swiss	440	17	44
#10 Rstd Chicken Brst w. Provolone	410	13	45
#11 Ham w. American	380	20	45
#12 Salami w. Provolone	480	25	45
#13 Peppered Pastrami Turkey Swiss	510	26	44
#14 Smoked Ham w. Swiss	445	17	45
#15 Salami & Pepperoni w. Prov.	510	27	45
#16 BLT Sandwich	520	30	43
#17 Tuna no Cheese	420	18	45
#18 Rst Beef & Turkey w. Provolone	420	14	45

Continued next page...

Updated Nutrition Data ~ www.CalorieKing.com
Persons with Diabetes ~ See Disclaimer (Page 24)

Port of Subs® cont... (Feb '10)

Figures Based on West Coast Outlets

Grillers: 5" Serving	C	F	Cb
BBQ Pork Griller	780	18	104
Grilled Chicken	520	13	58
Hot Pastrami	540	15	58
Italian	555	21	58
NY Steak & Cheese	615	18	57
***Tortilla Wrap:** Per Wrap, 12" Tortilla*			
Chicken Caesar	630	34	35
Turkey & Bacon Ranch	590	38	34
Tortilla (1)	200	7	27
Fresh Salads:			
Caesar Salad with Dressing: 6 oz	335	30	7
with Grilled Chicken, 13 oz	540	34	15
Chefs Salad w/ Oil & Vinegar, 11 oz	390	25	13
Garden Salad w/ Oil & Vinegar, 8 oz	95	5	10
Grilled Chicken w/ Oil & Vin. 13 oz	300	10	16
Macaroni Salad, 5 oz	330	22	28
Potato Salad, 5 oz	230	12	28
Tuna Salad w/ Oil & Vinegar, 11 oz	310	23	12
Dessert:			
Brownie, 5 oz	300	10	48

Pret A Manger® (Feb '10)

Sandwiches	C	F	Cb
Avocado & Parmesan	570	27	59
Balsamic Chicken & Avocado	500	20	64
Chicken & Bacon	460	13	58
Classic Turkey Club	520	21	59
Smoked Salmon	460	14	48
Slims: Avocado & Parmesan	285	14	30
Balsamic Chicken & Avocado	250	11	32
Chicken & Bacon	240	13	29
Classic Turkey Club	260	11	30
Baguettes:			
Chicken Mozzarella	500	16	68
French Brie & Basil	500	20	58
Roasted Beef Arugula & Parm.	580	16	65
Slims: Chicken & Bacon	230	13	29
Classic Turkey Club	260	11	30
Roasted Beef, Arugula & Parm.	290	8	28
Wraps: Jalapeno Chicken, Hot	400	21	46
Spicy Falafel Hot	540	24	61
Swedish Meatball Ragu, Hot	700	37	49
***Soup:** Per Medium 12 oz Serving*			
Angus Steak Chili with Beans	345	11	35
Moroccan Lentil	435	20	54
Souper Reuben	300	17	23
Veggie Split	330	5.5	29

Pret A Manger® cont... (Feb '10)

***Salads:** Per Pack, w/o Dressing*	C	F	Cb
Cobb & Greens	430	24	30
Grilled Chicken & Avocado	430	28	41
Grilled Chicken Caesar	400	16	24
Red, White & Greens	300	17	14
Bakery: Banana Cake	420	24	48
Carrot Cake	460	29	47
Chocolate Brownie	390	20	51
Chocolate Cake	470	19	71
Raspberry Bar	390	18	55

For Complete Menu ~ See CalorieKing.com

Pretzelmaker® (Feb '10)

Pretzels:	C	F	Cb
Bites: Small (1), 5.3 oz	450	11	80
Medium (1), 7½ oz	640	16	112
Large (2), 11½ oz	1020	26	176
Cinnamon Sugar, 6 oz	520	12	95
Pretzel Dog	440	27	34
Pretzels: Caramel Nut	390	7	74
Cinnamon Sugar	370	8	68
Garlic	350	7	64
Original	340	7	61
Parmesan	360	9	61
Plain	290	2	61
Ranch	240	7	63
***Sauces:** Per 1.5 oz Container*			
Caramel	140	0	35
Cheddar Cheese	70	5	6
Cream Cheese	200	20	4
Cream Cheese Icing,	180	9	22
Ketchup	20	0	4
Mustard	5	0	1
Nacho Cheese	80	5	7
Pizza	30	0.5	6
***Beverages:** Per 20 fl.oz*			
Breezer: Coffee	640	21	107
Mocha	620	20	106
Peach	650	20	117
Raspberry	650	20	117
Strawberry Banana	650	20	115
Lemonade: MCF, 20 fl.oz	160	0	92
MCF, 32 fl.oz	270	0	147
Diet Coke, 20 fl.oz	0	0	0

Qdoba (Jun '10)

Burritos: With 13" Flour Tortilla	C	F	Cb
Grilled Chicken	520	18	55
Ground Beef	570	25	55
Pulled Pork	490	13	64
***Signature Burritos:** With 13" Flour Tortilla*			
Ancho Chile BBQ	420	11	70
Grilled Vegetables	390	12	59
***Quesadillas:** With 13" Soft Flour Tortilla*			
Grilled Chicken	960	54	56
Shredded Beef	960	52	60
***3-Cheese Nachos:** With Meat & Tortilla Chips Only*			
Grilled Chicken	750	36	76
Ground Beef	800	43	76
Pulled Pork	720	31	85
***Tacos:** With Crispy Shell*			
Grilled Chicken (1)	120	6.5	8
Ground Beef (1)	140	9	9
Pulled Pork (1)	110	4.5	11
Shredded Beef (1)	120	5.5	10
***Taco Salads:** With Crunchy Tortilla Bowl*			
Grilled Chicken	595	2	44
Ground Beef	645	39	44
***Breakfast Items:** With 10" Flour Tortilla*			
***Breakfast Burrito:** With Spicy Chorizo, Egg & Potato*			
With 3-Cheese Queso Sauce	460	21	44
With Fajita Ranchero Sauce	400	15	43
Condiments: 3-Cheese Queso, 2 oz	100	8	3
Ancho Chile BBQ, 2 oz	90	2.5	16
Black Beans, 6 oz	210	1.5	35
Cheese, 1.5 oz	170	14	0
Cilantro Lime Rice, 6 oz	330	8	60
Fajita Vegetables, 2 oz	30	1.5	4
Grilled Vegetables, 3.5 oz	60	3.5	5
Guacamole, 3 oz	130	11	7
Mango Salsa, 4 oz	60	0	14
Pico de Gallo, 2 oz	10	0	1
Pinto Beans, 6 oz	190	1.5	34
Sour Cream, 2 oz	60	4	3

Quizno's Subs® (Jun '10)

Based on Quizno's Standard Portion Sizes. Figures may not apply for Baltimore, Boise, Cleveland, Denver, Des Moines, Raleigh, Springfield.

***Subs** Regular: With Cheese & Dressing Unless Indicated*

Every-Day Value Subs:	C	F	Cb
Ham & Swiss	770	44	63
Roast Beef & Cheddar	780	43	64
Tuna Melt	1220	94	60
Turkey & Cheddar	770	44	63

Quizno's Subs® cont... (Jun '10)

Based on Quizno's Standard Portion Sizes. Figures may not apply for Baltimore, Boise, Cleveland, Denver, Des Moines, Raleigh, Springfield.

***Subs (Cont):** Regular, w/Cheese & Dressing Unless Indicated*

Signature:	C	F	Cb
Baja Chicken	780	36	64
Bourbon Grille Steak	830	35	76
Chicken Carbonara	840	42	60
Double Cheese Cheesesteak	1030	63	65
Honey Mustard Chicken	830	41	66
Mesquite Chicken	790	39	61
Prime Rib and Peppercorn	930	53	66
Steakhouse Beef Dip	860	45	65
Torpedos: Beef Bacon & Cheddar	790	32	85
Italian	895	47	82
Pesto Turkey	675	24	85
Turkey Club	815	38	84
Bullets:			
Beef, Bacon & Cheddar	385	18	38
Italian	445	25	36
Pesto Turkey	330	13	38
Tuna Melt	525	37	35
Turkey Club	405	21	38
***Sammies:** With Cheese & Dressing Unless Indicated*			
Alpine Chicken	380	19	28
Bistro Steak Melt	395	24	30
Cantina Chicken, without Cheese	265	6	35
Italiano	410	25	28
Roadhouse Steak, without Cheese	250	4	38
Sonoma Turkey	380	23	29
Veggie	330	19	29
Kids Sammies:			
Cheesy	230	10	25
Ham & Cheese	200	6	25
Turkey & Cheese	200	6	26
***Soups:** Per Bowl*			
Broccoli Cheese	305	18	26
Chicken Noodle	155	3.5	25
Chili, with 2 Crackers	275	7	34
Tomato Basil	205	9	19
***Regular Salads:** With Flatbread & Dressing*			
Chicken Caesar	920	67	39
Classic Cobb	800	56	40
Honey Mustard Chicken	920	65	48
Raspberry Chipotle	710	30	70

Updated Nutrition Data ~ www.CalorieKing.com
Persons with Diabetes ~ See Disclaimer (Page 24)

Rally's/Checkers® (Jun '10)

Burgers/Sandwiches	C	F	Cb
Bacon Double Cheeseburger	650	42	32
Big Buford	670	40	41
Cheese Double Cheese	510	31	31
Chili Cheeseburger	320	15	30
Crispy Fish Sandwich	430	19	51
Rallyburger	390	22	32
Wings: Classic Honey BBQ, 5 pieces	390	17	18
Extra Hot, 5 pieces	355	21	2
Parmesan Garlic, 5 pieces	480	35	1
Fries:			
Chili Cheese Fries, 7.76 oz	550	34	48
French: Medium, 3.88 oz	350	21	36
Large, 4.41 oz	400	24	42

Ranch 1® (Jun '10)

	C	F	Cb
Sandwiches: Chicken & Cheese	390	12	39
Chicken Philly, 9.2 oz	410	13	40
Crispy Chicken, 11.4 oz	710	39	60
Crispy Spicy Chicken, 11.4 oz	545	17	68
Grilled Spicy Chicken, 10.3 oz	365	7	46
Ranch 1 Classic, 9.4 oz	685	47	37
Bowls: Chicken Teriyaki, 19.3 oz	505	7	78
Fajitas, Chicken, 10 oz	540	24	53
Chicken, Rice, 10.9 oz	275	6	28
Popcorn Chicken: Small, 5.5 oz	325	12	30
Large, 7.5 oz	420	15	38
Kids Meal, 2 oz	110	4	10
Salads: *Complete*			
Grilled Chicken Caesar, 13.2 oz	430	30	14
Mandarin Chicken, 19.3 oz	815	43	78
Southwest Chicken, 17.5 oz	745	50	44
Fries: Medium, 5.8 oz	380	21	43
Large, 8 oz	530	29	58
Kids Meal, 4 oz	280	15	31
Cheese: Regular, 9 oz	495	27	54
Large, 14 oz	755	42	80

Red Hot & Blue® (Jun '10)

BBQ Platters: *Without Sides*	C	F	Cb
Five Meat Treat	1165	85	15
Memphis Half Chicken	1510	103	11
Pulled Chicken	365	24	6
Pulled Pork	485	33	6
Smoked Sausage	950	67	36
BBQ Sandwiches: *Regular, Without Sides*			
Beef Brisket	415	17	36
Carolina Chopped Pork	460	23	34
Smoked Sausage	470	23	37
Ribs, Half Slab: Dry	1350	100	32
Sweet	1315	95	40
Wet	1260	95	26

Red Hot & Blue cont... (Jun '10)

Salads: *Without Dressing*	C	F	Cb
Grilled Chicken Caesar	755	45	45
RH & B Chopped Salad	935	55	54
Smokehouse Salad	770	44	44
Southern Fried Chicken	690	30	58
Soup: Corn Chowder, 1 bowl	320	17	22
Sides: BBQ Beans	215	4	37
Mashed Potatoes with Gravy	335	15	47
Potato Salad	510	32	46

Red Lobster® (Jun '10)

Lunch	C	F	Cb
Starters:			
Chilled Jumbo Shrimp Cocktail	120	0.5	9
Crispy Calamari & Vegetables	1520	97	115
Lobster, Crab & Seafood Mushrooms	380	21	20
Pan Seared Crab Cakes	280	14	13
Classics: *Per Lunch Portion*			
Cajun Chicken Linguini Alfredo	630	27	45
Crab Linguini Alfredo	560	25	47
Crunchy Popcorn Shrimp	280	14	26
LightHouse Menu, Grilled/Broiled: *½ Portion Serving*			
Main Lobster Meat, 1.6 oz	45	0.5	0
Rainbow Trout	220	10	6
Salmon	270	9	6
Tilapia	210	3	9
Signature Combinations:			
Admiral's Feast	1500	87	110
Seaside Shrimp Trio	1030	57	68
Ultimate Feast	620	30	29
Dinner			
Starters: Clam Strips	370	22	31
Lobster, Artichoke & Seafood Dip	1200	74	101
Mango-Jalapeno Shrimp Skewers	560	22	58
Parrot Isle Coconut Shrimp	590	33	54
Lobster & Crab Entrees:			
Lobster & Shrimp Pasta	1020	50	86
North Pacific King Crab Legs	390	3.5	2
Rockzilla	130	1.5	0
Snow Crab Legs Meat, 3.56 oz	160	1	0
Sides: Fries	330	17	40
Home-Style Mashed Potatoes	180	9	22
Garden Salad	90	3	13
Garden Salad with Shrimp	105	3	13
Dipping Sauces: *Per 1.5 oz*			
Cocktail Sauce	40	0	9
Sweet & Spicy Glaze	100	0	24
Tartar Sauce	190	19	6
100% Pure Melted Butter	350	38	2

For Complete Nutritional Data ~ see CalorieKing.com

Red Robin® (Jun '10)

Appetizers: As Served	C	F	Cb
Chili Chili Con Queso	1375	88	109
Creamy Artichoke & Spinach Dip	1115	60	101
Guacamole, Salsa & Chips	815	47	88
Just-in-Quesadilla	1070	55	69
Nachos: Chili	1955	132	130
With Chicken	2085	134	132
RR's Buzzard Wings	1075	84	4
Towering Onion Rings	1775	112	171
***Entrees:** With Sides, Dressings & Sauce*			
Arctic Cod Fish & Chips	1120	67	83
Clucks & Fries: Regular Style	1450	92	100
Buffalo Style	1695	121	100
Ensenada Chicken Platter	755	41	26
Grilled Chicken alla Caprese	645	34	35
Jumbo Shrimp & Slaw Plater	1255	56	148
Red's Rice Bowl	830	10	137
Shrimp & Cod Duo	1435	84	133
Steak Sliders(3)	1125	58	91
***Sandwiches & Burgers**: With Standard Components*			
Gourmet Burgers:			
A.1. Peppercorn	1025	59	70
Bacon Cheeseburger	1030	69	51
Bleu Ribbon	999	57	70
Burnin' Love	935	60	55
Cheeseburger	930	60	53
Guacamole Bacon	1045	64	54
Natural	570	24	51
Pub	955	55	57
Royal	1195	83	52
Sauteed 'Shroom	960	56	58
The Banzai	1035	62	68
Whiskey River BBQ	965	53	68
Other Favorite Burgers: Garden	560	23	73
Grilled Turkey	640	37	50
Lettuce-Wrap Your Burger	420	27	8
Sandwiches:			
Chicken: Blackened	695	34	52
Bruschetta	680	31	55
California	835	44	52
Crispy	910	54	70
Teriyaki	905	48	64
Other Favorite Sandwiches:			
Crispy Cod	605	29	61
Grilled Salmon	855	50	53
Wraps:			
Caesar's Chicken	850	43	69
Whiskey River BBQ Chicken	1110	62	84

Rita's® (Feb '10)

***Cream Ice:** Average All Flavors*	C	F	Cb
Kids, 7.5 oz	240	3	53
Regular, 12 oz	380	5	85
Large, 19 oz	600	8	134
***Italian Ice:** Average All Flavors*			
Kids, 7.5 oz	200	0	50
Regular, 12 oz	320	0	80
Large, 19 oz	500	0	126
***Sugar Free Ice:** Average All Flavors*			
Kids, 7.5 oz	90	0	30
Regular, 12 oz	130	0	46
Large, 19 oz	230	0	80
***Custard:** Average All Flavors*			
Kids, 4 oz	230	12	28
Regular, 5.75 oz	330	17	40
Large, 7.5 oz	430	22	52
***Gelati:** Per 10 oz*			
With Cream Ice: All Custard	420	14	71
Average Other Flavors	425	14	71
With Italian Ice, average all flavors	395	12	70
***Misto:** Per Regular, 15.5 oz*			
With Cream Ice, average all flavors	560	13	111
With Italian Ice: Chocolate	510	7	106
Vanilla	480	8	103
***Light M&Ms, Oreo Blendinis:** Per 11 oz*			
Chocolate	440	8	86
Mango-Peach/Pineapple	420	6	82

For Complete Nutritional Data ~ see CalorieKing.com

Robeks (Jun '10)

***Smoothies:** Per 12 fl.oz*	C	F	Cb
Acai Energizer	160	1	33
Cardio Cooler	245	1	45
Cranberry Quest	210	1	49
Dr. Robeks	185	1	42
Malibu Peach	180	0	44
Passionfruit Cove	195	1	46
Pomegranate Passion	190	0	46
Raspberrry Romance	210	0	50
Robeks Rejuvenator	220	1	51
Strawnana Berry	190	0	44
Venice Burner	225	1	48
Zen Berry	215	1	51
Light Smoothies: Banana-Mango	160	0	42
Pineapple-Mango	170	0	44
Raspberry-Banana	160	0	42
Strawberry-Pineapple	130	0	33

Updated Nutrition Data ~ www.CalorieKing.com
Persons with Diabetes ~ See Disclaimer (Page 24)

Rocky Rococo® (Feb '10)

Pastas: *Per Serving*	C	F	Cb
Can't Decide, 14 oz	465	9	77
Fettuccine w. Alfredo Sauce:			
Regular, 14 oz	460	14	66
Light, 7 oz	230	7	33
Spaghetti w. Meatballs: Reg., 15 oz	630	16	89
Light, 7.5 oz	315	8	45
Spaghetti w. Tomato Sauce: Reg.	470	4	87
Light, 7 oz	235	2	44
Pizzas: *Per Slice, 1/8 Pizza*			
Cheese	380	9	54
Garden	390	10	56
Pepperoni	425	13	54
Sausage	495	19	54
Sausage Mushroom	500	19	55
Sides			
Breadsticks: w. Marinara Sce (6)	420	7	72
w. Jalapeno Cheese Sauce (6)	530	18	72
Wheat Muffin (1)	200	4	38

Roly Poly® (Feb '10)

Wraps: *Per Small Whole Wheat Bread Wrap*	C	F	Cb
Baked Ham & Roast Pork:			
Italian Classic	335	12	32
Key West Cuban Mix	330	9	44
Peachtree Melt	325	11	28
Pork Melt	310	11	26
Porky's Nightmare	320	12	28
Chicken: Basil Cashew Chicken	330	10	30
Catalina Chicken Salad	320	11	28
Chicken Caesar	310	11	28
Chicken Cordon Bleu	310	11	26
Chicken Fajita	315	9	28
Chicken Popper	285	8	29
Cobb Salad	255	12	27
Delhi Chicken	325	12	33
Hickory Chicken	350	10	25
Oriental Chicken	270	4	29
Santa Fe Chicken	305	11	28
Seafood: Popeye's Tuna	305	4	31
Classic Tuna Melt	340	17	26
Texas Tuna Melt	310	12	30
Thai Hot Tuna	340	11	30
Tuna Luau	325	14	34

Round Table® Pizza (Feb '10)

Appetizers	C	F	Cb
Buffalo Wings, 6 pieces	420	30	6
Garlic Bread, 6 pieces	420	21	54
with Cheese, 6 pieces	600	36	54
Garlic Parmesan Twists, 3 pieces	510	15	78
Honey BBQ Wings 6 pieces	480	27	12
Pizzas *(Large 14"): Per Slice, 1/12 Pizza*			
Original Crust: Cheese	230	9	25
Chicken & Garlic Gourmet	250	11	25
Chicken Smokehouse	270	12	26
Gourmet Veggie	240	10	27
Guinevere's Garden Delight	220	8	26
Hawaiian	220	8	27
Italian Garlic Supreme	270	14	25
King Arthur Supreme	270	13	26
Maui Zaui, with Polynesian Sce	260	10	29
Montague's All Meat Marvel	290	15	25
Pepperoni	240	11	24
Smokehouse Combo	290	14	26
Pan Crust: Cheese	300	11	38
Chicken & Garlic Gourmet	340	13	39
Chicken Smokehouse	360	14	40
Gourmet Veggie	320	12	41
Guinevere's Garden Delight	300	10	39
Hawaiian	300	10	40
Italian Garlic Supreme	360	16	39
King Arthur Supreme	340	14	39
Maui Zaui with Polynesian Sce	340	12	43
Montague's All Meat Marvel	360	15	38
Pepperoni	320	13	38
Skinny Crust: Cheese	190	9	18
Chicken & Garlic Gourmet	220	11	18
Chicken Smokehouse	240	12	19
Gourmet Veggie	200	10	20
Guinevere's Garden Delight	180	8	19
Hawaiian	190	8	20
Italian Garlic Supreme	240	14	18
King Arthur Supreme	240	13	19
Maui Zaui with Polynesian Sce	220	10	22
Montague's All Meat Marvel	260	15	18
Pepperoni	210	11	18
Sandwiches:			
Chicken Club	800	43	59
Ham Club	740	40	60
RT Pizza	410	18	78
Turkey Club	720	38	59
Turkey Sante Fe	730	40	57

For Complete Nutritional Data ~ see CalorieKing.com

Rubio's Mexican Grill® (Feb '10)

Burritos: *Chips Not Included*	C	F	Cb
Baja: Grill Chicken	620	26	53
Steak	670	34	53
Bean & Cheese	700	33	75
Carnitas Rajas	740	39	75
Fish	710	40	71
Grilled Mesquite Shrimp	710	34	72
Grilled Veggie	630	29	73
Langostino	720	34	81
Mahi Mahi	700	42	49
Big Burrito Especial: Chicken	830	32	99
Steak	870	38	99
Health Mex: Chicken	500	10	70
Mahi Mahi	510	15	68
***Nachos*:** Grande	1270	78	112
Grande Chicken	1390	80	114
Grande Steak	1430	87	114
Quesadillas: Cheese	1070	67	85
Chicken	1190	69	87
Tacos			
Regular: Carnitas Rajas	210	11	23
Fish, Especial	330	20	30
Grilled Chicken	280	15	22
Grilled Mesquite Shrimp	230	12	22
Grilled Steak	220	10	22
Langostino Lobster	230	9	26
World Famous Fish	270	14	29
Grilled Gourmet: Chicken	360	21	23
Garlic Herb Shrimp	360	22	23
Portobello & Poblano	310	19	25
Steak	370	23	23
Health Mex: Chicken	150	1.5	21
Mahi Mahi	160	4	21
Street: Carnitas	100	5	9
Chicken	100	4	9
Steak	120	6	9
Salads: *Includes Dressing/Sauce*			
Chicken Chipotle Ranch	520	35	24
Chicken Chopped	570	33	34
Chicken Fiesta	590	46	13
Chicken Grilled Grande Bowl	700	33	61
***Wrapsalads*:** *Includes Dressing/Sauce*			
Chicken Chipotle Ranch	770	42	65
Chicken Chopped	800	40	72
Chicken Fiesta	830	53	53
Salsas: *Per 1 oz*			
Picante	20	1	2
All Other Varieties	5	0	1
Desserts			
Brownie, 3 oz	430	22	57
Churro, 1.6 oz	170	8	22

Ruby Tuesday® (Feb '10)

	C	F	Cb
Appetizers: *Per ¼ Order without Sides or Sauce*			
Asian Dumplings	115	5	11
Cheddar Fries	335	20	25
Fried Mozzarella	180	11	11
Jumbo Lump Crab Cake	70	4	3
Southwestern Spring Rolls	175	10	14
Thai Phoon Shrimp	190	13	11
Burgers & Sandwiches: *Per Serving*			
Handcrafted Burgers:			
Alpine Swiss Burger	1400	99	68
Bison Bacon Cheeseburger	1180	78	64
Boston Blue Burger	1600	113	83
Brewmaster Burger	1395	99	73
Ruby's Classic Burger	1340	98	64
Smokehouse Burger	1610	114	86
Prime Burgers Triple Prime	1445	115	45
Triple Prime Cheddar	1385	110	45
Triple Prime Havarti	1465	116	45
Sandwiches:			
Avocado Turkey Burger	1235	81	62
Bella Turkey Burger	1126	69	67
Buffalo Chicken Burger	1130	67	74
Chicken BLT	1135	66	74
The Ultimate Chicken	1220	67	60
Turkey Burger	1000	61	62
Fork-Tender Ribs: *Per Serving*			
Asian, Half	545	32	18
BBQ, Half	485	24	26
Memphis, Half	460	29	6
Ribs & Louisiana Fried Shrimp	910	41	64
Premium Seafood: *Per Serving*			
Asian Glazed Salmon	600	41	9
Crab Cake Dinner	270	17	10
Creole Catch	280	13	2
Herb Crusted Tilapia	400	24	9
Lobster Ravioli	885	55	57
New Orleans Seafood	410	23	3
Parmesan Shrimp Pasta	1215	66	94
Salmon Florentine	775	56	9
Quesadillas: *Per Serving*			
Buffalo Shrimp	1465	89	87
California Club	1365	91	42
Cheeseburger Quesadilla	1495	102	61
Chicken Quesadilla	1090	70	41
Southwestern	1575	107	68
Steak: *Per Serving*			
Handcrafted Steak:			
Cowboy Sirloin	650	31	21
Peppercorn Mushroom Sirloin	490	20	12
Petite Sirloin	350	18	1
Rib Eye	1100	94	1
Shrimp Scampi & Steak	745	34	39
Steak (7 oz) & Lobster Tail	460	21	1

Updated Nutrition Data ~ www.CalorieKing.com
Persons with Diabetes ~ See Disclaimer (Page 24)

Ruby Tuesday® cont... (Feb '10)

Smart Eating Choices: Per Serving	C	F	Cb
Grilled Chicken Salad	505	27	5
Chicken Bella	420	14	9
Grilled Chicken Wrap	445	16	40
Plain Grilled: Chicken	260	3	0
Petite Sirloin	250	7	0
Salmon	420	26	0
Sugar Snap Peas	115	6	6
Turkey Burger Wrap	660	33	45
White Bean Chicken Chili	235	8	21
***Salad Sensations:** Per Serving*			
Asian Salmon Spinach Salad	640	29	35
Avocado Shrimp Salad	545	32	28
Carolina Chicken Salad	1150	70	48
Club House Salad	920	59	21
Santa Fe Chicken Salad	675	35	30
Southwestern Beef Salad	1135	81	48
***Dressings & Sauces:** Per 1 oz*			
Asian BBQ Sauce	60	3	7
Asian Sesame Sauce	85	5	8
Balsamic Vinaigrette Dressing	35	3	4
BBQ Sauce	50	0	13
Blue Cheese Dressing	180	19	1
Boston BBQ Sauce	40	0	10
French Dressing	120	11	6
Honey Mustard Dressing	90	8	5
Italian Dressing	60	6	2
Marinara Sauce	20	1	1
Parmesan Cream Sauce	65	6	2
Ranch Dressing	100	11	1
Signature Parmesan Dressing	150	16	1
Spicy Southwestern Ranch Dressing	110	12	1
Thousand Island Dressing	70	7	3
Signature Sides			
Baked Potato: Plain	280	2	46
Loaded Baked Potato	590	29	48
Creamy Mashed Cauliflower	135	8	9
White Cheddar Mashed Potatoes	130	7	15
Onion Straws	300	21	20
Piping-Hot Fries	400	18	50
Rice Pilaf	225	7	33
Sauteed Baby Bellas	100	4	10
Succotash	250	16	13
Desserts			
Blondie for One	625	27	86
Double Chocolate Cake	900	40	124
Italian Cream Cake	990	56	108
Cookie: Chocolate Chip	320	15	40
White Choc. Macadamia Nut	340	20	38

For Complete Menu ~ see CalorieKing.com

Runza® (Feb '10)

Sandwiches	C	F	Cb
BBQ Chicken Sandwich, grilled	390	9	46
Buffalo Chicken Sandwich, grilled	440	13	36
Cheese Sandwich	560	21	66
Deluxe Chicken, crispy	480	19	51
Original Sandwich	500	17	65
Polish Dog	420	26	30
Smothered Chicken, grilled	380	10	41
Swiss Cheese Mushroom	590	25	68
Burgers			
Junior: Cheeseburger	330	17	28
Cheeseburger Runza	310	14	30
Swiss Mushroom	380	21	26
Legendary: ¼ lb Chseburger Runza	430	21	32
½ lb Double Chseburger Runza	640	32	37
¼ lb Bacon Cheeseburger	510	29	36
¼ lb Legend Supreme	770	37	62
¼ lb Swiss Cheese Mushroom	450	25	36
Sides			
French Fries: Small, 3.1 oz	280	15	31
Medium, 4.55 oz	410	23	46
Large, 6.9 oz	630	35	70
Frings, 6.3 oz	540	28	64
Onion Rings: Medium, 4.1 oz	370	20	41
Large, 6.5 oz	590	32	66
Onion Ring Dip, 2.1 oz	90	6	4
***Salads:** No Dressing*			
Sweet Berry Chicken	410	16	20
Tossed Salad w. Crispy Chicken	440	27	29
Tossed Salad w. Grilled Chicken	280	13	13
***Dressing**:* Asian Sesame Ginger, 2.4 oz	300	26	14
Fat-Free Hidden Valley Ranch	60	0	15
Raspberry Vinaigrette, 2 oz	25	0	6
***Soups:** Per Bowl*			
Boston Clam Chowder	320	23	33
Broccoli Cheese	360	27	35
Cauliflower Cheese	330	26	32
Chicken Noodle	170	5	21
Homemade Chili	310	10	26
Potato w. Bacon	310	20	40
Vegetable Cheese	330	22	28
Wisconsin Cheese	430	35	36
***Kids Meals:** Includes Small Fries*			
Mini Corn Dogs (5)	550	32	56
Chicken Strips (2)	460	25	42
Desserts & Drinks			
Chocolate Chip Cookie (1)	310	16	34
Shakes: Cappuccino, reg., 12 f.loz	470	18	65
Vanilla, regular, 12 fl.oz	470	16	69
Pepsi Runza Slushie, med., 18 fl.oz	220	0	60

Ryan's® Grill, Buffet & Bakery (Feb '10)

Main Courses: Sides Not Included	C	F	Cb
BBQ Ribs, 3.6 oz	180	12	7
BBQ Chicken, 2.75 oz	150	6	9
Carved Turkey Breast, 2 oz	90	3.5	0
Chicken Fried Steak 2.2 oz	210	13	15
with gravy, 2.6 oz	220	13	16
Chicken Pot Pie, 4.4 oz	290	18	24
Fried Breaded Catfish, 6.3 oz	340	16	12
Fried Fish (1), 1.6 oz	90	5	4
Fried Shrimp (11)	150	8	16
Fried Tilapia, 0.9 oz	70	2.5	4
Grilled Chicken Breast, plain, 4 oz	180	4	0
Grilled Pork Chop: Plain (1), 3 oz	170	9	0
BBQ; Teriyaki, avg., 1 chop	190	10	4
Grilled Teriyaki Chicken Thighs, 1 oz	60	2.5	4
Macaroni and Cheese, 3.5 oz	120	2.5	19
Meat Lasagne, 6.15 oz	250	11	22
Meatloaf, 2 oz	100	6	6
Mexican Casserole, 4.4 oz	190	9	21
Pizza: Cheese, 1 slice, 3 oz	200	8	21
Pepperoni, 1 slice, 3 oz	250	13	21
Rotisserie Chicken: Breast, 4.8 oz	280	13	0.5
Leg, 2.65 oz	120	9	0.5
Thigh, 4.3 oz	250	16	1
Sirloin Steak, 3 oz	180	9	0
Spaghetti, 3 oz	130	2.5	23
Spaghetti Sauce with Meat, 2 oz	140	8	10
Taco Meat, 1.4 oz	70	4	3
White Turkey with gravy, 4.23 oz	90	2	4
Sides: Baked Potato, plain, 6.35 oz	180	0	31
Baked Beans, 3.88 oz	90	1	20
Breaded Fried Okra, 3 oz	220	12	28
Brussel Sprouts, 2.8 oz	40	2	6
Corn Cobbet (1) 2.68 oz	90	3	11
Garlic Mashed Potatoes, 3 oz	90	4	11
Glazed Baby Carrots with Sce, 1.9 oz	60	3	7
Gr. Vegetables with Broccoli, 1.75 oz	40	3	2
Pinto Beans, 3.25 oz	70	1	14
Rice Pilaf, 1.5 oz	60	1	12
Steamed Cabbage with Bacon, 1.75 oz	60	5	2
Yellow Squash with Onions, 1.75 oz	40	3.5	2
Desserts: Cheesecake, plain, 1 sl.	370	19	45
Ice Cream Cone (flat bottom)	15	0	3
Key Lime Pie, 1 slice, 2.65 oz	280	12	39
Lemon Creme Cake, sugar free, 1 sl.	170	15	9
Cookies: Oatmeal Raisin (1)	120	5	16
Sugar Cookie (1)	120	5	17

7-Eleven® (Dec '09)

Breakfast	C	F	Cb
Big Eats: *Per Sandwich*			
Sausage, Egg & Chese Biscuit	500	30	41
Egg, Ham & Cheese Croissant	300	25	25
Sausage, Egg & Cheese Muffin	380	23	25
Roller Grill Items: *Per Item*			
Hot Dogs: Big Bite, ¼ lb	360	34	2
Biggest Big Bite, ⅓lb	480	45	3
Bratwurst Sausage (1)	370	34	4
Breakfast Bite Sausage (1)	250	21	2
Buffalo Chicken Bite (1)	170	14	11
Cheese & Jalapeno Taquito (1)			
Cheeseburger Bite (1)	440	38	2
Sauces			
Casa Buena Chedd. Chse, Med., 2oz	110	9	5
Hot, 2 oz	110	9	4
Casa Buena Prem. Chili, 1 oz	15	0.5	2
Sandwiches			
Big Eats: *Per Sandwich*			
Smkd Tky w/ Jack Chse/Wheat Bread	460	22	42
With Southwest Mayo	540	26	49
Ham & Havati Chse on Onion Roll	420	15	43
Egg Salad On White Bread	520	29	42
Tuna Salad On Wheat Bread	450	1	48
Turkey & Cheddar On Wheat Sub	280	6	37
Turkey & Swiss On Pita Bread	460	14	64
Bakery Stix™ Treats: *Per Stick (3.5 oz)*			
Grilled Cheese	270	11	30
Ham & Cheese	280	12	32
Pepperoni & Cheese	340	18	30
Salads			
Tuna Macaroni Salad, 8 oz	270	8	29
Reser's Coleslaw, 3½ oz	130	7	17
Reser's Macaroni Salad, 3½ oz	220	15	20
Reser's Potato Salad, 3½ oz	200	10	19
Donuts: Blueberry Cake (1)	330	22	31
Chocolate Iced (1)	250	11	35
Glazed (1)	250	16	24
Jelly (1)	420	16	66
Sour Cream Donut (1)	450	19	65
Brownies: Original, 5 oz	570	28	83
Peanut Butter Cup Brownie, 4.4 oz	560	20	55
Walnut Brownie, 5 oz	600	31	78
16 fl.oz size	10	0	2
20 fl.oz size	14	0	3
Beverages			
Cold			
French Vanilla Iced Cappuccino	140	3	26
Hot			
Cafe Select Coffee: 12 fl.oz	8	0	2
Hershey's: S'Mores Cocoa, 8 fl oz	200	7	36
Take 5, 8 fl oz	190	6	34
Peppermint Patty Cocoa, 8 fl oz	180	3	36

Continued next page...

Updated Nutrition Data ~ www.CalorieKing.com
Persons with Diabetes ~ See Disclaimer (Page 24)

7-Eleven® cont... (Dec '09)

Fountain Drinks (Fig. Assume ⅓ Ice)	C	F	Cb
Coca-Cola/Pepsi/Dr.Pepper/7Up:			
Gulp, 20 oz	195	0	51
Big Gulp, 32 oz	310	0	82
Super Gulp, 44 oz	430	0	112
Double Gulp, 64 oz	625	0	163
Diet Coke/Diet Pepsi, 16 oz	1	0	0
Slurpees: Average All Flavors,			
12 oz size	95	0	24
22 oz size	175	0	44
28 oz size	220	0	56
40 oz size	315	0	80
Hawaiian Punch; Dr Pepper, avg.,			
12 oz size	180	0	48
22 oz size	330	0	88
28 oz size	420	0	112
40 oz size	600	0	160

Saladworks® (Feb '10)

Salads: *Per Container*	C	F	Cb
Autumn Harvest	310	12	43
Bently	245	10	11
Buffalo Blue	250	7	24
Chicken Caesar	285	4	19
Cobb	270	16	13
Fire Roasted Cabo Jack	370	18	31
Garden Deluxe	240	2	92
Greek	190	10	19
Mandarin Chicken	230	7	37
Nuevo Nicoise	230	5	73
Sophie's Salad	310	14	35
Tivoli	430	20	74
Focaccia Fusion: BLT	345	13	32
Chicken Monterey	385	12	35
Fajitalicious	380	12	33
Ham Continental	395	11	38
Turkey Continental	375	10	36
Turkey Ranch	365	10	33
Soup: *Per 3.5 oz Container*			
Butternut Squash	80	4.5	11
Chicken & Sausage Gumbo	110	6.5	8
Chicken Chili	135	5	20
Chicken Orzo	180	3.5	15
Garden Fresh Pea	110	2	15
Italian Wedding	110	7	9
Maryland Crab	75	0	12
New England Clam Chowder	205	11	17
Rst Corn Tom. w/ Smoked Cheddar	215	16	9
Tomato Bisque	160	8	13
Vegetarian Chili	160	0	25
Zesty Italian Lentil & Sausage	130	5.5	20

Samurai Sam's® (Feb '10)

Teriyaki Rice Bowls: *Includes White Rice & Veggies*	C	F	Cb
Dark Chicken: Regular	550	10	80
Large	820	14	125
Steak: Regular	530	8	79
Large	800	11	122
Shrimp: Regular	420	1.5	78
Large	650	2	121
Spicy Steak & Broccoli: Regular	540	8	83
Large	830	11	130
Sweet & Sour Dark Chicken: Regular	550	10	82
Large	830	14	128
Veggie: Regular	360	0.5	81
Large	560	1	126
Teriyaki Wraps: *Includes White Rice & Veggies*			
White Chicken	640	11	96
Steak	650	14	94
Veggie	510	9	95
Sides: California Roll (1)	260	1	46
Crab Ragoon (3)	210	12	20
Gr. Chicken & Vegetable Eggroll (1)	140	4.5	17

Sandella's Flatbread Cafe (Feb '10)

Wraps	C	F	Cb
Buffalo Chicken	455	17	53
Chicken Fajita	445	13	54
Pacific Chicken	420	11	56
Pesto Turkey	480	18	58
Sweet & Spicy Chicken	355	4	55
Paninis			
Chicken Delicato	535	22	51
Spinach, Ham & Swiss	510	19	53
Turkey & Mozzarella	495	19	54
Tuscan Chicken	580	25	56
Quesadillas			
California	410	16	53
Chicken Fajita	385	8	52
Mediterranean	470	24	55
Grilled Flatbread			
Aloha	570	20	70
Brazilian Chicken	460	15	51
Pesto Chicken	665	33	57
Spinach & Bacon	680	41	52
Vegetarian	685	19	61
Chopped Salads			
Aloha	295	11	36
Greek	305	9	18
Rice Bowls			
Black Bean & rice	705	7	133
Chicken Fajita	630	9	102

For Extra Menu Items ~ see CalorieKing.com

Sbarro's® (Dec '09)

Entrees	C	F	Cb
Baked Ziti w. Sauce	700	41	43
Chicken Parmigiana	520	22	16
Meat Lasagna	650	37	36
Spaghetti w. Sauce	820	28	120
***Pizza:** Per Slice (Thin Crust)*			
Cheese	460	13	60
Pepperoni	730	37	61
Sausage	670	31	60
Supreme	630	27	63
***Stuffed Pizza:** Per Slice*			
Spinach & Broccoli	790	34	89
Pepperoni	960	42	89

Schlotzsky's® (Feb '10)

	C	F	Cb
***Oven-Toasted Sandwiches:** Per Medium Sandwich*			
Angus: Beef & Provolone	760	29	81
Corned Beef Reuben	910	40	80
Corned Beef	580	13	78
Pastrami Reuben	910	39	80
Pastrami & Swiss	905	36	83
BLT	560	21	74
Chicken & Pesto	570	14	73
Chicken Breast	515	6	78
Chipotle Chicken	550	14	68
Dijon Chicken	575	11	79
Homestyle Tuna	565	16	73
Santa Fe Chicken	620	15	76
Smoked Turkey Breast	520	9	77
Smoked Turkey Reuben	895	38	84
Turkey & Guacamole	565	13	82
Turkey Bacon Club	785	32	77
Original Style: The Original	770	34	78
Cheese	790	38	76
Ham & Cheese	735	27	80
Turkey	830	35	80
Panini: Classic Swiss & Tomato	625	26	63
Grilled Chicken Romano	570	16	62
Italiano	735	32	67
Mozzarella & Portobello	485	15	63
Smoked Ham Crostini	645	23	67
Smoked Turkey & Guacamole	600	21	69
Wraps: Asian Chicken	535	12	80
Feta & Portobello	620	39	55
Grilled Chicken & Guacamole	690	36	60
Homestyle Tuna	455	17	55
Parmesan Chicken Caesar	555	21	61

Schlotzsky's® cont... Feb '10)

***8" Pizzas:** Per Pizza*	C	F	Cb
BBQ Chicken & Jalapeno	715	16	99
Baby Spinach Salad	455	7	80
Bacon, Tomato & Portobello	620	23	75
Combination Special	640	25	76
Double Cheese	595	21	74
Fresh Tomato & Pesto	555	19	73
Grilled Chicken & Pesto	685	22	75
Mediterranean	560	20	74
Pepperoni & Double Cheese	685	30	74
Smoked Turkey & Jalapeno	655	21	78
Thai Chicken	725	23	85
Vegetarian Special	540	17	74
***Salads:** Without Dressing/Croutons Unless Indicated*			
Baby Spinach & Feta	115	7	6
Caesar Salad with Croutons	105	5	10
Chicken Salad	290	15	12
Garden Salad	50	1	12
Greek Salad	135	8	13
Gr. Chicken Caesar with Croutons	220	8	12
Ham & Turkey Chef Salad	255	13	14
Pasta Salad	70	3	12
Potato Salad	240	13	29
Turkey Chef Salad	310	18	14
***Kid's Meals:** Without Cookie or Drink*			
Cheese Pizza	480	13	73
Cheese Sandwich	395	15	48
Ham & Cheese Sandwich	425	16	49
Pepperoni Pizza	525	17	73
Turkey Sandwich	300	5	49
Desserts			
Brownie	415	22	54
Carrot Cake	715	42	80
New York Style Cheesecake	350	23	30
Cookies: Chocolate Chip	160	8	22
Fudge Chocolate Chip	160	8	22
Oatmeal Raisin	150	6	22
Sugar	160	7	22
White Choc Macadamia	170	9	21

Second Cup® ~ *see CalorieKing.com*

Updated Nutrition Data ~ www.CalorieKing.com
Persons with Diabetes ~ See Disclaimer (Page 24)

Shakey's® (Feb '10)

Pizzas (12"): Per 1/10 Pizza	C	F	Cb
Cheese: Pan Crust	185	6	26
Thin Crust	150	6	18
Firehouse: Pan Crust	255	12	27
Thin Crust	220	12	19
Garden Veggie: Pan Crust	185	6	27
Thin Crust	150	5	19
Margherita: Pan Crust	175	5	26
Thin Crust	135	4.5	18
Rustic Garlic Chicken: Pan Crust	190	5.5	26
Thin Crust	155	5.5	18
Shakey's Special: Pan Crust	210	6.5	31
Thin Crust	195	10	18
Texas BBQ Chicken: Pan Crust	205	5	29
Thin Crust	170	5	21
Ultimate Meat: Pan Crust	280	14	26
Thin Crust	245	13	18
Additional Toppings: Beef	35	3	0
Cheese	15	1	0.5
Chicken	15	0.5	0
Ham	10	0.5	0
Pepperoni	25	2.5	0
Sausage	45	4	0.5
Sharables: *Per Serving*			
Chicken Strips (5)	620	31	48
Mojo Potatoes (5)	215	11	25
Mojo Supreme, serves 4-6	1950	120	160
Shakey's Spicy Wings (6 pces)	495	29	27
Shakey's Famous Chicken: *Per Piece*			
Fried Chicken: Breast	475	26	16
Leg	170	19	6
Thigh	350	24	10
Wing	130	9	3.5

Sheetz® (Feb '10)

M.T.O Breakfast: Plain Bagel, Cheese if Indicated, without Condiments or Dressing	C	F	Cb
Shmagels: Bacon	530	27	53
Egg & American **Cheese**	440	19	50
Ham & Provolone	525	21	55
Shmiscuits: Bacon	540	35	39
Egg & American Cheese	450	27	36
Ham & Swiss Cheese	550	30	41
Sausage & American Cheese	625	44	36
Shmuffins: Bacon	410	25	29
Egg & American **Cheese**	320	17	26
Ham	310	11	30
Sausage & Cheddar **Cheese**	495	34	26
Steak	395	16	27

Sheetz® cont... (Feb '10)

M.T.O Cold Subz: Per 6" White Sub w/o Cheese/Toppings or Condiments Unless Indicated	C	F	Cb
American Cheese	350	11	45
BLT	445	19	48
Chicken Salad with Tomatoes	500	23	55
Italian	365	10	47
Rst Beef w/ Lettuce, Tom., Olives., On.	310	5	50
Tuna Salad w. Lettuce, Tom., Pickles	465	18	57
Turkey & Provolone	395	12	48
M.T.O® Hot Subz: *Per 6" White Sub*			
Chicken & American Cheese	470	15	45
Meatball with Marinara Sauce	385	13	49
Pepperoni	440	20	45
Steak & Swiss Cheese	535	19	47
M.T.O Deli Ciabata: *Without Cheese Unless Indicated*			
Chicken Salad	480	25	51
Deli Combo with Provolone Cheese	475	23	45
Ham & Swiss Cheese	410	15	46
Italian w/ Lettuce, Tomato & Onion	450	4	45
Tuna Salad w/ Lettuce, Tom., Pickles	455	20	54
Turkey w/ Provolone, Lettuce & Tom.	395	14	47
M.T.O Hot Dogz: *Without Cheese*			
Deli Dogz with Ketchup & Mustard	285	15	26
Hot Dogz with Chili & Onions	310	19	27
M.T.O Nachos:			
Nachos Bueno w. Nacho Cheese	515	23	65
M.T.O Saladz: *W/o Cheese/Dressing Unless Indicated*			
Chef Salad with Shredded Cheese	250	12	13
Crispy Chicken w/ Shredded Cheese	370	16	31
Garden Salad w/ Shredded Cheese	130	8	8
Grilled Chicken	145	4	7
Steak Salad	210	8	8
Taco Salad	355	10	38
Sides			
Fryz: Bag, 3.2 oz	160	6	23
Cup, 5.1 oz	260	10	36
Cheese, 14.4 oz	670	32	81
Smokehouse, 15.3 oz	985	53	103
Coffeez™: *Per 16 fl.oz*			
Hot Chocolate, medium	250	4	52
Cupo'ccino®: *Per Medium (16 fl.oz)*			
Capo'ccino: Creme Burlee	280	8	50
Fat-Free French Vanilla	140	0	34

Shoney's® (Dec '09)

Breakfast	C	F	Cb
Off The Grill:			
Bacon, Egg & Cheddar Croissant	790	57	30
Sirloin Steak & Eggs	580	36	3
Platters: Pancakes, with Bacon	665	11	110
with Sausage Patties	775	21	110
Skillets: Big Biscuit	980	56	93
Fiesta	1030	76	42
Sunrise Special	1470	62	191
Lunch/Dinner:			
Starters: Angus Steak Chili	620	37	50
Chicken Enchilada Soup	445	22	50
Chicken Strips	1270	84	87
Onion Rings	980	69	102
Burgers: *Without Sides*			
All American	1160	93	40
BBQ Bacon Cheeseburger	1470	117	45
Classic	1360	111	40
Mushroom Swiss	1195	89	42
Chicken: *Without Sides*			
Sandwiches: Blackened Chicken	720	36	40
Grilled Chicken Sandwich	720	36	40
Croissant, Chicken Salad	645	33	39
Classic Sandwiches: *Without Sides*			
Philly Cheese Steak	1140	74	61
Reuben	835	45	44
Slim Jim	695	36	57
Turkey Club	1250	83	60
Croissant, BLT	580	48	26
Entrees: *With Standard Sides*			
Chicken: Blackened w BBQ Sauce	585	18	39
with Honey Mustard	785	44	33
Chicken Strips	1320	88	91
Grilled with BBQ Sauce	585	18	39
with Honey Mustard	650	46	22
Fish: Fish & Chips Basket	1310	74	102
Fish Sandwich, without sides	1190	63	105
Grilled Salmon	515	34	27
Pan-Blackened Catfish Fry	915	60	66
Southern Catfish Fry	1465	78	137
Pasta: Baked Spaghetti	1460	54	145
Lasagna: Half Portion	730	44	58
Full Portion	1140	65	93
Skillets:			
Artichoke & Crabmeat Casserole	1410	80	134
Lemon Chkn w. Mshrm & Rice	1220	67	91
Slow-Cooked Pot Roast	835	45	57

Shoney's® cont... (Dec '09)

Entrees (Cont): *With Standard Sides*	C	F	Cb
Steak:			
Half-O-Pound	1325	103	62
Porterhouse Steak, 16 oz	2170	136	97
Ribeye, 10 oz	1485	90	97
Smothered Liver & Onions	775	46	48
Steakhouse Sirloin, 8 oz	1380	83	97
T-Bone, 12 oz	1725	110	100
Salads: *Entrée Size*			
Fried Chicken	1100	70	93
Grilled Chicken	1060	56	70
Salmon	870	60	49
Kid's Menu:			
Cheeseburger	790	56	41
Fish Wrap	490	32	25
Grilled Cheese	450	32	24
Mac & Cheese	965	54	83
Sides:			
Baked Potato, plain	225	0	51
Biscuit (1)	190	9	23
Fries: Chili Cheese Fries	680	42	61
French	520	30	56
Homefries	120	6	15
Fruit Bowl	60	0	15
Garlic Grecian Bread, 1 slice	330	24	23
Grits	395	2	86
Loaded Potato Mix	115	13	8
Mashed Potatoes	240	11	31
Onion Rings	490	35	51
Toast, dry	130	2	23
Wild Rice	150	4	25
Desserts:			
Apple Crisp	810	38	81
Hot Fudge Cake	710	30	101
Key Lime Cheesecake	830	58	74
Pies: Peanut Butter	570	35	57
Strawberry, 1 slice	350	13	53
Whole Pie	2095	80	319
Sundaes: Banana Split	545	21	93
Hot Fudge	535	25	68
Peach	370	17	46
Strawberry	375	17	47

Updated Nutrition Data ~ www.CalorieKing.com
Persons with Diabetes ~ See Disclaimer (Page 24)

Sizzler® (Feb '10)

Burgers & Sandwiches:	C	F	Cb
Burgers: Mega Bacon Chseburger	1010	61	48
Sizzler Burger: ⅓ lb	620	30	47
½ lb	760	40	47
Sandwiches: Crispy Chicken	590	27	61
Grilled Chicken Club	665	31	48
Malibu Chicken	645	32	57
Hot Entrees: *Without Sides, Dipping Sauces & Condiments Unless Indicated*			
Chicken: Hibachi Chkn Breast (1)	200	7	7
with Hibachi Sauce, 1 oz	245	7	17
Lemon-Herb Chicken Breast	215	11	1
with Lemon Herb Sauce, 1 oz	260	15	2
Malibu Chicken Patty, each	305	20	10
with Malibu Sauce, 1.5 oz	570	15	10
Seafood: Gr. Salmon w/ Rice Pilaf	530	20	40
Fish 'n Chips	1035	49	111
Fisherman's Platter	820	34	82
Gr. Shrimp Fettuccine Alfredo	985	55	64
Shrimp: Grilled Skewers (2)	545	26	42
Shrimp Fry (12)	435	12	48
Shrimp, Shrimp, Shrimp	970	41	92
Steaks: Classic, 8 oz	320	14	2
Classic Trio	700	32	32
Porterhouse, 18 oz	1365	107	1
Rib Eye, 12 oz	950	62	1
Steak & Grilled Shrimp Skewers	640	27	43
Ultimate Sizzlin' Trio	1410	86	74
Prepared Salads: *Per 4oz Serving w/out Dressing*			
Ambrosia	125	4	22
Caesar	50	4	2
Carrot Raisin	110	6	12
Creamy Cole Slaw	70	4	6
Greek	45	4	2
Macaroni	225	12	27
Potato	325	27	18
Seafood	160	11	11
Salad Dressings: *Per 2 Tbsp, 1 oz*			
Honey Mustard	110	8	9
Italian, Low Fat	40	3	6
Ranch	115	12	1
Signature Blue Cheese	105	11	1
Thousand Island	95	9	5

Sizzler® cont... (Feb '10)

Salad Bar Items:	C	F	Cb
Bacon Bits, 2 oz	110	6	6
Cottage Cheese, 2 oz	50	2	2
Eggs, Chopped, 2 oz	50	4	0
Garbanzo Beans, 2 oz	50	0	8
Kidney Beans, 2 oz	50	0	8
Peas, 2 oz	30	0	6
Turkey Ham, 2 oz	75	6	2
Sides: *Without Condiments/Toppings*			
Baked Potato	265	4	51
Brocoli, 5 oz	50	0	7
Cheese Toast, 1 slice	235	19	13
French Fries, 5 oz	285	13	42
Rice Pilaf, 5 oz	225	4	39
Smashed Red Potatoes, 6 oz	160	6	24
Soups: *Per 6 oz Bowl*			
Broccoli Cheese	305	19	28
Chicken Noodle	100	2	14
Clam Chowder	325	18	35
French Onion	55	2	6
Menudo	70	2	7
Minestrone	70	1	14
Dessert Bar: Chocolate Syrup, 1 oz	90	0	21
Choc/Vanilla Soft Serve, 4 oz	135	4	24
Strawberry Topping, 1 oz	70	0	18
Whipped Topping, 1 Tbsp	10	1	1

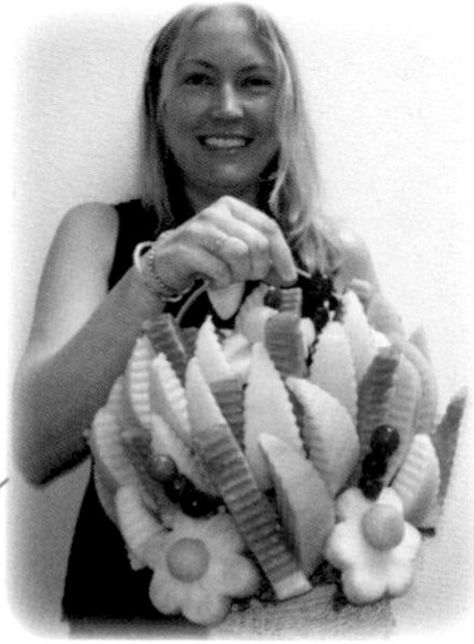

Balance eating out with fruit and veggies
(EdibleArrangements.com)

Skyline Chili® (Feb '10)

Burritos:	C	F	Cb
All Chili Burrito	560	30	37
All Chili Deluxe Burrito	650	35	45
Meals: *Per Regular Serving*			
Black Bean & Rice, 3-Way	800	40	74
Black Bean & Rice, 4-Way	810	40	77
Black Bean & Rice, 5-Way	880	40	89
Black Bean & Rice, Spaghetti	490	12	79
Bowls:			
Chili	270	16	6
Chili Bean	270	12	17
Chili Cheese	440	30	6
Coney	870	69	9
Loaded Chili	580	40	18
Vegetarian Black Beans & Rice	320	9	46
Chili Spaghetti:			
Regular	450	18	43
with Beans & Onions	530	17	64
with Beans	520	17	61
Coneys: Regular with Cheese	340	22	17
without Cheese	220	12	17
Steamed Potatoes:			
Plain	310	0	72
Cheddar	740	41	72
Chili	440	8	74
Sour Cream	570	27	72
Salads: *Without Dressing*			
Buffalo Chicken Salad	150	7	7
Classic Chicken Salad	150	7	8
Garden Salad	80	5	6
Greek Chicken Salad	170	8	9
Greek Salad	60	3.5	5
Southwestern Chkn w/ Tortilla Chips	760	44	65
Wraps: *Without Dressing*			
Buffalo Chicken	520	21	55
Classic Chicken	510	21	55
Greek Chicken	510	21	54
Southwest Chicken	670	30	65
Sides:			
Cheese	230	19	1
Chili	130	8	3
Crackers, 1 bowl	100	3	20
French Fries	630	33	79

For Complete Nutritional Data ~ see CalorieKing.com

Smoothie King® (Feb '10)

Fruit Smoothies: *Per 20 fl.oz Cup*
Figures Include Turbinado. Without Turbinado, deduct 100 calories and 23 carbs.

	C	F	Cb
Build Up, High Protein Smoothies:			
Almond Mocha	365	9	42
Banana	320	9	32
Chocolate	365	9	42
Lemon	370	9	44
Pineapple	320	9	29
Get Energy: Acai Adventure	435	5	92
Go Goji	435	0	104
Green Tea Tango	280	3	52
Indulge: Banana Boat	525	12	97
Pina Colada Island	600	10	110
Snack Right: Banana Berry Treat	365	0	86
Berry Punch	360	0	91
Fruit Fusion	355	1	76
Grape Expectations	550	0	133
Stay Healthy: Cranberry Cooler	495	0	120
Cranberry Supreme	555	1	130
Mangosteen Madness	385	0	94
Orange Ka-BAM	465	0	117
Trim Down: Angel Food	355	0	84
Blackberry Dream	365	1	88
Island Impact	310	0	73
MangoFest	285	0	72
Muscle Punch	365	1	84
Passion Passport	395	0	96
Peach Slice	315	0	72
Pineapple Pleasure	280	0	67
Raspberry Collider	340	0	86
Raspberry Sunrise	390	0	95
Slim-N-Trim: Chocolate	295	2	57
Orange Vanilla	215	1	46
Strawberry	375	1	84
Strawberry Kiwi Breeze	375	0	90
Youth Fountain	255	0	61
The Shredder: Chocolate	310	3	36
Strawberry	355	1	56
Youth Fountain	255	0	61

32 fl.oz Cup: Multiply 20 fl.oz figures by 1.5
40 fl.oz Cup: Multiply 20 fl.oz figures by 2

Continued next page...

Updated Nutrition Data ~ www.CalorieKing.com
Persons with Diabetes ~ See Disclaimer (Page 24)

Smoothie King® cont... (Feb '10)

Kids Kup Smoothies	C	F	Cb
Berry Interesting	275	0	69
Choc-A-Laka	245	3	45
Gimme-Grape	265	0	64
Smarti Tarti	200	0	49

Snappy Tomato (Feb '10)

***Pizza:** Per Slice, ⅛ of Pizza*	C	F	Cb
Buffalo Grilled Chicken	250	8	32
Cheese Pizza	220	7	30
Hawaiian Pizza	370	18	33
Meat Topper	430	23	31
Pepperoni Pizza	340	17	31
Ranch Pizza	370	21	31
Snapperoni Pizza	390	22	31
Supreme Pizza	340	17	32
Veggie Pizza	240	8	33
***Oven Baked Hoagie Sandwiches:** W/o Toppings, Sauce/Dressing*			
Grilled Chicken	490	11	71
Steak & Cheese	670	28	73
***Snappetizers:** Without Sauce*			
Snappy Wings (2), 3 oz	150	5	12

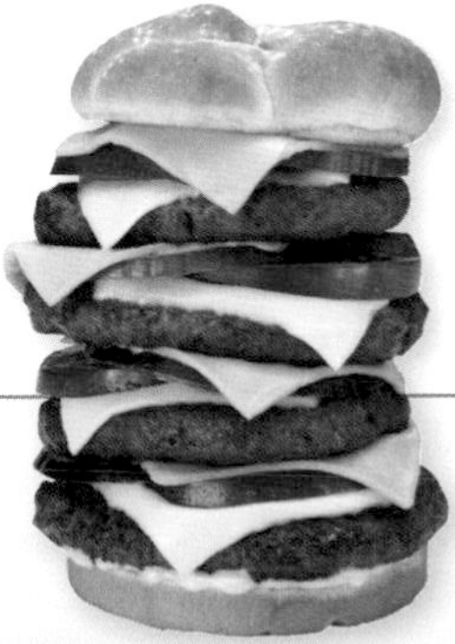

*This **Quadruple Bypass Burger®** is offered by Heart Attack Grill in Chandler, Arizona.*

With some 5000 calories, it contains 2 lbs beef, 4 fried eggs, 8 slices cheese, mayo and garnish – all in a large bun dipped in pure lard.

Definitely not for anyone with a heart!

(Photo: Ken Epstein)

Sonic Drive-In® (Feb '10)

Burgers	C	F	Cb
Sonic Burger w. Mayonnaise	650	37	55
Sonic Burger w. Mustard	560	26	54
Sonic Cheeseburger w. Mayo	720	42	56
Sonic Cheeseburger w. Mustard	620	31	55
Sonic Bacon Cheeseburger	780	48	57
Super Sonic Chseburger: w. Mayo	980	64	58
w. Mustard	890	53	57
Jr. Burger	310	15	30
Sandwiches/Coneys/Wraps			
Coney: Extra-Long Chili Cheese (1)	660	39	55
Corn Dog (1)	210	11	23
Toaster Sandwiches: Chkn Club	740	46	55
Bacon Cheeseburger	670	39	52
Wraps: Crispy Chicken	490	23	49
Grilled Chicken	390	14	39
Fritos Chili Cheese	670	39	66
Chicken			
Chicken Strip Dinner (4)	930	43	100
Jumbo Popcorn Chicken:			
Small, no Sauce, 4 oz	380	22	27
Large, no Sauce, 6 oz	560	32	41
***Salads:** No Dressing*			
Crispy Chicken	340	19	24
Grilled Chicken	250	10	12
***Dressings:** Per 2 oz Serving*			
Honey Mustard	180	16	10
Italian Fat-Free	40	0	10
Light Ranch	110	5	14
Original Ranch	190	20	2
Sides			
French Fries: Plain, medium, 4 oz	330	13	48
w. Cheese, medium, 4.75 oz	420	21	51
w. Chili & Cheese, med., 7.1 oz	490	27	54
Mozzarella Sticks, no sauce, 4.95 oz	440	22	40
Onion Rings, medium, 5½ oz	440	21	55
Tater Tots: Plain, medium, 2.45 oz	200	13	20
Cheese Tots, medium, 3.4 oz	300	21	22
Chili Cheese Tots, med., 5.5 oz	370	27	26

Continued next page...

Sonic Drive-In® cont... (Feb '10)

Breakfast	C	F	Cb
Burritos: Bacon, Egg & Cheese	450	27	38
Sausage, Egg & Cheese	480	31	38
SuperSonic	570	36	48
French Toast Sticks: with Syrup (4)	580	31	70
without Syrup (4)	500	31	49
Breakfast Sandwiches			
CroiSonic: Bacon	510	36	29
Sausage	600	46	29
Toaster: Bacon, Egg & Cheese	530	32	40
Sausage, Egg & Cheese	620	42	40
Desserts: *Per Regular*			
Banana Split	420	9	80
Vanilla Cone	180	6	30
Vanilla Dish	240	9	36
Cream Pie Shakes: *Regular*			
Banana	590	19	98
Chocolate	660	19	114
Coconut	580	20	93
Strawberry	620	19	106
CreamSlush: *Regular*			
Blue Coconut	430	13	76
Lemon-Berry	460	12	85
Floats: *Regular*			
Diet Coke; Diet Dr Pepper	220	8	33
Coca-Cola	290	8	54
Fruit Smoothies: Strawb., reg.	500	0	124
Strawberry-Banana, regular	460	0	113
Shakes: *Regular*			
Chocolate	540	16	89
Banana; Vanilla, average	470	16	76
Pineapple; Strawberry, avg	500	16	80
Single Topping Sundaes: *Regular*			
Choc.	410	13	67
Hot Fudge	440	18	63
Pineapple	370	13	58
Sonic Blast: *Regular*			
Butterfinger	580	22	88
M&M's	600	24	88
Reese's Peanut Butter Cups	560	19	89
Drinks: Barq's Root Beer, 20 fl.oz	190	0	52
Cranberry Juice: Regular	170	0	46
Large, 20 fl.oz	210	0	56

For Complete Nutritional Data ~ see CalorieKing.com

Souper Salad® (Feb '10)

Soups: *Per 5 oz Serving*	C	F	Cb
Adobe Rice & Chicken	100	5	10
Black Bean	80	2	11
Cherokee Joe's Cornbread	70	1.5	13
Chicken Noodle with Stars	40	2.5	2
Chicken Tortilla	60	2	7

Souper Salad® cont... (Feb '10)

Soups: *Per 5 oz Serving*	C	F	Cb
Holiday Harvest	90	6	5
Mama Mia Chicken	80	3	8
Minestrone	70	1	13
Mr. B's Hot & Sour Chicken	60	1.5	8
Pasta Tortellini	100	3.5	14
Red French Onion, without Croutons	40	1	6
Seafood Bisque	120	8	8
Spicy Meatballs with Rice	100	4.5	10
Vegetable Lentil	70	0	16
Vegetarian Vegetable	50	0.5	11
Signature Salads: *Per ⅓ Cup*			
Broccoli Cauliflower Coleslaw	80	6	6
California Chicken	80	6	4
Fisherman's Kettle	120	8	9
Marinated Mushrooms	60	7	1
Pasta de Garden	80	5	8
Red Potato	50	3.5	5
Roasted Vegetables	20	1.5	2
Santa Fe Corn	100	3.5	13
Tuna Skroodle Pasta	130	9	10
Bread			
Blueberry Bread, 1 piece	110	2	22
Cheese Drop Biscuit, 1 piece	70	3	8
Cornbread, 1 piece	130	3.5	23
Garlic Breadstick, 1 stick	130	4.5	18
Gingerbread, 1 piece	130	4.5	22

For Complete Nutritional Data ~ see CalorieKing.com

Souplantation® (Feb '10)

Soups: *Per Cup*	C	F	Cb
Low Fat: Chicken Tortilla	100	3	11
Classical Minestrone	120	2	20
Vegetable Medley	90	1	14
Regular Soup: *Per Cup*			
Chesapeake Corn Chowder	290	17	30
Cream of Mushroom	290	24	15
Irish Potato Leek	260	16	23
Marvellous Minestrone w/ Bacon	220	8	31
Minestrone w/ Italian Sausage	220	12	17
New Mexican Corn	200	10	19
Vegetarian Harvest	200	10	23
Breads: Sourdough	150	0.5	27
Buttermilk Cornbread, 1 piece	140	2	27
Focaccia: Garlic Asiago	160	8	19
Old World Greek	190	9	24
Tossed Salads: *Per Cup*			
Aztec Taco with Turkey	130	9	7
Caesar Salad Asiago	270	22	10
Won Ton Chicken Happiness	170	9	15

Continued next page...

Souplantation® cont... (Feb '10)

Hot Tossed Pastas: Per Cup	C	F	Cb
Bruschetta	260	4	41
Creamy Bruschetta	360	16	43
Garden Vegetable with Meatballs	310	10	44
Italian Vegetable Beef	290	9	43
Vegetarian Marinara with Basil	260	4	44
***Prepared Salads:** Per ½ Cup*			
Aunt Doris' Red Pepper Slaw	70	0	18
Baja Bean & Cilantro	180	3	29
BBQ Potato	170	9	21
Carrot Raisin	90	3	17
Dijon Potato with Garlic Dill Vinegar	150	12	9
Greek Couscous w/ Feta & Pinenuts	210	10	25
Oriental Ginger Slaw with Krab	70	3	8
Southern Dill Potato	120	3	20
Thai Noodle with Peanut Sauce	190	10	19
Zesty Tortellini	230	15	20
***Dressing & Croutons:** Per 2 Tbsp*			
Balsamic Vinaigrette	180	19	1
Blue Cheese Dressing	130	13	3
Honey Mustard Dressing	150	13	8
Fat Free	25	0	7
Italian Dressing, Fat-Free	45	0	10
Ranch Dressing	150	15	4
Fat Free	50	0	2
Thousand Island Dressing	90	9	3
Croutons, Garlic Parmesan, 5 pces	80	5	6
Muffins: Chocolate Brownie	180	8	26
Fruit Medley Bran	130	0.5	29
Georgia Peach Poppyseed	150	6	20
Tangy Lemon	140	4	24
Wildly Blue Blueberry	140	5	22
***Desserts:** Per ½ Cup*			
Apple Cobbler	360	10	67
Apple Medley	70	0	18
Banana Royale	80	0	20
Rice Pudding	110	2	20
Vanilla Pudding	150	4	27
Cookies & Cake:			
Choc. Chip Cookie, small	75	3	10
Chocolate Lava Cake, ½ cup	330	8	62
Syrup/Topping: Choc. Syrup, 2 T	110	3	20
Granola Topping, 2 Tbsp	110	4	16

For Complete Nutritional Data ~ see CalorieKing.com

Southern Tsunami® (Dec '09)

Sushi: Per Pack	C	F	Cb
Blue Crab Roll, 8.85 oz	455	14	63
Classic Miso Roll, 10.8 oz	465	9	64
California Roll w/ Brown Rice, 9.5 oz	305	7	53
Cream Cheese Roll, 9.8 oz	530	20	64
Crunchy Shrimp Roll, 10.3 oz	520	20	69
Dragon Roll: (Seawater Eel), 10.15 oz	470	14	72
Eel Roll (Freshwater Eel), 9.9 oz	505	16	69
Eel Roll (Sea Eel), 9.9 oz	450	11	71
M&M Roll: Shrimp & Avocado, 7.55 oz	335	5	62
Tuna & Cucumber, 7.87 oz	320	1	60
Marina Plate, 7.7 oz	380	7	57
Meteor Special, 9.26 oz	395	3	73
Nigiri: Fish Roe, 1 piece,1.35 oz	60	0	10
Fresh Salmon, 1 piece, 1.3 oz	70	1	9
Fresh Water Eel, 1 piece, 1.5 oz	100	4	11
Octopus, 1 piece, 1 oz	60	1	9
Sea Eel, 1 piece, 1.5 oz	85	3	11
Shrimp, 1 piece, 1 oz	45	0	9
Smoked Salmon, 1 piece, 1.87 oz	95	1	16
Tilapia, 1 piece, 1.13 oz	50	1	9
Tuna, 1 piece, 1 oz	50	0	7
Yellowtail, 1 piece, 1.2 oz	55	1	9
Ocean Crab Roll, 10 oz	415	8	66
Orange Roll, 10.55 oz	405	6	71
Rainbow Roll, 12.45 oz	500	8	70
Spicy Roll: Salmon, 9.82 oz	485	14	64
Baby Shrimp, 10 oz	420	8	68
Tuna, 10 oz	460	9	64
Tempura Roll, 11.1 oz	540	11	87
Tsunami Roll, 9.15 oz	470	12	74
Vegetable Combo: 12 pieces, 9.4 oz	355	6	68
Roll n' Wrap: Avocado Salad, 5 oz	200	9	30
Smoked Salmon Salad, 4 oz	180	8	20
Combinations: Fullmoon, 9.9 oz	435	12	69
Seaside: Tuna & Salmon, 8.4 oz	410	4	63
Tuna, Salmon, Shrimp, Eel, 6.9 oz	395	7	59
Shoreline, 11.23 oz	480	7	82
Stardust, 12.4 oz	555	9	103

Spaghetti Warehouse® (Feb '10)

Appetizers: *Per Serving*	C	F	Cb
Bruschetta	550	37	48
Garlic Cheese Bread	1330	90	81
Mozz. Fritta w/ Tom. Sce & Ranch	930	60	66
Stuffed Mushrooms	310	19	14
Toasted Ravioli w/ Tomato Sauce	980	46	106
Meals: *Without Soup, Salad or Bread*			
Baked Penne	780	37	81
Chicken Alfredo	760	25	76
Chicken Florentine	990	47	91
Chicken Tettrazini	690	19	85
Fettuccini Alfredo	600	24	76
Four Cheese Manicotti	810	41	70
Seafood Mediterranean	680	26	84
Shrimp Alfredo	700	25	78
Spaghetti: With Beer Chili	450	8	75
with Italian Sausage	670	18	82
with Marinara Sauce	400	4	76
with Meatballs	770	27	91
with Meat Sauce	500	8	83
Feasts: *Per Serving*			
Fettuccini	1430	80	120
Lasagna	1650	96	109
Spaghetti	1270	62	122
Ultimate Italian	1500	76	120

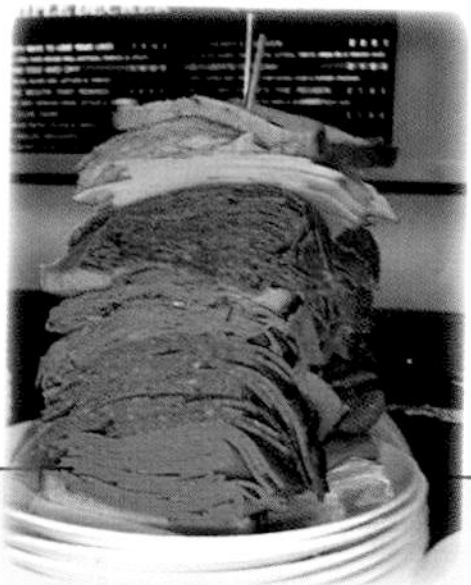

This Triple Decker (Carnegie Deli, New York) contains up to 3 lb meat and 8 oz cheese ~ approx. 4000 calories and 300 grams fat.
Note: Only half the sandwich is shown – the other half is hidden behind!
Carnegie's Challenge: Eat one Triple Decker . . . get the second one free!

Starbucks® (Apr '10)

Kid's Drinks & Others: *Per 12 fl.oz unless indicated*	C	F	Cb
Apple Juice	190	0	48
Apple Juice, Steamed, 8 fl.oz	110	0	28
Hot Chocolate, 2% Milk w/ Whip	290	13	39
White Hot Choc., 2% Milk w/ Whip	380	15	48
Figures Based on 16 fl.oz Grande w/o Whip			
Brewed Coffee			
Caffe Misto (Au Lait): W/ Whole Milk	130	7	9
With Nonfat Milk	70	0	10
With Soy Milk	100	3	12
Espresso Hot			
Caffe Americano	15	0	3
Caffe Latte: With Whole Milk	220	11	18
With Nonfat Milk	130	0	19
With Soy Milk	170	4.5	23
Caffe Mocha: WithWhole Milk	290	12	40
With Nonfat Milk	220	2.5	42
With Soy Milk	250	6	45
Cappuccino: With Whole Milk	140	7	11
With Nonfat Milk	80	0	12
With Soy Milk	110	3	15
Caramel Macchiato: W/ Whole Milk	270	10	34
With Nonfat Milk	190	1	35
With Soy Milk	230	5	38
Cinn. Dolce Latte: With Whole Milk	290	10	39
With Nonfat Milk	210	0	41
With Soy Milk	250	4	44
Cinn. Dolce Latte, With Sugar-Free Syrup:			
With Whole Milk	210	11	17
With Non-Fat Milk	130	0	19
With Soy Milk	170	4.5	24
Espresso: 1 doppio, 2 fl.oz	10	0	2
1 solo, 1 fl.oz	5	0	1
Con Panna, 1 fl.oz	30	2.5	2
Espresso Iced			
Caffe Americano	15	0	3
Caffe Latte: With Whole Milk	150	7	12
With Nonfat Milk	90	0	13
With Soy Milk	120	3	17
Caffe Mocha: With Whole Milk	220	8	35
With Nonfat Milk	170	2.5	36
With Soy Milk	200	4.5	38
White Choc. Mocha: W/ Whole Milk	360	11	55
With Nonfat Milk	310	6	55
With Soy Milk	330	8	58
Espresso Truffle	250	11	34

Continued next page...

Updated Nutrition Data ~ www.CalorieKing.com
Persons with Diabetes ~ See Disclaimer (Page 24)

Starbucks® cont... (Apr '10)

Figures Based on Grande (16 fl.oz)
Without Whip Unless Indicated

	C	F	Cb
Frappuccino Blended Coffee:			
Caffe Vanilla	310	3	67
Caramel	270	3.5	53
Cinnamon Dolce	260	3	52
Coffee	240	3	48
Espresso	190	2.5	38
Java Chip	340	8	64
Mocha	260	3.5	54
White Chocolate Mocha	300	4.5	59
Frappuccino Blended Creme:			
Cinnamon Dolce	320	2	64
Double Chocolaty Chip	400	8	75
Mint Chocolaty Chip	400	6	80
Pumpkin Spice	360	2.5	71
Strawberries & Creme	440	2.5	92
Tazo: Chai	330	2	67
Green Tea	380	2.5	78
Vanilla Bean	350	2.5	72
Frappuccino Light Blended Coffee:			
Caffe Vanilla	190	1	42
Caramel	160	1.5	30
Cinnamon Dolce	140	0.5	29
Coffee	130	0.5	25
Java Chip	200	4.5	36
Mocha	140	1	29
Tazo Iced Tea Drinks: *Per 16 fl.oz*			
Black/Green/Passion Shaken	80	0	21
Black/Grree/Passion Lemonade	130	0	33
Vivanno Smoothies: *Per 16 fl.oz*			
Chocolate with 2% Milk	270	4.5	48
Orange Mango with 2% Milk	260	2	51
Strawberry with 2% Milk	280	1.5	56
Drink Extras:			
Caramel Drizzle, 0.13 oz	15	0.5	2
Flavored Syrup: 0.25 oz	20	0	5
Sugar-Free, 0.25 oz	0	0	0
Mocha Sauce, 0.5 oz	25	0.5	6
Sweetened Whipped Cream:			
Grande/Venti, Cold, 1.2 oz	110	11	3
Grande/Venti, Hot, 0.8 oz	70	7	2

Starbucks® cont... (Apr '10)

Breakfast Specialities:	C	F	Cb
Bacon, Gouda on Artisan Roll	380	20	31
Egg White, Spinach, Feta Wrap	280	9	33
Egg White/Turkey Bacon S'wich	340	10	47
Ham, Cheddar on Artisan Roll	370	16	32
Oatmeal, 1.3 oz	140	2.5	25
with brown sugar, 0.5 oz	190	2.5	38
Sandwiches, Panini & Wraps:			
Chicken & Vegetable Wrap	290	9	36
Egg Salad	490	22	54
Tarragon Chicken Salad	480	11	62
Tuna Melt Panini	390	12	49
Turkey & Swiss with Mayo	390	13	36
Bars & Brownies: Blueberry Oat Bar	370	14	47
Double Chocolate Brownie	410	24	46
Marshmallow Dream Bar	210	4	43
Rich Toffee Pecan Bar	380	22	42
Cookies: Chocolate Chunk	360	17	50
Outrageous Oatmeal	370	14	56
Starbucks Indulgent	320	19	40
Croissants: Butter	310	18	32
Chocolate	300	17	34
Reduced Fat Coffee Cakes:			
Banana Chocolate Chip	390	7	79
Cinnamon Swirl	340	9	62
Very Berry	350	10	58
Starbucks Classic Coffee Cake	420	19	59
Muffins: Apple Bran	350	9	64
Blueberry Streusel	360	11	59
Low Fat Red Raspberry	340	6	65
Zucchini Walnut	490	28	52
Scones: Blueberry	460	22	61
Maple Oat Pecan	470	20	64
Petite Vanilla Bean	140	5	21
Sweet Rolls & Danishes:			
Apple Fritter	420	20	59
Cheese Danish	420	25	39
Classic Glazed Old-Fashioned Donut	420	21	57
Double Iced Cinnamon Roll	490	20	70
Glazed/Choc. Old-Fashioned Donut	420	21	57
Morning Bun	350	16	45
Parfaits: Strawb. & Blueb. Yogurt	300	3.5	60
Greek Yogurt & Honey	290	12	43

Ice Cream & Ice Cream Bars ~ See Page 35, 38
For Bottled Drinks ~ See Page 39

Steak Escape® (Feb '10)

Sandwiches & Burgers	C	F	Cb
7" Sandwiches: Cajun Chicken	410	5	58
Classic Italian Sub	470	11	60
Vegetarian	310	1	65
Turkey Club	380	2	62
Wild West BBQ	455	6	60
12" Sandwiches: Cajun Chicken	630	10	80
Classic Italian Sub	760	22	85
Vegetarian	440	2	93
Turkey Club	580	3	88
Wild West BBQ	730	12	84
Kids Sandwiches: Chicken	205	7	29
Ham	185	1	31
Steak	210	3	29
Turkey	185	1	31
Salads			
Grilled Side: Salad	40	0.5	8
w. Chicken	175	5	11
w. Ham/Turkey	130	2	8
w. Steak	185	6	11
Sides			
Fresh Cut Fries:			
Kids Meal Fries, 3 oz	250	13	34
12 oz cup	500	26	67
16 oz cup	650	34	87
25 oz cup	920	48	123
32 oz cup	995	52	134
Loaded French Fries:			
Bacon & Cheddar, 10.85 oz	905	44	88
Ranch & Bacon, 10.85 oz	1045	71	84
Kids Chicken Tenders (2)	240	11	21
Portions: Chicken, 8 oz	240	0	8
Ham, 6 oz	150	1	6
Steak, 8 oz	260	0	10
Turkey, 6 oz	150	1	6
Smashed Potatoes: Plain, 13.8 oz	245	0	53
w. Chicken, 20 oz	385	4	56
w. Ham, 20 oz	340	2	59
w. Steak, 20 oz	395	5	56
w. Turkey, 20 oz	340	2	59

For Complete Nutritional Data ~ see CalorieKing.com

Steak 'n Shake® (Jan '10)

Sandwiches & Burgers	C	F	Cb
Cheddar 'n Bacon Steakburger	570	28	39
Frisco Melt Sandwich	980	72	42
Grilled Cheese & Bacon Sandwich	750	54	41
Grilled Chicken Breast Sandwich	240	7	29
Original Dbl Steakburger w. Cheese	410	21	26
Original Single w. Cheese	310	15	26
Philadelphia Steakburger	595	32	44
Triple Steakburger	450	22	26
Turkey Melt Sandwich	915	64	47
Sides:			
Chicken Fingers, without fries	260	18	14
Chili 3-Way	825	45	65
Chili 5-Way	1120	69	74
Chili Deluxe, 6 oz cup	540	38	21
Fries:			
French: Regular, 5 oz	450	23	57
Large, 7.25 oz	645	34	82
Cheddar Cheese, regular, 9 oz	615	36	64
Salads: *Without Dressing:*			
Apple Walnut Gr. Chicken	335	10	38
Beef Taco	1000	69	66
Classic Grilled Chicken	465	25	23
Fried Chicken	700	53	20
Soups: *Per 6 fl.oz Cup, without Crackers or Toppings*			
Chicken Gumbo	80	2	14
Chicken Noodle	80	1.5	10
Broccoli & Cheese	90	4.5	10
Vegetable Beef	60	1.5	12
Breakfast: Bacon Bagel	460	17	51
Biscuit & Sausage Gravy	655	38	59
Classic Stack O' Cakes (4)	320	4	62
Cheddar Scrambler	1150	80	72
Sourdough Sausage Melt	1040	85	35
Sourdough Steakburger Melt	810	57	33
Desserts: Outrageous Parfait	830	43	103
Berry Berry Cobbler a la mode	650	29	92
Brownie Fudge Sundae	862	44	112
Strawberry Shortcake	575	27	76
Shakes: *Per Regular*			
Banana, Mocha, Vanilla, avg.	720	22	116
Chocolate	745	22	122
Chocolate Mint, large	930	29	148
Frozen Yogurt Vanilla	695	16	126
Fruit & Frozen Yogurt, Strawberry	545	13	97
Orange Freeze	685	20	113

Updated Nutrition Data ~ www.CalorieKing.com
Persons with Diabetes ~ See Disclaimer (Page 24)

Subway® (Apr '10)

6" Sandwiches (6g Fat or Less)	C	F	Cb
Figures based on 9-grain wheat bread and toppings: lettuce, tomato, onion, green peppers and cucumbers. ***Cheese, oil or mayo not included.***			
Black Forest Ham	290	4.5	47
Oven Roasted Chicken Breast	320	4.5	49
Roast Beef	310	4.5	46
Subway Club	320	5	47
Sweet Onion Chicken Teriyaki	380	4.5	60
Turkey Breast	280	3.5	47
Turkey Breast & Black Forest Ham	300	4	48
Veggie Delite	230	2.5	45
6" Toasted Sandwiches: *Figures based on 9-grain wheat bread, lettuce, tomato, onion, green peppers, cucumbers and cheese.* ***Oil or mayo not included.***			
Big Philly Cheesesteak	520	18	53
BLT	360	13	45
Chicken & Bacon Ranch	570	28	49
Italian B.M.T.	450	20	48
Meatball Marinara	580	23	70
Spicy Italian	520	28	47
Subway Melt	380	11	49
The Feast	540	22	50
Tuna	530	30	46
Flatbread Sandwiches (8g Fat or Less): Figures based on flatbread, lettuce, tomatoes, onions, green peppers and cucumbers. *Cheese, oil or mayo not included.*			
Black Forest Ham	320	7	47
Oven Roasted Chicken Breast	350	7	48
Roast Beef	340	8	45
Subway Club	350	8	47
Sweet Onion Teriyaki	410	7	59
Turkey Breast	310	6	47
Turkey Breast & Black Forest Ham	330	7	47
Veggie Delite	260	5	44
Low-Fat Footlong Sandwiches: *Figures based on 9-grain wheat bread, lettuce, tomato, onion, green peppers and cucumbers.* ***Cheese, oil or mayo not included.***			
Black Forest Ham	570	9	94
Oven Roasted Chicken Breast	640	9	97
Roast Beef	630	9	91
Subway Club	640	10	95
Sweet Onion Chicken Teriyaki	760	9	120
Turkey Breast & Black Forest Ham	570	7	94
Veggie Delight	460	4.5	90

Subway® cont... (Apr '10)

4" Mini Sandwiches:	C	F	Cb
Kids Pak Figures based on 9-grain wheat bread, lettuce, tomatoes, onions, green peppers.			
Black Forest Ham	180	2.5	31
Roast Beef	200	3	30
Turkey Breast	190	2.5	31
6" Breakfast Omelet Sandwiches*: Figures based on regular egg and 9-grain bread*			
Double Bacon, Egg & Cheese	520	25	47
Egg & Cheese	420	18	46
Steak, Egg & Cheese	490	20	48
Western Egg & Cheese	460	19	48
Salads (6g Fat or Less)			
Includes lettuce, tomato, onions, green peppers, olives, cucumber. ***No Dressing or Croutons.***			
Black Forest Ham	110	3	12
Oven Roasted Chicken Breast	130	2.5	10
Roast Beef	140	3.5	10
Subway Club	140	3.5	12
Sweet Onion Chicken Teriyaki	200	3	25
Turkey Breast	110	2	12
Turkey Breast & Ham	120	3	12
Veggie Delite	50	1	10
Sandwich Components: *For 6" Sub or Salad*			
Cheese: Cheddar, 2 triangles, 0.5 oz	60	5	0
Processed American, 0.4 oz	40	3.5	1
Pepperjack; Provolone, 0.5 oz	50	4	0
Shredded Monterey Blend, 0.5 oz	50	4.5	1
Swiss, 0.5 oz	50	4.5	0
Meats: Bacon, 2 strips, 0.3 oz	45	3.5	0
Chicken Strips, 2.5 oz	80	1.5	0
Ham, 2 oz	60	2	2
Roast Beef, 2.5 oz	80	2.5	1
Seafood Sensation, 2.5 oz	190	16	7
Subway Club, 3 oz	90	2.5	2
Tuna, 2.5 oz	260	24	0
Sauces & Dressings:			
Chipotle Southwest, 1½ Tbsp	100	10	1
Honey Mustard, Fat-Free, 1½ Tbsp	30	0	7
Mayonnaise: 1 Tbsp, ½ oz	110	12	0
Light, 1 Tbsp, ½ oz	50	5	0.5
Mustard, Yellow or Deli Brown. 2 tsp	5	0	0.5
Olive Oil Blend, 1 tsp	45	5	0
Ranch Dressing, 1¼ Tbsp	110	11	1
Sweet Onion, Fat-Free, 1¼ Tbsp	40	0	9

Continued next page...

Subway® cont... (Apr '10)

Soups: Per Bowl	C	F	Cb
Chicken & Dumpling	170	5	23
Chicken Tortilla	110	1.5	11
Chili Con Carne	340	11	35
Chipotle Chicken Corn Chowder	140	3	22
Cream of Potato with Bacon	240	13	26
Fire-Roasted Tomato Orzo	130	1	24
Golden Broccoli & Cheese	180	11	16
Minestrone	90	1	17
New England Style Clam Chowder	150	5	20
Roasted Chicken Noodle	80	2	12
Rosemary Chicken & Dumpling	90	1.5	14
Spanish Style Chicken with Rice	110	2.5	16
Tomato Garden Vegetable w. Rotini	90	0.5	20
Vegetable Beef	100	2	17
Wild Rice with Chicken	230	11	26
Cookies & Desserts			
Apple Slices, 1 packege, 2.5 oz	35	0	9
Chocolate Chip Cookie, 1.6 oz	210	10	30
Dannon Light & Fit Yogurt, 6 oz	80	0	16
Oatmeal Raisin Cookie	200	8	30

Sweet Tomatoes®

~ Same Menu & Data as Souplantation (See Page 253) ~

Swiss Chalet® (Feb '10)

	C	F	Cb
Starters:			
Garl. Chse Loaf, w/o Cheese	650	35	74
Chalet Chicken Wings (8), w/ sauce	550	34	23
Cheese Perogies (7)	420	10	69
Caesar Salad with Dressing	420	37	16
Burgers/Sandwiches/Wraps: *Without Sides*			
Bacon Cheese Burger,w/o garnish	890	54	46
Hamburger without garnish	730	49	44
Veggie Burger without garish	430	13	51
Chicken on a Kaiser, dark meat	510	14	42
Chicken Quesadilla, w/o sour cream	590	18	73
Rotisserie Chicken: *Meat Only*			
Double Leg with Skin	630	38	4
Half Chicken, with Skin	610	31	5
Quarter Chicken: Leg, without Skin	220	10	0
Leg meat with Skin	310	19	2
Breast meat without Skin	180	3.5	0
Breast meat with Skin	300	11	3
Chicken Pot Pie, 1 pie	550	34	63
Chicken Stir-Fry: with Rice	750	30	89
without Rice	430	26	26
From the Grill: *Without Sides*			
BBQ Ribs: Half Rack	650	42	6
Full Rack	1300	85	11

Swiss Chalet® cont... (Feb '10)

Entree Salads:	C	F	Cb
Bacon Ranch	530	37	22
Chalet Chopped	440	27	29
Spinach Chicken Salad, w/o tortilla	170	2	14
Dressing/Sauce:			
Caesar Dressing, ½ oz	90	9	1
Chalet Dressing, 1 Tbsp, ½ oz	80	7	3
Chalet Dipping Sauce, 3.5 oz	25	0.5	5
Greek Dressing, ½ oz	70	7	1
Sides: Baked Potato, 10 oz	220	0	48
Gravy, 4 oz	45	1.5	7
Mashed Potatoes, 5 oz	150	4	27
Sauteed Mushrooms, 6 oz	220	16	11
Seasoned Rice, 6 oz	240	3.5	48
Desserts/Pies: Apple Pie	440	19	65
Caramel Fudge Cheesecake	660	41	68
Chocolate Lava Cake	430	23	53
Coconut Cream Pie	540	33	57
Cranberry Raspberry Yogurt	110	2	22
Lemon Meringue Pie	400	11	73
Old Fashioned Fudge Cake	720	44	81
Pecan Pie	590	29	79

Taco Bell® (May '10)

Burritos	C	F	Cb
Regular:			
½ lb Combo	450	18	52
½ lb Nacho Crunch	520	25	54
7-Layer	510	18	68
Cheesy Bean & Rice	480	21	60
Fresco Style: Bean	340	8	56
Supreme: Chicken	340	8	50
Steak	330	8	49
Grilled Stuft:			
Beef	700	30	79
Chicken	650	24	77
Steak	640	24	76
Supreme: Beef	420	15	52
Chicken	390	12	51
Steak	380	12	51
Chalupas			
Baja: Beef	410	26	31
Chicken	390	23	29
Steak	380	23	29
Nacho Cheese: Beef	370	22	31
Chicken	340	18	0
Steak	330	19	30

Continued next page...

Updated Nutrition Data ~ www.CalorieKing.com
Persons with Diabetes ~ See Disclaimer (Page 24)

Taco Bell® cont... (May '10)

Gorditas:	C	F	Cb
Baja: Beef	340	18	30
Chicken	320	15	29
Steak	310	15	28
Nacho Cheese: Beef	290	14	31
Chicken	270	10	30
Steak	260	11	29
Supreme: Beef	300	13	31
Chicken	270	10	29
Steak	270	11	29
Nachos: Regular	330	21	31
BellGrande	770	42	78
Supreme	440	24	42
Tacos:			
Crunchy Supreme	200	12	15
Double Decker	330	13	38
Supreme	360	15	41
Soft Taco: Beef	210	9	21
Grilled Steak	250	14	20
Ranchero Chicken	270	14	21
Supreme, Beef	240	11	24
Fresco Style: Crunchy	150	7	13
Soft: Beef	180	7	22
Grilled Steak	160	4.5	21
Ranchero Chicken	170	4	22
Specialities:			
Crunchwrap, Supreme	540	21	71
Enchiritos: Beef	370	17	35
Chicken	350	14	34
Steak	340	14	33
MexiMelt	280	14	23
Pizza, Mexican, 7.5 oz	540	30	47
Quesadillas: Chicken	520	28	41
Steak	510	28	40
Taco Salads: Chicken Ranch	910	54	71
Chipotle Steak	900	57	70
Fiesta: With Shell	770	41	75
Wthout Shell	460	24	41
Express with chips	660	34	67
Tortada, Bacon Ranch	570	24	57
Volcano: Burrito	800	42	81
Nachos	1000	62	89
Taco	240	17	14
Sides			
Cheesy Fiesta Potatoes, 4.75 oz	270	16	28

Taco Bell® cont... (May '10)

Sides (cont)	C	F	Cb
Guacamole, 1½ oz	70	6	4
Mexican Rice, 3 oz	130	3.5	21
Pintos 'n Cheese	180	6	19
Salsa, 1½ oz	10	0	2
Sour Cream, Reduced Fat, 1½ oz	60	4	4
Why Pay More!™			
Burritos: Bean	370	10	55
Beefy 5 Layer	550	22	69
Caramel Apple Empanada	310	15	39
Cheese Roll-Up	200	10	19
Cinnamon Twists	170	7	26
Crunchy Taco,	170	10	12

Note: Nutritional data for New York residents may vary slightly. Please check Taco Bell website

Taco Cabana® (Feb '10)

Burritos	C	F	Cb
Bean & Cheese	730	35	77
Black Bean	450	8	82
Stewed Chicken	660	25	73
Flameante Chicken: *Per Serving*			
¼ Chicken Dark Dinner	920	41	82
¼ Chicken White Dinner	770	22	81
½ Chicken Dinner	1220	54	83
Sizzling Fajitas: Chicken Dark	700	21	92
Chicken White	710	20	93
Steak	730	24	93
Tacos:			
Crispy: Beef	180	10	11
Chicken	160	7	13
Soft: Bean & Cheese	300	14	31
Beef	230	9	21
Black Bean	200	4	34
Carne Guisada	190	5	20
Chicken	210	7	23
Sides: *Per Serving*			
Black Beans	80	0	14
Borracho Beans	110	3	16
Guacamole, small	110	9	7
Queso, small	200	15	5
Refried Beans	250	13	24
Rice	120	0.5	25
Salsa, all types, 1 oz	10	0	2
Ranch, 1 oz	35	4	1
Sour Cream, 3 oz	160	14	3
Tortillas: 6" Flour	120	3	19
6" Table Corn	70	1	11

Taco Del Mar® (Feb '10)

	C	F	Cb
Mondito Refried Burritos: *Per Burrito. Includes Tortilla, Rice, Beans, Meat & Salsa Unless Indicated*			
Beef, 11 oz	**555**	**19**	71
21.7 oz	**1070**	**36**	134
Cheese, w/o meat, 9.75 oz	**460**	**13**	69
Chicken, 11 oz	**545**	**17**	70
21.7 oz	**1030**	**32**	131
Fish,w/ Cabbage & White Sauce	**505**	**21**	61
Pork, 11 oz	**545**	**18**	71
Enchiladas: Per Enchilada. *Include Tortilla, Meat, Cheese, Rice, Beans, Sauce, Lettuce & Salsa Unless Indicated*			
Beef, 23.4 oz	**1030**	**37**	115
Cheese, w/o meat, 19.8oz	**820**	**27**	112
Chicken, 23.4 oz	**990**	**33**	113
Pork, 23.4 oz	**990**	**35**	114
Nachos & Chips: *Includes Chips, Cheese, Beans, Salsa, Sour Cream & Guacamole*			
Nachos, refried, 1 tray, 16.75 oz	**1190**	**65**	110
Chips & Salsa only, 1 tray 7 oz	**590**	**27**	78
Quesadillas: *Per Quesadilla. Includes Tortilla, Meat, Cheese & Salsa Unless Indicated*			
Beef, 12.45 oz	**800**	**37**	66
Cheese, w/o meat, 9.95 oz	**710**	**35**	63
Chicken, 12.45 oz	**770**	**33**	64
Pork, 12.45 oz	**770**	**35**	65
Tacos: Per Taco. *Includes Shell, Meat, Cheese, Lettuce & Salsa Unless Indicated*			
Hard: Beef; Chicken avg., 4.75 oz	**265**	**14**	17
Fish, 4.6 oz	**270**	**15**	23
Pork, 4.75 oz	**260**	**14**	17
Soft: Beef; Chicken avg., 5.8 oz	**270**	**10**	28
Fish, 5.7oz	**270**	**11**	34
Pork, 5.8 oz	**260**	**10**	28
Taco Salads, Refried: *Includes Shell, Beans, Lettuce, Meat, Cheese, Salsa, Sour Cream & Guacamole Unless Indicted*			
Beef, 21 oz	**930**	**49**	75
Chicken, 21 oz	**900**	**45**	73
Pork, 21 oz	**900**	**46**	74
Sides: Black Beans, 4.25 oz	**140**	**2**	24
Refried, 4.25oz	**160**	**3.5**	24
Pinto, 4.25 oz	**90**	**0**	20
Rice & Pinto, 11 oz	**320**	**3**	66
Rice & Black Bean, 11 oz	**370**	**5**	69
Rice & Refried Beans, 11oz	**390**	**7**	69
Sauce: Enchilada, 3 oz	**35**	**0**	7
Guacamole, 0.75oz	**40**	**3.5**	2
Desserts: Per 1			
Brownie, Oreo, 3.25 oz	**400**	**17**	59
Cookies: White Choc. Macadamia	**270**	**16**	30
Average all flavors, 2.5 oz	**240**	**12**	21

Taco John's® (Feb '10)

	C	F	Cb
Burritos: Super Burrito	**450**	**18**	54
Meat & Potato Burrito	**500**	**23**	58
Chicken & Potato Burrito	**470**	**19**	56
Crunchy Chicken & Potato Burrito	**600**	**28**	65
Bean Burrito	**360**	**9**	56
Beefy Burrito	**440**	**20**	45
Beef Grilled Burrito	**600**	**32**	52
Combination Burrito	**400**	**14**	50
Chicken Grilled Burrito	**590**	**29**	50
Tacos:			
Soft Shell Taco	**220**	**11**	21
Taco Bravo	**340**	**13**	40
Taco Burger	**270**	**12**	28
10 Grams of Fat or Less:			
Crispy	**180**	**10**	13
Chili, without Cheese	**160**	**6**	17
Soft Shell without Cheese	**190**	**8**	20
Specialties: Taco Salad w/o dressing	**520**	**33**	37
Chicken Taco Salad w/o dressing	**480**	**27**	35
Crunchy Ckn Taco Salad w/o dressing	**660**	**40**	47
Super Nachos: Small	**450**	**27**	38
Regular	**810**	**48**	74
Super Potato Oles: Small	**620**	**39**	53
Regular	**1030**	**65**	87
Quesadilla Melt: Cheese	**440**	**23**	43
Fajita Beef	**540**	**28**	49
Fajita Chicken	**510**	**23**	47
Crunchy Chicken w/o sauce	**450**	**27**	24
Snacks: Chips & Queso	**430**	**25**	43
Buffalo Chicken Snackarito	**290**	**15**	27
Cini-Sopapilla Bites	**210**	**5**	37
Ranch Chicken Snackarito	**240**	**12**	23
Sides: Potato Oles: Small	**430**	**26**	45
Medium	**600**	**36**	62
Large	**770**	**46**	80
Kid's Meal portion	**290**	**18**	31
Refried Beans: with cheese	**320**	**6**	47
without cheese	**260**	**1.5**	47
Mexican Rice	**250**	**6**	45
Condiments: Nacho Cheese, 3 oz	**120**	**9**	5
Salsa, 2 oz	**20**	**0**	4
Sour Cream, 2 oz	**120**	**12**	2
House Dressing, 1.5 oz	**70**	**7**	2
Ranch Dressing, 1.5 oz	**140**	**16**	3
Desserts: Apple Grande	**270**	**12**	39
Choco Taco	**390**	**20**	48
Churro	**190**	**7**	15

Taco Mayo® (Feb '10)

	C	F	Cb
Burritos			
Bean	495	16	71
Beef	490	23	41
Super Burrito, Beef	540	23	57
Super Chicken	405	16	39
Melts			
Tamale	615	34	50
Tostada	525	32	35
Quesadillas			
Chicken	675	37	46
Fajita Chicken	700	39	47
Fajita Steak	725	40	47
Tacos			
Crispy Taco, Beef	160	10	10
Soft Taco: Beef	230	11	17
Chicken	185	6	16
Salads			
Acapulco: Chicken Salad	680	50	35
Steak	705	51	35
SalsaLita Steak	305	8	33
Taco Steak	445	25	30
Sides			
Mexicali Rice	160	1	36
Refried Beans	295	9	43
Potato Locos, Small	380	24	36

Taco Time® (Feb '10)

	C	F	Cb
Burritos			
Beef, Bean & Cheese	490	17	55
Chicken B.L.T.	690	39	43
Big Juan: Chicken	580	16	70
Ground Beef	630	23	73
Casita: Chicken	490	17	42
Ground Beef	540	24	46
Crisp Burrito: Chicken	380	17	33
Ground Beef	430	21	36
Pinto Bean	360	14	47
Soft Burrito: Meat	430	16	43
Pinto Bean	370	10	54
Soft Veggie	520	17	73
Tacos			
Soft Tacos: *Per 7 oz*			
Chicken	360	9	40
Ground Beef	420	16	43
Jr Soft Taco, 5.3 oz	310	13	28
Super Soft Wheat Taco: Beef	590	23	63
Chicken	535	16	59
Other Favorites: Cheddar Melt	250	12	25
Nachos Grande	930	43	96
Tostada: Bean	230	13	21
Chicken	320	13	22
Ground Beef	375	20	25

Taco Time® cont... (Feb '10)

	C	F	Cb
Sides			
Cheddar Fries, med. 7 oz	500	35	39
Mexi Fries®, medium, 6 oz	390	26	38
Mexi-Rice, 3.5 oz	80	0.5	17
Stuffed Fries, medium, 7 oz	460	28	42
Refritos with Chips, 6 oz	230	7	29
Salads:			
Regular: Chicken Taco, 9.5 oz	310	13	22
Ground Beef Taco, 9 oz	370	20	24
Tostada Delight: Chicken, 9 oz	450	19	35
Ground Beef, 9 oz	490	26	36
Salsas, Sauces & Dressings			
Chipotle Ranch Dressing, 1 oz	170	18	1
Guacamole, 1 oz	50	4.5	2
Salsa Fresca, 1 oz	10	0	2
Desserts: Churro: Plain	210	16	17
with Cinnamon & Sugar	250	16	27
Crustos	290	6	58
Empanada, average	240	7	41

Target Food Court (Feb '10)

	C	F	Cb
Entrees:			
Beef Hot Dog	380	23	27
Bratwurst	400	24	27
Chicken Tenders	220	8	18
Italian Sausage	440	29	27
Jalapeno & Cheddar Sausage	410	26	26
Kids: Chicken Nuggets	180	12	9
Hot Dog	330	19	28
Macaroni & Cheese	310	12	39
Mini Beef Hot Dogs	320	15	34
Sandwiches: Ham & Cheddar	460	14	48
Pita Melts, average	240	10	23
Turkey & Provolone	440	12	51
Turkey Club	570	27	44
Salads: California	600	32	44
Chicken Caesar	560	36	19
Soups: Broccoli & Cheese	190	11	16
Chicken Noodle	130	1	18
Snacks: French Fries	230	9	33
Nachos with Cheese & Jalapenos	530	25	67
Popcorn	300	16	32
Yogurt Parfait	300	8	50
Treats: Blueberry Muffin	410	18	56
Brownie	340	15	45
Chocolate Chip Cookie	510	26	68
Cinnamon Roll	480	20	65
Pretzels: Bavarian with Butter	490	6	93
Cheddar	540	15	87
Smoothies: Mango	220	0	54
Strawberry	250	0	62

For Complete Nutritional Data ~ see CalorieKing.com

TCBY® (Feb '10)

Soft Serve Frozen Yogurt: Per ½ Cup	C	F	Cb
Average all flavors	110	2	23
Golden Vanilla	120	2	23
Peanut Butter Cup	130	1.5	26
No Sugar Added, Fat Free:			
Average all	90	0	24
Chocolate	80	0	23
No Sugar Added:			
White Chocolate Macadamia	90	0	24
Sorbet: *Per ½ Cup*			
Classic Tart	90	0	21
Mango	110	0	26
Orange; Strawberry Kiwi	100	0	24
Raspberry	100	0	25
Hand-Scooped Frozen Yogurt			
Butter Pecan: Child, 2 oz	120	6	14
Small, 4 oz	240	12	28
Medium, 6 oz	360	17	42
Large, 8 oz	470	23	56
Chocolate Chocolate: Child, 2 oz	90	2.5	15
Small, 4 oz	190	5	30
Medium, 6 oz	280	8	45
Large, 8 oz	380	10	60
Cookies & Cream: Child, 2 oz	110	3.5	17
Small, 4 oz	210	7	33
Medium, 6 oz	320	10	50
Large, 8 oz	420	13	67
Mocha Almond: Child, 2 oz	110	4	17
Small, 4 oz	230	8	33
Medium, 6 oz	340	12	50
Large, 8 oz	450	16	67
Strawberries & Cream: Child, 2 oz	90	2	15
Small, 4 oz	170	4	30
Medium, 6 oz	260	6	45
Large, 8 0z	350	8	60
Vanilla Bean: Child, 2 oz	90	2.5	14
Small, 4 oz	180	5	29
Medium, 6 oz	270	8	43
Large, 8 oz	370	10	58
No Sugar Added Hand-Scooped			
Choc. Chocolate Swirl: Child, 2 oz	70	0	16
Small, 4 oz	130	0.5	32
Medium, 6 oz	200	1	49
Large, 8 oz	270	1.5	65
Vanilla Fudge Brownie: Child, 2 oz	80	1.5	17
Small, 4 oz	160	3	34
Medium, 6 oz	240	4.5	51
Large, 8 oz	310	6	69

Teriyaki Stix® (Feb '10)

Bowls:	C	F	Cb
Chicken	705	8	111
with Vegetables	735	8	118
Curry	705	16	110
Orange Chicken	770	16	113
Veggie	590	0.5	134
Sandwiches: *Without Cheese or Dressing*			
Ham	185	2	30
Roast Beef	260	3	43
Stacked Club	725	17	96
Turkey	270	2.5	44
Smoothies: Jungle Mist	270	0	73
Raspberry Razzle	215	0	57
Watermelon Wave	270	0	71

The Taco Maker® (Feb '10)

Burritos	C	F	Cb
Regular: Bean	405	16	52
Beef	365	12	44
Chicken	505	20	44
Crispy: Bean	400	26	31
Beef	245	5	41
Soft Shell: Beef	365	13	45
Chicken/Turkey, avg.	435	18	46
Max: ½ lb Beef	420	18	51
Nachos: *Per Regular*			
Cheese	300	23	7
Grande Deluxe: Beef	440	32	13
Chicken	510	37	13
Guacamole	505	40	16
Tacos: *Per Regular*			
Beef	90	5	3
Chicken	140	9	25
Plates:			
Burrito Grande: Beef	430	17	53
Chicken	500	21	53
Fajita Dinner			
Beef/Chicken, avg.	800	39	71
Fiesta Dinner:			
Beef	550	23	54
Chicken	765	36	54
Quesadilla Dinner, Cheese	1100	62	95
Taco Salads: *Without Dressing*			
Beef	740	42	49
Chicken	550	23	45
Fries: Regular	150	6	21
Baked Potatoes			
Papa Taco: Bean	270	4	54
Beef	445	19	54
Chicken	520	24	54
Potato, Bacon & Cheese	523	27	52
Turkey	505	23	56

Updated Nutrition Data ~ www.CalorieKing.com
Persons with Diabetes ~ See Disclaimer (Page 24)

ThunderCloud Subs® (Feb '10)

Subs: Small, with Standard Toppings	C	F	Cb
Classic: BLT	405	17	40
Roast Beef	290	6	40
Smoked Chicken	295	4	40
Turkey	280	4	41
Hot Subs: Meatball	650	32	56
Hot Pastrami	430	13	41
Signature Subs: Club	480	19	43
California Club	510	23	45
N.Y. Italian	570	30	42
Office Favorite	850	46	81
Texas Tuna	700	45	44
Veggie Delite, with Hummus	360	10	53

Tim Hortons® (Feb '10)

Breakfast:	C	F	Cb
Country Buns:			
Whole Wheat (1)	240	1	46
White (1)	240	1	49
Sandwiches: Bagel BELT	450	14	58
Bacon, Egg & Cheese	420	23	34
Egg & Cheese	370	19	34
Sausage, Egg & Cheese	540	35	35
Hashbrowns, 1.65 oz	100	5	12
Lunch:			
Sandwiches: BLT	450	18	53
Chicken Salad	380	9	55
Egg Salad	390	13	52
Ham & Swiss w/ Tim's Own Dress.	440	12	56
Toasted Chicken Club	460	7	70
Turkey Bacon Club w/ Mustard	440	8	63
***Soups:** Per 10 oz Bowl*			
Beef Stew	235	8	25
Chicken Noodle	120	2	18
Chili	300	16	18
Cream of Broccoli	160	9	16
Creamy Field Mushroom	150	3	28
French Onion	230	9	26
Hearty Potato Bacon	250	13	23
Hearty Vegetable	70	0	14
Minestrone	120	4	24
Split Pea with Ham	150	2.5	27
Turkey & Wild Rice	120	1.5	21
Vegetable Beef Barley	110	1.5	21

Tim Hortons® Cont... (Feb '10)

Bagels:	C	F	Cb
Plain	260	1.5	52
Blueberry; Cinnamon Raisin	270	1	55
Everything	280	2	53
Onion	260	1.5	52
Poppy Seed	270	2	53
***Timbits:** Low-Fat*			
Cake: Chocolate Glazed	70	2.5	10
Old Fashion Plain	70	5	5
Sour Cream Glazed	90	4.5	12
Filled, all varieties	60	2	10
Yeast: Apple Fritter	50	1.5	9
Honey Dip	60	15	9
***Baked Goods:** Per Serving*			
Cookies:			
Caramel Chocolate Pecan	230	11	32
Chocolate Chunk	230	9	35
Oatmeal Raisin Spice	220	8	35
Peanut Butter	280	16	27
Triple Chocolate	250	13	31
Donuts:			
Cake: Chocolate Glazed	260	10	39
Old Fashioned Plain	260	19	20
Pumpkin Spice	260	11	38
Sour Cream Plain	270	17	27
Filled: Blueberry	230	8	36
Boston Cream	250	9	38
Canadian Maple	260	9	41
Strawberry	230	8	36
Honey Cruller	320	19	37
Yeast: Apple Fritter	300	11	49
Desserts:			
Low Fat Yogurt: Creamy Vanilla	160	2.5	32
Strawberry	150	2.5	28
Beverages:			
Cafe Mocha, 10 fl.oz	180	8	27
Cappuccino: Eng. Toffee, 10 fl.oz	220	6	40
French Vanilla, 10 fl.oz	240	7	39
Iced Original:			
with Small Milk, 10 fl.oz	180	1.5	39
with Small Cream, 10 fl.oz	300	15	41
Coffee w/med. sugar/cream, 10 fl.oz	75	3.5	9
Hot Chocolate, 10 fl.oz	240	6	45

T.J. Cinnamons® (Feb '10)

Bakery	C	F	Cb
Cinnamon Roll, 5.25 oz	505	10	73
Cinnamon Twist (1), 2½ oz	260	14	33
Pecan Sticky Bun: (1), 6.5 oz	690	22	91
4-Pack	2750	90	363
Sticky Bun Smear w/ Pecans, 1¼ oz	180	12	18
T.J. Cream Cheese Icing, 1 oz	115	5	18
Beverages: *Per 12 fl.oz Serving*			
Mocha Chill: w/o Whipped Cream	265	4	46
with Whipped Cream	305	7	47

Togo's Eatery® (Feb '10)

Sandwiches: *Regular 6" Roll*	C	F	Cb
Chef's Creations: BBQ Ranch Chkn	750	27	88
Chipotle Rst Beef w/ Provolone	990	49	66
Pacific Cobb	710	36	68
Pastrami Reuben w/ Swiss	990	55	67
Cold: *Includes Standard Sides & Mayo Unless Indicated*			
Albacore Tuna	660	28	73
Black Forest Ham & Cheese	670	31	67
Chicken Salad w. Almonds	650	29	74
Roast Beef & Avocado	720	29	70
The Italian with Canola Oil	860	43	71
Turkey & Avocado	640	26	74
Turkey Bacon Club	680	32	68
Hot: BBQ Beef	670	19	85
Chicken	630	20	72
Hot Pastrami	750	33	69
Meatball	690	27	78
Sicilian Chicken	710	28	73
Vegetarian: Avocado & Cheese	740	40	73
Avocado & Cucumber	560	25	75
Egg Salad & Cheese	750	39	70
Salad Wraps: *Includes Whole Wheat Wrap, Standard Toppings & Dressing*			
Asian Chicken w/ Asian Dressing	670	32	74
BBQ Chkn Ranch w/ Buttmlk Rnch	630	26	77
Cobb w/ Blue Cheese	680	36	63
Farmer's Market w/ Bals. Vinaig.	440	14	72
Santa Fe Chicken w/ Spicy Pepitas	800	44	75
Salads: *Per Full Salad, without Dressing*			
Asian Chicken	200	9	17
BBQ Chicken Ranch	230	3.5	31
Chicken Caesar	210	6	17
Cobb	330	20	12
Taco, includes shell	600	39	36

Tropical Smoothie Cafe® (Feb '10)

Breakfast:	C	F	Cb
Wraps: Early Bird	615	24	68
Western	635	28	57
Lunch:			
Bistro Sandwiches: *Without Cheese & Sauce*			
Cranberry Walnut Chicken Salad	735	40	71
Hummus Veggie	670	26	84
The Italian	460	16	38
Turkey Bacon Ranch	430	13	37
Turkey Guacamile	595	14	75
Ultimate Club	525	19	43
Wasabi Roast Beef	375	11	33
Toasted Wraps: Buffalo Chicken	625	26	60
Jamaican Jerk Chicken	625	17	79
King Caesar	605	29	56
Sesame Chicken	805	23	113
Totally Turkey	615	25	55
Salads: *Includes Standard Dressing*			
Cranberry Walnut Chicken	475	38	20
Sesame Chicken	580	19	73
Thai Chicken	500	11	74
TSC Signature	350	13	37
Low Fat Smoothies: *With Turbinado*			
Blimey Limey	470	0	117
Blue Lagoon	330	1	80
Hawaiian Breeze	380	0	92
Island Fever	420	0.5	103
Rockin Raspberry	425	0.5	103
Strawberry Beach	450	0	109
Sunrise Sunset	410	0.5	100
Supercharged: *With Turbinado*			
Health Nut	530	7	92
Lean Machine	470	0.5	115
Muscle Blaster	485	3	91
Peanut Paradise	690	18	99
Stress Defender	465	0	112
Simply Indulgent Smoothies: *With Turbinado*			
Beach Bum	565	5	125
Chocolate Chiller	555	7	117
Peanut Butter Cup	720	21	123
Tropi-Colada	510	5.5	115

With Splenda, deduct 200 calories & 50g carbs

Updated Nutrition Data ~ www.CalorieKing.com
Persons with Diabetes ~ See Disclaimer (Page 24)

Tubby's® (Feb '10)

Subs: Per Regular Sandwich	C	F	Cb
Burger Subs: Big Tub	670	56	55
Burger Special	900	59	59
Cheeseburger	910	60	59
Pizza Burger	930	60	62
Taco Burger	825	47	67
Deli Subs: Club Sub	700	41	53
Ham & Cheese	570	30	54
Tubby's Famous	665	39	55
Turkey & Cheese	625	32	51
Turkey Club Sub	850	39	83
Specialty Subs: BLT	635	42	50
Cold Veggie	460	14	66
Italian Sausage	730	45	56
Tuna	415	18	47
Veggie Stir Fry	650	27	89
Chicken Subs:			
Chicken & Broccoli	550	23	56
Chicken & Cheddar	545	23	54
Chicken Club Sub	705	41	53
Chicken Fajita Sub	445	12	57
Grilled Chicken	345	5	52
Steak Subs:			
Mushroom Steak	835	26	52
Pepper Steak	710	46	52
Pizza Steak	985	57	85
Steak & Cheese	825	56	51
Steak Special	745	46	58

Uno Chicago Grill® (Feb '10)

Appetizers:	C	F	Cb
Pizza Skins, ⅓ pizza, 5 oz	480	31	39
Roasted Vegetable Quesadilla (1)	300	13	36
Shrimp & Crab Fondue, 3.3 oz	220	16	13
Burgers: *Without Sides*			
BBQ w/ Bacon & Cheddar (2)	1400	92	64
Sliders (2)	1200	80	52
Uno Burger (2)	1080	72	48
Entrees: *Without Side or Breadstick*			
Baked Stuffed Chicken (2)	360	18	6
Chicken Milanese (2)	860	58	42
Chicken Thumb Platter (2)	480	18	34
Fisherman's Platter (2)	1540	110	148
Smoke, Sizzle & Splash: *Without Sides or Breadstick*			
Baked Haddock (2)	580	17	6
Lemon Basil Salmon	480	34	0
The Chop House Classic	520	18	0
Flatbread Pizza: *Per ⅓ pizza*			
Mediterranean	280	15	29
Pepperoni, Gluten-Free Crust	340	15	41
Spicy Chicken	350	16	34

For Complete Nutritional Data ~ see CalorieKing.com

Villa Pizza® (Dec '09)

Pizza (18"): Per Slice (⅙ Pizza)	C	F	Cb
Neapolitan: Cheese	525	19	60
Sausage and Cheese	675	32	61
Pepperoni and Cheese	635	29	60
Stuffed: Meat	880	42	83
Spinach and Mushroom	790	35	87
Sicilian: Deluxe	945	39	105
Stromboli:			
Sausage and Cheese	880	44	83
Pepperoni and Cheese	745	33	83
Pasta & Italian Specialties:			
Baked Ziti	680	35	63
Meat Lasagna	1235	81	86
Spinach and Cheese Lasagna	1065	60	88
Spaghetti	2710	122	349
Chicken Francais	225	11	4
Chicken Cacciatore	780	68	11
Italian Sausage and Peppers	645	64	3
Sauteed Fresh Vegetables	465	43	19
Salads:			
Caesar	110	8	7
Fresh Mozzarella	310	22	10
Greek	155	11	9

Vocelli Pizza® (Feb '10)

Pizze: Per Slice (⅛ Pizza)	C	F	Cb
Grande Cheese	260	6	38
Grande Pepperoni	410	20	38
Gourmet: *Per Slice (⅛ Pizza)*			
Deluxe	390	16	40
Meat Magnifico	490	25	38
Philly Steak	360	13	38
Panini: *Per Sandwich*			
Chicken	900	38	81
Italian	910	42	77
Vegetarian	750	31	83
Insalata: *Per Plate*			
Antipasta	630	50	16
Chicken Caesar	220	4.5	4
Mediterranean	270	18	20
Tuscany Chicken	350	16	15
Antipasti: Croutons, 1 package	30	1	5
Bruschetta, 1 slice	150	8	14
Buffalo Wings (10)	560	39	3
BBQ Wings (10)	610	33	26
Pepperoni Sticks, 2½ slices	470	26	36
Dressings: *Per 2 oz Packet*			
Blue Cheese	230	25	2
Italian	200	21	4
Ranch	260	28	2

Wahoo's Fish Taco® (Feb '10)

Bowls: W/ White Rice & Blk Beans	C	F	Cb
Blackened Chicken	860	15	127
Charbroiled Chicken	860	15	126
Charbroiled Fish	930	22	126
Teriyaki Fish	930	22	127
***Classic Burrito,** A la Carte:*			
Carne Asada	480	19	53
Carnitas	605	25	54
Charbroiled/Blackened: Fish, av.	545	23	53
Chicken, average	495	18	52
Mushroom	405	16	55
Shrimp	400	16	53
Veggie w/ White Rice & Black Beans	635	19	98
***Tacos,** A la Carte:*			
Blackened Chicken	185	5	22
Carne Asada	180	5	22
Carnitas	235	8	23
Veggie w/ White Rice & Black Beans	215	4	36
Sides: Brown Rice	350	7	64
White Beans	285	3	54
***Salads:** Chips Not Included*			
Blackened Chicken	415	22	14
Carne Asada	400	23	16
Charbroiled Fish	485	29	14

For Complete Nutritional Data ~ see CalorieKing.com

WAWA® (Feb '10)

Breakfast	C	F	Cb
Bagels: Plain	290	1	60
with Butter	490	23	60
Cinnamon Raisin	290	1	63
with Cream Cheese	410	13	62
Everything	310	6	56
Croissant, Plain	280	14	35
Muffins: Banana Walnut	670	34	83
Blueberry	610	30	78
Chocolate Chip	680	34	86
Corn	640	29	87
Bowls: *Per Bowl, without Syrup*			
Creamed Chipped Beef On Rye	340	11	51
Pancake: Without Syrup	330	10	56
with Bacon	370	12	57
with Sausage	490	24	57
with Turkey Sausage	420	16	67
Scrambled Egg: with Bacon	370	25	9
with Sausage	490	36	10
Ciabatta Melts: *On Shorti Rolls without Extras*			
Scrambled Eggs: With Bacon	530	20	58
with Beef Cheesesteak	640	22	60
with Ham & Swiss	570	19	60
Italian Style	640	26	60

WAWA® cont... (Feb '10)

Breakfast (Cont)	C	F	Cb
Sizzlis: *Without Hashbrowns*			
Bagels: Bacon, Egg & Cheese	360	14	42
Pork Roll, Egg & Cheese	400	16	43
Sausage, Egg & Cheese	500	26	43
Biscuit, Sausage, Egg & Cheese	620	40	47
Croissant, Sausage, Egg & Chse	500	36	26
Lunch:			
Bagel Sandwiches: *With Plain Bagel, w/o Toppings*			
BLT	390	8	62
Chicken Salad	630	29	66
Ham	380	4	62
Roast Beef	410	3	62
Cold Hoagies: *On Shorti Roll w/ithout Toppings*			
Egg Salad	820	36	90
Tuna Salad	580	36	48
Turkey	280	4	44
Soups: *Per Medium Serving*			
Cream of Broccoli	250	15	22
Maryland Crab	120	1	20
Minestrone	140	3.5	23
Sides: *Per Medium Serving*			
Chili	260	8	33
Macaroni & Cheese	460	21	50
Mashed Potatoes	530	33	52
Meatballs in a Cup	360	25	20
Shephard's Pie	470	27	41
Stuffing	400	23	42
Dinner:			
Cold Hoagies: *On Shorti Roll without Toppings*			
Egg Salad	540	32	46
Turkey	320	5	46
Hot Dogs: *Without Toppings, Mustard or Sauce*			
Regular	230	15	21
Big Bacon Cheese Dog	640	40	41
Kielbasa	310	17	21
Hot Hoagies: *On Shorti Roll without Toppings*			
Beef Cheesecake	360	8	42
Chicken Cheesecake	340	6	42
Homestyle Roast Beef	420	12	46
Meatballs w/ American Cheese	660	36	60
Sides: *Per Medium Serving*			
Creamy Tortellini with Bacon	420	25	33
Soups: *Per Medium Serving*			
Italian Wedding	150	5	18
Loaded Potato	410	26	28
Toasted Flatbreads: Pepp. Pizza	750	42	59
Salsa Chicken	560	19	58
Turkey Quesad. w/ Sour Cream	520	18	61
Beverages: Per 24 oz			
Hot Cappuccinos: Original	370	13	63
English Toffee	340	9	63
Smoothie, Strawberry Banana	450	3.5	104

Updated Nutrition Data ~ www.CalorieKing.com
Persons with Diabetes ~ See Disclaimer (Page 24)

Wendy's® May '10)

Burgers & Sandwiches	C	F	Cb
Burgers: ¼ lb Single	**470**	21	43
½ lb Double, with Cheese	**750**	42	44
¾ lb Triple with Cheese	**1030**	62	44
Baconator, Double	**980**	62	46
Double Stack	**360**	18	27
Jr. Bacon Cheeseburger	**310**	16	26
Jr. Cheeseburger Deluxe	**300**	14	29
Sandwiches: Chicken Club	**630**	30	56
Crispy Chicken	**350**	15	38
Homestyle Chicken	**460**	16	53
Spicy Chicken	**470**	16	55
Ultimate Chicken Grill	**340**	7	41
French Fries: Kid's, 2.5 oz	**210**	10	28
Small, 4 oz	**330**	15	45
Medium, 5 oz	**410**	19	56
Large, 6.5 oz	**540**	25	73
Chicken Nuggets, 5 piece	**230**	14	13
Boneless Chicken Wings:			
Honey BBQ	**570**	18	69
Spicy Chipotle	**500**	20	48
Sweet & Spicy Asian	**540**	18	62
Nugget Sauce: Barbecue	**45**	0	11
Heartland Ranch	**120**	12	3
Garden Sensations Salads:			
Chicken BLT with Homestyle Chicken	**470**	27	23
With Honey Dijon Drssng & Croutons	**790**	53	42
Chicken Caesar with Grilled Chicken	**180**	4	8
With Caesar Dressing & Croutons	**490**	32	20
Mandarin Chkn w/ Almonds & Noodles	**370**	16	31
With Oriental Sesame Dressing	**540**	25	51
Caesar Side, w/o Dressing or Croutons	**70**	4	4
Side Salad without Dressing	**35**	0	8
Sides:			
Hot Stuffed Baked Potatoes:			
Bacon & Cheese	**460**	13	67
Broccoli & Cheese	**330**	2	69
Sour Cream & Chives	**320**	4	63
Chili Large, 16 oz	**330**	10	32
Mandarin Orange Cup, 5 oz	**90**	0	21
Frosty: Choc/Van., small, average	**310**	8	52
Frosti-cino, small	**380**	11	63
Frosty Shakes: Choc. Fudge, large	**540**	13	94
Strawb/Vanilla, large, average	**510**	13	89
Twisted Frosty: Chocolate/Vanilla	**480**	16	77
M&M's, Chocolate/Vanilla, average	**555**	19	87
Oreo, Chocolate/Vanilla	**440**	14	72

For Complete Nutritional Data ~ see CalorieKing.com

Wienerschnitzel® (Feb '10)

Hot Dogs: *With Standard Bun*	C	F	Cb
Original: BBQ Bacon	**380**	21	33
Chili	**300**	14	31
Chili Cheese	**350**	18	31
Deluxe	**280**	13	30
Pastrami	**420**	24	30
Plain	**270**	13	27
Stadium	**280**	13	30
Corn Dogs: Regular	**250**	17	15
Mini (6)	**320**	22	22
Burgers: Original	**290**	9	29
Chili	**310**	9	29
Chili Cheese	**350**	13	29
Deluxe: Hamburger	**400**	19	33
Cheeseburger	**450**	23	33
Double Chili Cheese	**560**	24	35
Pastrami	**510**	26	30
Sandwiches: Chicken Deluxe	**430**	21	37
Italian Sausage	**350**	17	31
Pastrami	**580**	34	36
Polish Sausage	**490**	29	39
Sides: Chili Cheese Fries	**540**	38	39
Fries: Regular	**300**	22	25
Large	**430**	31	35
Jalapeno Poppers (3)	**210**	11	21
Breakfast:			
Biscuit: Egg, Bacon, Cheese	**440**	25	36
Egg, Sausage, Cheese	**540**	34	40
Burrito: Egg, Bacon, Cheese	**490**	25	39
Egg, Sausage, Cheese	**590**	34	43
French Toast Sticks	**490**	29	49
Syrup, 1.1 oz	**120**	0	31
Desserts:			
Cones: Plain, 6 oz.	**300**	11	49
Chocolate Dipped, 6 oz.	**490**	29	57
Floats: Mountain Dew, Root Beer avg.	**440**	12	84
Tropicana Strawberry Lemonade	**450**	12	82
Freezees: Butterfinger	**620**	24	100
Oreo; M&M	**630**	25	99
Reese's Peanut Butter Cup	**630**	26	97
Sundaes: Caramel, Hot Fudge avg.	**400**	15	65
Chocolate	**390**	14	64
Pineapple; Strawberry	**370**	14	59
Shakes, avgerage all flavors	**650**	23	110
Drinks: *16 fl.oz, without ice*			
Lipton Raspberry Iced Tea	**180**	0	45
Mountain Dew	**230**	0	61
Mug Root Beer	**210**	0	57
Pepsi	**200**	0	55

Whataburger® (Feb '10)

Burgers/Sandwiches	C	F	Cb
Justaburger	290	15	26
Whataburger: Burger	620	30	58
w. Bacon & Cheese	780	43	59
Double Meat	870	49	58
Triple Meat	1120	68	58
Jr.	300	15	28
Sandwich: Grilled Chicken	470	19	49
Whatacatch	450	24	44
Whatachick'n	550	27	57
French Fries: Small, 3 oz	320	18	36
Medium, 4½ oz	480	27	56
Large, 6 oz	640	36	73
Onion Rings: Medium, 4.27 oz	400	25	37
Large, 6.4 oz	600	38	56
Chicken Strips (2)	300	16	22
Salads: *Without Dressing*			
Chicken Strips Salad	350	16	33
w/ Shredded Cheddar Cheese	520	29	34
Garden Salad	50	0	11
w/ Shredded Cheddar Cheese	220	13	12
Grilled Chicken Salad	220	7	18
w/ Shredded Cheddar Cheese	390	20	19
Dressing: *Per 2 oz*			
Buttermilk Ranch	310	33	3
Honey Mustard	250	21	15
THOUSAND ISLAND	150	13	0
Malts:			
Chocolate; Strawb.: Small, 15.75 oz	670	15	123
Medium, average, 25.25 oz	1045	25	188
Vanilla: Small, 15.75 oz	600	17	98
Medium, 25.25 oz	940	27	155
Shakes			
Chocolate; Strawb.: Small, 15.75 oz	630	16	111
Medium, average, 25.25 oz	995	26	171
Vanilla: Small, 15.75 oz	560	17	87
Medium, 25.25 oz	890	28	139
Breakfast: Cinnamon Roll	390	9	71
Hash Brown Sticks (4)	200	12	20
Texas Toast, 1 slice	150	7	20
Biscuit: Plain	300	17	32
w. Bacon	350	20	32
w. Gravy	560	33	54
w. Sausage	540	37	32
Honey Butter Chicken	560	34	50
Biscuit Sandwich: w. Egg & Chse	450	28	33
w. Bacon, Egg & Cheese	500	32	33
w. Sausage, Egg & Cheese	690	49	33

Whataburger® cont... (Feb '10)

Breakfast (Cont)	C	F	Cb
Breakfast On A Bun: w. Bacon	360	21	25
w. Sausage	550	38	25
Breakfast Platter (Biscuit/Eggs/Hash Brown):			
w. Bacon	730	45	93
w. Sausage	920	63	93
Pancakes: Plain (3)	540	7	104
w. Bacon	580	11	104
w. Sausage	780	28	104
Taquito: w. Bacon & Egg	380	21	27
w. Bacon, Egg & Cheese	420	24	27
w. Potato & Egg	430	23	57
w. Potato, Egg & Cheese	470	27	57
w. Sausage & Egg	410	24	27
w. Sausage, Egg & Cheese	450	28	27
Dessert: Hot Apple Pie, 3 oz	230	11	29

White Castle® (Feb '10)

Sandwiches & Burgers	C	F	Cb
Cheeseburger	170	9	15
Double	300	17	23
Whitecastle Hamburger	140	7	14
Double	250	13	22
Sandwiches:			
Chicken Ring with Cheese	200	10	19
Chicken Breast with Cheese	195	7	21
Chicken Supreme	230	10	21
Fish with Cheese	185	8	19
Surf & Turf with Cheese	390	22	28
Sides			
Chicken Rings: 6 rings, 3.9 oz	300	20	17
9 rings, 5.8 oz	460	30	25
Clam Strips, 4 oz	250	22	5
Fish Nibblers, 4.1 oz	280	16	24
French Fries,4.3 oz	355	26	24
Mozzarella Cheese Sticks, 3 sticks	250	14	22
Onion Chips, 4 oz	480	23	62
Onion Rings Homestyle, 3.4 oz	400	21	49
Sauces & Condiments: *Per Packet*			
Ketchup, 0.3 oz	10	0	3
Lemon Juice, 0.1 oz	5	0	0
Mayonnaise, 0.3 oz	70	7	0
Ranch Dressing, 1 oz	150	17	1
Sauce: BBQ, 0.3 oz	15	0	3
Cheese, 1.5 oz	130	10	6
Seafood, 1 oz	30	0	7
White Castle Zesty Zing, 1 oz	120	11	4

Updated Nutrition Data ~ www.CalorieKing.com
Persons with Diabetes ~ See Disclaimer (Page 24)

Winchell's® (Feb '10)

Baked Products	C	F	Cb
Donuts: *Per Donut*			
Cake Donuts, Chocolate Iced	240	10	36
Old Fashioned, Glazed	410	17	60
Jelly Filled:			
Apple with Cinnamon Crumb	450	18	65
Raspberry with Glaze	480	15	78
Strawberry with Sugar	460	15	74
Raised Round: Choc. Iced; Glazed	220	9	31
Sugared	230	9	34

WingStreet (Feb '10)

Chicken	C	F	Cb
Crispy Bone In Wings: *Per 2 Pieces*			
All American, 1.7 oz	170	13	7
Buffalo, Mild/Med./Hot, 2.3 oz	210	13	14
Cajun, 2.3 oz	210	13	15
Garlic Parmesan, 2.3 oz	280	23	8
Bone Out Wings: *Per 2 Pieces*			
All American, 2.15 oz	190	10	11
Buffalo, Mild/Medium, 2.8 oz	220	11	18
Cajun, 2.8 oz	220	10	19
Garlic Parmesan, 2.75 oz	280	20	12
Traditional Wings: *Per 2 Pieces*			
All American, 1.4 oz	80	5	0
Buffalo, Medium/Hot, 2 oz	120	6	7
Cajun, 2 oz	110	6	8
Garlic Parmesan, 2 oz	180	16	1
Sides: Apple Pies, 2 pies, 3.7 oz	360	18	47
Fried Cheese Sticks (4), 3.4 oz	310	19	25
Taters, ½ order, 8 oz	790	52	74

Woody's Bar-B-Q (Feb '10)

Entrees	C	F	Cb
½ Chicken	840	56	0
Baby Back Ribs, ½ Rack, 14 ribs	520	40	2
Beef Prime Rib, 3 oz	230	19	1
Chicken Breast: 1 piece	250	14	4
Spicy Breaded, 1 piece	200	8	14
Chicken Tenders, 2 pieces	190	7	18
Chicken Wings, 2 pieces	210	13	4
Homestyle Meat Loaf, 4 oz	340	26	10
Hot Dog	330	28	8
Pulled Pork, ½ cup	250	19	4
Sausage, 5 pieces	260	16	20
Shrimp, 6 shrimp	180	1	33
Spare Ribs, ½ slab, 4 oz	270	21	0

For Complete Nutritional Data ~ see CalorieKing.com

Yoshinoya® (Feb '10)

Bowls: *Without sauce unless indicated*	C	F	Cb
Beef Bowl®: Regular	685	27	81
Large	970	38	116
Beef Bowl® w/ Vegetables, regular	605	20	84
Beef & Chicken Combo, large	995	30	131
Chicken Bowl: Regular	610	12	94
Large	910	17	140
Chicken Bowl w/ Teriyaki Sce, reg.	740	12	125
Shrimp Bowl: Grilled	505	3	96
with Seafood Sauce	635	3	126
Vegetable Bowl, regular	390	2.5	86
Kids: Beef	350	11	49
Chicken	360	7	53
Soups: Chicken Vegetable	70	1.5	7
Clam Chowder	210	7	34
Miso Soup	60	1.5	8
Salad, Chicken	360	14	14
Garden	50	0	9
Macaroni	350	21	37
Sesame Wings, 6 pieces	420	27	2

Z Pizza® (Feb '10)

Pizzas: *Small 10", Per ⅙ Slice*	C	F	Cb
Berkeley Soy Cheese Veggie	180	8	19
California	150	6	19
Casablanca	190	9	18
Greek	150	6	17
Italian	180	8	17
Mexican	180	7	19
Napoli	180	8	18
Provence	160	7	20
Santa Fe	180	7	20
Thai	170	6	19
Tuscan	160	7	18
ZBQ	170	5	21
Sandwiches: Hot Meatball Sub	670	34	45
Pollo Latino Sandwich	350	11	38
Supersub	460	23	34
Turkey Breast Sandwich	400	14	35
Z-Tuna Sandwich	670	32	68
Calzones: Meat Calzone	770	37	77
Veggie Calzone	750	27	102
Salads: *Small w/o Dressing*			
Arugula	260	20	14
Caesar Side	200	17	8
California	100	6	10
Pear and Gorgonzola Salad	530	44	25
ZBQ Salad	220	11	17

Zaxby's (May '10)

Zappetizers	C	F	Cb
Onion Rings, without Sauce	625	41	55
Spicy Fried Mushroom without Sauce	430	28	37
Tater Chips, 5.6 oz	800	53	76
***Meal Dealz:** Without Sauce or Drink*			
Big Zax Snak	765	34	78
Buffalo Wings	740	39	53
Nibbler with Zac Sauce	1295	66	126
***Most Popular:** As Served*			
Chicken Finger Plate: Regular	1055	50	91
Large	1590	73	147
Wings & Things: Regular	1140	57	80
Sandwich Baskets: I*ncludes Fries*			
Cajun Club	1185	57	107
Zaxby's Club	1215	68	102
***Wings & Fingerz:** As Served*			
Buffalo Chicken Fingerz: 5 pieces	425	20	8
10 pieces	845	40	18
Buffalo Wings: 5 pieces	370	23	0
10 pieces	735	46	1
Boneless Wings w/o Sauce, 5 pieces	390	20	29
Chicken Fingerz, 5 pieces	420	20	8
10 pieces	840	40	17
Zax Kidz:			
Kiddie Cheese, without drink	435	20	55
Kiddie Finger, without drink	390	17	34
***Zalads:** With Texas Toast, w/o Dressing Unless Indicated*			
Blue Zalad: With Blackened Fillet	590	27	36
With Buffalo Fingerz & Sauce	755	39	45
Caesar Zalad:			
With Chicken Fingerz, w/o T. Toast	665	34	31
With Grilled Fillet, without T. Toast	515	23	24
House Zalad: With Grilled Fillet	610	29	35
with Chicken Fingerz	760	40	42
Zensation, without Texas Toast	840	39	77
***Salad Dressings:** Per 1.23 oz Packet*			
Blue Cheese	180	19	2
Honey French	150	12	9
Honey Mustard	150	3	6
Lite Vinaigrette	50	2	7
Mediterranean	140	14	4

Zaxby's Cont... (May '10)

***Salad Dressings(Cont):** Per 1.23 oz Pkt*	C	F	Cb
Ranch	160	16	2
Thousand Island	230	24	3
Sides:			
Celery Basket, 2.6 oz	5	0	2
Cole Slaw, 2.75 oz	115	8	10
Crinkle Fries, 8 oz	590	25	84
Texas Toast, 3 wedges, 1.4 oz	145	6	20

Zero's Subs® (May '10)

Oven Baked 6" Subs: *Includes Wheat Bread and Standard Sides Unless Indicated*	C	F	Cb
BLT	410	19	48
BLT, without Mayo	330	12	43
Cosmo Vegetarian	470	23	46
Cosmo Vegetarian Deluxe	490	25	48
without Cheese, Oil & Vinegar	235	3	47
Grilled Veggie	395	14	52
Grinder	555	31	48
Grinder, Multigrain	560	32	50
without Cheese, Oil & Vinegar	400	18	49
Ham & Cheese	440	19	44
without Cheese, Oil & Vinegar	285	5	43
Hot Italian Sausage	665	37	45
Meatball & Cheese	565	30	50
without Cheese	465	22	50
Pepperoni & Cheese	545	31	42
without Cheese	345	15	41
Philly Chicken & Cheese	400	10	48
without Cheese	320	4	45
with Mushroom & Green Peppers	410	10	49
Philly Steak without Cheese	410	15	46
Philly Steak & Cheese	490	21	48
with Mushroom & Green Peppers	500	21	50
Roast Beef & Cheese	460	19	45
without Cheese, Oil & Vinegar	305	5	45
The Club	515	23	44
without Cheese, Oil & Vinegar	360	10	43
Tuna & Cheese	520	26	47
without Cheese, Oil & Vinegar	365	12	46
Turkey & Cheese	455	17	44
without Cheese, Oil & Vinegar	300	3	43

Updated Nutrition Data ~ www.CalorieKing.com
Persons with Diabetes ~ See Disclaimer (Page 24)

Notes on Cholesterol

- **Cholesterol** is a white waxy substance produced mainly by our liver. It is also found in animal food products. Plant foods have no cholesterol.
- **Cholesterol is essential to life.** It is a structural part of every body cell wall and is the building block for vitamin D, sex hormones, and bile acids which help in the digestion of dietary fats.
- **The body makes sufficient cholesterol** for its needs and does not rely on cholesterol in the diet. Dietary fats have a major influence on blood cholesterol levels - more so than dietary cholesterol.
- **A high blood cholesterol level increases** the risk of atherosclerosis - the thickening of arteries that can reduce or block blood flow to the heart, brain, eyes, kidneys, sex organs and other body parts.

  This in turn increases the risk of heart attack, stroke, blindness, kidney failure, impotence and other blood circulatory problems.

  Other risk factors which increase the risk of atherosclerosis include high blood pressure, smoking, obesity and uncontrolled diabetes.

Heart Attack Warning Signals

Many victims die before reaching the hospital by ignoring warning signals and delaying medical help.

Symptoms vary and commonly include:

- **Chest pain,** vice-like squeezing or burning sensation in center of the chest or between the shoulder blades, or in the mid-back. Pain may even feel like severe indigestion.
- **Pain** may be felt in the arms, shoulders, neck or jaw.
- **Shortness of breath** often occurs with or before chest discomfort.
- **Other signs,** with or without pain, include a cold sweat, nausea or light-headedness.

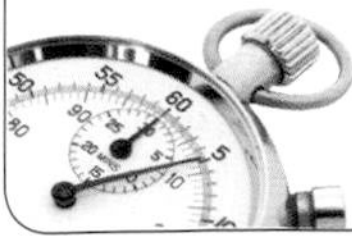

If you experience any of the above symptoms call IMMEDIATELY for medical help. Every minute counts.

***Call 9-1-1** or your emergency number*

Blood Cholesterol

CHECK YOUR RISK!

Total Cholesterol Level (mg/dl) ▼		*Risk of Heart Attack* ▼
240 and above	~	High Risk
200 - 239	~	Borderline/High
Below 200	~	Desirable

- **Know your cholesterol level, particularly if there is a family history of heart disease or stroke. If level is high, see your doctor.**

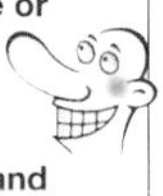

- **All adults should have their cholesterol, HDL and triglycerides tested at least every 5 years.**

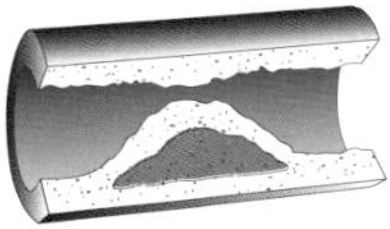

▲ **Atherosclerosis can clog arteries and impede blood flow to the heart or other body organs.**

▼ **A thrombus (blood clot) can form on unstable, festering athero-sclerotic plaque and rapidly block blood flow. A heart attack or stroke can result.**

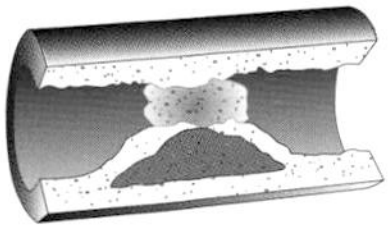

Fats & Cholesterol Guide

The amount and type of dietary fat has the greatest influence on blood cholesterol levels.

Fats in food are a mixture of 3 basic types: saturated, monounsaturated, and polyunsaturated. Animal fats are mainly saturated while plant oils and fish oils are mainly mono- and polyunsaturated.

Saturated fats have subgroups known as long-chain, medium-chain, and short-chain fats. Most of the long chain fats raise blood cholesterol, and increase the risk of blood clots and thrombosis leading to artery blockage.

Long-chain saturated fats are found mainly in full-cream milk, cheese, butter, cream, fatty meats and sausages, and processed foods.

Monounsaturated fats tend to more selectively lower 'bad' LDL cholesterol and maintain the protective 'good' HDL cholesterol in the bloodstream – but only if they replace saturated fats in the diet.

Foods rich in monounsaturates include canola and olive oils, canola margarine, peanuts, and avocados.

Polyunsaturated fats consist of two main classes. **Omega-6** polyunsaturates tend to lower blood cholesterol. Rich sources include safflower, sunflower and corn oils.

Omega-3 polyunsaturated fats can lower blood cholesterol; significantly lower blood triglycerides; and reduce the rise of thrombosis, heart arrythmmia, and artery spasm.

Best practical omega-3 sources include canola oil and margarine, soybean oil and fish.

A balanced intake of the two omega classes is important for optimal health. For most Americans, slightly increasing omega-3 intake would help attain a more ideal balance.

Trans fats from hydrogenated vegetable oils and shortenings should also be avoided. They are common in commercial baked and fried food products such as cakes, muffins, pastries, doughnuts, fried snacks and french fries.

Note: All fats are high in calories and need to be limited for weight control.

DIETARY FATS COMPARISON

■ Saturated Fat ■ Monounsaturated Fat

Polyunsaturated Fats:

□ Linoleic (Omega-6) ■ Alpha-Linolenic (Omega-3)

OILS — **PERCENTAGE CONTENT**

OILS	Saturated Fat	Monounsaturated Fat	Linoleic (Omega-6)	Alpha-Linolenic (Omega-3)
CANOLA OIL	7	63	20	10
LINSEED/FLAX OIL	9	19	17	55
SAFFLOWER OIL	9	14	77	
GRAPESEED OIL	10	22	68	
SUNFLOWER OIL	11	23	66	
CORN OIL	14	32	52	2
OLIVE OIL	14	76	10	
SOYBEAN OIL	15	23	54	8
PEANUT OIL	19	45	34	2
COTTONSEED OIL	26	16	58	
PALM OIL	51	39	10	

SPREADS & FATS

Saturated Fat includes 'Trans Fats' — □ WATER CONTENT

SPREADS & FATS	Saturated Fat	Monounsaturated Fat	Linoleic (Omega-6)	Alpha-Linolenic (Omega-3)	Water Content
LIGHT MARGARINE	14	14	21		51
CANOLA MARGARINE	18	45	12	6	19
POLYUNSATURATED MARG	24	20	36		20
BUTTER	57	18	2		24
LARD	41	47	12		
BEEF FAT	44	37	4		15

GOOD SOURCES OF OMEGA-3 FATS

Plant Sources	Omega-3 Fats (Grams)
Canola Oil, 1 Tbsp, ½ fl.oz	1.5g
Flaxseed Oil, 1 Tbsp	8g
Soybean Oil, 1 Tbsp	1.2g
Canola Margarine, 1 Tbsp, ½ oz	1g
Soybeans, cooked, ½ cup, 4 oz	0.5g
Walnuts, ½ oz	0.5g

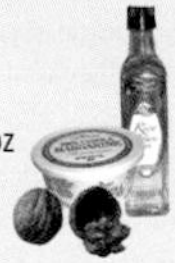

FISH - *Per 4 oz Serving*

High Content: Salmon (Chinook), Tuna,	3g
Trout (Lake), Sardines, Herring, Mackerel	3g
Medium Content:	
Salmon, (Pink/Red/Coho), 4 oz	2g

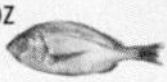

Fair Content: *Per 4 oz Serving*

Bass, Catfish, Cod, Grouper, Hake, Halibut, Kingfish, Perch, Pollock, Shark, Trout (Rainbow), Tuna, Crab, Oysters, Blue Mussels, Shrimp, Squid } **0.5-1g**

How Much Is Needed?

As little as 1-2 grams daily of omega-3 fats may benefit general health. High doses of fish-oil supplements should only be taken as directed by your doctor.

Dietary Cholesterol

Cholesterol in food varies in its effect on blood cholesterol level (BCL) from person to person. Much depends on the amount and type of fat and fiber eaten at the same meal.

Any elevating effect of dietary cholesterol on BCL is more likely to occur when the diet is high in saturated fat. Little elevation, if any, generally occurs when dietary fats are balanced in favor of monounsaturated and polyunsaturated fats (including omega-3 fats).

For example, while fish does contain cholesterol, the omega-3 fats can prevent any increase in BCL. Conversely, a meal containing no cholesterol but rich in saturated fat may result in a significant increase in BCL.

Consequently, the need to be overly-concerned about dietary cholesterol is being de-emphasized in favor of the approach of limiting total fat, saturated fat, and trans fat in particular – and substituting unsaturated fats.

The liver usually cuts back its own cholesterol production in response to cholesterol in the diet. Many people can consume normal amounts of high-cholesterol foods without concern.

However, it is difficult to identify just who is at risk - the so-called 'hyper-responders'. Because over 50% of Americans have a BCL above ideal levels, the **American Heart Association** advises all Americans to be prudent and limit their cholesterol intake to less than 300mg daily, as well as to adopt a heart-healthy diet.

This limitation still allows the inclusion of most foods that are regularly eaten – even the overly-maligned egg.

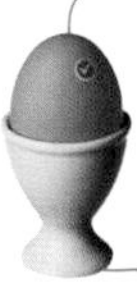

Eggs contain a modest 5 grams of fat per large egg, barely 2 grams of which are saturated, the rest being mono-unsaturated and polyunsaturated.

By comparison, a cup of whole milk has 8g fat of which almost 5g is saturated.

CHOLESTEROL COUNTER

Cholesterol is found only in foods of animal origin. Plant foods contain no cholesterol.
AHA recommends limiting dietary cholesterol to less than 300mg/day.

	Chol mg
Meat - Average all types:	
Lean Meat, cooked, 4 oz	70
Fatty Meat, cooked, 4 oz	105
Fat, thick strip, 2 oz	35

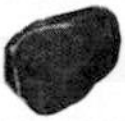

Note: While lean meat and fat have similar amounts of cholesterol, choose lean meat to limit fat intake.

	Chol mg
Chicken/Turkey, average, 4 oz	90
Organ Meats: Liver, fried, 4 oz	500
Brains, beef, pan fried, 3 oz	1700
Sausages: Frankfurter, 1.5 oz	25
Salami, 2 slices, 2 oz	40
Bacon: 3 slices, cooked, 1 oz	20
Fish: Fish fillets, average, ckd, 4 oz	70
Tuna/Salmon, canned, 3 oz	30
Scallops, 9 medium, 3 oz	30
Shrimp, 12 large, raw, 3 oz	130
Oysters, raw, 6 medium, 3 oz	45
Lobster, Crab, raw, 3 oz	80
Eggs (Chicken), 1 large	210
1 medium	180
Egg White, *Egg Beaters*	0
Milk/Yogurt: Whole, 1 cup, 8 fl.oz	35
1% Milk, 1 cup	10
Skim/Non-fat, 1 cup	5
Soy Milk, Tofu, Tempeh	0
Cheese: Natural/Hard/Cream, 1 oz	30
Cottage, lowfat, 4 oz	5
Ricotta, part skim, 4 oz	25
Fats: Butter, 2 Tbsp, 1 oz	60
Margarine, Oils (vegetable)	0
Mayonnaise, 1 Tbsp	10
Cream: Heavy, whipping, 2 T, 1 oz	40
Half & Half/Sour, 2 Tbsp, 1 oz	10
Ice Cream: Regular, ½ cup, 4 fl.oz	30
Fruit, Vegetables, Avocados	0
Nuts, Seeds, Grains	0
Coffee, Tea, Soda, Beer, Wine	0

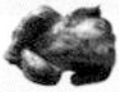

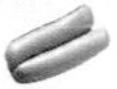

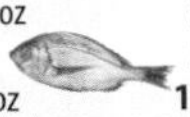

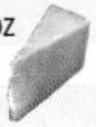

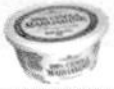

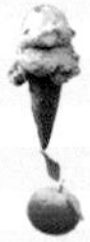

For Comprehensive Food Listings ~ see CalorieKing.com

DIETARY HINTS TO LOWER BLOOD CHOLESTEROL

1. **Maintain a healthy weight.**
If overweight, lose weight with a low-fat meal plan and daily exercise.

2. **Reduce saturated fat intake by:**
(a) eating less dairy fat. Choose low-fat or fat-reduced varieties of milk, yogurt, soy drinks, cheese, and ice cream.
(b) replacing saturated fats with fats and oils rich in monounsaturated and polyunsaturated fats. Choose vegetable oils such as canola, olive, sunflower and soybean. Avoid solid frying fats.

Take Control and *Benecol* (spreads) contain plant stanol esters which can lower total and LDL cholesterol.

(c) eating less fat from meat and poultry. Choose lean cuts of meat and skinless chicken. Go easy on lunch meats, salami and fatty sausages. Enjoy fish.

(d) eating less saturated and trans fats from baked and fried fast-foods. Avoid deep-fried foods. Avoid donuts, cakes, pastries and cookies unless made with healthier fats and oils.

3. **Increase your soluble fiber intake.**
Foods rich in soluble fiber include beans, lentils, chick peas, hummus, nuts, seeds, psyllium-seed husks and psyllium-fiber supplements. Oat bran, rice bran and barley are also good sources, as are fruit, veggies and avocados. (*See Fiber Guide - Page 276-281*).

4. **Eat more soy bean products** such as: soy drinks, tofu, tempeh (cultured soy beans), soy flour and soy vegetarian foods. Soy protein in place of animal protein can significantly decrease high blood cholesterol levels as well as 'bad' LDL cholesterol and blood triglycerides while 'good' HDL cholesterol is maintained. For best results, eat at least 25g of soy protein per day (from 3-4 servings).

5. **Eat more fruit, vegetables, and whole grains** in place of high-fat foods.
Aim for 2 fruits and 5 servings of vegetables per day. They also contain valuable antioxidants.
The fat of avocados (and most nuts) is mainly unsaturated and can lower blood cholesterol levels.

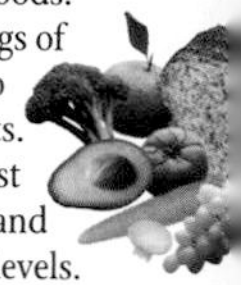

6. **Limit cholesterol to 300mg per day.**
(Extra Notes ~ See Previous Page)

7. **Avoid brewed unfiltered coffee**
(espresso; plunger-style). Several cups per day may raise blood cholesterol. Filtered coffee is fine.

8. **Spread your food intake over the day.**
Have 5-6 small meals per day rather than just 2-3 large meals. Nibbling, versus gorging, favors lower blood cholesterol.

ALCOHOL - WINE

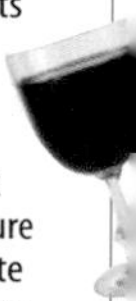

Alcohol is a mixed bag. Moderate amounts of 1-2 drinks daily appear to reduce the risk of heart attack and ischemic stroke in older persons.

However, larger amounts increase the risk of high blood pressure, obesity, heart failure and hemorrhagic stroke, and can aggravate hypertriglyceridemia: as well as many other health hazards. *(See Alcohol Guide – Page 25)*

The speculative benefits of moderate alcohol intake have been overstated in the media. The overriding harmful effects of excess alcohol do not allow its recommendation for any aspects of health promotion.

Fruit, Vegetables & Tea Also Protect:
Red wine and red grapes (more so than white) contain antioxidants which may help protect cholesterol in the blood from becoming oxidized.

Many fruits, vegetables, grains, nuts and tea also contain protective antioxidants.

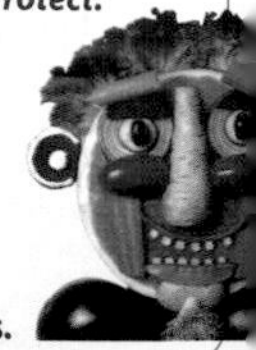

How Fats Affect Blood Flow

Fats in the diet affect more than blood cholesterol levels.They can also strongly influence blood clot formation and thrombosis, as well as blood flow and ultimate oxygen delivery to body parts and organs.

While advanced atherosclerosis can impede blood flow to the heart and other organs, it is thrombosis (complete blockage by blood clots) or arterial spasm which commonly results in a heart attack or stroke.

Plant and fish oils rich in omega-3 fats lessen the risk of blood clots, thrombus formation, and artery spasm by reducing platelet stickiness and adhesion to artery walls. This reduces the risk of atherosclerotic plaque becoming unstable and reactive.

Omega-3 fats also improve blood flow by reducing blood viscosity and increasing the flexibility of red blood cells (RBC) that need to flex and twist on themselves in order to squeeze through tiny narrow capillaries often half their diameter.

A diet high in saturated fats has the opposite effect by stiffening RBC membranes and increasing blood viscosity, thereby hindering blood flow. The stiffening of the RBC membrane also reduces its ability to release vital oxygen to body cells and take up carbon dioxide.

Stiff red blood cells may also form aggregates that resemble coin stacks. In narrow blood vessels, this further impedes blood flow and impairs oxygen release through the much-lessened surface area of red blood cell membranes exposed to blood. (Smoking, lack of exercise, and stress can have similar adverse effects on thrombosis, red blood cell flexibility, and blood flow.)

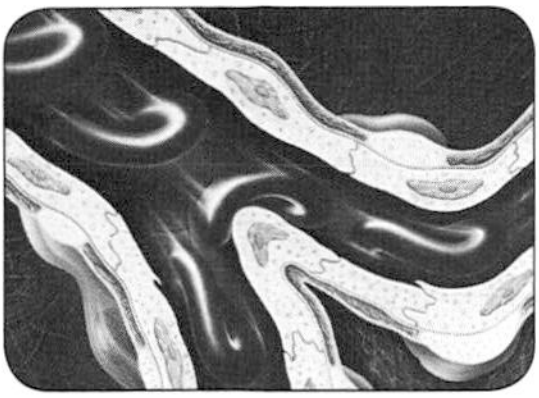

▲ Picture of Healthy Blood Flow

Flexible red blood cells twist and slide through tiny capillaries - often half the diameter of red blood cells.

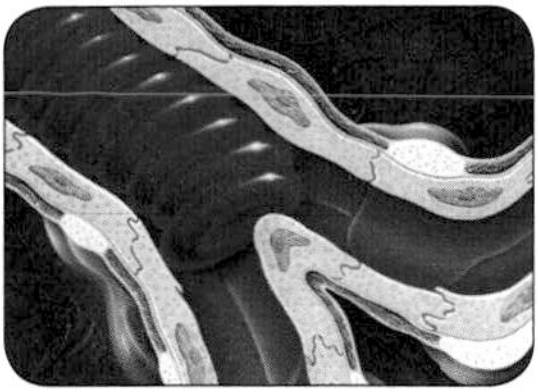

▲ A Not-So-Healthy Picture!

Red blood cells have lost their flexibility and ability to twist and slip through capillaries. They are stacked up, thereby impeding blood flow.

A diet high in saturated fats can contribute to this picture - as can smoking, lack of exercise, and stress.

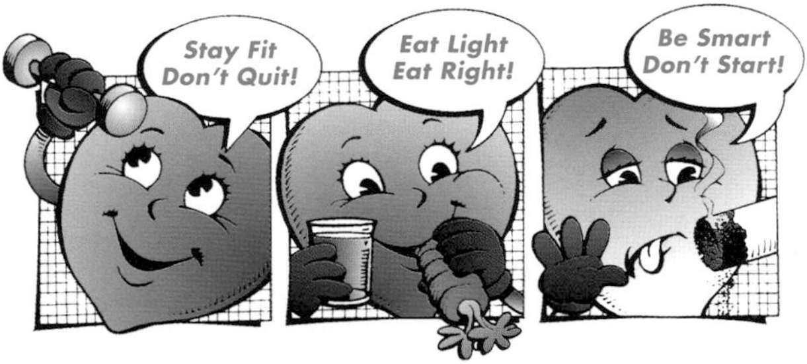

Fiber Guide

Introduction

Fiber is the general term for those parts of **plant** food that we cannot digest (although bacteria in the large bowel partly digests fiber through fermentation). It is not found in foods of animal origin (meats, dairy products).

Fiber promotes intestinal health, bowel regularity, can benefit diabetes and blood cholesterol levels, and may help prevent colon cancer. High-fiber foods also assist weight control.

Most Americans don't eat enough fiber - less than 20 grams/day - instead of a healthier **25 to 35 grams/day.**

Fiber promotes good health, and better control of diabetes and cholesterol.

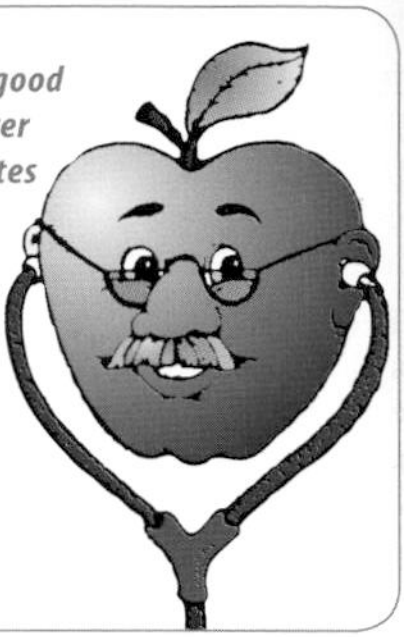

'An apple a day keeps the doctor away.' ... it just might!

Types of Fiber

Plant foods contain a mixture of different fibers in varying proportions. Insoluble and soluble fiber categories are based on their solubility in water. All types of fiber are beneficial to the body.

- **Insoluble fibers** (cellulose, hemi-celluloses, lignin) make up the structural parts of plant cell walls.

  Best food sources are wheat bran, corn bran, rice bran, whole-grain cereals and breads, beans and peas, nuts, seeds, and the skins of fruits and vegetables.

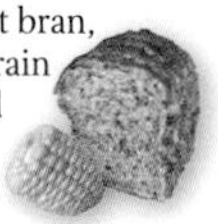

These fibers absorb many times their own weight in water. They create a soft bulk and hasten the passage of waste products through the intestines.

They promote bowel regularity, and aid in the prevention and treatment of uncomplicated forms of **constipation, diverticulosis and hemorrhoids.**

The risk of colon cancer may also be reduced by fiber's diluting effect on potentially harmful substances.

- **Soluble fibers** (pectin, gums, mucilages) are found mainly within plant cells, soy milk (whole bean) and products.

Types of Fiber (Cont)

Best Sources of Soluble Fiber: Fruits and vegetables, oat bran, barley, beans and peas, prunes, psyllium and flax seed.

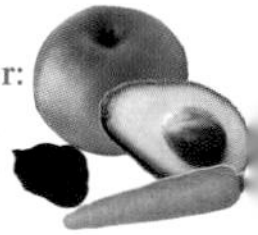

These fibers form a gel which slows both stomach emptying and the absorption of sugars from the intestines. **This helps to control blood sugar levels.**

Weight control is also aided by the slower emptying of the stomach and the feeling of **fullness provided by soluble fiber.**

Some soluble fibers can lower **blood cholesterol** by binding bile acids and excreting them. More body cholesterol must then be broken down to supply bile acids for emulsification of dietary fats. **Rice bran, while not high in soluble fiber, can also lower blood cholesterol.**

- **Resistant starch** is that part of starchy foods (approx. 10%) which is tightly bound by fiber and resists normal digestion. Friendly bacteria in the large bowel ferment and change the resistant starch into short-chain fatty acids, which are important to bowel health and may protect against colon cancer.

Starchy foods include bread, cereals, rice, pasta, potatoes and legumes.

Fiber & Weight Control

Fiber can assist weight control in several ways. Fiber-rich foods such as fresh fruit and vegetables, potatoes and whole-grain bread contain few calories for their large volume (due to their low-fat, high-water content).

Their bulk fills the stomach and satisfies the appetite much sooner than fiber-depleted foods. The extra chewing time also contributes to satiety, and gives the stomach time to register a feeling of fullness. Excessive calories are less likely to be consumed.

Fiber-depleted foods and drinks are more concentrated in calories; e.g. fats, sugar, candy, soft drinks, fruit juices, alcohol. They require little or no chewing. Large amounts with excessive calories can be consumed before the appetite is satisfied.

Example: Whereas one fresh apple might satisfy the appetite, an apple juice drink with the equivalent sugars and calories of 2-3 apples only minimally satisfies the appetite. (See illustration below.)

High-fiber foods fill the stomach. Fewer calories are consumed.

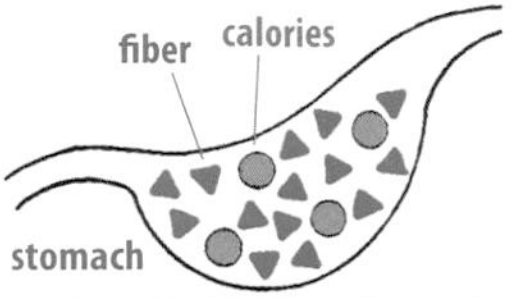

Low-fiber foods are more concentrated in calories. More food must be eaten to fill the stomach.

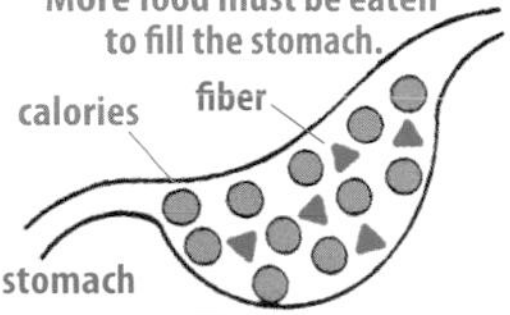

EFFECTS OF REMOVING FIBER FROM FOOD

2-3 pieces of fresh fruit produces 1 glass of fruit juice. The removal of fiber concentrates the sugar and calories.

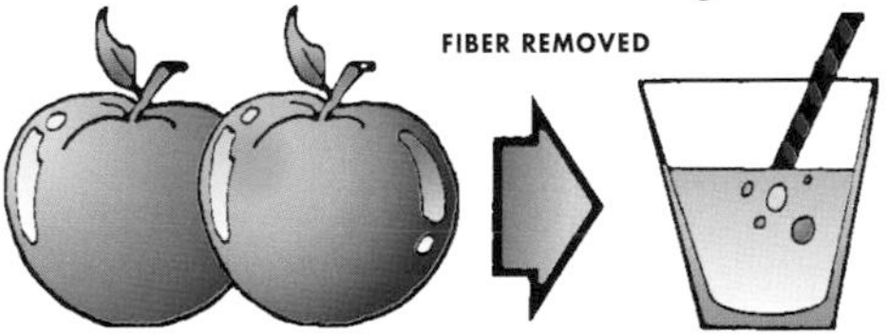

Fresh Fruit		Fruit Juice
High Fiber	↔	Negligible Fiber
Low Calorie Density	↔	High Calorie Density
Long Eating Time	↔	No Eating Time (Drink)
Satisfies Hunger	↔	Does Not Satisfy Hunger
Sugar Slowly Absorbed	↔	Sugar More Quickly Absorbed
Less Insulin Required	↔	More Insulin Required

Constipation

Constipation can reasonably be defined as a failure to have a bowel movement at least every second day – and just as importantly, without straining or pain.

Typically, constipated stools are too hard, too narrow and too small.

The **main cause** is simply a lack of dietary fiber. Other contributing factors include insufficient fluids, too little exercise, emotional stress, gastrointestinal disease, lack of proper dentition to chew high-fiber foods, and some medications (e.g. some antacids, antidepressants, pain medications).

Note: Check with your doctor to rule out any underlying medical problem – especially if you have a change in bowel habits in middle-age or later years.

DESIRABLE FIBER INTAKE

Adults: 25-35gm per day
Children (under 18): Age + 5gm
Example: 6-year old (6 + 5)= 11gm

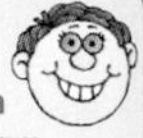

SAMPLE FOOD QUANTITIES

For 35 Grams of Fiber/Day

		Fiber
	Breakfast Cereal (higher-fiber)	5g
plus	4 slices whole-grain Bread	6g
plus	3 servings fresh Fruit	9g
plus	1 medium Potato (w. skin)	4g
or	1 cup Brown Rice	
or	½ cup whole-grain Pasta	
plus	3-4 servings Veggies/Salad	6g
plus	1 cup Bean Soup	5g
or	¼ cup Baked/Soy Beans	
or	½ cup Corn/Peas/Lentils	
or	1¼ oz Almonds (natural)	
or	3 medium Figs	

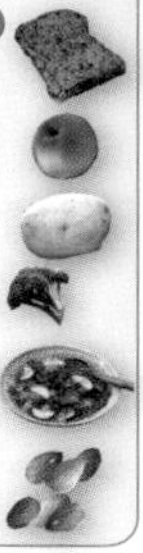

HINTS TO INCREASE FIBER AND AVOID CONSTIPATION

1. **Breakfast is an important** contributor to daily fiber intake. Eat high-fiber breakfast cereals (bran-based cereals, oatmeal etc.). Add 1-2 tablespoons of unprocessed bran.

   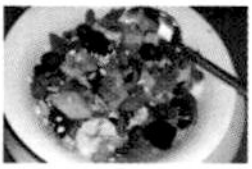

   Dried fruits, chopped nuts, soy grits, and seeds are also excellent additions to cereals.

   Note: **A gradual increase in fiber will prevent bloating, gas or pain. People intolerant to bran may benefit from psyllium-based fiber supplements and cereals.**

2. **Drink adequate water daily.** Fiber works by absorbing many times its own weight in water.

3. **Eat whole-grain breads,** or fiber-enriched breads. They have over double the fiber of regular white bread.

   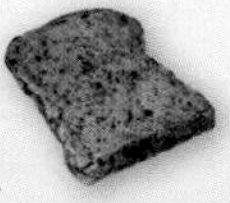

4. **Enjoy fruit as fresh fruit** with skin rather than as fruit juice. Enjoy whole-grain pasta, barley, brown rice, nuts and seeds.

5. **Eat more vegetables,** salads and legumes – especially cooked beans, lentils, potatoes with skins, avocado, broccoli, brussels sprouts, cabbage, carrots, celery, and peas.

   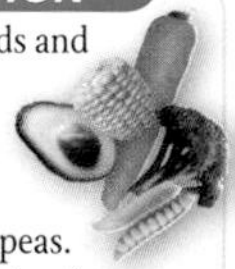

6. **Add bran** (barley/rice/wheat) or soy grits to soups, casseroles, yogurt, desserts, cookies, cakes. Also use whole-meal flour or soy flour in place of white flour. Use nuts, seeds, and ground linseed.

7. **Snack** on fresh or dried fruits, carrot or celery sticks, popcorn, nuts or seeds, whole-grain crackers, high-fiber bars (low-fat). Limit amounts if overweight.

8. **Exercise regularly** to strengthen abdominal muscles and stimulate the gut. Keep up water intake, especially in warm weather.

9. **Avoid** indiscriminate and regular use of harsh laxatives. They can overstimulate the intestinal muscles and may make normal bowel activity impossible. It may take several weeks to restore normal bowel function.

FOODS WITH ZERO FIBER

- **Dairy Products (Milk, Cheese, etc)**
- **Meats, Poultry, Fish, Eggs**
- **Fats/Oils, Sugar/Syrups**

(Only foods of plant origin contain fiber.)

Breakfast Cereals

	Fiber
General Mills:	
Basic 4, 1 cup, 2 oz	3
Cheerios (Honey Nut; Multigrain), 1 c., 1 oz	3
Multi-Bran Chex, 1 cup, 2 oz	7
Oatmeal Crisp Almond, 1 cup, 2 oz	4
Raisin Nut Bran, 1¼ cup, 2 oz	5
Total, average all types, ¾ cup, 1 oz	3
Wheat Chex, 1 cup, 2 oz	5
Wheaties ¾ cup, 1 oz	3
Health Valley:	
Amaranth Flakes, ¾ cup, 1 oz	4
Crunches & Flakes, ¾ cup, 1.9 oz	4
Fiber 7 Flakes, ¾ cup, 1 oz	4
Golden Flax, ¾ cup, 1.9 oz	6
Granola (Low-Fat),⅔ cup, 2 oz	6
Healthy Fiber Flakes, ¾ cup, 1.1 oz	4
Oat Bran Flakes, all types, ¾ cup, 1 oz	3
Oat Bran O's, ¾ cup, 1 oz	3
Real Oat Bran, ½ cup, 1.7 oz	5
Kellogg's: All-Bran, ½ cup, 1.1 oz	10
All-Bran w. Extra Fiber, ½ cup, 1 oz	13
All-Bran Bran Buds, ⅓ cup, 1.1 oz	13
Corn Flakes, Fruit Loops, Smacks 1 cup, 1 oz	1
Cocoa/Rice Krispies Treats, 1¼ cup, 1 oz	0
Complete: Wheat Bran Flakes, ¾ c., 1 oz	5
Oat Bran Flakes, ¾ cup, 1.1 oz	4
Corn Pops, 1 cup, 1.1 oz	0.5
Cracklin' Oat Bran, ¾ cup, 1.7oz	6
Frosted Mini Wheats, 24 bisc., 2 oz	5
Granola w. Raisins, ⅔ cup, 2.1 oz	3
Nutri-Grain Cereal Bars, 1 bar, 1.3 oz	1
Raisin Bran, 1 cup, 2.1 oz	7
Smart Start, Strong Heart, Cinnamon Raisin, 1 cup, 1.8 oz	4
Special K, 1 cup, 1.1 oz	0.5

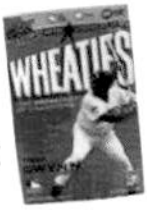

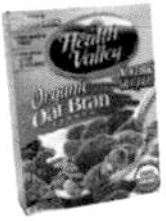

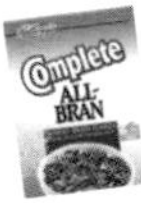

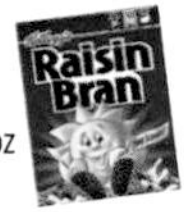

Fiber ~ Fiber (grams)

Breakfast Cereals (Cont)

	Fiber
Kashi: GoLEAN Cereal, 1 cup, 1.8 oz	10
GoLEAN Crunch!, 1 cup, 1.9 oz	8
GoLEAN Bars, avg. (1)	4
Good Friends: Original, 1 cup, 1.9 oz	12
Cinna-Raisin Crunch, 1 cup, 1.8 oz	8
Heart to Heart, ¾ cup, 1.2 oz	5
7 Whole Grain Pilaf, ½ cup, cooked, 5 oz	6
7 Whole Grain Puffs, 1 cup, 0.7 oz	1
Quaker: Cap'n Crunch, ¾ cup, 1 oz	1
100% Natural Granola, avg., ½ cup, 1.8 oz	3
Crunchy Corn Bran, 1 cup, 1 oz	5
Life Cereal, ¾ cup, 1.1 oz	2
Oat Bran, ½ cup, 1.4 oz	6
Oatmeal, average, 1 packet	3
Post: 100% Bran, ⅓ cup, 1 oz	9
Alpha Bits, 1 cup, 1 oz	3
Blueberry Morning, 1 cup, 1.9 oz	2
Cocoa/Fruity Pebbles, 1 cup, 1 oz	3
Cranberry Almond Crunch, 1 cup, 1.8 oz	3
Fruit & Bran, 1 cup, 1.9 oz	6
Grape-Nuts, ½ cup, 2 oz	6
Great Grains, ⅔ cup, 1.9 oz	4
Honey Bunches of Oats, ¾ cup, 1.1 oz	2
Shredded Wheat & Bran, ½ cup, 2 oz	6

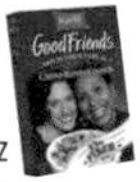

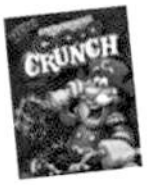

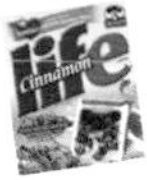

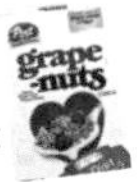

Brans & Supplements, Metamucil

Oat Bran: 1 Tbsp (level)	1
⅓ cup, (5⅓ Tbsp), 1 oz	5
Rice Bran, raw. ¼ cup, 1 oz	6
Wheat Bran (unprocessed):	
Raw, 1 Tbsp	1.5
2 Tbsp (level), ¼ oz	3
¼ cup, (4 Tbsp), ½ oz	6
Wheat Germ: Raw, ¼ cup, 1 oz	4
Psyllium Seed Husks, 2 Tbsp	8
Fibersure, 1 heaping tsp	5
Metamucil: Orange, 1 rnd Tbsp, 11g	3
Fiber Wafers (2)	6

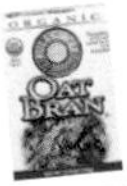

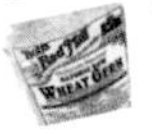

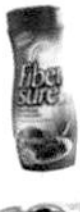

Hot Cereals, Oatmeal

Bulgur (cracked Wheat), ckd, 1 cup	8
Corn/Hominy Grits, dry, 3 Tbsp, 1 oz	0.5
Cream of Wheat, cooked, ¾ cup	1
Oatmeal (uncooked ⅓ cup), ckd, ⅔ cup	3

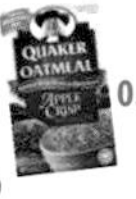

Fiber Guide

Breads & Crackers

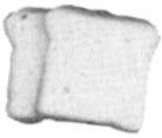

	Fiber
Bread: White, 1 slice, 1 oz	0.6
Whole-wheat, 1 slice, 1 oz	1.5
Whole-grain, 1 slice, 1 oz	2
Rye, Pumpernickel, 1 oz	1.5
Bagel/Roll/Bun, 1 medium, 2 oz	1.5
Pita, whole wheat, 6½" pocket	4.5
Crackers: Graham, average, 2	0.4
Saltine, 4 crackers	0.4
Crispbreads (Rye), average, 2	4
Matzo 1 board, 1 oz	1
Rice Cakes, average, 1 cake	0.3
Tortilla: Regular, 6"	0.5
Whole-wheat, 6"	1.3

Barley, Pasta, Rice & Flours

Barley, pearled, raw, ¼ cup, 1.7 oz	8
Rice: White, cooked, 1 cup	0.6
Brown, cooked, 1 cup	3.5
Rice-A-Roni, average, 1 cup, prepared	1.5
Spaghetti/Noodles: Cooked, 1 cup	2
Whole-Wheat, cooked, 1 cup	4
Flour: Wheat, All-purpose, 1 cup, 4½ oz	3.5
Whole-Wheat, 1 cup, 4½ oz	15
Cornmeal, stone ground, 1 cup, 4½ oz	13
Carob Flour, 1 cup, 3½ oz	41
Rye Flour, 1 cup, 3½ oz	15
Soy Flour: Defatted, 1 cup, 3½ oz	17
Full-fat, raw, 1 cup, 3 oz	8
Soy Meal, defatted, 1 cup, 4½ oz	14

Frozen Entrees & Dinners

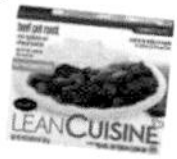

Average All Brands: *Per Serving*	
Beans/Chili base, average	6-10
Potato/Pasta base, average	4-6
Vegetable base, average	3
Meat/Chicken base, average	2-3
Pizzas, ¼ large, average	3
Vegetarian Soy Burgers, 1 pattie	4

Soups

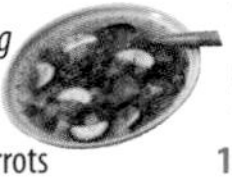

Chicken Noodle, 1 cup	0.5
Tomato Soup, average, 1 cup	0.5
Vegetable Soup, average, 1 cup	3
Health Valley: *Per 1 Cup Serving*	
Black Bean; Minestrone	8
Tomato	1
5-Bean Vegetable; Lentil & Carrots	10
Mushroom Barley; Vegetable	4
Split Pea	8

Fast Foods & Restaurants

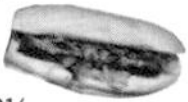
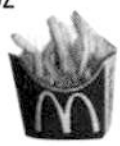
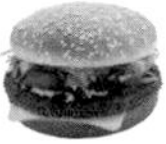
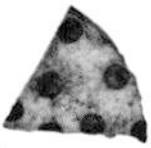
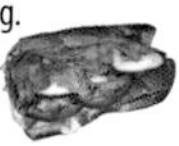

	Fiber
Hamburgers: Small, average	1.5
Large/Whopper, average	2.5
Hot Dog, Regular	1.5
French Fries: Small serving, 2½ oz	2.5
Regular/Medium, 3½ oz	3.5
Chicken Nuggets, 6 pack	0.5
Chicken Sandwich, average	2
Taco, average	4
Sundaes, Shakes, Soft Drinks	0
Arby's: Baked Potato w. Broc. & Cheese	8
Roast Beef Sandwich, regular	2
Denny's: Grilled Chicken Salad, no bread	4
Classic Burger, no fries	4
Club Sandwich, no fries	2
Grilled Chicken Sandwich, no fries	4
Domino's **(12"):** Classic/Thin, 1 slice	1
Deep Dish, 1 slice	3
Feast Pizza, Classic/Thin, 1 slice	2
McDonald's: Big Mac	3
Hamburger; Quarter Pounder	1
Egg McMuffin	2
Grilled Chicken Caesar Salad	3
Pizza Hut: *Per 1 Slice, Medium*	
Pan Pizza: Cheese, Pepperoni	1
Supreme	2
Thin 'n Crispy, Supreme	2
Hand-Tossed, average all varieties	2
Subway: Sandwich, white roll, avg.	4
w. Honey Wheat Roll, average	3.2
Footlong w. Wheat Roll, average	8
Salads, average	4

Cakes, Cookies, Snack Bars

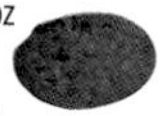
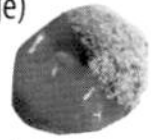
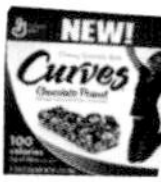

Apple/Fruit Pie, 1 serving, 4 oz	2
Cake: w. plain flour, 1 serving, 3.4 oz	1.5
w. whole-wheat flour, 1 serving	3
Carrot Cake, 1 serving, 1.2 oz	2
Cookies, oatmeal, (3 small/1 large)	1
Donuts, Medium, 1.7 oz	0.7
Fruit Cake, 1 serving, 1½ oz	2
Fig Bars, 1 cookie, ½ oz	0.7
Muffins, Oat Bran (2 small, 1 large), 4 oz	5
Granola Bars, average, 1 bar	2
Atkins Advantage Bars, average	7
Clif Bars, 2.5 oz	5
Curves, Chocolate Peanut Bar, 25g	5
Fi-Bar Chewy & Nutty 1 bar	1
Health Valley: Fruit/Granola Bars	3
Cereal Bars	1
Luna Bars, avg., 1.7 oz	3
Special K, Protein Meal Bar, 1.6 oz	5

Chocolate, Chips, Popcorn

	Fiber
Cheese Balls/Curls/Twists	1
Chocolate, Hard Candy, 1 oz	0
Chocolate with nuts/fruit, 2 oz bar	1.5
Mars Bar, 1.8 oz	1
Potato Chips, corn chips, 1 oz	1
Popcorn, 3 cups	3
Pretzels, Twists (6)	1

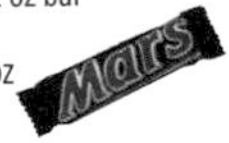

Nuts, Seeds

	Fiber
Almonds: Natural, 25 nuts, 1 oz	3.5
Blanched (skins removed), 1 oz	3
Cashews, Filberts, Pecans, 1 oz	1.7
Peanuts, Mixed Nuts, Coconut, 1 oz	2.5
Peanut Butter, 2 Tbsp, 1 oz	2
Pistachio Nuts, dried, shelled, 1 oz	3
Walnuts, Black/English, dried, 1 oz	2
Seeds: Amaranth, 2½ Tbsp, 1 oz	3.5
Flax Seeds, 3 Tbsp, 1 oz	7
Psyllium Seed Husks, 5 Tbsp, 1 oz	20
Quinoa Seeds, 3 Tbsp, 1 oz	1.7
Sesame Seeds, whole, 1 oz	3.4
Sesame Butter/Tahini, 2 Tbsp, 1.1 oz	1.4
Sunflower kernels, ¼ cup, 1 oz	3.8
Teff Seeds, 1 oz	3.8

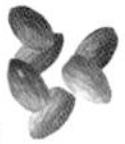
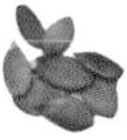

Fruit – Fresh

	Fiber
Apples: 1 medium, 5½ oz (whole)	
with skin + core	3.7
with skin, no core	3.2
without skin, no core	1.7
Apricots, 2 medium, 4 oz	1.5
Avocado, average, ½ medium	6.7
Banana, 1 medium, 6 oz (w. skin)	3
Blueberries, raw, ½ cup, 2½ oz	1.7
Cherries, sweet, raw, 8 fruits, 1.6 oz	1
Grapefruit, average, ½ fruit, 10 oz	1.4
Grapes, 1 medium bunch, seedless, 7 oz	2
Kiwifruit, 1 medium, 2.7 oz	2.3
Mango, 1 medium, 11 oz (whole)	1.6
Melons, Cantaloupe, 4 oz (edible)	1
Nectarine, 1 medium, 4 oz	1.9
Olives, average all types, 7 jumbo, 2 oz	1.5
Oranges, 1 medium (7-8 oz w. skin)	
5½ oz (peeled)	3.8
Passionfruit, 2 medium, 2½ oz	5
Peaches, 1 large, 6 oz	2
Pears, raw, 1 medium, 6 oz	4.5
Pineapple, 1 slice, 3 oz	1.2
Plums, 2 medium, 6 oz	1.8
Strawberries, 6 medium/3 large, 2 oz	1
Watermelon, 4 oz (edible)	0.5

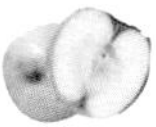
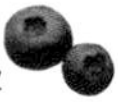
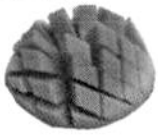
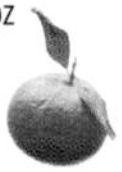
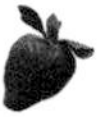

Fruit – Dried, Juice

	Fiber
Dried Fruit: Apricots, 8 halves, 1 oz	2.2
Dates (3 med); Raisins (2 Tbsp), 1 oz	1.5
Figs, 3 medium, 1½ oz	5
Prunes, 4 medium, 1 oz	2
Fruit Juice: Orange/Apple etc, 1 glass	<0.5
Prune Juice, 5 oz	1.4
Carrot Juice, 8 oz	1.8

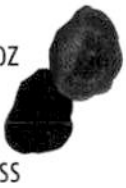

Vegetables

	Fiber
Asparagus, 4 medium spears	1.3
Bean Sprouts, ½ cup, 2 oz	1
Beans: Snap/Green, ½ cup, 2 oz	2
Baked Beans in Tom Sce, ½ c, 4½ oz	5
Dried Beans, ckd, average, ½ cup	7
Beets, ckd, slices, ½ cup, 3 oz	1.7
Broccoli, cooked, ½ cup, 3 oz	2.4
Brussels Sprouts, ckd, ½ cup, 3 oz	3.5
Cabbage: White, ckd, ½ cup, 2½ oz	1
Red, ckd, ½ cup, 2½ oz	2
Carrots, 1 medium (7½"), ½ cup, 3 oz	2.5
Cauliflower, cooked, 3 flowerets, 2 oz	1.5
Celery, raw, diced, 1 cup, 3½ oz	1.6
Chick Peas (Garbanzos), ckd, ½ c., 3 oz	6.5
Corn, kernels, ckd, ½ cup, 2½ oz	2.5
Cream-style, ½ cup, 4½ oz	1.5
Cucumber/Lettuce/Mushrooms, 2 oz	0.5
Eggplant, raw, sliced, ½ cup, 1½ oz	2
Lentils, cooked, ½ cup, 3½ oz	8
Mixed Vegetables, frozen, cooked, ½ cup	3
Onions, Raw, 1 medium, 4 oz	1.5
Spring Onions, chop., ¼ cup, 1 oz	0.7
Peas: Green, Raw, 2½ oz	3.7
Cowpeas (Black-eyed), ckd, ½ cup	10
Split Peas, ckd, ½ cup, 3½ oz	8
Peppers, sweet, raw, 1 large, 6 oz	3
Potatoes: 1 medium, with skin, 5 oz	4
without skin	2.5
½ cup mashed, 3½ oz	1.5
French Fries, small, 2.6 oz	3
Spinach, cooked, ½ cup, 3 oz	2.2
Squash: Summer, cooked, ½ cup, 3 oz	2.5
Winter, cooked, ½ cup, 3½ oz	2.4
Tomatoes: 1 medium, 4½ oz	1.5
Tomato Sauce, 1 cup	0.3
Soybean Products: Miso, ½ c., 5 oz	7.4
Tempeh, cooked, 1 piece, 3 oz	2
Tofu, ½ cup, 4.4 oz	0.4
Salads: Side Salad, average	1
Bean Salad, ½ cup	5
Coleslaw, ½ cup	1
Potato Salad, ½ cup	2

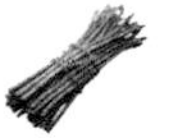
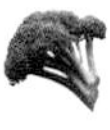
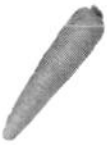
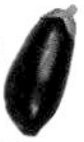
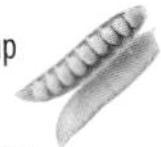
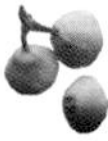
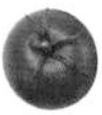

Protein Guide

General Notes

- **Protein has many important body functions.** It builds and repairs muscle, and is the basis of our body's organs, hormones, enzymes, and antibodies to fight infection.
- **Protein is also an emergency fuel** in the absence of sufficient carbohydrate and fats. For this reason, weight loss should be gradual so as to preserve protein levels in muscle, the heart and other body organs.
- **It is easy to obtain sufficient protein,** even if vegetarian. **Plant proteins are not inferior to animal proteins.** In fact, eating more soy and other plant proteins, and less animal protein, may help to build stronger bones and prevent osteoporosis, and may help to control blood cholesterol levels.
- **When changing to a vegetarian diet,** include soybeans, and other beans, soy milk drinks (calcium-enriched), lentils, tofu, tempeh, nuts and whole-grain breads and cereals. Milk, yogurt, cheese and eggs can enhance nutrient intake.

Protein & Muscle

- Although muscles are built of protein, protein is not a special fuel for working muscle cells – carbohydrates and fats are.
- In fact, a diet high in protein (and fat) and low in carbohydrate can significantly reduce the performance of endurance sports athletes. **Carbohydrates** are the best fuel for muscles exercised for long periods.
- Any **extra protein** required by athletes and body-builders can easily be obtained from the extra food eaten to satisfy hunger and energy needs.
- Remember, **excessive protein** intake will not build bigger muscles. Any excess is converted and stored as fat. Excess protein can also strain the kidneys, which excrete the waste products of protein metabolism.

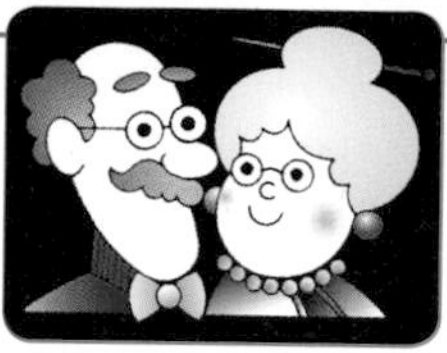

Elderly people (and dieters) must eat sufficient food to ensure adequate protein intake.

Inadequate protein leads to a drop in immune response with greater susceptibility to illness and infections. Muscle strength and muscle mass also drop.

Protein needs are easily met with sensible eating. Athletes who eat enough food for their energy needs can obtain sufficient protein.

RECOMMENDED DAILY PROTEIN INTAKE ~ HEALTHY RANGE ~

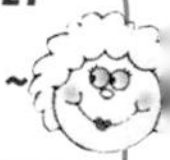

(Lower figure is RDA)

		PROTEIN
Children:	1-3 yrs	13g-26g
	4-8 yrs	19g-38g
	9-13 yrs	34g-64g
Males:	14-18 yrs	52g-120g
	19+	56g-120g
Females:	14+	46g-110g
Pregnancy:		71g-120g
Breastfeeding:		71g-120g

Note: On lower-calorie diets, aim for higher amounts of protein within the Healthy Range.

Iron & Anemia Guide

- **Iron deficiency** is one of the most common nutritional deficiencies in women. The risk is increased in dieters who do not eat well-balanced meals. Chronic shortage of iron leads to anemia.
- **Women** between 11 and 50 years of age are at greater risk because of the monthly loss of menstrual blood. Pregnancy, growth, and endurance sports also demand extra iron.
- **In red blood cells**, iron combines with protein to form **hemoglobin** – the red pigment which carries oxygen in the blood. A lack of iron limits the production of hemoglobin and consequently the amount of vital oxygen delivered to body cells.

Note: A blood test will tell you if your Hb and Iron stores (ferritin) are adequate. (Iron stores can be low even when Hb is normal.)

- **Vitamin C** (in fruits/veggies/salads) enhances absorption of 'non-heme' iron in bread, cereals, milk, vegetables, nuts, eggs and iron supplements. Small amounts of meat, fish or poultry also help. (They contain 'heme' iron).
- **Iron absorption is lessened** by up to 60% when high calcium foods are consumed with iron-rich main meals. Tea, coffee, phytates (in bran) and oxalates lessen absorption of non-heme iron.
- **For infants to 1 year**, use iron-fortified milk/soy formula if not breast-feeding. Introduce iron-fortified baby cereals at 4-6 months.

Note: Iron deficiency in children (even without anemia), can result in lethargy, irritability, repeated infections, and developmental problems.

Iron Supplements

- **Most people** can obtain adequate iron from their diet. **A wide variety** of animal and plant foods contain iron. (See Iron Counter)
- **Iron supplements** are only recommended for women with heavy menstrual blood losses or during pregnancy (if tests show a low-iron status), endurance athletes with low blood ferritin (iron stores) and for persons with diagnosed anemia. Check with your doctor.
- While the 5 mg of iron in multi-vitamin/mineral supplements is safe for most people, large amounts can be toxic, (especially for persons with hemochromatosis iron-overload condition).

ANEMIA SYMPTOMS

Anemia reduces the amount of oxygen carried in the blood. The body tissues become starved of oxygen. Symptoms include:

- **Pale skin; brittle fingernails (may turn up into spoon shape)**
- **Excessive tiredness or fatigue**
- **Breathlessness**
- **Feeling of malaise and irritability**
- **Always feel cold**
- **Decrease in attention span**

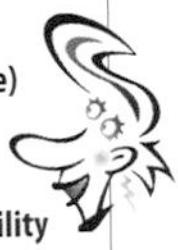

Note: Other medical conditions may also cause similar symptoms. Check with your doctor.

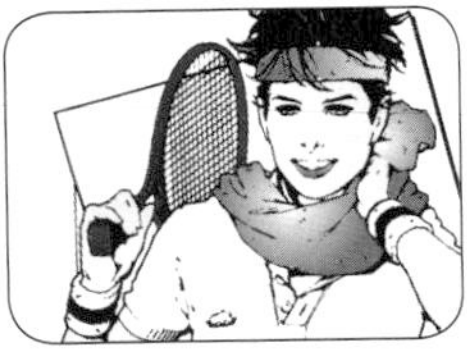

A nutritious diet with adequate iron is important - particularly for women and athletes.

RECOMMENDED DAILY IRON INTAKE (mg)

			Iron
Infants (0-6 mths):			
	Breast-fed	~	**0.5mg**
	Bottle-fed	~	**3mg**
	6-12 mths	~	**11mg**
Children:	1-11 yrs	~	**7-10mg**
Males:	12-18 yrs	~	**11mg**
	19+ yrs	~	**8mg**
Females:	12-18 yrs	~	**15mg**
	19-50 yrs	~	**18mg**
	51+ yrs	~	**8mg**
	Pregnancy	~	**27mg**
	Breast-feeding	~	**12-16mg**

Protein & Iron Counter

Pro ~ Protein (grams)

Iron ~ Iron (mg)

Meat

	Pro	Iron
Steak: Average all cuts, lean (no fat)		
Small (4 oz raw/3 oz ckd)	23	2.3
Medium (6 oz raw/4¼ oz ckd)	34	3.4
Large (10 oz raw/7¼ oz ckd)	57	5.7
Roast Beef, lean, 2 slices, 3 oz	24	2.5
Ground Beef patty, lean, ckd, 3 oz	21	2
Lamb chop, broiled, 3 oz	22	1.5
Liver, cooked, 3 oz	23	5.5
Veal cutlet, 1 medium	23	1
Pork, cooked, lean, 3 oz	24	1
Bacon, 3 medium slices	6	0.3
Ham, roasted, 2 pieces, 3 oz	18	1
Ham, luncheon, 2 slices, 1½ oz	7	0.3
Pastrami *(Oscar Mayer)*, 3 sl., 1¾ oz	10	1.3
Sausages: Bologna, 2 sl., 2 oz	7	1
Braunschweiger, 2 sl., 2 oz	8	5.3
Pork link, thick, 2 oz	6	0.5
Frankfurter, 1⅓ oz	5	0.5
Salami, hard, 3 slices, 1 oz	7	0.5
Vegetarian *(Boca Burger)*, 1 pattie	13	2

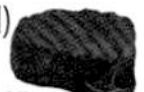
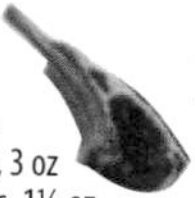
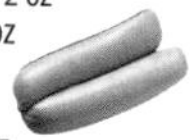

Chicken/Turkey *(Without Skin)*

	Pro	Iron
Chicken, ckd; Breast, Roasted, 4 oz	36	1.5
Leg/Thigh,Roasted, 2 oz	14	0.5
½ Whole Chicken	60	2.5
Drumstick, Rstd, 1 med., 3 oz	13	0.5
Turkey, cooked: Light meat, 3 oz	28	2
Dark meat, lean, 3 oz	24	2

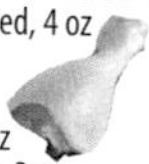

Fish

	Pro	Iron
Fresh Fish: *Per 4 oz, cooked*		
Cod, Flounder/Sole, Pollock	28	0.5
Catfish, Haddock, Halibut, M/Mahi	28	1.3
Ocean Perch, Swordf., Orange Roughy	28	1.3
Canned Fish: Tuna, Light, 3 oz	25	1.5
White, 3 oz	23	0.5
Salmon, pink, 3 oz	17	0.7
Salmon, red, 3 oz	17	1
Sardines, 3 whole (3"), 1¼ oz	9	1
Anchovies, 1 can, 1½ oz	13	2
Shellfish: Crabmeat, 3 oz	17.5	0.7
Clams, raw, 4 large/9 sml, 3 oz	11	12
Crayfish, cooked, 3 oz	20	2.7
Lobster, cooked, 3 oz	17	0.5
Oysters, raw, 6 medium, 3 oz	7	5
Scallops, 2 lge/5 small, 1 oz	5	0
Shrimp, raw, 6 large, 1½ oz	8.5	1
Fish Products: Fish Sticks, 4 sticks	10	0.5
Fish Portions, in batter, 4 oz	13	0.6
Gefilte Fish, 1 medium ball, 2 oz	8	1

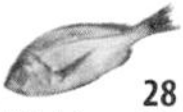
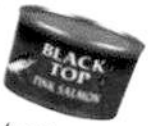

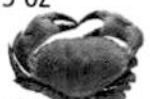
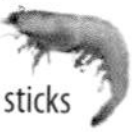

Eggs

	Pro	Iron
1 Large Egg, whole	6	0.7
Egg Yolk	3	0.7
Egg White	3	0
Omelet: Plain, 2 eggs	13	1.7
Ham & cheese	17	3
Egg Substitutes (liquid):		
Egg Beaters, ¼ cup, 2 oz	4.5	1
Better 'n Eggs/Scramblers, ¼ cup, 2 oz	6	0.7

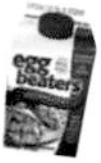

Milk, Yogurt, Ice Cream

	Pro	Iron
Milk: Whole: 2%, 1 cup	8	0
Low-Fat (1%); Fat-Free, 1 cup	8.5	0
Chocolate Milk, 1 cup	8	0.6
Thick Shake, Chocolate, 10 oz	9	1
Vanilla, 10 oz	11	0.3
Soymilk (fortified), average, 1 cup	7	1
Soy Dream Enriched, shelf-stable, 1 cup	7	8
Yogurt: Plain, 6 oz	10	0
Fruit flavors: 6 oz	8	0.3
8 oz	11	0.5
Ice Cream: Rich, ½ cup	2	0
Regular, Vanilla, ½ cup	2.5	0
Sherbet, ½ cup	1	0
Custard, baked, ½ cup	7	0.5

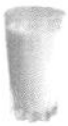
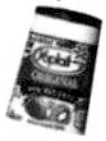
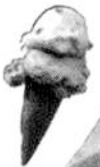

Cheese

	Pro	Iron
Hard Cheeses, average, 1 oz	7	0.2
Cottage Cheese, ½ cup	13	0.3
Cream Cheese, avg., 1 oz	2	0.3
Ricotta, part skim, ½ cup	14	1

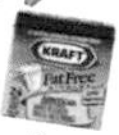

Bread, Bagels, Biscuits

	Pro	Iron
Bread (w. enriched flour): 1 slice, 1 oz	2	1
4 thin slices, 4 oz	8	4
4 thick slices, 6 oz	1.2	6
Bagel, plain 2 oz	6	1.5
Biscuits, 1 oz	2	0.7
Pita Bread, 1 pita, 1½ oz	4	1
Pumpernickel, 1 slice, 1 oz	3	1

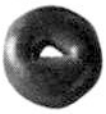

Infant/Baby Foods

	Pro	Iron
Infant Formula Milk:		
Enfamil/Gerber/Similac		
Regular/Low Iron , 5 fl.oz	2.2	0.2
With Iron, 5 fl.oz	2.2	1.8
Isomil/Nursoy/ProSobee	3	1.8
Baby Cereals:		
Average all brands		
Dry, 4 Tbsp, ½ oz	1	7
Jars (w. fruit), 4½ oz	1	7

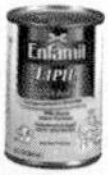

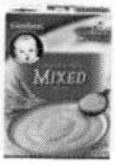

Breakfast Cereals

	Pro	Iron
Hot Cereals, cooked:		
Bulgur, cooked, 1 cup, 5 oz	9	2
Oatmeal: Reg., non-fortified, 1 cup	6	1.5
Instant, fortified, avg., 1 pkt	4	8
Quaker, all flavors, ½ cup	5	18
Corn/Hominy Grits: 1 cup	3	1.5
Quaker: Reg., 3 Tbsp, 1 oz	2	0.8
Instant White, 1 packet	2	8
Cream of Wheat, 1 cup	4	10
Brands ~ Ready-To-Eat		
Arrowhead: Average all varieties, 1 oz	3	1
General Mills: Basic 4, 1 cup, 2 oz	4	4.5
Cheerios, Original, 1 cup, 1 oz	3	8
Cocoa Puffs, 1 cup, 1 oz	1	4.5
Kix, 1⅓ cups, 1 oz	2	8
Multi-Bran Chex, 1 cup, 2 oz	4	16
Country Corn Flakes, 1 cup, 1.2 oz	2	8
Total Raisin Bran, 1 cup, 2 oz	3	18
Wheaties ¾ cup, 1 oz	3	8
Health Valley: Oat Bran O's, ¾ cup, 1 oz	3	0.7
Amaranth Flakes, ¾ cup, 1 oz	3	0.7
Bran Flakes w. Raisins, ¾ cup, 1.1 oz	5	1.5
Low-Fat Granola, ⅔ cup, 2 oz	5	1.4
Real Oat Bran Alm. Crunch, ½ cup, 1.7 oz	6	0.7
Golden Flax, ¾ cup, 1.9 oz	6	1
Kashi: Friends, 1 cup, 1.9 oz	5	1.8
GoLean Crunch!, 1 cup, 1.9 oz	9	1.8
7 Whole Grain Flakes, 1 c., 1.8 oz	6	1.4
Kellogg's: All-Bran: ½ cup, 1 oz	4	4.5
Complete Oat Flakes, ¾ cup, 1.1 oz	3	18
Cocoa Krispies, ¾ cup, 1 oz	1	4.5
Corn Flakes, 1 cup, 1 oz	2	8
Low-fat Granola w. Raisins ⅔ c., 2.1 oz	4	2
Product 19, 1 cup, 1 oz	2	18
Raisin Bran, 1 cup, 2 oz	7	4.5
Rice Krispies, 1¼ cup, 1.2 oz	2	9
Smart-Start Healthy Heart, 1 c., 1.8 oz	6	4.5
Special K: Regular, 1 c., 1.1 oz	6	8
Protein Plus, ¾ cup, 1 oz	10	8
Post: Raisin Bran, ⅔ cup, 2 oz	4	11
Grape Nuts, ½ cup, 2 oz	6	16
Quaker: Crunchy Corn Bran, 1 cup, 1 oz	2	8
100% Natural Granola, ½ cup, 1.7 oz	5	1.4
Life, ¾ cup, 1.1 oz	3	8
Cap'n Crunch, ¾ cup, 1 oz	1	4.5
Oat Bran, ½ cup, 1.4 oz	7	2.7

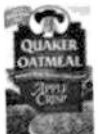

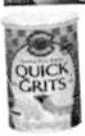

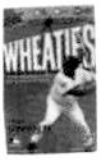

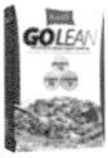

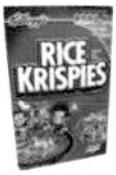

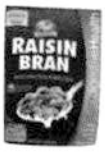

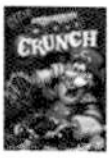

Brans & Wheatgerm

	Pro	Iron
Oat Bran, raw, 1 Tbsp	2	0.5
Rice Bran, raw, 2 Tbsp	1	1
Wheat Bran, unprocessed, 2 T.	1	1
Wheat Germ, 2 Tbsp, ½ oz	4	1.3

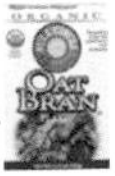

Grains & Flours, Yeast

	Pro	Iron
Amaranth, ½ cup, 3.4 oz	14	7
Barley, ½ cup, 3.2 oz	12	2
Buckwheat Flour: Whole-groat, 1 cup	15	2.7
Carob Flour, 1 cup, 3.6 oz	5	3
Corn Flour, 1 cup, 4 oz	11	2
Corn Meal, 1 cup, 4½ oz	8	3.5
Flour: White, 1 cup, 5.6 oz	9	6
Whole-grain, 1 cup, 4¼ oz	16	5
Millet, whole-grain, 1 cup, 3½ oz	12	7
Rye Flour: Dark, 1 cup, 4½ oz	18	6
Light, 1 cup, 3½ oz	9	1
Soy Flour, full fat, 1 cup, 3 oz	29	5.5
Yeast: Brewers, 2 Tbsp, ½ oz	8	1.5
Nutritional Yeast Flakes *(Red Star),* 1 heaping Tbsp, ½ oz	8	0.8

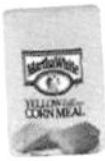

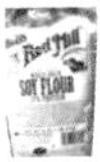

Rice, Spaghetti, Macaroni

	Pro	Iron
Rice: Brown/White, average 1 cup cooked, 6½ oz	5	1
Spaghetti/Macaroni/Noodles (enriched):		
Cooked, 1 cup, 4½ oz	7	2
Canned: in Tomato Sce, ½ c	2	0.5
w. Meatballs, 1 cup, 8 oz	10	2
Macaroni & Cheese, 1 c., 9 oz	8	1

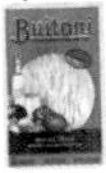

Soups

	Pro	Iron
With Noodles/Vegetables, 1 c.	3	0.5
With Meat/Beans/Peas, 1 c.	8	1.5

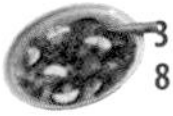

Fruit

	Pro	Iron
Fresh/Canned:		
Average, all types 1 medium/2 small fruit	1	0.5
Avocado, ½ medium	2	1
Dried Fruit: Apricots, 8 halves, 1 oz	1	1.3
Dates, 6 dates, 2 oz	1.5	0.7
Figs, 4 medium figs, 2 oz	2	1.7
Prunes, 5 medium, 1½ oz	1	1
Raisins, 1 oz	1	0.7
Fruit Juice: Average, 1 cup	0.5	0.5
Prune Juice, 6 fl.oz	1	2.5
Tomato Juice, 1 cup, 8 fl.oz	1.5	1

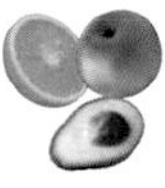

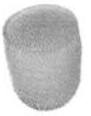

Vegetables	Pro	Iron
Beans: Snap/green, ½ cup, 2 oz	1	0.8
Dried: Average all types, cooked, ½ cup	7	2.5
Baked Beans, ½ cup 4½ oz	5	2
Bean Sprouts, mung, 1 c., 4 oz	3	1
Broccoli, 3raw, ½ cup, 1½ oz	1.5	0.7
Cabbage; Cauliflower, raw, 1 c. 3 oz	1.5	0.6
Corn, raw, ½ cup kernels, 3 oz	2.5	0.3
1 ear trimmed to 3½"	2	0.4
Lentils, cooked, ½ cup, 3½ oz	9	3.3
Mushrooms, raw, ½ c., sliced	1	0.3
Peas: Green, raw, ½ c., 2½ oz	4	1.2
Split Peas, cooked, 1 cup, 7 oz	16	2.5
Potatoes, cooked:		
1 medium, with skin, 5 oz	3.3	2
without skin, 4 oz	2.3	1
French Fries, small, 2.6 oz	2	1
Potato Salad, ½ cup, 4 oz	3.5	2.5
Pumpkin, ½ cup mashed, 4.3 oz	1	1
Seaweed, kelp, 1 oz	<1	2.5
Spinach, cooked, ½ cup, 3 oz	2.7	3.5
Squash, ckd, all types, ½ cup	1	0.3
Tomatoes, 1 medium, 4½ oz	1	0.6
Vegetables, mixed, ckd, 1 cup	2.5	0.7
Soybeans, cooked, ½ cup, 3 oz	14	4.4

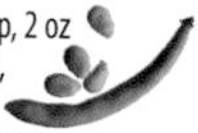
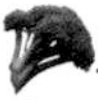
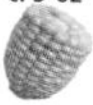

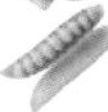
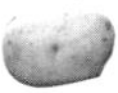
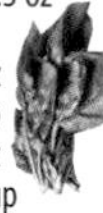

Tofu, Tempeh, Miso	Pro	Iron
Tofu, raw, firm, ½ cup, 4½ oz	10	1.5
Tempeh, ½ cup, 3 oz	16	2
Miso, ½ cup, 5 oz	16	4
Miso Soup, 1 cup	3	0.4
Soybean Protein (TVP), 1 oz	18	3

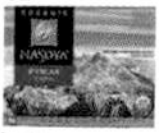

Cakes, Pastries, Pies (Made with enriched flour)	Pro	Iron
Carrot w. cream cheese frosting, 4 oz	4	1.3
Cheesecake, 1 piece, 4 oz	6	0.5
Chocolate, 1 piece, 2 oz	2	2
Fruitcake, 1 piece, 3 oz	4	2
Plain, 1 piece, 3 oz	4	1.2
Croissant, plain, 2 oz	5	2
Danish Pastry, 1 pastry, 2¼ oz	4	1.3
Donuts, average, 2 oz	4	1.2
Muffins, average, 1 med., 1½ oz	3	1
Pancakes, 4" diam., two, 2 oz	4	1
Pies: Fruit, 1 piece, 5½ oz	4	1.5
Pecan, 1 piece, 5 oz	7	4.5
Puddings, average, ½ cup, 4½ oz	4	0.3
Waffles, 1 large, 2½ oz	7	1.5

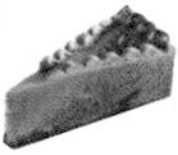
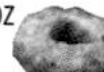
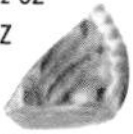

Peanut Butter	Pro	Iron
Regular: 2 Tbsp, 1.1 oz	8	0.5
Peter Pan Plus, 2 Tbsp, 1.1 oz	8	4.5

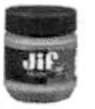

Sugar, Honey, Jam	Pro	Iron
Sugar: White	0	0
Brown, 1 Tbsp	0	0.3
Molasses: Light/Med., 1 Tbsp	0	1
Blackstrap, 1 Tbsp, ¾ oz	0	3
Corn Syrup, 1 Tbsp, ¾ oz	0	1
Honey, Jams, Jelly	0	0.2

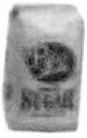
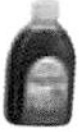

Candy, Chocolate, Carob	Pro	Iron
Candy, sugar-based	0	0
Chocolate: Plain, 2 oz bar	4	0.8
with nuts, 2 oz bar	6	0.8
Carob, plain, 2 oz	6	0.7

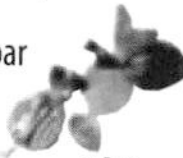

Cookies, Crackers, Chips	Pro	Iron
Cookies, average, 4 cookies	2	1
Crackers, Graham, 2½" sq., (2)	1	0
Rice Cakes, average, one	1	0
Corn/Potato Chips, 1 oz	2	0.3

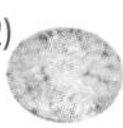

Nuts & Seeds	Pro	Iron
Nuts: Almonds, shelled, 20-25 nuts	6	1
Brazil Nuts, 7-8 medium nuts, 1 oz	4	1
Cashews, 12-16 nuts, 1 oz	5	1.5
Macadamias, 1 oz	2	0.5
Peanuts, dry rsted, 40 nuts, 1 oz	6	0.6
Pecans, 24 halves, 1 oz	2	0.5
Walnuts, 15 halves, 1 oz	4	0.7
Seeds: Sesame Seeds, dry, 1 Tbsp	2	0.6
Pumpkin Kernels, dry, hulled, 1 oz	7	4.2
Sunflower Seeds, dried, hulled, 1 oz	6	2
Tahini, 1 Tbsp, ½ oz	2.5	1.4

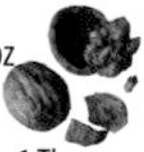

Granola & Food/Protein Bars	Pro	Iron
Granola Bars, avg., 1 bar, 2 oz	2	0.5
Anytime Health,		
Meal Bars, 80g	20	0.5
Snack Bars, 50g	12	0.3
Balance Bars, Orig. 1.76 oz	14	4.5
Bariatrix Proti-Bars (1), 1.4 oz	15	0.7
Dr Soy Protein Bars, 1.76 oz	11	18
GeniSoy Protein Bar, 1.6 oz	15	6.3
Jenny Craig Bars, 1.8 oz	4	3.6
Met-Rx "Big 100", 3.5 oz	27	7.2
Myoplex Carb Sense Bar, 2.5 oz	26	2
Optifast Peanut Butter, 1.59 oz	8	0.5
PowerBar: Harvest	10	4.5
Performance Bar, 2.3 oz	10	6.3
ProteinPlus, 1 bar, avg., 2.75 oz	24	8
Slim-Fast: High Protein Meal, 1.7 oz	15	2.7
Optima Meal, 2 oz bar	8	2.7
Special K: Protein Meal, 1.6 oz	10	1.8
Protein Snack, 0.9 oz	4	0.7

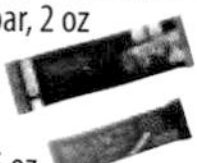
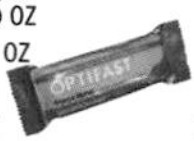
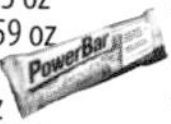
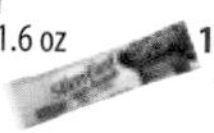

High Protein Drinks

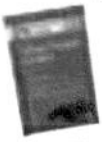
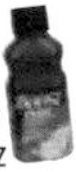

	Pro	Iron
Anytime Health:		
Whey Protein Isolate,		
All flavors, 1 oz	25	0
Atkins Shakes, 11 fl.oz can	18	2.7
Boost High Protein, 8 oz	10	3.5
Carnation Instant Breakfast, 10 oz	13	4.5
Curves Protein Drink, 2 scoops, dry	15	18
dotFIT: FirstString, 4 scoops, 5.2 oz	42	2.5
Meal Replacement,		
Chocolate, 2 scoops, 2.2 oz	20	3.2
WheySmooth, Choc., 2 scoops, 2.2 oz	40	1.8
Ensure Plus, 8 oz can	13	2.3
Gatorade: Nutrition Shake, 11 oz	20	1.8
Protein Recovery Shake, 11 oz	20	0
GeniSoy Shake, 1 scoop, 1.2 oz	14	3.6
Kashi GoLean Shake, 2 sc., 2.1 oz	21	2.7
Met-Rx RTD 40	40	4.5
Myoplex, Original Nutrition Shake, 1 pkt	42	5.4
Optifast 800, made up, 8 fl oz	14	3.6
Resource (Novartis) Standard, 8 fl.oz	15	4.5
Slim-Fast Shakes: Meal, 11 oz can	10	2.7
High Protein, 11 oz can	15	2.7
Optima, 11 oz can	10	2.7
Special K2O Protein Water, 16 fl.oz	5	0
Walgreens Slim For Less, 11 oz can	10	2.7
Weider Mass 1000, 4 scoops, 7 oz	34	6

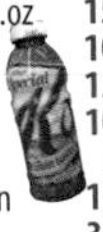

Coffee, Tea, Soda

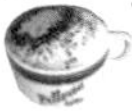
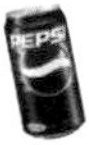

	Pro	Iron
Coffee, Coffee Substitutes, 1 cup, 8 fl.oz	0	0
Coffee w. 2 oz milk, 1 cup, 8 fl.oz	2	0
Caffe latte, large, 16 fl.oz	12	0
Cappuccino, large, 16 fl.oz	8	0
Frappuccino, avg., 16 fl.oz	6	0
Hot Chocolate,		
with milk, 1 cup, 8 fl.oz	8	1.2
Soft Drinks/Soda	0	0
Tea (all types)	0	0

Beer, Wine, Spirits

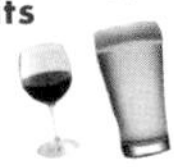

	Pro	Iron
Beer, 12 fl.oz	1	0
Wines, red/white, 1 glass	0	0.4
Spirits/Liquor	0	0

Fast-Foods/Burgers

	Pro	Iron
Pancakes: Average all outlets, 3	8	2
Shakes, Chocolate, 16 fl.oz	12	0.4
Sundaes: Average all outlets	7	0.3
Arby's: Roast Beef Sandwich, regular	20	4.6
Chicken Club Salad	32	3.8
Roast Beef Sandwich, Super	21	3.8
Burger King: Whopper S/wich	29	5.4
Bacon Double Cheeseburger	32	4.5
BK Big Fish Sandwich	24	4.5

Fast Foods/Burgers (Cont)

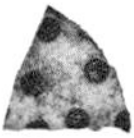
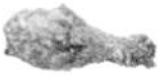
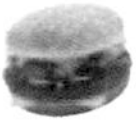
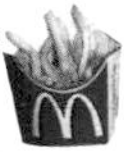

	Pro	Iron
Carl's Jr:		
Famous Star Hamburger w/ Cheese	27	2
Charbroiled Chicken Club Sandwich	39	3
Super Star Hamburger w/ Cheese	47	3
Domino's Pizza: Deep Dish (12")		
Beef, 2 slices	10	2.2
Cheese, 2 slices	12	1.8
Pepperoni, Sausage, 1 sl.	10	1.8
KFC: Original, Breast	42	1
Crispy Strips, 3 strips	33	1.8
Snacker, Regular	15	2.7
McDonald's: Big Mac	25	4
Cheeseburger	15	2.5
Chicken McNuggets (6)	14	1
Crispy Chicken Classic Burger	28	3.5
Filet-O-Fish	15	2
Hamburger	12	2.5
Quarter Pounder w. Cheese	29	4
French Fries: Small, 2.5 oz	3	0.5
Large, 5.4 oz	6	1.5
Salads w. Chicken, average	30	2
Triple Shake, average, 16 fl.oz	16	1
Breakfast: Egg McMuffin	18	3
Bacon, Egg & Cheese McGriddles	15	2.5
Sausage Burrito	12	2.5
Sausage McMuffin w. Egg	21	3.5

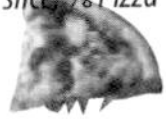
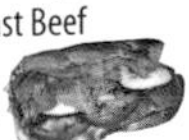
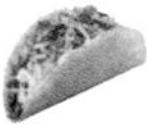

	Pro	Iron
Pizza Hut: *Per Medium, 1 slice, 1/8 Pizza*		
Thin 'n Crispy, Supreme	10	1
Pan Pizzas, average	11	2
Hand Tossed, Pepperoni	10	1.5
Fit n' Delicious, Ham/Pineapple/Tomato	7	1
Subway (6" Subs): Roast Beef	26	4.5
Meatball Marinara	24	7.2
Roast Chicken Breast	23	2.7
Subway Club	26	3.6
Sweet Onion Chicken Teriyaki	26	3.6
Taco Bell: Bean Burrito	12	2.7
Chicken Quesadilla	28	1.8
Chicken/Steak Enchirito	21	1.8
Gordita Baja Beef	13	2.7
Steak Burrito Supreme	18	2.7
Taco Supreme	11	1
Wendy's: ¼ lb Single Burger	27	6.8
Chicken Club	37	3.6
Jr Hamburger	13	2.7

High Blood Pressure

Many American adults have hypertension (high blood pressure), and are unaware of it. It is generally symptomless, so **have your blood pressure checked annually** – particularly if it runs in the family.

Untreated hypertension overworks the heart, damages arteries and promotes atherosclerosis. This in turn greatly increases the risk of heart disease, stroke, blindness, kidney disease and impotence. The earlier hypertension is detected, the sooner it can be brought under control.

BLOOD PRESSURE CLASSIFICATION

For Adults Age 18 & Older ~ Not Acutely Ill or on Medication (American Heart Association)

	DIASTOLIC		SYSTOLIC
Normal ➤	Below 80	and	Below 120
Prehypertension ➤	80-89	or	120-139
Hypertension:			
Stage 1 ➤	90-99	or	140-159
Stage 2 ➤	100 or more	or	160 or more

HYPERTENSION DAMAGES ARTERIES & PROMOTES ATHEROSCLEROSIS

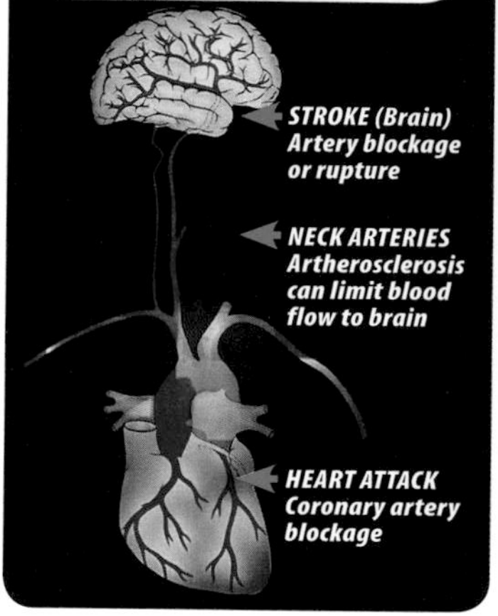

Treating Hypertension

Prehypertension (in the chart above) means you don't have high blood pressure now but are likely to develop it in the future.

You can take steps to lessen the risk by adopting healthy lifestyle habits such as:

- reducing sodium intake
- eating adequate fruit and vegetables
- losing weight if overweight
- limiting alcohol to 2 drinks or less daily
- quitting smoking
- exercising regularly, managing stress.

Stage 1 hypertension can often be treated with the above lifestyle changes.

Stage 2 hypertension usually requires drug therapy. However, salt restriction, abstaining from alcohol, and the above lifestyle changes will improve the success of drug therapy, and enable smaller drug doses to be prescribed.

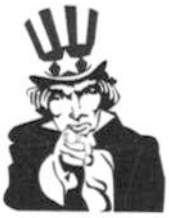

STROKE
KNOW THE WARNING SIGNS

Stroke is a medical emergency!
If you notice one or more of these signs, call 9-1-1 or your doctor immediately.

These signs may be signalling a possible stroke or transient ischemic attack:

- **Sudden weakness** or numbness in your face, arm, or leg on one side of your body
- **Sudden confusion,** trouble speaking or understanding
- **Sudden trouble seeing,** in one or both eyes
- **Sudden trouble walking,** dizziness, loss of balance or coordination
- **Sudden severe headache** - 'a bolt out of the blue' – with no apparent cause

Salt & Sodium

- **Sodium is a mineral element** most commonly found in salt (sodium chloride). It also occurs naturally in much smaller amounts in animal and plant foods, and water – normally sufficient for our needs without having to add salt to our diet.
- **Sodium is required** for nerve and muscle function, as well as to balance the amount of fluid in our tissues and blood.

  Sodium acts like a sponge to attract and hold fluids in body tissues.
- **Excess sodium** can cause water retention, and increase the risk of developing hypertension. Very high salt intake may also increase the risk of stomach cancer.
- **Too little sodium** may cause low blood pressure (hypotension), and decrease blood flow to the heart, brain and kidneys - especially during exercise. (A certain blood volume is required to sustain the blood pressure needed for adequate blood flow in the capillaries).

Salt-Sensitive Persons

- **Normally, our kidneys** excrete excess dietary sodium. The thirst we feel after a salty meal is the body calling for water to dilute the sodium, and enable the kidneys to flush out excess sodium.
- **However, 'salt - sensitive'** persons (up to 50% of adults) tend to retain excess sodium (above approximately 3000mg daily) instead of excreting it. Such persons are more likely to develop hypertension and would benefit most from sodium restriction. Assume you are susceptible if there is a family history of hypertension.
- **Although not everyone will benefit, all Americans are being asked to moderate their salt and sodium intake** as a public health measure – particularly because so many do not know whether or not they have hypertension, and also because we do not know just who is salt-sensitive.

SAFE SODIUM LEVELS

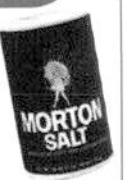

The American Heart Association recommends a **maximum sodium intake of 2300mg per day** for adults with normal blood pressure. However, people who consume **less than 1500mg sodium** have the lowest blood pressure levels.

Persons with hypertension and kidney ailments are usually restricted to as little as **1000mg sodium per day**. Your doctor will discuss the correct sodium level for you.

Persons with Menière's Disease (chronic attacks of vertigo, dizziness, hearing loss, imbalance), often benefit from lower sodium intake of less than 2000mg/day, as well as even distribution of food and fluids over the day (to prevent fluctuations in body fluids and pressure in the inner ear). Also avoid caffeine and MSG. Limit sugar and alcohol.

further info: www.CalorieKing.com

FINDING HIDDEN SODIUM

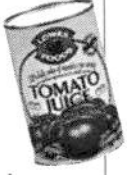

On average, **less than one third of our sodium intake comes from the salt shaker.** The rest is hidden in processed foods that have salt added during manufacture.

Sodium compounds added to food or medicinals can also contribute significant sodium.

Sodium bicarbonate in particular is widely used in antacid tablets (such as Alka Seltzer) and powders. Sodium bicarbonate contains 27% sodium by weight. Each gram contributes 270mg sodium. Large amounts of sodium can be unwittingly consumed – up to 600mg per tablet. (See Antacids ~ Page 293)

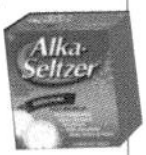

Example: 2 Alka-Seltzer Tablets = 1000mg sodium

Other sodium compounds include monosodium glutamate (MSG), sodium ascorbate, sodium nitrite, and sodium citrate.

ALCOHOL DANGER

Excessive alcohol intake contributes to hypertension. Susceptible persons should limit alcohol intake to 1-2 drinks per day.

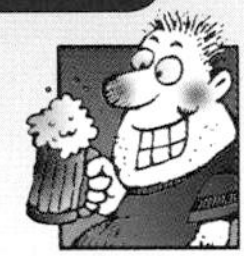

Salt Sodium Guide

Sodium accounts for only 40% of the weight of salt (sodium chloride). Examples:
1 gram (1000mg) Salt has 400mg Sodium
1 teaspoon (5g) Salt has 2000mg Sodium

HINTS TO REDUCE SODIUM

- **Cut down use of the salt shaker.** Start with an easy 50% cut in sodium by using Lite Salt (*Morton*) or *Cardia* Salt. Then gradually cut back until you can leave the salt shaker off the table. Sea salt is still high in sodium.
- **Use fresh herbs,** and salt-free seasonings to add flavor to food.
- **Choose low-sodium,** sodium-free, and reduced-sodium products in place of regular, salted products.
- **Check food labels for sodium levels.** FDA Guidelines for sodium descriptors are:
  - **Reduced Sodium:** At least 25% less sodium than the original product
  - **Low Sodium:** 140 mg or less/serving
  - **Very Low Sodium:** 35mg or less/serving
  - **Sodium Free:** Less than 5mg/serving
  - **No Salt Added:** Made without the salt normally added, but still contains the sodium that is a natural part of the food
- **Use reduced-sodium breads,** butter and margarine. Regular varieties contain up to 2% salt. This is considered high in view of their significant contribution to our diet.
- **Go easy on salty condiments and sauces** such as ketchup, mustard, soy sauce, spaghetti sauces, and salad dressings. Use low-sodium varieties.
- **Limit pizzas and salty fast-foods.** Check ***CalorieKing.com*** food database.
- **Avoid salty snack foods** such as potato chips, corn chips, salted nuts, pretzels and cheesy-flavored snacks. **Choose unsalted** popcorn, nuts or seeds. Eat more fruit.
- **Don't salt children's food** to your taste.
- **Avoid antacids with** sodium bicarbonate (such as *Alka-Seltzer*). They are high in sodium. Look for low-sodium alternatives.

FOODS HIGH IN SODIUM

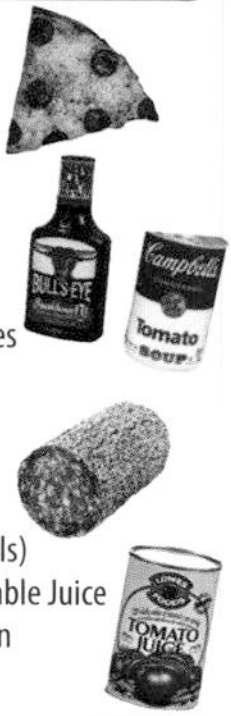

- Cheese, Butter, Margarine
- Pickles, Sauerkraut, Olives
- Condiments, Sauces
- Salad Dressings
- Canned vegetables/salads/beans
- Deli Salads (with dressing)
- Frozen/Packaged Meals/Entrees
- Soups: Canned/dry; bouillon cubes
- Meats: Ham, bacon, sausage, luncheon meats, smoked meats
- Canned Fish (in brine/salt)
- Sea Salt, Garlic/Celery Salt
- Snack Foods (potato chips, pretzels)
- Tomato Juice (Canned), V8 Vegetable Juice
- Fast Foods: Pizza, Burgers, Chicken
- *Alka-Seltzer* Antacid

MODERATE SODIUM

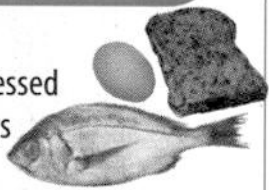

- Bread (Reduced Salt)
- Meat, Fish, Poultry - Unprocessed
- Milk, Yogurt, Soy Drinks, Eggs
- Peanut Butter
- Breakfast Cereals (less than 200mg/serving)
- Chocolate Candy, Fruit/Nut Bars
- *Reduced Sodium & Low Sodium* Products

FOODS LOW IN SODIUM

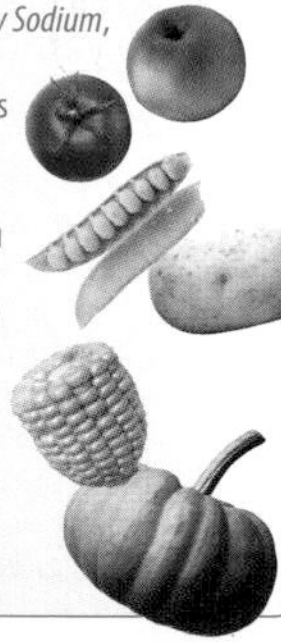

- Products labelled *Very Low Sodium*, or *Sodium Free*
- Fresh fruits and vegetables
- Canned and Dried Fruits
- Potatoes, Rice, Pasta
- Dried Beans & Lentils, Tofu
- Nuts & Seeds (unsalted)
- Corn & Popcorn (unsalted)
- Pepper, Spices, Herbs
- Jam, Honey, Syrup
- Candy, Gum
- Hard & Jelly Candy
- Coffee, Tea, Alcohol
- Fresh Fruit Juices, Water

The American Heart Association recommends a sodium intake of **less than 2300mg/day**

Milk & Dairy Products

	Sodium
Milk: Whole/lowfat/skim, average	
1 cup, 8 fl.oz	120
Whole, low sodium, 1 cup	5
Choc Milk *(Hershey's)*, 1 cup	130
Soy Milk, 8 fl.oz	30
Buttermilk, cultured, 8 fl.oz	250
Dry/Powder, skim, ¼ cup, 1 oz	110
Yogurt, with fruit average, 8 oz	130
Cheese: Bleu, 1 oz	330
Parmesan, 1 oz	450
Kraft Cheddar, 2% milk, 1 oz	230
Philadelphia Cream Cheese, 1 oz	90
Process Cheese., average, 1 oz	430
Swiss, 1 oz	40
Cottage Cheese, ½ cup, 4 oz	450
Ricotta Cheese, ½ cup, 4 oz	150

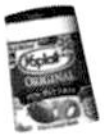

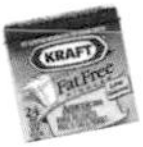

Ice Cream, Frozen Yogurt

Icecream, average, ½ cup	50
Frozen Yogurt, ½ cup	50

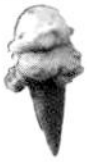

Fats/Oils

Butter/Margarine:	
Regular, 2 Tbsp, 1 oz	230
Unsalted, reg., 2 Tbsp, 1 oz	5
Mayonnaise, aver., 2 Tbsp, 1 oz	160
Oils/Lard/Drippings	0
Cream, average, 1 Tbsp	5
Coffee-Mate: Powdered, 1 tsp	2
Liquid, 1 Tbsp	5

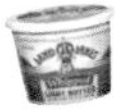

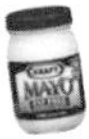

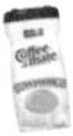

Eggs

Whole, 1 large	70
Omelet, 2 egg, plain	220
w. cheese	400
Egg Beaters: Original, ¼ cup	115
Flavors, average, ¼ cup	230

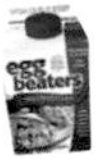

Meats

Meat, average all types, cooked (Beef/Lamb/Veal/Pork), 4 oz	80
Corned Beef, cooked, 3 oz	800
Bacon, cooked, 2 sl., ½ oz	270
Ham, 3 oz	1100

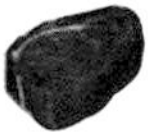

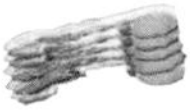

Chicken & Turkey

Chicken/Turkey, cooked, unsalted, 4 oz	80
Stuffing Mixes, average., ½ cup	500

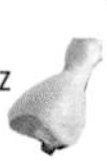

Sodium ~ **Sodium (mg)**

Sausages & Meats

	Sodium
Bologna, 1 oz	280
Frankfurter, 2 oz	640
Ham, chopped, ¾ oz slice	290
Liverwurst (Braunschweiger), 1 oz	320
Pepperoni, 5 slices, 1 oz	570
Salami, cooked, 1 oz	350
dry/hard, 1 oz	600
Sausage, 1 oz link	220
Pork, 2 oz patty	260
Spam: Classic, 2 oz	790
25% Less Sodium, 2 oz	580
Turkey Roll, 1 oz	160

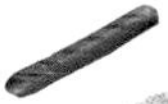

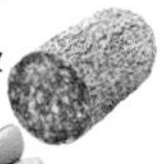

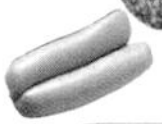

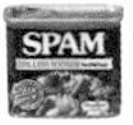

Fish: Fresh Fish, average, plain

Cooked, 4 oz (no bone)	60
Broiled w. butter, 4 oz	150
Breaded & fried, 4 oz	320
Fish fillets, batter-dipped 3 oz	350
Fish sticks, 1 oz stick	160
Gefilte Fish (w. broth), 1 pce, 1½ oz	220
Herring, pickled, 2 pces, 1 oz	260
Lobster, meat only, 4 oz	180
Oysters, fresh, 6 med., 3 oz	95
Salmon: Canned, 3 oz	460
No Salt Added, 3 oz	65
Smoked fish, average, 3 oz	650
Tuna: Canned, regular, 3 oz	330
No Added Salt, 3 oz	40
Spicy Flavored, 5 oz can	550

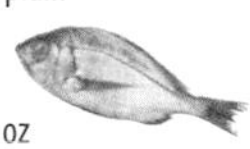

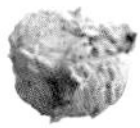

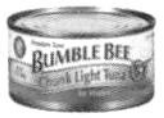

Entrees & Meals

Frozen Meals, average	600-900
Lean Cuisine, average	700
Stouffer's, average	580
Dinners, average	900-1200
Side Dishes, average	400-600
Pizza, frozen, ¼ large, 6 oz	800-1200
Microwave Cup Meals	900-1200
Cup O'Noodles, average	1500

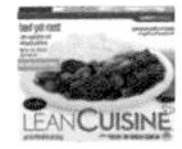

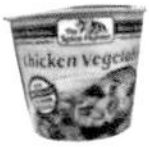

Fast-Foods & Restaurants

Cheeseburger	750
Chicken Dinner (3 piece)	2200
Chicken Nuggets w. Sauce	800
Fish/Chicken Sandwich	1000
French Fries, small, 2½ oz	150
Hamburger: Regular	500
Large with cheese	1100
Hot Dog (Frankfurter)	800
Pizza, 2 medium slices	1200
Shake, chocolate	250
Taco	400

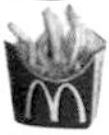

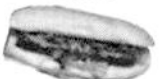

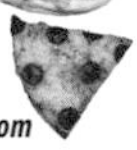

Extra Listings ~ see CalorieKing.com

Sodium ~ Sodium (mg)

	Sodium
Soups: Condensed, 1 c., 8 oz	800-1000
Low Sodium	70
Chicken Noodle, 1 cup	900
Bouillon Cube, average	950
Cup-A-Soup: Average	850
Lite, average	450
Soup Mixes, average, 1 cup	900

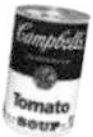

Condiments, Sauces, Dressings

	Sodium
A-1 Sauce, 1 Tbsp	280
Barbecue Sauce, 1 Tbsp	130
Bragg Liquid Aminos, 1 tsp	220
Chili Sauce, 1 Tbsp	230
Ketchup: Tomato, 1 Tbsp	180
Low Sodium, 1 Tbsp	20
Mayonnaise, 1 Tbsp	80
Mustard, 1 tsp	70
Pizza Sauce, ½ cup	700
Salad Dressings, 2 Tbsp, 1 oz	160-400
Spaghetti Sauce, ½ cup	500
Soy Sauce: 1 Tbsp	900
Lite *(Kikkoman)*, 1 Tbsp	600
Sweet & Sour, ½ cup	250
Tabasco, 1 tsp	25
Vinegar, Lemon Juice	0
Worcestershire, 1 Tbsp	200
Tomato: Sauce, 1 cup	1200
Paste/Puree (salted), ½ cup	1000
No Salt Added, ½ cup	25

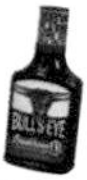

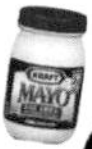

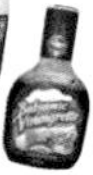
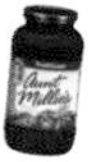
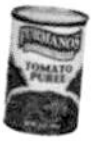

Salt & Salt Substitutes

	Sodium
Table Salt: 1 teaspoon, 6g	2400
Single Serve package, 1 g	400
Cardia Salt, 1 teaspoon	1080
Lite Salt *(Morton)*, 1 teaspoon, 6g	1200
Morton **Salt Substitute**	5
No Salt **Salt Substitute,** 1 teaspoon	5
Garlic/Seasoned Salt 1 teaspoon, 4g	1300
Sea Salt, 1 teaspoon, 5g	2250

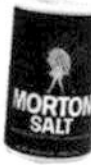

Seasonings, Herbs & Spices

	Sodium
Baking Powder, 1 tsp, 3g	340
Baking Soda (Sodium bicarb), 1 tsp, 3g	810
Accent (Flavor Enhancer), 1 tsp	600
Chili Powder, 1 tsp, 3g	25
Curry Powder	0
Lemon Pepper *(Lawry's)*, 1 tsp	340
Meat Tenderizer, 1 tsp, 5g	1750
MSG (Monosodium glutamate), 5g	500
Mrs Dash Blends/Marinades	0
Pepper, Mustard (dry), 1 tsp	1
Yeast, Nutritional, 1 Tbsp	10

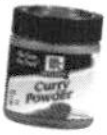

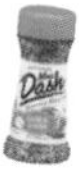

Breakfast Cereals

	Sodium
Kellogg's:	
All-Bran, ½ cup, 1 oz	80
Special K, 1 cup, 1.1 oz	220
Corn Flakes, 1 cup, 1 oz	200
Just Right, ¾ cup, 2 oz	240
Mini Wheats Frosted, 24 bisc., 1.8 oz	5
Health Valley Cereals, 1 serving	5
Quaker: Cap'n Crunch, ¾ cup, 1 oz	200
Crunchy Corn Bran, ¾ cup, 1 oz	230
100% Natural Granola, ½ cup, 1 oz	15
Puffed Rice/Wheat, 2 cups, 1 oz	1
General Mills: Total, ¾ cup, 1 oz	190
Oatmeal: Regular, ¾ cup	1
Instant *(Quaker)*, ⅔ cup (1 pkt)	270

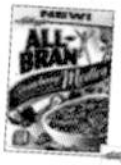

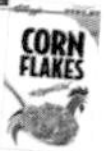

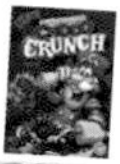

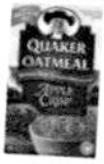

Breads, Bagels, Crackers

	Sodium
Bread: Average all types, 1 oz	140
Low Sodium, 1 oz	10
Bagels: Plain, 2 oz	200
Sara Lee, 3 oz	500
Biscuits, average, 1 oz	180
Bun/Roll, 1 medium, 1½ oz	200
Crackers: Saltine, 2 crackers	70
Low Salt *(Premium)*, 2	25
Graham, 2 regular	50
Croissant, average, 2 oz	280
Rice Cakes, average	25
Ritz **Crackers,** Low-Sodium, 1 oz	60
Ry-Krisp Crispbread, Sesame, 2	100

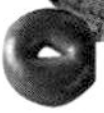
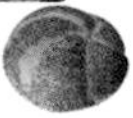
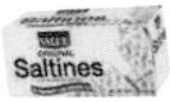

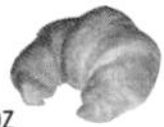

Cookies, Cakes, Desserts

	Sodium
Cookies: Average, 2-3 cookies, 1 oz	100
Mrs Fields', average, 2½ oz	180
Baked Custard, ½ cup	100
Brownie, ¼ oz piece	75
Cake, average, 3 oz piece	250
Cinnamon Sweet Roll, 2 oz	250
Danish, Apple	250
Donut, average	150
Muffins: 1 medium, 2 oz	150
Pancakes, 3 x 4"	360
Pie, average ⅙ of 9" pie	300
Pudding: Average, ½ cup	160
Jell-O (Mix), Instant, ½ cup	400
Waffles:	
Home-made, 7", 2½ oz	350
Frozen: Average, 1¼ oz	260
Aunt Jemima, avg, 2½ oz	565

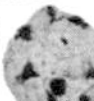
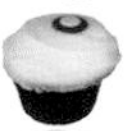
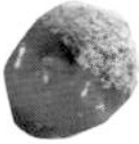
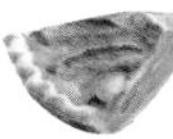
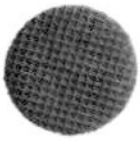

Fruit & Juices

	Sodium
Fresh Fruit, average all types, 1 serving	1
Dried/Canned Fruit, ½ cup	1
Fruit Juice: Fresh, sqz'd, 6 fl.oz	1
Commercial, aver., 6 fl.oz	20
Carrot Juice *(Ferraro's)*, 8 fl.oz	230
Tomato Juice *(Campbell's)*, 6 fl.oz	570
Low Sodium (No Salt Added)	20
V8 Vegetable *(Campbell's)*, 6 fl.oz	600
(No Salt Added), 6 fl.oz	45

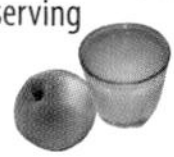
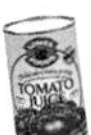

Vegetables

Fresh/Frozen (No Salt Added): *Per ½ Cup*	
Asparagus, Bean Sprouts, Corn	3
Beets, Carrots, Celery, ½ cup	40
Broccoli, Cabbage, Cauliflower	10
Cucumber, Green Beans, Mushroom, Okra	3
Onions, Peas, Potato, Pumpkin, Squash	3
Peppers, Hot Chili, raw, each	3
Spinach, Turnips, ½ cup, ckd	40
Tomato, 1 medium, 5 oz	10
Canned: Asparagus, 4 spears	300
Beans, baked in tomato sauce	450
Beets, ½ cup, 3 oz	240
Corn Kernels, ½ cup, 3 oz	190
Creamed, ½ cup, 4½ oz	330
Mushrooms w. butter sce, 2oz	550
Peas, ½ cup, 3 oz	250
Sauerkraut, ½ cup, 4 oz	750

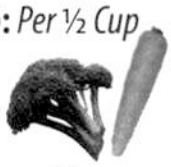
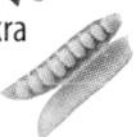
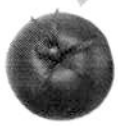
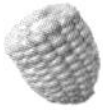
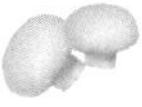

Pickles, Olives

Olives, pickled: Green, 1 large	90
Ripe/black, 1 large	40
Pickles: Bread & Butter, 4 sl., 1 oz	200
Dill, 1 pickle, 2½ oz	900
Sweet, 1 gherkin, ½ oz	130

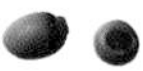
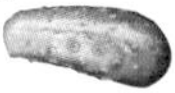

Soybean Products

Miso (Soy Paste), ¼ c., 2½ oz	2500
Soybean Protein Isolate, 1 oz	280
Tempeh, ½ cup, 3 oz	5
Tofu, average, ½ cup, 4 oz	5

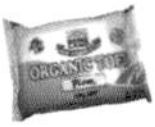

Jam, Honey, Syrups

Jam/Jelly, 1 Tbsp	2
Honey/Maple Syrup, 1 Tbsp	1
Log Cabin Syrup, 1 fl.oz	35
Lite, 1 fl.oz	90

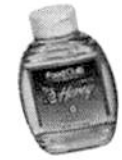

Peanut Butter

Peanut Butter: Regular, 2 Tbsp, ½ oz	190
Low Sodium *(Jif)*, 2 Tbsp	65
Unsalted *(Trader Joe's)*, 2 Tbsp	5

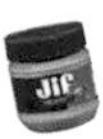

Snacks, Nuts

	Sodium
Cheese Balls/Curls, 1 oz	280
Corn/Tortilla Chips, average, 1 oz	220
Granola bars, average, 1 bar	80
Nuts: Plain, unsalted, 1 oz	1
Lightly salted, 1 oz	80
Salted or Honey Roasted, 1 oz	160
Popcorn: Plain (unsalted), 1 cup	1
Flavored, average, 1 cup	60
Salt added, 1 cup	180
Potato Chips: Plain, 1 oz	160
Flavored, average, 1 oz	250
Pretzels, regular, 3, 1 oz	450

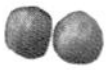
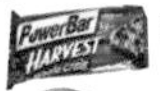

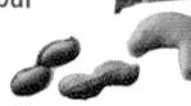
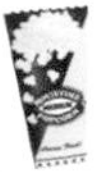
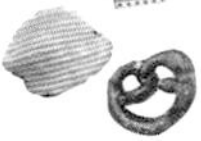

Candy, Chocolate

Chocolate, milk, 1 oz	30
Fudge, chocolate, 1 oz	55
Candy Bars, average, 1½ oz	60
Hard Candy, Jelly Beans, 1 oz	10
Licorice, 1 oz	30

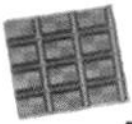
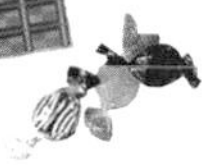

Beverages, Alcohol

Coffee (& Substitutes), Tea, 1 cup	1
Cocoa, dry, plain, 1 Tbsp	0
Mix, average, 1 envelope	120
Quik *(Nestle)*, 2 tsp	35
Soft Drinks, average, 8 fl.oz	20
Mineral Water, Perrier, 8 fl.oz	5
Gatorade Thirst Quencher, 8 fl.oz	110
Water: Average, 1 cup, 8 fl.oz	5
Drier regions, 1 cup	20+
Alcohol: Beer, average, 12 fl.oz	15
Wines, average, 4 fl.oz	10
Spirits (distilled), 1½ fl.oz	1

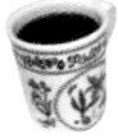
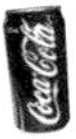

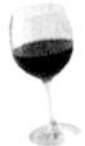

Antacids – Alka-Seltzer

	Sodium
Alka-Seltzer *(Per Tablet):*	
Alka-Seltzer P.M., 1 tablet	500
Original (Light Blue Box)	570
Extra Strength (Dark Blue Box)	590
Flavored Lemon/Lime & Cherry	500
Antacid (yellow Box)	310
Gelatine Capsule, 1	0
Alka-Mints, chewable	0
Bromo Seltzer, ¾ capful	760
Rolaids, All types	0
Tums, Regular/Extra Strength	0
Sodium Bicarbonate (27% sodium), 1g	270

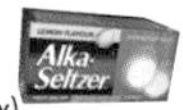

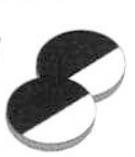
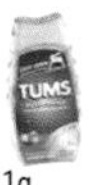

Index C

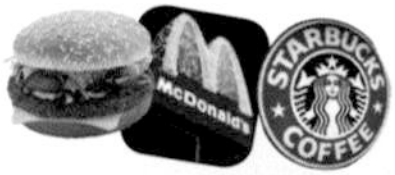

FAST-FOOD RESTAURANTS INDEX
~ SEE PAGE 182 ~

FAST-FOODS INDEX ~ PAGE 182 ~

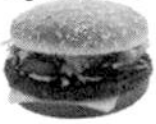

FAST-FOODS INDEX ~ PAGE 182 ~

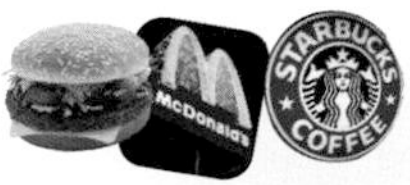

FAST-FOOD RESTAURANTS INDEX
~ SEE PAGE 183 ~

Index T - Z